# Color Atlas of Embryology

Ulrich Drews

176 color plates by Astried Rothenburger and Rüdiger Gay

1995
Georg Thieme Verlag Stuttgart · New York
Thieme Medical Publishers, Inc. New York

Ulrich Drews, M.D.
Anatomy Institute, University of Tübingen
Österbergstraße 3, 72074 Tübingen

Color plates by Gay + Rothenburger
Alexanderstraße 104, 70180 Stuttgart

Translated by David B. Meyer, Ph.D.
School of Medicine
540 East Canfield Avenue, Detroit, MI 48201

*Library of Congress Cataloging-in-Publication-Data*

Drews, Ulrich.
[Taschenatlas der Embryologie, English]
Color atlas of embryology / Ulrich Drews; color plates by Astried Rothenburger and Rüdiger Gay; translated by David B. Meyer.
p. cm.
Includes bibliographical references and index.
1. Embryology -- Atlases. I. Title.
[DNLM: 1. Embryology -- atlases. QS 617 D776t 1995a]
QM602.D7413 1995
611'.013'0222 -- dc20
DNLM/DLC
for Library of Congress 95-298

This book is an authorized translation of the German edition published and copyrighted 1993 by Georg Thieme Verlag, Stuttgart, Germany.
Title of the German edition: Taschenatlas der Embryologie


Thieme Medical Publishers, Inc., 381 Park Avenue South, New York, NY 10016
Typesetting by Götz, D-71636 Ludwigsburg
Printed in the United States of America by King Printing

ISBN 3-13-100321-9 (Thieme, Stuttgart)
ISBN 0-86577-544-3 (TMP, New York)

## Preface

The Color Atlas of Embryology is the product of an extraordinarily intense interaction between the author and illustrators. The design of each plate was perfected by Astried Rothenburger and Rüdiger Gay in collaboration with the author, enhancing the didactic effectiveness associated with a color atlas. The juxtaposition of the text and illustrations, as well as the corresponding headings, can be comprehended at a glance.

New topics are introduced by easily understandable overview plates, followed by detailed plates. This "window technique" allows a general orientation before the reader delves into more specific details. The student can use the overviews as introduction or as summaries and reviews for recapitulation and *test preparation*. The relevance of the individual plates is explained briefly in the introduction to the corresponding chapter.

Embryology, as a branch of anatomy, is a medical discipline. At the same time, it is concerned with the scientific question of how genetic information is processed during differentiation. The justifiable attempt to streamline medical education has led to curriculum restrictions in embryology, at the expense of the understanding of molecular biological correlations. In this atlas, therefore, the scientific background information has been included. However, it is presented apart from the information necessary for medical study. It thus can be called upon for understanding, but need not be worked through in an obligatory manner. The medically relevant knowledge, has been subdivided into human reproduction, a detailed description of the stages of human embryonic development, and the development of organ systems (see the table on the inside cover page). The three large portions of the book, "Human Development" (Chapter 2), "Scientific Foundations" (Chapter 3), and "Organ Systems" (Chapter 4–9) are correlated by crossreferences. Malformations are discussed in connection with the organ systems and in Chapter 10.

Chapter 2, "Human Development," is based on the classic material from the Carnegie collection and from embryos of the Blechschmidt collection. In 1983, I had the opportunity to become personally acquainted with the great embryologist, Erich Blechschmidt, at his home in Glottertal near Freiburg. I hope that his enthusiasm for morphogenesis is revealed in the nature of the presentation, as well as the fascination with the uniqueness of the prenatal development of man, that he made clear.

My special thanks go to Astried Rothenburger and Rüdiger Gay for their productive collaboration, as well as Thomas Bruhns, upon whose graphic reconstructions the following plates are based: in Chapter 2 plates 2.7A, 2.9, 2.11 to 2.15, 2.19, and 2.39; in Chapter 3 plate 3.20; in Chapter 4 plates 4.5B, 4.7A, 4.9B, 4.11, 4.19, 4.20, and 4.21B, as well as in Chapter 6 plates 6.2B, 6.3C, 6.6, 6.8, and 6.10 for heart development. Gesine Bachmann collaborated on the plates for comparative embryology. Petr Raikhmann set up the model for intestinal rotation (plate 7.7) with the Softimage program. I thank my colleague F. Degenhardt from Hannover for coordinating his ultrasound illustrations with the embryological preparations on plates 2.2, 2.32, and 2.37. I thank Anna Drews for reading and editing the proofs and Ute Drews for her collaboration in writing and putting together the text.

Rottenburg, Summer 1993 Ulrich Drews

The English translation was prepared by David B. Meyer and revised by K. Tamussino (Chapter 1) and S. Bieger. My thanks go to Dr. C. Bergmann at Thieme and the translators. On this occasion I would like to thank the Thieme publishing house, in particular Achim Menge, who initiated and supported the production of the atlas of embryology over many years.

## Contents in Brief

**Table of Contents**

# Chapter 1: Reproduction

**Introduction** ........ 1

## Germ Cells

1.1 **Life Cycle** ........ 4

A. The life cycle passes through a haploid phase in the gametes and a diploid phase in the embryo and the individual

B. "Sexuality" in Bacteria is the basis of sexuality and life cycle in higher organism

1.2 **Cell Cycle** ........ 6

A. The cell cycle with meiosis and the cell cycle with cell fusion at fertilization complement each other

B. In male gametes, differentiation starts after meiosis. In female gametes, it starts in the prophase of the first maturation division

1.3 **Chromosomes** ........ 8

In a mitotic cell cycle, chromosomes form euchromatin and heterochromatin, go through DNA synthesis, and condense in metaphase

1.4 **Meiosis** ........ 10

In meiosis, the homologous chromosomes pair and exchange genes in prophase of metaphase I

1.5 **Fertilization** ........ 12

Fertilization starts with the acrosome reaction of the spermatozoon and ends with the activation of the oocyte

1.6 **Overview: Human Germ Line** ........ 14

Germ cells arise in the embryonic yolk sac, differentiate in the gonads, and pass on the genome as gametes

## Pregnancy and Delivery

# Chapter 2: Human Development

## Fetal Membranes and Placenta

### *Chorionic Vesicle*



### *Placenta*

# Chapter 3: General Embryology

# Chapter 4: Nervous System

*Cerebellum*



*Cerebrum*

## Chapter 5: Sense Organs

# Chapter 6: Heart and Vessels

*Vascular System*

# Chapter 7: Gastrointestinal Tract

# Chapter 8: Urogenital System

# Chapter 9: Head

# Chapter 10: Causes of Malformations

# Chapter 1: Reproduction

## Introduction

**1.1 Life Cycle.** In organisms with sexual reproduction, a maternal and a paternal set of chromosomes are united within a single cell, enabling an exchange of genes in the diploid organism. In the next reproductive cycle, the diploid set of chromosomes is again reduced to a haploid set. In Fungi and primitive plants, haploid and diploid cells constitute organisms with equal rights in the life cycle of the species.

The human life cycle similarly passes through a haploid and a diploid phase, the haploid phase being confined to the germ cells. A sperm cell thus corresponds to an independent unicellular organism (→ 3.0). From this perspective, the continuity of species resides in the germ cells; the diploid organism serves only to pass on the species' DNA. As exemplified by the bacterial sex factor, recombination and passing on of chromosomal genes are fundamental molecular principles that already exist in bacteria.

**1.2 Cell Cycle.** The cell cycle refers to the events occurring in the life of a dividing cell. These consist of a $G_1$ phase, followed by DNA replication (S phase), leading into the $G_2$ phase with duplicated chromosomes, which finally segregate in mitosis. Meiosis represents a cell cycle with a single S-phase and two cell divisions, resulting in the formation of four haploid gametes. Diploidy is restored at fertilization by means of a cell cycle with cell fusion.

As with other cell lines with *stem cells,* the germ cells go through a phase of proliferation and a phase of differentiation (→ 3.28). In germ cells, the proliferative phase occurs during embryonic development and is separated from the differentiative phase by a resting stage. Differentiation does not start before puberty and is preceded by the meiotic divisions.

In oocytes the basic pattern is modified. Meiosis already begins during embryonic development and is arrested in prophase of the first meiotic division. The "resting stage" (dictyate) comprises a true resting phase between the embryonic period and puberty and a highly active phase of differentiation during oogenesis. This modification reduces the number of mature ova, in which considerably more is invested than in spermatozoa. The coupling of the second meiotic division with fertilization is probably a protective mechanism that prevents the parthenogenetic development of the oocyte.

**1.3 Chromosomes.** The schematic illustration of chromosome structure in the mitotic cell cycle facilitates an understanding of meiosis. The representation of chromosomes as X-shaped structures is due to the microscopic technique employed to visualize chromosomes. Chromosomes are arrested in metaphase by colchicine. At this stage the chromatin fibers are duplicated and condensed. They have already separated from each other and are held together only in the centromere region, forming an X-shape.

**1.4 Meiosis.** The two essential processes occurring during meiosis are pairing of homologous chromosomes and recombination between chromatin strands. Exchange of DNA between paired chromatids occurs before the sites of "crossing over" (chiasmata) become visible under the light microscope. Crossovers are adhesive points between the nucleoproteins of chromosomes and are secondary to the actual DNA recombination event (although they had been interpreted as true breakage sites by early light microscopists).

"*Lampbrush chromosomes*" arise when chromosomes in the prophase of the first meiotic division, which have already become condensed for cell division, are uncoiled at genetic loci that are necessary for differentiation of the oocyte (maternal factors for embryonic development). Although transcription normally occurs only in $G_1$, these loci can thus be transcribed in $G_2$ phase.

**1.5 Fertilization.** For about 100 years, events occurring during fertilization could only be studied in marine animals with external fertilization, such as sea urchins. The use of appropriate physiological salt solutions has made it possible to carry out fertilization of eggs from mammals (i.e., organisms with internal fertilization) in vitro. In vitro fertilization is a medical treatment for infertility, for example in cases of inflammatory closure of the fallopian tubes.

**1.6 Germ Line.** The "germ line" concept was formulated by Nußbaum in 1886 and dates back to the observation that the primordial germ cells do not arise in the "germinal epithelium" of the gonad (→ 8.6). In amphibian oocytes, a cytoplasmic region that gives rise to germ cells can already be delimited at the oocyte stage. This cytoplasmic region contains mRNA that is partitioned to prospective germ cells by cleavage divisions. The mRNA that determines the differentiation of germ cells was transcribed in lampbrush chromosomes, and is therefore a "maternal factor" for embryonic development in amphibians. In mammalian and human development, these genes are not "switched on" until the third week, when germ cells arise in the yolk sac. The germ cells resemble the stem cells of the blood and are not unique in comparison with other determined cell lines.

**1.7 Male Genital Organs.** The description of these organs is centered on the path taken by sperm and on the function of the male glands in producing ejaculate. The representation of the prostate emphasizes the clinically important distinction between *prostatic hypertrophy* and *prostatic carcinoma.* In prostatic hypertrophy, the increased estradiol produced with age leads to the proliferation of periurethral glands, which displaces the actual androgen-dependent glandular tissue of the capsule and obstructs urinary flow. Prostatic carcinoma arises in the androgen-dependent glandular tissue itself.

**1.8 Spermatogenesis.** The *Sertoli cells* of the testis correspond to the *follicular epithelial cells* of the ovary. In the ovarian cycle, follicular epithelial cells develop into granulosa cells (→ 1.11). Sertoli cells and granulosa cells respond to FSH. The *Leydig cells* of the testis correspond to the *theca cells* of the ovary; these cells are stimulated by LH. The Leydig cells produce testosterone, which is converted into estradiol by the Sertoli cells. By analogy, the theca cells produce androgens that are converted into estradiol by granulosa cells.

**1.9 Waves of Spermatogenesis.** A standardized staging system is essential for the evaluation of spermatogenesis in the case of hormonal or genetic disturbances. The sequence of stages in the seminiferous epithelium results from waves of spermatogenesis. These waves are due to clones of spermatocytes synchronously undergoing spermatogenesis, with the daughter cells linked to each other by syncytial bridges.

**1.10 Female Genital Organs.** The description of these organs is centered on the physiology of sperm ascension and the prerequisites for fertilization in the ampulla of the fallopian tube. The significance of collagen for the closure of the vaginal part of the cervix (portio) during pregnancy and its loosening by relaxin at the onset of parturition is addressed in Plate 1.17. The physiological irritations at the portio and the overgrowth tendency of the vaginal squamous epithelium are significant factors in the development of epithelial carcinoma of the cervix.

**1.11 Oogenesis.** The size of the group of about 10–15 primordial follicles that constitutively begin oogenesis (i.e., without hormonal stimulation), may correspond to the original litter size of a mammal. In humans, the cycle is controlled by the dominant follicle, which initially profits from the hormone production of the remaining tertiary follicles of the group, but then induces their degeneration. In the case of an artificially induced ovulation, the dominant follicle as well as the remaining tertiary follicles can ovulate, so that multiple pregnancies can occur.

**1.12 Ovulation.** The oocyte is released from the ovary into the body cavity and picked up by the ciliated Fallopian tube, which is ontogenetically related to renal excretory ducts (→ 8.1). The evolutionary preservation of this primitive mechanism is explained by the fact that ovulation is a central step in the reproduction of a species and therefore permits no fundamental change. The hormonal control of ovulation, in contrast, is becoming more and more finely tuned by evolutionary selection, for example in regulating the exact movements of the Fallopian tube as an oocyte is collected.

**1.13 Menstrual Cycle.** The original hierarchy in the control of the *sexual cycle* begins in the pineal gland, in which the circadian rhythm originally is coupled to the length of the day and night by means of pineal light receptors (→4.23). The seasonal rhythm regulated by the lengths of the days and nights can be uncoupled from exogenous light stimuli and converted to an endogenous rhythm. The cyclic activities of the rhythm-generating center in the central nervous system (CNS) induce cyclic FSH and LH secretion from the pituitary gland and thus determine the maturation of the follicles and the cyclic reappearance of sexual receptivity (estrus). In the estrus phase, ovulation is subject to another central feedback mechanism: it is coordinated with mating behavior via the LH peak. In humans, regulation by external stimuli is further reduced. Ovulation is triggered independently of external influences by the dominant follicle itself, via an estrogen peak, which secondarily induces the LH peak. The induction of the LH peak and thus of ovulation can be inhibited by exogenously supplied steroid hormones (*ovulation inhibitors*). In a cycle without ovulation, the corpus luteum is absent. The decidua fails to differentiate in the second half of the cycle. The falling off of hormone levels at the end of the cycle leads to sloughing off of the endometrium.

**1.14 Endometrium.** The function of the endometrium is to nourish the fertilized oocyte and to implant the embryo. Its glands produce a nutrient-rich mucosal film in which the free blastocyst swims. In the compact zone, connective tissue cells are transformed into nutrient-rich decidual cells that can be phagocytized by the penetrating trophoblast cells. After menstruation or curettage, the endometrium regenerates from the basal zone, which contains the undifferentiated glandular ends and contracted stumps of spiral arteries embedded in the trabeculae of the smooth musculature of the myometrium.

**1.15 Course of Pregnancy.** Embryonic development has different implications for the clinican than for the embryologist. Until the conclusion of implantation, the embryo produces no signs of pregnancy. Defective implantations do not prevent menstruation but can lead to a prolonged and delayed menstruation. Up to the 10th week, pregnancy and embryonic development goes nearly unnoticed and has few effects on the mother. Clinically, pregnancy is the long period during which the fetus develops and influences the psychological and physical well-being of the mother. For the embryologist, in contrast, the major events occur in the embryonic period in early pregnancy.

**1.16 Gravidarium (Pregnancy Calculator Wheel).** A pregnancy can be precisely dated and a birth date calculated by means of a gravidarium. Because the gestation period, like all biological processes, is subject to a natural fluctuation, this calculation is only an estimate. To avoid ambiguity between lunar and calendar months, obstetricians date pregnancies in weeks. The weeks of pregnancy are calculated from the last menstruation so that a discrepancy of two weeks exists with respect to the true age of the embryo.

**1.17 Hormone Levels.** During pregnancy the hormone levels in the mother are profoundly changed. Steroid hormone metabolism is determined by the placenta and the fetal adrenal gland. Hormone levels are thus clinically important indicators in the course of pregnancy.

**1.18 Birth.** The difficulty associated with birth in humans is due to the size of the fetal head, which results from the development of the brain. The painful birth process is one of the key stimuli for the development of the mother-child bond.

# Germ Cells

## 1.1 Life Cycle

### A. Life Cycle in Diploid Organisms

Sexual reproduction is based on an alternation between the *haploid* and *diploid phase* of the life cycle. In the diploid phase, cells contain two sets of chromosomes, whereas in the haploid phase, only one set is present.

The diploid organism arises by the union of haploid gametes at **fertilization** (**A1**). The gametes fuse to form a diploid **zygote** (**A2**). The zygote grows by mitotic cell division to form the **embryo** (**A3**) and ultimately the diploid **individual** (**A4**). Early in embryonic development, the *germ cells* become segregated from the remaining *somatic cells* as a separate cell line. The germ cells multiply by mitosis in the gonads and undergo meiotic divisions (meiosis **A5**).

In *mitosis* (**A4**) all chromosomes of the diploid set duplicate and segregate into two identical daughter cells. In *meiosis* the duplication is followed by *pairing* and *recombination* of the homologous chromosomes. (Homologous chromosomes are the corresponding chromosomes that were contributed to the zygote by the two haploid gametes.) By means of two meiotic divisions, four haploid **gametes** (**A6**) arise without additional DNA synthesis. These gametes contain novel combinations of the homologous chromosomes in the diploid parent.

The normal **individual** (**A7**) consists of diploid somatic cells that withdraw from the life cycle upon death and are not reproduced in the next generation. Only the germ cells function in the passing on and the recombination of genetic information. The development of germ cells separately from the somatic cells is referred to as the *germ line*. Germ cell proliferation and differentiation take place in the gonads of diploid individuals, where there is protection from external influences. In mammals, not only fertilization but also fetal development is moved to the protected interior of the female sexual organs.

### B. "Sexuality" in Bacteria

Sexuality may have originated as a mechanism of gene recombination, as exemplified in bacteria by the modified mode of infection used by bacteriophages.

**1. Infection.** Bacteria possess a ring chromosome of DNA. Bacteriophages are viral parasites of bacteria that can inject their DNA into a bacterial cell through a *sex pilus*. Inside the bacterium, synthesis of viral proteins proceeds until the bacterium undergoes lysis.

**2. Transfection.** Alternatively, after injection into the bacterium, the viral DNA may remain in the form of a ring-shaped *plasmid*. These plasmids often encode important genetic information for bacteria, such as resistance to antibiotics. Plasmids are passed on to other bacteria by transfection, a modified mode of infection involving the sex pili, which are encoded by the plasmid.

**3. Conjugation.** If the plasmid is integrated into the bacterial ring chromosome, the entire ring chromosome can be transferred to another bacterium of the same species via the sex pili. The homologous ring chromosomes pair, and *crossing over* and *recombination* of genes can occur.

In the ensuing cell division, unequal daughter cells are generated. One of the two daughter cells carries the genes encoding the sex pili, i.e., the "male *determinants* " necessary for conjugation. This mechanism corresponds to the species-specific adhesion of sperm to the zona pellucida, leading to the fusion of sperm with the membrane of the oocyte (→ 1.14 A4).

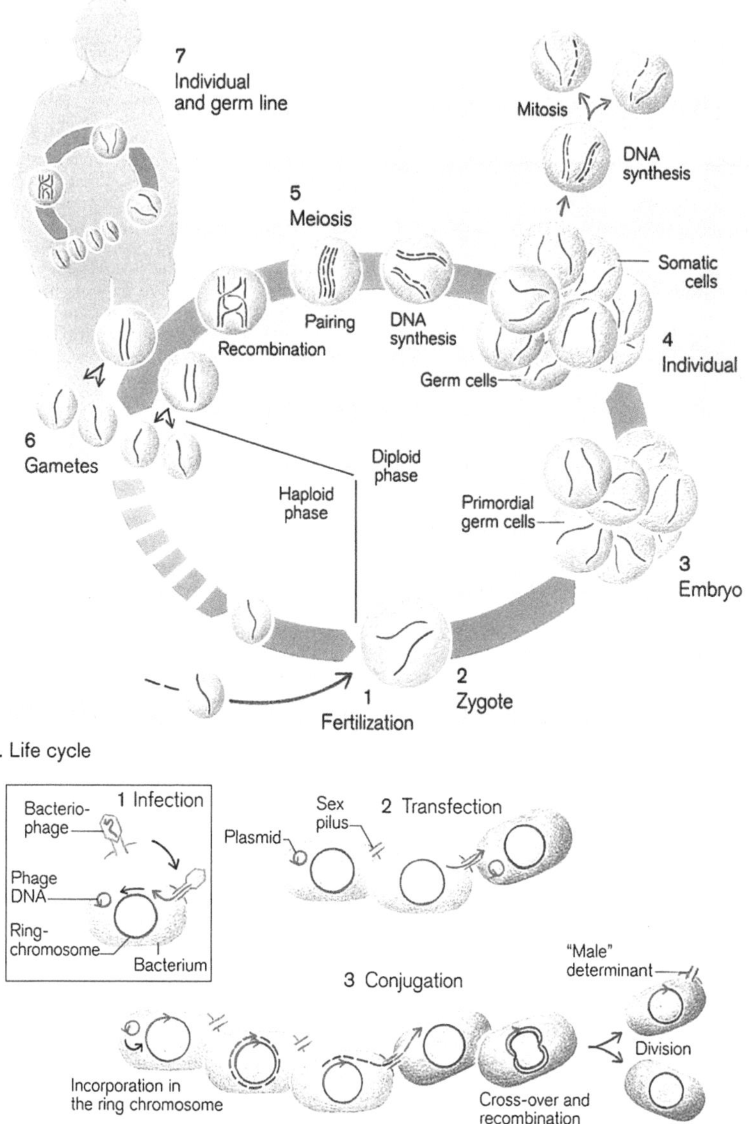
7
Individual
and germ line
Mitosis
DNA
synthesis
5
Meiosis
Somatic
cells
Pairing
DNA
synthesis
Recombination
4
Individual
Germ cells
6
Gametes
Diploid
phase
Haploid
phase
Primordial
germ cells
3
Embryo
2
Zygote
1
Fertilization
1 Infection
Bacterio-
phage
Phage
DNA
Ring-
chromosome
Bacterium
Sex
pilus
2 Transfection
Plasmid
"Male"
determinant
3 Conjugation
Division
Incorporation in
the ring chromosome
Cross-over and
recombination

A. Life cycle

B. "Sexuality" in bacteria

## 1.2 Cell Cycle

### A. Cell Cycle in the Germ Line

**1. Mitotic Cell Cycle.** A mitotic cell division begins with the *S-phase* (DNA synthesis) in which DNA and structural proteins of the chromosomes are replicated. After a brief $G_2$ *phase*, the cell automatically proceeds with mitosis (M). In *prophase* of mitosis, the chromosomes become visible. In *metaphase*, they become organized at the mitotic spindle. The chromatids are separated and segregated to opposite cell poles prior to reconstitution of the 46 chromosomes in the nuclei of the daughter cells. Homologous chromosomes are independent of each other in the mitotic cell cycle.

**2. Meiotic Cell Cycle.** Meiosis consists of a cell cycle with one S-phase and two cell divisions (meiotic divisions). In prophase of the first meiotic division, the homologous chromosomes pair and undergo recombination. In the pairing process, the 46 individual chromosomes form 23 pairs of chromosomes, each containing 4 DNA strands, since the chromosomes were replicated prior to synapsis (pairing). Through the two meiotic divisions, in which *Metaphase I* and *Metaphase II* follow each other without S-phase, the chromosomes are ultimately distributed to four gametes, each of which contains 23 nonreplicated chromosomes (1.1 A5).

**3. Cell Cycle with Cell Fusion.** To restore the diploid state, meiosis must be followed by cell fusion. After the fusion of the *haploid gametes* (fertilization), two *pronuclei* arise in which the two sets of 23 chromosomes are replicated in an S-phase. The replicated chromosomes are arranged on a common spindle, which thus contains 46 replicated, unpaired chromosomes. This is the spindle of the *first cleavage division*.

### B. Development of Male and Female Gametes

The development of germ cells comprises a phase of *proliferation* (mitotic divisions), *meiosis*, and the *differentiation* of the gametes. A *resting stage* is present between the embryonic period and puberty. Male germ cells rest as mitotic spermatogonia. Female germ cells pass through the resting stage and through differentiation in prophase of the first meiotic division.

**1. Spermatogenesis.** Sperm are small, motile cells that are produced in extravagant numbers. The stem cell of spermatogenesis is the *spermatogonium*. After puberty, spermatogonia proliferate in the seminiferous tubules of the testis. The last mitotic division produces *primary spermatocytes*, each of which give rise to two *secondary spermatocytes* by the first maturation division. The second maturation division yields four *spermatids* that differentiate into *spermatozoa*.

**2. Oogenesis.** The stem cells of oogenesis are called *oogonia*. Because only few mature ova are necessary, the majority of oogonia die during development. Oogonia undergo a phase of mitotic multiplication and enter into prophase of the first meiotic division during embryonic development. After pairing of homologous chromosomes, meiosis is arrested in the **dictyate stage**. During the ovarian cycle, growth and differentiation of oocytes take place while the oocytes remain in prophase of the first meiotic division. Transcription reaches maximum levels in the paired chromosomes, as structural constituents of the oocyte and mRNA for the young embryo are synthesized. The haploid state is ultimately produced when meiosis resumes. A series of unequal divisions takes place, during which the differentiated oocyte is preserved and the superfluous chromosomal sets are expelled as polar bodies containing minimal volumes of cytoplasma. The *first polar body* is expelled shortly before ovulation, whereas the *second polar body* is shed after fertilization.

S
G1
G2
M
1
Cell cycle
with mitosis
Prophase
Metaphase
Daughter
cells
S
G1
G2
Fertilization
(cell fusion)
Cleavage
Pronuclei
S
G1
DNA
synthesis
G2
M
2
Cell cycle
with meiosis
Prophase
Metaphase I
Metaphase II
Gametes
3
Cell cycle
with cell fusion

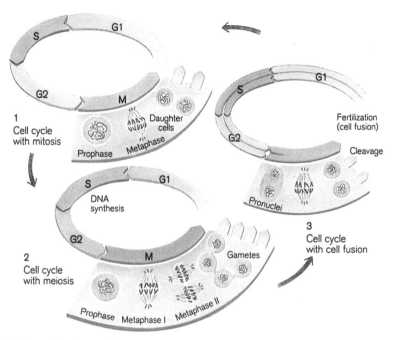

A. Cell cycle in the germ line

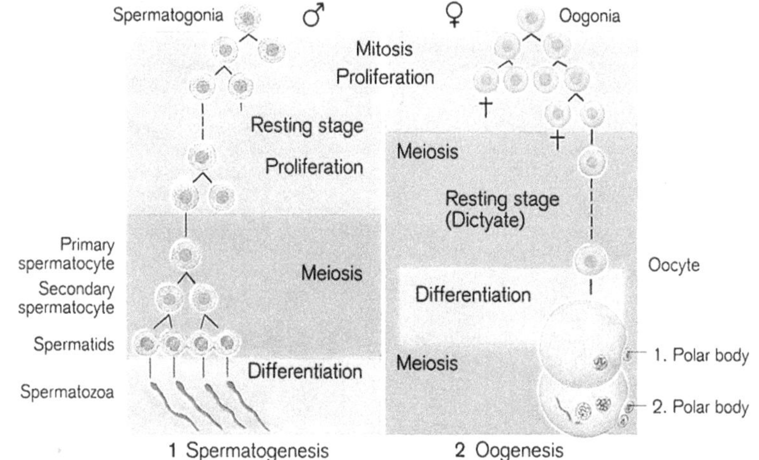


B. Development of male and female germ cells

## 1.3 Chromosomes

### A. Chromosome Structure

**1. DNA Double Helix.** Genetic information is encoded in the sequence of four nucleotides in a DNA double helix. The DNA spiral is 2 nm thick. Its morphological structure was revealed indirectly by X-ray crystallography.

**2. Nucleosome.** The DNA strand of a chromosome is wound in spirals around a chain of nucleosomes, which consist of basic nuclear proteins, the *histones* . The DNA filament makes 2 1/2 turns around each nucleosome. Nucleosomes are closely linked to each other by a small connecting protein that also belongs to the histone family (H1). Preparation of chromatin for electron microscopy, however, leads to the stretching of chromatin strands so that nucleosomes resemble beads on a 10 nm-thick string.

During the evolution of eukaryotes, histones have remained highly conserved. These basic nucleoproteins are contrasted with the acidic nucleoproteins, which include enzymes such as DNA and RNA polymerases and other acidic regulatory proteins that determine the functional state of DNA (not shown).

**3. Transcription.** During transcription in the G1-phase of the cell cycle, the nucleosomes break down into their histone subunits. The coding and noncoding strands of the DNA double helix separate; mRNA molecules are transcribed from the coding (template) strand by *RNA-polymerase*. The double helix and the nucleosome structure are regenerated behind the transcription site.

**4. Euchromatin and Heterochromatin.** In transciptionally active regions of chromatin, the nucleosome chain is dispersed in the nucleoplasm (*euchromatin*). In regions in which transciption does not occur, the nucleosome chain is wound into a superhelix (*heterochromatin*).

**5. DNA Synthesis.** During replication of DNA in the S-phase of the cell cycle, nucleosomes again break down into their histone subunits. Replication of the two DNA strands by *DNA polymerase* produces a chromosome with two chromatin fibers, the DNA strands of which are wound around nucleosomes. The 46 unpaired chromosomes (2n), with a DNA content of 2c, thus give rise to 46 unpaired replicated chromosomes (2n) with a DNA content of 4c. Replicated chromosomes are not transcribed (exception: lampbrush chromosomes in oogenesis, → 1.4 A4b).

**6. Superhelix.** Chromosome condensation into a superhelix (35 nm) during prophase of mitosis resembles the process of heterochromatin formation.

At metaphase, the *condensed chromatin fibers* thicken into irregular loops inside a framework of structural proteins, forming the two chromatids (1000 nm) of the metaphase chromosome.

**7. Metaphase Chromosomes.** The free arms of an X-shaped (metacentric) chromosome are the separated *chromatids*, which are connected only in the region of the *centromere*, and which give rise to the chromosomes of the daughter cells in anaphase of mitosis. In the region of the centromere, the chromosome is attached to the spindle fibers (*microtubules*). The point of attachment consists of structural proteins and is called the *kinetochore*.

**8. Chromosome Complement of Humans.** The representation and classification of chromosomes in a chromosome complement is always based on the condensed, replicated metaphase chromosomes, since chromosomes are only visible in this state under the light microscope. Cells are lysed by treatment with a hypotonic salt solution, then are dropped onto a slide. Well-spread chromosomes are stained and photographed. The chromosomes can then be cut out of the photograph and aligned according to size in a karyotype.

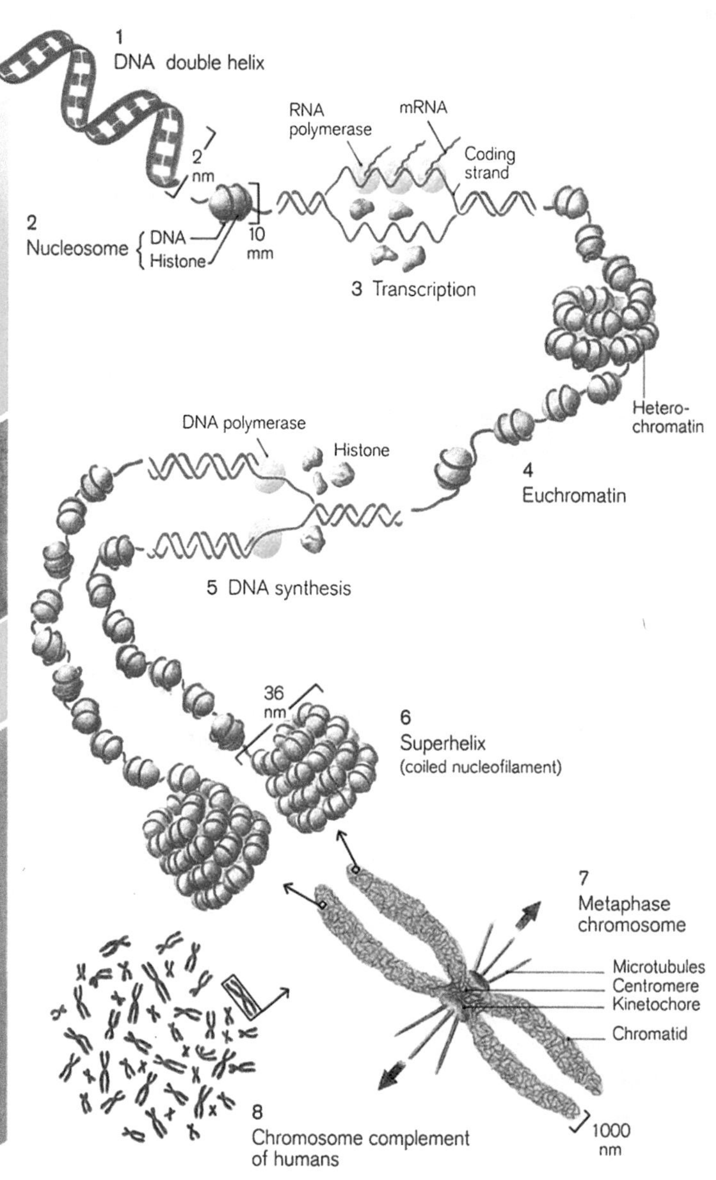


A. Structure of chromosomes

# 1.4 Meiosis

## A. Chromosomes in Meiosis

Pairing of homologous chromosomes and recombination of genes occur in prophase of the first meiotic division (**Prophase I**). The protracted prophase is divided into four stages based on the light microscopic appearance of the chromosomes:

**1. Leptotene** (slender). Chromosomes are visible in the nucleus as slender filaments, with their ends anchored in the nuclear membrane. The adhesive points are grouped in a region of the nuclear membrane opposite the *centriole* (bouquet arrangement). The chromatin filaments of the 46 chromosomes are still tightly intertwined. As the chromosomes condense, the linkages are cut by specific DNAses and the integrity of the chromosome strands is restored by other enzymes (ligases).

**2. Zygotene** (paired). While continuing to unravel and condense, the homologous chromosomes pair (synapse), forming *synaptonemal complexes*. Each chromosome is schematically represented as a double line, although the replicated chromatin strands still cannot be recognized at this stage as individual chromatids. During the zygotene phase, recombination of genes by crossing-over takes place. When the paired chromosomes are spread and contrasted with electron-dense metal atoms, a central strand and two lateral elements, connected by banded structures, can be distinguished by electron microscopy (**2a**). The central filament and the lateral elements are composed of glycoproteins. The condensed and replicated nucleoprotein fiber of each homologous chromosome is arranged on a *lateral element*. The crossed-over loops representing sites of crossing-over are hypothetical.

In spermatogenesis, the X and Y chromosomes pair along the short arm. This pairing occurs in the "*sex vesicle*" (**2b**) which can be recognized light microscopically in the nucleus of spermatocytes. In spreads of metaphase I chromosomes, the sex chromosomes exhibit a tandem arrangement due to the end-to-end pairing.

**3. Pachytene** (short and thick). The chromosomes are maximally condensed. Cross-overs are still not visible. The paired chromosomes begin to separate from each other. In spermatogenesis, the primary spermatocytes persist longest in the pachytene stage (→ 1.8 A3).

**4. Diplotene** (doubled). Four individual chromatids (tetrads) and crossovers (*chiasmata)* become visible. A chiasma indicates where crossing-over has occurred. The homologous chromosomes no longer adhere to each other at the centromere, but remain connected at the chiasmata (**4a**). In oocytes, the first meiotic division is arrested at the diplotene stage *(dictyate*) and the chromosomes decondense. At the end of the resting phase, genetic loci necessary for maturation of the oocyte are activated as the oocyte begins differentiation in the ovarian cycle. Loops of DNA are unfolded from the nucleosome chains of the paired chromosomes and transcription takes place. In amphibia, the loops of these *lampbrush chromosomes* can be viewed under the light microscope (**4b**).

**Metaphase I.** As the centromeres of the recombined homologous chromosomes separate further, the chiasmata move to the ends of the chromosomes (terminalization). This results in the formation of a typical ring structure or double-cross structure of meiosis I chromosomes. The first meiotic division gives rise to two daughter cells with *23 replicated chromosomes.*

**Metaphase II.** The second meiotic division immediately follows the first,without or with only a brief decondensation of chromosomes. As in mitosis, the chromosomes are separated last in the region of the *centromere*. Cytoplasmic bridges are preserved between the spermatids (as between the ova and polar bodies) ( → 1.8 A1).

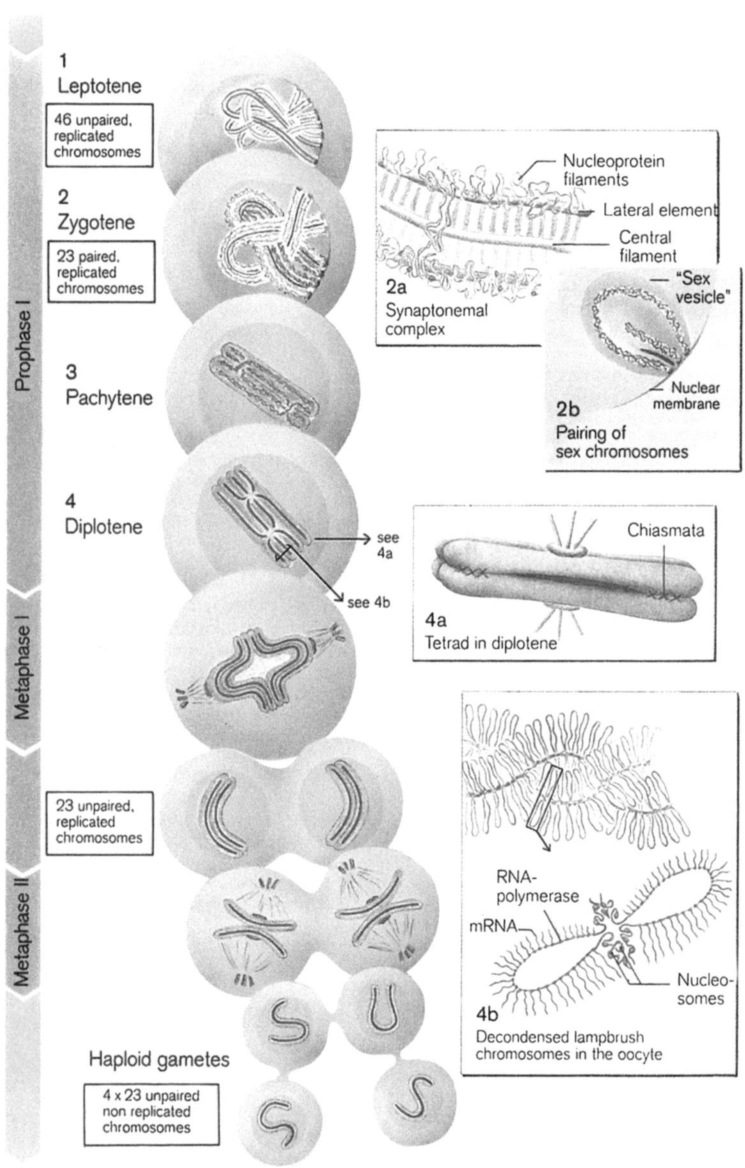

Prophase I
Metaphase I
Metaphase II
1
Leptotene
46 unpaired, replicated chromosomes
2
Zygotene
23 paired, replicated chromosomes
3
Pachytene
4
Diplotene
see 4a
see 4b
23 unpaired, replicated chromosomes
Haploid gametes
4 x 23 unpaired non replicated chromosomes
Nucleoprotein filaments
Lateral element
Central filament
2a
Synaptonemal complex
"Sex vesicle"
Nuclear membrane
2b
Pairing of sex chromosomes
Chiasmata
4a
Tetrad in diplotene
RNA-polymerase
mRNA
Nucleo-somes
4b
Decondensed lampbrush chromosomes in the oocyte

A. Chromosomes in meiosis

# 1.5 Fertilization

## A. Stages of Fertilization

**1. Acrosome Reaction.** The *acrosome* of the sperm head contains hydrolyzing enzymes that are necessary for the penetration of the *corona radiata* and *zona pellucida*. The enzymes, in part, are firmly linked to the inner membrane of the acrosome. The acrosome corresponds to a large lysosome covering the apex of the cell nucleus. The acrosome reaction occurs shortly before contact with the oocyte. The cell membrane and the external membrane of the acrosome fuse with one another at many points (**1a**). The zones of fusion develop pores, through which the contents of the acrosome are released. The perforated remains of the membrane are cast off as the corona radiata is penetrated (**1b**). The basal segment of the acrosome remains intact at the equator of the spermatozoon, forming a membranous sac. At this point, the inner membrane of the acrosome covers the sperm head and is fused posteriorly with the original cell membrane (**1c**).

**2. Adhesion of Sperm.** The corona radiata consists of follicular epithelium, which plays a role in *chemotaxis* of sperm and in the induction of the acrosome reaction. The spermatozoon penetrates the corona radiata in a few seconds with powerful tail movements and then adheres for several minutes to the zona pellucida. This adhesion is species-specific, utilizing a mechanism similar to a receptor-ligand interaction.

**3. Penetration of Zona Pellucida.** After the adhesion phase, the spermatozoon penetrates the zona pellucida within a few minutes. It passes through the zona pellucida at an angle and meets the cell membrane of the oocyte tangentially.

**4. Fusion of Cell Membranes.** Small vesicles (*cortical granules*) lie under the cell membrane of the mature oocyte. Contact of the spermatozoon induces a circulating excitatory potential at the cell membrane of the oocyte, leading to exocytosis of the vesicles by a chain reaction. The vesicles release their contents into the perivitelline space between the zona pellucida and the oocyte cell membrane. Factors are liberated that modify the structure of glycoproteins of the zona pellucida, so that it is impenetrable to further spermatozoon (zona pellucida reaction). Contact of the spermatozoon with the oocyte cell membrane induces three processes: (1) The *zona pellucida reaction* is initiated, preventing the penetration of additional spermatozoa (*block to polyspermy*) (2) The block of metaphase II in the oocyte is removed (3) The metabolism of the oocyte is activated. Embryonic development begins.

As the sperm head penetrates the oocyte, the tail flagellum beats so powerfully that the oocyte is set into slight rotation and the tail of the spermatozoon slips completely into the perivitelline space. The strength of the flagellar stroke subsides suddenly. While the sperm head decondenses and swells to form the male pronucleus, the entire tail flagellum, which beats intermittently, is taken up into the oocyte, where it disintegrates. The oocyte is covered with a dense coat of microvilli (**4a**). (Only the plasma membrane region above the metaphase II chromosomes of the oocyte is free of villi and bulges out like a hillock.) The sperm head dips into the villi at the oocyte surface. In the postacrosomal segment, the sperm cell membrane fuses with the oocyte cell membrane (**4b**) and is incorporated into the oocyte membrane. Sperm head, neck, and tail sink into the oocyte yolk (**4c**).

**5. Second Meiotic Division.** At ovulation, the oocyte is arrested in metaphase II. Fertilization releases the block and the second polar body is expelled.

**6. Pronuclei.** The chromosomes of the spermatozoon and oocyte (haploid sets) decondense and form the female and male pronuclei.

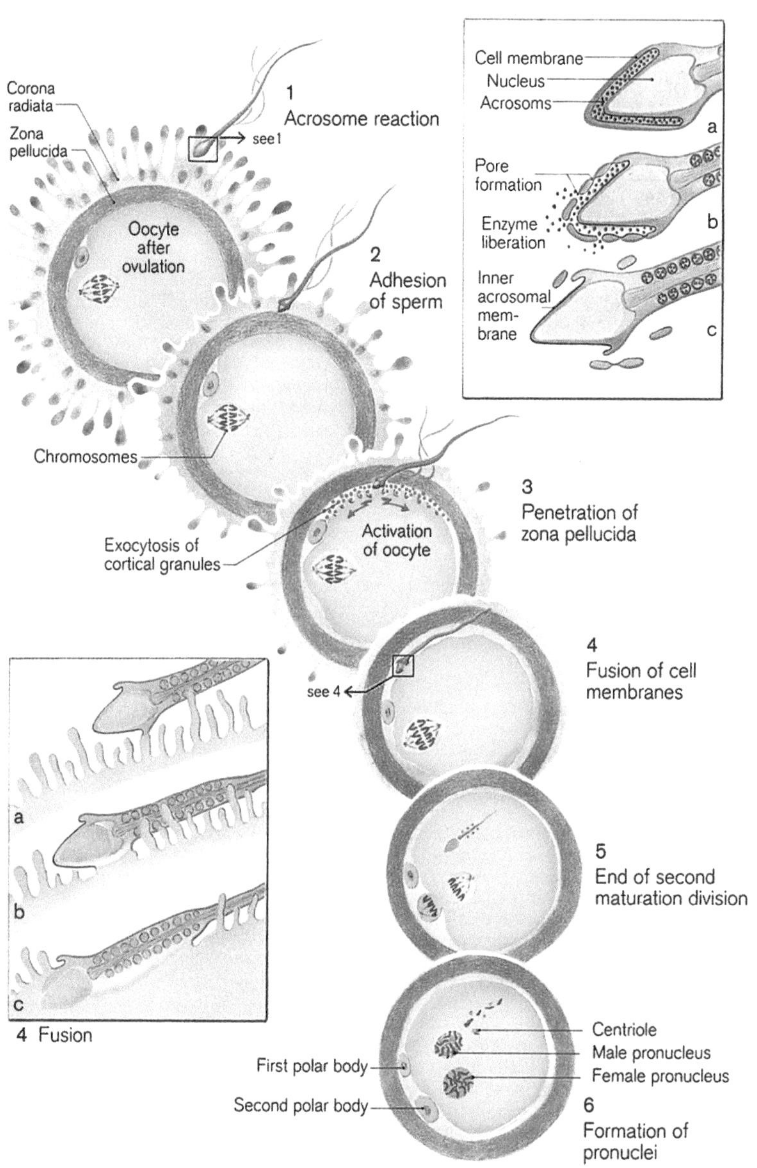


A. Fertilization

## 1.6 Overview

### A. Human Germ Line

**Zygote and Early Embryo.** In the zygote and early embryo, each cell can give rise to either somatic or germ cells. Each blastomere of the zygote can give rise to an individual embryo when raised separately. The further development of each cell depends entirely on its future position in the embryo. The primordial germ cells can first be identified in the yolk sac in the 4th week (→ 8.6). They are induced there, together with the stem cells of the blood. On the basis of their high content of alkaline phosphatase(as in other mammals) they can also be identified histochemically in the human embryo.

**Migration of Primordial Germ Cells.** In the 4th week, the primordial germ cells migrate from the yolk sac to the indifferent gonadal anlage via the dorsal mesentery. During their migration, they multiply by mitotic division.

**Colonization of the Gonadal Anlage.** The germ cells proliferate further in the coelomic epithelium of the indifferent gonadal anlage.

**Sexual Differentiation.** Sex determination occurs in the somatic cells of the gonadal anlage. If a Y chromosome is present, a testis develops from the indifferent anlage; if no Y chromosome is present, an ovary is formed.

**Germ Cells in the Embryonic Period.** The number of *oogonia* reaches its maximum (7 million) in the 5th month. Following proliferation, the oogonia begin the first meiotic division (meiosis I). Follicular cells envelop the oogonia, forming primordial follicles in which the first meiotic division is arrested. Outside of the primordial follicles, the oogonia die. In the *anlage of the testis*, the primordial germ cells are incorporated into the testis cords as atogonia and enter into a resting phase.

**Germ Cells at the Time of Birth.** In the *ovary*, the oocytes rest in the primordial follicles, arrested in prophase of the first meiotic division (dictyate stage). In the *testis*, the spermatogonia rest as mitotic cells in the compact testis cords.

**Differentiation at Puberty.** In the *ovary*, there are still about 40 000 oocytes present. In each cycle, a group of ova begins differentiation. The paired chromosomes decondense (*lampbrush chromosomes*) and mRNA necessary for initiation of embryonic development is transcribed and stored in the cytoplasm of the oocyte (maternal factors). The first meiotic division is completed shortly before ovulation with the expulsion of the first polar body. The second meiotic division (meiosis II) is arrested in metaphase II. Ovulation takes place at this stage.

In the *testis*, the spermatogonia resume proliferation at puberty. The meiotic divisions and differentiation into sperm follow a fixed number of mitotic divisions.

**Fertilization.** Contact with a sperm releases the block of metaphase II. The second meiotic division proceeds, ending with the expulsion of the second polar body.

**Zygote.** After the formation of the pronuclei, embryonic development begins with the formation of a new zygote.

**Regulation of the Law Protecting Embryos.** According to the German embryo protection law of 13 December 1990, all diagnostic and therapeutic manipulations of the human germ line are prohibited. In the mammalian embryo (from fertilization to implantation), each cell of the zygote, and later on of the embryoblast has the potential to develop into a germ cell. Therefore, no diagnostic or therapeutic measure may be carried out, in particular after in vitro fertilization prior to implantation. Diagnostic tests by means of chorionic biopsy are permitted only after implantation.

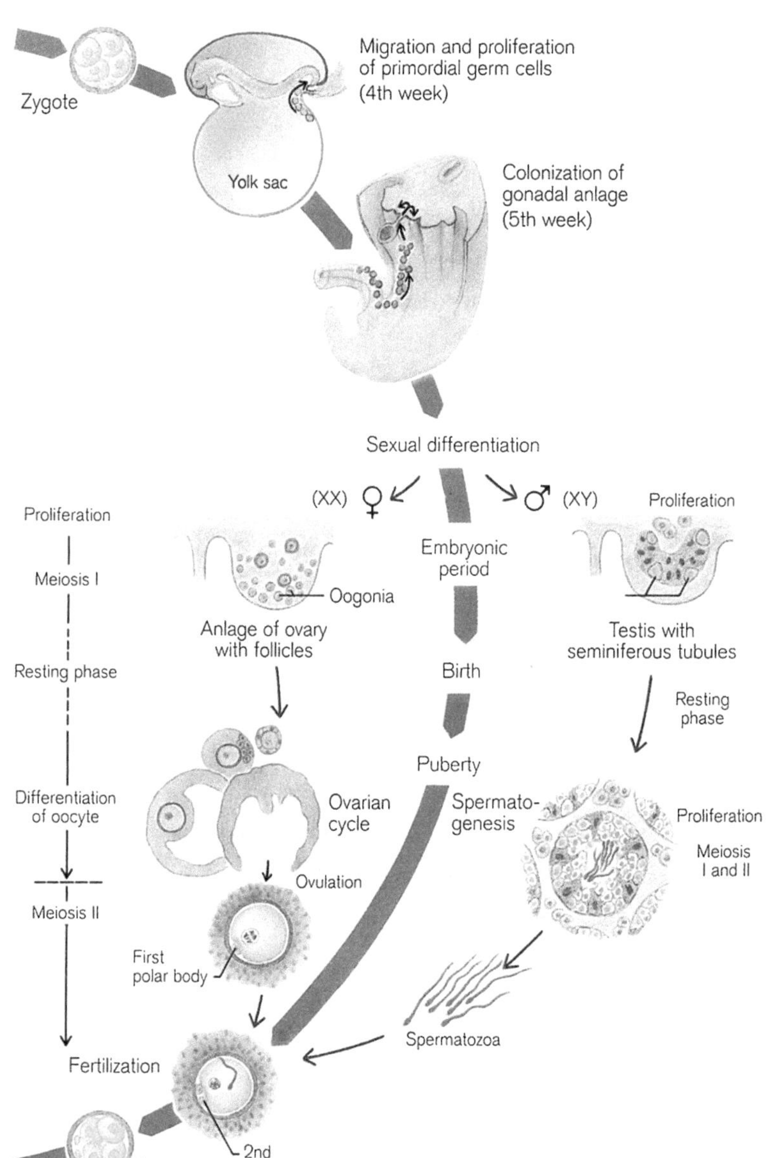
Zygote
Migration and proliferation of primordial germ cells (4th week)
Yolk sac
Colonization of gonadal anlage (5th week)
Sexual differentiation
(XX) ♀
♂ (XY)
Proliferation
Meiosis I
Resting phase
Differentiation of oocyte
Meiosis II
Fertilization
Oogonia
Anlage of ovary with follicles
Embryonic period
Birth
Puberty
Proliferation
Testis with seminiferous tubules
Resting phase
Ovarian cycle
Ovulation
First polar body
Spermato-genesis
Proliferation
Meiosis I and II
Spermatozoa
Zygote
2nd polar body

A. Human germ line

# Male Organs

## 1.7 Male Genital Tract

### A. Anatomy of Male Genital Organs

**1. Testes and Epididymides.** Sperm develop in the *seminiferous tubules* of the testis. These tubules are derived from the U-shaped testis cords and open at both ends into the *rete testis*. Each convoluted tubule forms a testicular lobule or segment. These segments are separated from one another by irregular connective tissue *septa* emanating from the compact testicular capsule (*tunica albuginea*). Together with fluid produced by the Sertoli cells, sperm are transported passively to the *rete testis* and then, via 10–20 efferent ductules, into the epididymis. 90% of the fluid secreted by the testis is resorbed in the epididymis. The *principal cells* in the convoluted duct of the epididymis (**1a**) possess branched cell processes (stereocilia) and are responsible for the nourishment and maturation of the sperm. The sperm are transported further by the peristaltic action of *fibromyocytes* lying closely apposed to the epithelium. In the epididymis, they first acquire the ability to move independently. In the tail of the epididymis (*cauda*), the duct of the epididymis widens; sperm are stored here and resorbed if not ejaculated. Transport through the epididymis takes 10–14 days.

**2. Prostate and Seminal Vesicle.** Before opening into the *urethra*, the *vas deferens* widens to form the *ampulla* and is joined by the excretory duct of the *seminal vesicle*. The prostate consists of glands located directly beneath the urethral epithelium (*periurethral glands* ) that increase and become enlarged after the age of 40 (prostatic hypertrophy) and of tubuloalveolar glands extending into the rigid stroma of the prostate, which is permeated by smooth muscle cells.

**3. Bulb and Urethra** (sagittal section). The urethra of the penis is surrounded by the *corpus spongiosum*, which is thickened proximally to form the bulb. The *bulbourethral glands* open into the bulb, and submucosal *urethral glands* open into the roof of the urethra (**3a**).

**4. Composition of the Ejaculate**

**Preliminary Secretion:** Before ejaculation (in the plateau phase), the *bulbourethral glands* and the *urethral glands* secrete a clear, alkaline secretion that may contain sperm that have become sequestered in the urethral glands (**3a**).

**Ejaculate:** The *first fraction* of the ejaculate is derived from the prostate and contains few sperm. The prostatic secretion is acidic and rich in citric acid and acid phosphatase. The *middle fraction* is the main fraction and consists of a mixture of aqueous (*tail of the epididymis*, site of sperm storage) and gelatinous (*ampulla*) secretions and the majority of sperm. The *terminal fraction* is purely gelatinous and is produced by the *seminal vesicle*. The secretion of the seminal vesicle is alkaline and rich in fructose and prostaglandins. As a whole, the ejaculate is alkaline (4–6 ml, 40–250 million sperm, pH 7.2–7.8); it coagulates within one minute after thorough mixing and becomes fluid again after 20–30 minutes. (In rodents, the secretions of the prostate lobes and the seminal vesicle produce a vaginal plug which retains the sperm in the vagina).

**Sexual exitation.** Erection of the penis is triggered by tactile stimuli of erogenous zones or centrally by psychogenic stimuli. The pads in the arterial arm of the cavernous bodies relax and the arteriovenous anastomoses open, causing the cavernous spaces in the cavernous bodies to fill. Since the pressure in the corpus spongiosum is lower than that in the corpora cavernosa, the urethra remains open. Ejaculation is induced by pulsating contractions of the vas deferens and of the muscles of the pelvic floor. According to Masters and Johnson, four phases of sexual excitement can be distinguished: (1) **E**xcitation (psychic), **P**lateau phase (parasympathetic), (3) **O**rgasm (sympathetic) and (4) **R**egression (EPOR).

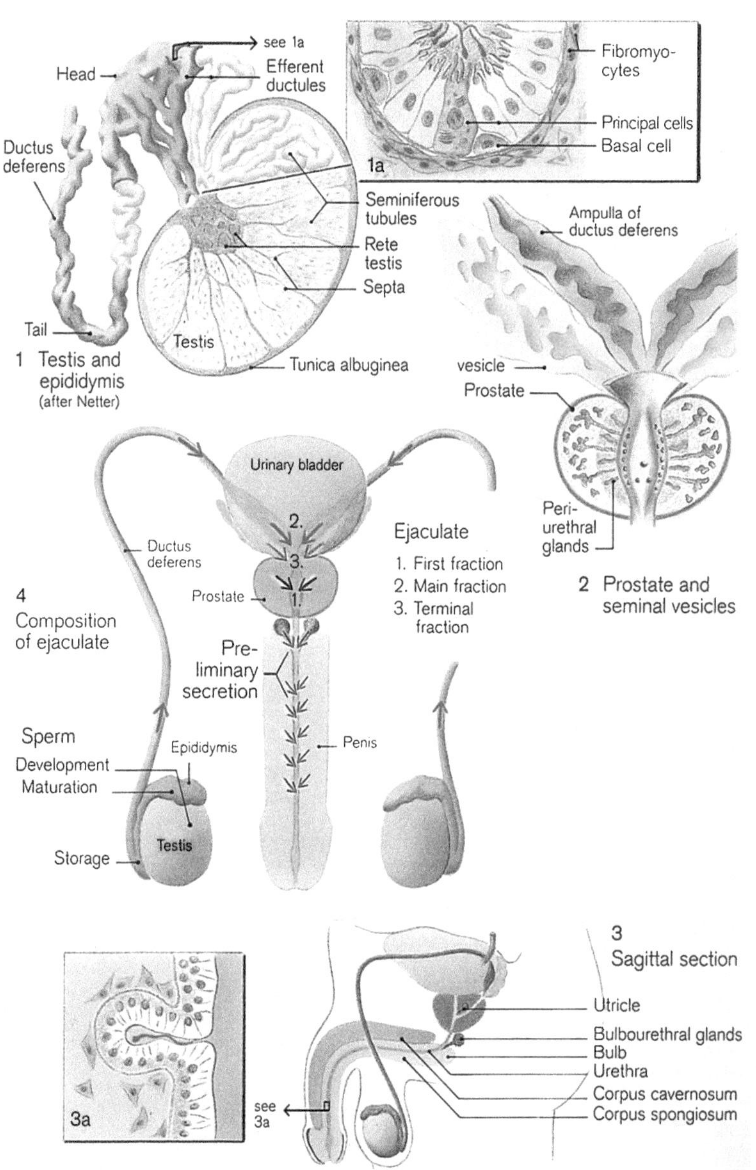
see 1a
Head
Efferent ductules
Ductus deferens
Fibromyocytes
Principal cells
Basal cell
1a
Seminiferous tubules
Rete testis
Septa
Tail
Testis
1 Testis and epididymis
(after Netter)
Tunica albuginea
Ampulla of ductus deferens
vesicle
Prostate
Peri-urethral glands
2 Prostate and seminal vesicles
Urinary bladder
Ductus deferens
Prostate
Ejaculate
1. First fraction
2. Main fraction
3. Terminal fraction
4
Composition of ejaculate
Pre-liminary secretion
Sperm
Development
Maturation
Storage
Epididymis
Testis
Penis
3
Sagittal section
Utricle
Bulbourethral glands
Bulb
Urethra
Corpus cavernosum
Corpus spongiosum
3a
see 3a

A. Male genital organs

## 1.8 Spermatogenesis

### A. Development of Leydig Cells and Seminiferous Tubules

**Embryonic Period.** In the testis anlage, the primordial germ cells colonize the testis cords, which are the anlage of the seminiferous tubules. They consist of *Sertoli cells* (supporting cells) interspersed basally with light staining spermatogonia. In the 12–20th embryonic week, the Leydig cells (interstitial cells) of the testis produce large amounts of testosterone, which is necessary for the differentiation of the male sexual organs and the male phenotype. During fetal life and early childhood, the seminiferous tubules remain in the resting stage. The *Leydig cells* regress and cannot be distinguished histologically from other connective tissue cells.

**Puberty.** At puberty, *luteinizing hormone* (LH) from the pituitary gland stimulates the Leydig cells while *follicle stimulating hormone* (FSH) stimulates the Sertoli cells. Testosterone levels rise. *FSH* and *testosterone* (T) induce spermatogenesis. The seminiferous tubules develop a lumen, enlarge, elongate, and complete a testicular segment (lobule) with many convolutions (→ 1.7 A1). Enlargement of the testis is caused by the multiplication and differentiation of the germ cells; the number of Sertoli cells remaining constant. Testis size is therefore a direct measure of spermatogenetic activity.

**Cooperation of Sertoli and Leydig cells.** Sertoli cells take up testosterone produced by the Leydig cells and transform it into *dihydrotestosterone (DHT)* by 5α-reductase action and into *estradiol* ($E_2$) by aromatase action. Both hormones are then secreted, together with an androgen-binding protein, into the seminal fluid.

### B. Spermatogenesis

The epithelium of the seminiferous tubules is formed by the *Sertoli cells,* which nourish and regulate the development of the male gametes. Sertolicell nuclei are lobed and possess one or two distinct nucleoli. The germ cells lie densely crowded in the deep invaginations of the Sertoli cells. During development, they advance toward the lumen of the seminiferous tubules.

**Spermatogonia.** The *spermatogonia* resume mitotic activity in puberty. All spermatogonia remain in contact with the basement membrane of the seminiferous tubules. The *basal compartment* containing the spermatogonia is separated from the *adluminal compartment* by special tight junctions between the Sertoli cells. The daughter cells of the last spermatogonial generation detach from the basement membrane and enter the adluminal compartment, becoming primary spermatocytes.

**Meiosis.** In the adluminal compartment, the primary spermatocyte enters prophase of the first meiotic division. The *leptotene* and *pachytene stages* are followed by formation of the spindle of the first meiotic division (metaphase I). Since the daughter cells (secondary spermatocytes) immediately begin the second meiotic division (metaphase II), a secondary spermatocyte with decondensed chromatin can rarely (in many species never) be observed.

**Spermiogenesis.** Spermatids emerge as daughter cells from the second meiotic division and differentiate into sperm: *The cell nucleus condenses* . A vesicle of the Golgi apparatus gives rise to the acrosomal vesicle, which caps the condensed cell nucleus, and forms the *acrosome.* The centriole develops into a flagellum with 9x2+2 microtubules. *Mitochondria* accumulate at the neck of the sperm and form a ring around the central filament. Excess cytoplasm is cast off as a residual body and may remain attached to the tail filament of the sperm. After detaching from the Sertoli cells, the sperm are transported passively with the fluid current. They become mobile only in the female genital tract.

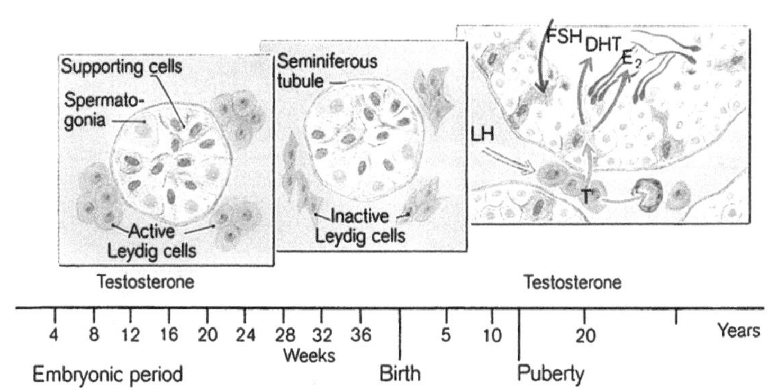


A. Development of Leydig cells and seminiferous tubules

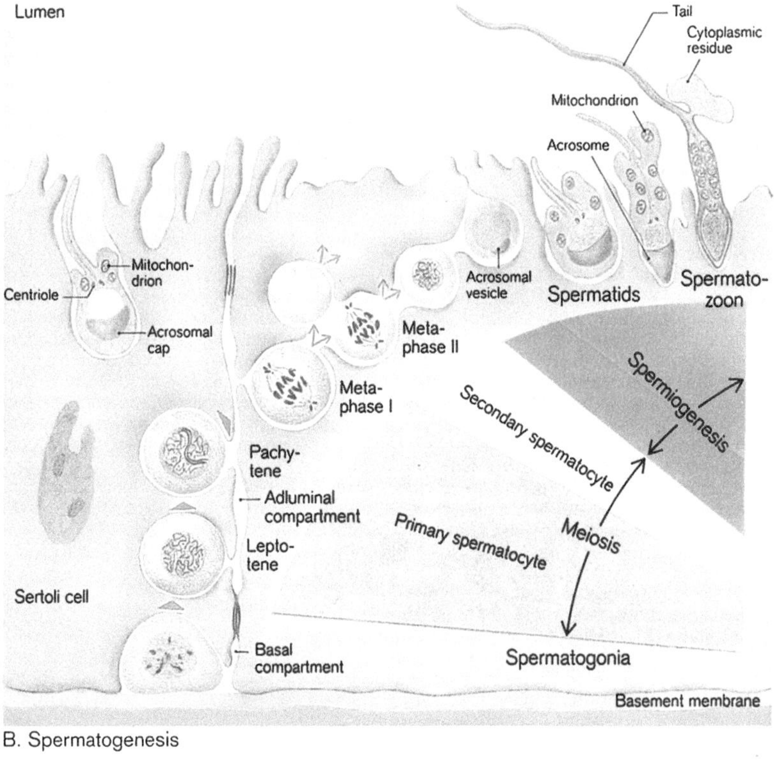

B. Spermatogenesis

## 1.9 Wave of Spermatogenesis

### A. Spermatogenetic Wave and Classification of Stages

**1. Syncytium Formation.** During the mitotic divisions of the spermatogonia, cytoplasmic bridges remain between the daughter cells and are also preserved during the meiotic divisions. The descendents of a single stem cell thus form a large syncytium in which the developmental steps of spermatogenesis are synchronously completed. Because of syncytial formation, spermatocytes and spermatids in the same stage always reside together in groups within the seminiferous epithelium. The successive groups of syncytial germ cells progressing through stages of differentiation form the *spermatogenetic wave*.

A spermatogonium goes through six predetermined mitotic divisions. The daughter cells exhibit differences in nuclear structure and stainability, so that one can distinguish four generations of type A spermatogonia, one intermediate type, and one type B. From the clone of spermatogonia, one daughter cell (Type A4) ceases development and reverts to a resting spermatogonium. In this way, a constant number of stem cells are preserved and the germinal epithelium is not exhausted.

**2. Spermatogenetic Wave.** After stimulation of spermatogenesis by FSH, the spermatogonia along the seminiferous tubules begin development successively, producing a wave of succeeding developmental stages of spermatogenesis. Each developmental stage involves all the daughter cells of a spermatogonium connected in a syncytium (represented as one cell). The temporal and spatial organization of the spermatogenic wave is functionally linked to the seasonal sexual activity of a species.

**a Shark:** In the simplest case, for example in the shark, a new wave at any site in the germinal epithelium begins only after the mature sperm of the preceding wave have been released into the lumen. In a cross-section of the tubule, therefore, only spermatocytes or spermatids of one developmental stage are seen.

**b Mouse:** In other species (e.g., rodents) the waves of spermatogenesis overlap, so that two developmental stages of spermatocytes and one or two developmental stages of spermiogenesis are superimposed in the germinal epithelium.

**c Human:** Whereas in rodents the same combination of spermatocytes and spermatids is present everywhere in a tubular cross-section, in humans several areas with different combinations lie side by side, so that an organization in the sense of a spermatogenic wave is not recognizable. Reconstruction of serial sections shows, however, that waves of spermatogenesis can also be demonstrated in humans. They are arranged in overlapping spirals.

**3. Stages in Human Germinal Epithelium.** For histological evaluation of spermatogenesis, the combinations of spermatocytes and spermatids appearing in the germinal epithelium are defined by a classification of stages. In the mouse, stages I–XII are distinguished; in the human, stages I–VI. A given segment of the germinal epithelium in the seminiferous tubules passes successively through all the stages. A sequence of stages is called a cycle of the germinal epithelium. If one arranges the stages I–VI of the germinal epithelium in a cross section of the seminiferous tubule and connects the successive developmental stages of spermatogenesis with a line, a spiral is formed that begins with the spermatogonia at the basement membrane and ends with the sperm in the lumen. The spiral represents the spermatogenetic wave. A cycle in the germinal epithelium lasts 32 days in the human. The time of development from spermatogonium to sperm is about 90 days.

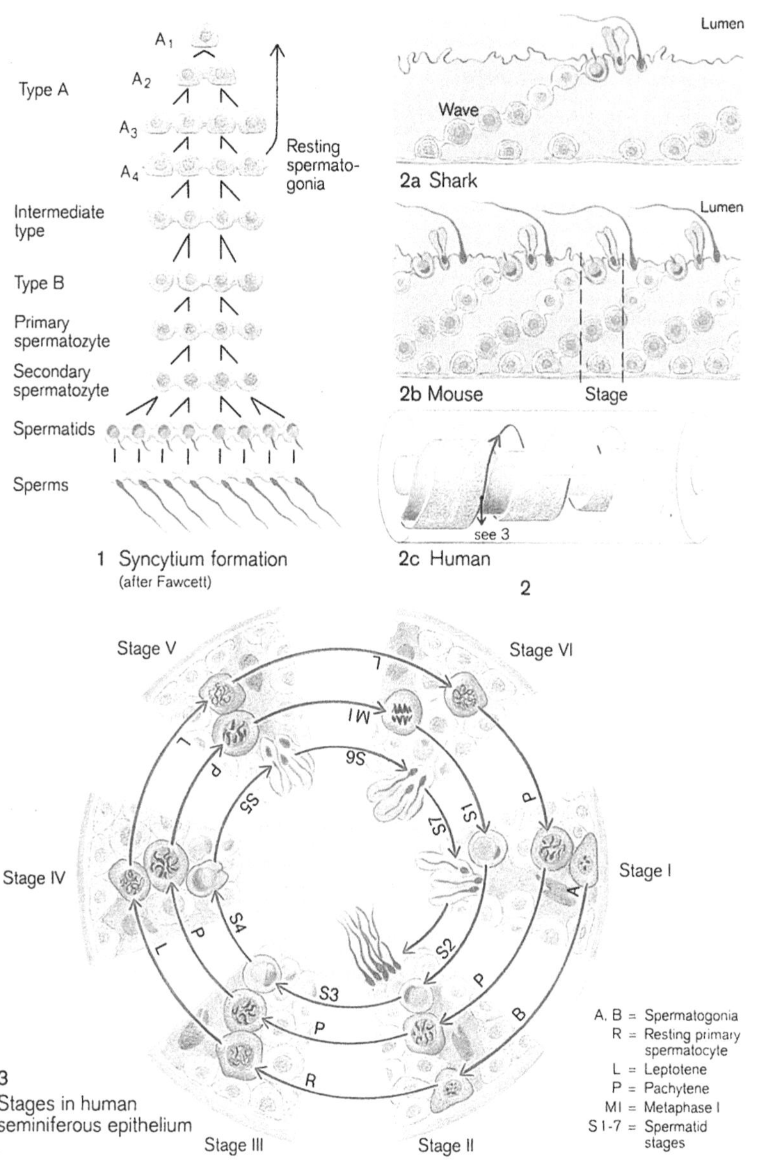


A. Spermatogenic wave and classification of stages

# Female Organs

## 1.10 Female Genital Tract

### A. Anatomy of Female Genital Organs

**1. Uterine Tube.** The uterine tube begins at the uterus-tube angle with a narrow segment, the **isthmus (1a)**, in which the mucosal folds are arranged in a longitudinal direction and the epithelium possesses few ciliated cells. The distal segment is broadened to form the **ampulla (1b)** where the mucous membrane forms a network of delicate folds in which the **ciliated cells (1c)** are in greater number than the mucus secreting cells. Fertilization occurs here. The ampulla is continuous with a funnel-shaped segment *(infundibulum)*, which opens into the body cavity and is surrounded by fimbriae. The cilia beat in the direction of the uterus and produce a **fluid current (1d)** close to the epithelium, which flows toward the isthmus. From the isthmus, which is functionally closed, the fluid returns in the direction of the ampulla as a central current. The laminar flow close to the epithelium is utilized for egg transport and the axial current is responsible for sperm transport.

**2. Uterus.** The wall of the uterus consists of smooth muscle ( *myometrium*), a mucosal lining (*endometrium*), and a peritoneal covering (*perimetrium*), which is continuous laterally with the broad ligament. The uterus projects into the vagina with the inferior segment of its neck (cervix uteri) forming the vaginal part of the cervix (portio vaginalis cervicis).

**3. Cervix.** The amount of smooth muscle cells are reduced in the cervix. The vaginal part consists of taut collagen connective tissue that firmly occludes the cervix during pregnancy. The *cervical canal* is functionally plugged by mucosal closure at the internal and external cervical os, as well as by the consistency of the cervical mucus (**3a**). Under the influence of progesterone, the *cervical mucus* solidifies and becomes impenetrable to sperm (nonspinnable). Under the influence of estrogen, it becomes more fluid (spinnable). Spermatozoa can swim upward in small fluid streams. Several spermatozoa can reach the uterine tube a few minutes after ejaculation. This rapid transport may be due to the contractions of the uterus during orgasm and not to the intrinsic motility of the spermatozoa. In the second phase, the spermatozoa colonize the *cervical glands* and ascend from there into the uterus within 4–7 hours. Spermatozoa can survive in the cervical glands for up to 48 hours and remain capable of fertilization (**3b**).

**4. Vagina.** The noncornified, squamous epithelium of the vagina contains much glycogen. It continues over the vaginal part of the cervix and borders the mucosa of the cervix at the external os of the uterus (**3b**). When the external os is patulous, it grows over the single layered cervical epithelium and ties off the cervical glands. Cysts can then develop (Nabothian cysts). In humans, the cyclic changes in the vagina are slight. An acidic milieu with a Ph of 5.7 prevails in the vagina and is not beneficial for the sperm. However, it can be buffered for about 50 minutes by the alkaline seminal fluid. After intercourse, 99% of the sperm are lost here. Only a few sperm arrive at the cervix from the briefly coagulated seminal fluid and are able to ascend further.

**5. External Genitalia.** The cavernous bodies of the clitoris (corpora ischiocavernosa) correspond to the corpora cavernosa of the penis. The cavernous bodies at the base of the labia minora (corpora bulbospongiosa) correspond to the corpus spongiosum that surrounds the male urethra (→ 8.9). Neuronal control and phases of sexual stimulation occur as in the male (EPOR). During the excitatory phase, the cavernous bodies fill up. The vagina enlarges and elongates, and a transudation of fluid takes place through the vaginal epithelium. The uterus becomes erect, so that the vaginal part of the cervix is placed into the middle of the vaginal roof ("tenting"). During orgasm, vagina and uterus contract.

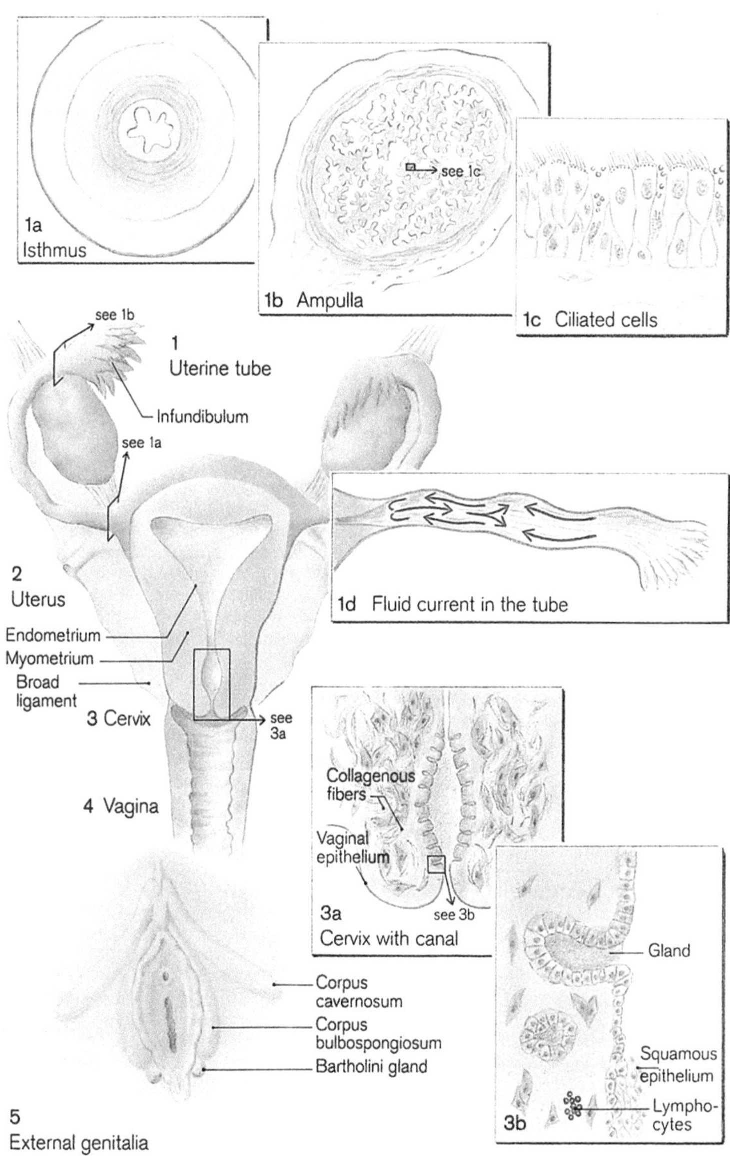
1a
Isthmus
1b Ampulla
see 1c
1c Ciliated cells
see 1b
1
Uterine tube
Infundibulum
see 1a
2
Uterus
Endometrium
Myometrium
Broad
ligament
3 Cervix
see
3a
4 Vagina
1d Fluid current in the tube
Collagenous
fibers
Vaginal
epithelium
3a
Cervix with canal
see 3b
Gland
Squamous
epithelium
Lympho-
cytes
3b
Corpus
cavernosum
Corpus
bulbospongiosum
Bartholini gland
5
External genitalia

A. Female genital organs

# 1.11 Oogenesis

## A. Prenatal Oogenesis

**1. Proliferation.** Oogonia multiply by *mitotic division* in the cortical zone of the embryonic ovary. The number of oogonia reaches its maximum in the 5th month with about $7 \times 10^6$. The proliferating oogonia form clusters and cords that are designated as *egg balls* (→ 8.6). Already in the 15th week, individual oogonia, which have reached the corticomedullary border of the ovary, enter into prophase of the first maturation division.

**2. Formation of Primordial Follicles.** From the 20th week, individual ova at the corticomedullary border of the ovary become surrounded by a single layer of *follicular epithelial cells*. Peripherally, proliferation and transition into meiosis continue, and without being arrested by follicular cells, end with cell death.Thus, the total number of oogonia drastically decreases.

**3. Arrest of the First Maturation Division.** The follicular epithelial cells form a **m**eiosis **i**nhibiting **s**ubstance (**MIS**) by means of which the first maturation division is arrested. The paired chromosomes decondense and enter a resting phase (dictyate) that can last up to 40 years.

**4. Follicular Growth.** Beginning before birth, continuously individual primordial follicles start to grow. Without FSH stimulation, they perish. After puberty, one follicle (the dominant follicle) matures up to ovulation in each cycle. Of the 7 million oocytes in the fetus, approximately 50 000 remain at puberty, and only about 400–500 of these are ovulated.

## B. Ovarian Cycle

**1. Constitutive Follicular Growth.** After puberty, individual primordial follicles begin to grow regularly without hormonal stimulation. The ova become enlarged; the follicular epithelium becomes cuboidal (*primary follicle*), then stratified (*secondary follicle*). The follicular epithelial cells sit on an external basal membrane, while the zona pellucida apically forms around the oocyte. Intercellular spaces in the epithelium coalesce and form a follicular cavity (*tertiary follicle*).

**2. Hormone Production.** *FSH receptors* appear on the follicular epithelial cells and *LH receptors* on the adjacent cells of the interstitium (theca interna). On the 7th day of the cycle, the level of gonadotropic hormones from the pituitary increases. Under the influence of *FSH* (follicle stimulating hormone) and *LH* (luteinizing hormone), the theca interna synthesizes estradiol ($E_2$) and the follicular epithelial cells (granulosa cells) synthesize progesterone (Pr) and estradiol ($E_2$), which arise by aromatization of androgens from the theca.

**3. Dominant Follicle.** All tertiary follicles are stimulated first and thus contribute to hormone production. However, between the 7th and 14th day of the cycle, they perish (with the exception of the dominant follicle). Additional *$E_2$ receptors* appear on the granulosa cells of the dominant follicle. The estradiol of the theca induces a further wave of proliferation in the granulosa cells and with it, an elevation of estradiol production in the dominant follicle (self stimulation).

**4. Ovulation.** The rise in the estradiol level elicits the LH peak (→ 1.13). In the preovulatory stage, *LH receptors* are likewise developed on the granulosa cells of the mature follicle. Ovulation occurs only when this last maturation step of the tertiary follicle coincides with the *LH peak*.

**5. Corpus Luteum.** After ovulation, the ruptured follicle is transformed into a corpus luteum. The vascular connective tissue of the theca interna perforates the basal membrane of the granulosa and penetrates between the granulosa cells. The inward budding of the vessels contributes to the sudden elevation of progesterone and estradiol after ovulation. If implantation does not take place, the corpus luteum degenerates at the end of the cycle (*luteolysis*) and leaves behind a connective tissue scar in the ovary (*corpus albicans*).

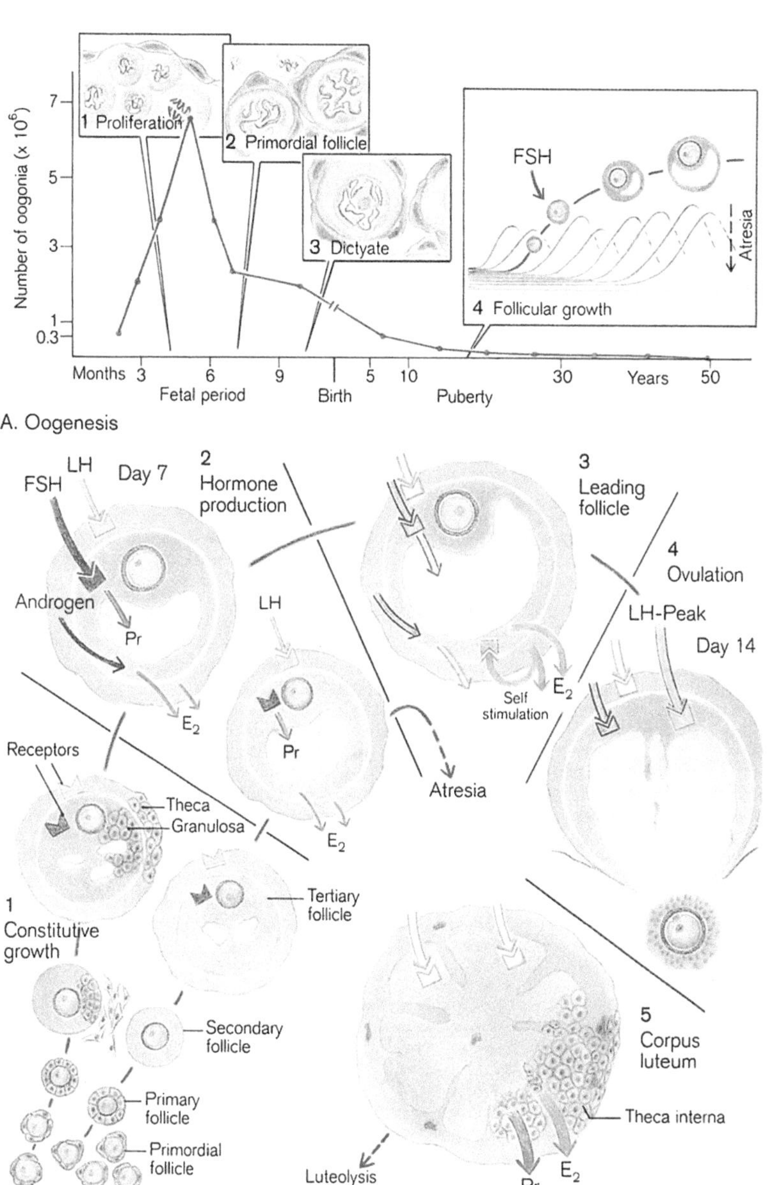

Number of oogonia (x $10^6$)
7
5
3
1
0.3
1 Proliferation
2 Primordial follicle
3 Dictyate
FSH
Atresia
4 Follicular growth
Months 3
6
9
5
10
30
Years
50
Fetal period
Birth
Puberty
A. Oogenesis
FSH
LH
Day 7
2
Hormone production
3
Leading follicle
4
Ovulation
Androgen
Pr
LH
LH-Peak
Day 14
$E_2$
Self stimulation
Pr
Receptors
Atresia
Theca
Granulosa
$E_2$
Tertiary follicle
1
Constitutive growth
Secondary follicle
5
Corpus luteum
Primary follicle
Theca interna
Primordial follicle
Luteolysis
Pr
$E_2$
B. Ovarian cycle

## 1.12 Ovulation

### A. Ovary with Preovulatory Follicle

In the adult ovary, the primitive arrangement of the embryonic gonad is still recognizable, with a cortical and medullary zone. The compact medulla is connected to the hilus and contains vessels and the remains of the *rete ovarii,* which corresponds to the rete testis. The *primordial follicles*, as well as the constitutively developing *primary, secondary*, and *tertiary follicles*, lie in the cortex. Between the cortical zone and the peritoneal covering lies a connective tissue layer (*tunica albuginea* of the ovary), which corresponds to the tunica albuginea of the testis (enlarged inset). From the 7th day of the cycle, a group of primary follicles begin to mature. Only one of these follicles, the dominant follicle, goes on to ovulate; the others become atretic.

Shortly before ovulation, the amount of *follicular fluid* increases so strongly in the dominant follicle, that it bulges the surface of the ovary like a ball. The preovulatory follicle has a diameter of 2.5 cm and is easily recognized by ultrasound. Peritoneal epithelium and connective tissue are stretched out thinly, together with the follicular wall. Fluid seeps out through the follicular wall. The enzymatic loosening of the follicular wall leads to a strengthening of the fluid stream, until finally the oocyte with the *cumulus oophorus* and a cloud of loose granulosa cells is flushed out into the uterine tube. The cells of the cumulus oophorus become the *corona radiata* (→ 1.5), which surrounds the oocyte.

**1. Maturation of the Oocyte.** During the growth of the oocyte in the tertiary follicle, the follicular epithelial cells send cell processes into the cytoplasm of the oocyte. Protein and yolk precursors synthesized in the liver are passed into the oocyte by exocytosis and apocrine detachment of vesicles. At the same time, the *zona pellucida* is formed around the oocyte. Composed of glycoproteins, it is penetrated by cell processes from the follicular epithelial cells. Internally, the microvilli of the oocyte project into the zona pellucida. The oocyte grows to a diameter of 120 to 150 µm.

**2. Effects of the Preovulatory LH-Peak.** The rise in LH before ovulation (→ 1.13) has the following effects: (1) The follicular epithelial cells (granulosa cells) retract their cell processes from the oocyte and zona pellucida. In addition, the oocyte becomes detached from the zona. This allows a *perivitelline space* to arise, into which the microvilli of the oocyte project. (2) The lampbrush chromosomes in the cell nucleus pull in their loops, condense, and the first maturation division ends. The spindle is aligned radially and the *first polar body* is expelled into the perivitelline space. (3) After a brief decondensation of chromosomes, the *second maturation division* begins, which is arrested in metaphase. The egg is now a secondary oocyte (→ 1.2B).

**3. The Oocyte in Ovulation.** The graafian follicle ruptures and the secondary oocyte is flushed out. The second maturation division continues after fertilization with the expulsion of the second polar body. In the absence of fertilization, the oocyte perishes within 24 hours.

### B. Movements of the Uterine Tube and Ovary

Before ovulation, the tube receives an increased blood supply and shows increased motility. The infundibular fimbria is positioned closely above the follicle site and collects the oocyte immediately. By rotating around the axis of the *suspensory ligament* of the ovary and the *ovarian ligament* , the ovary turns the mature follicle toward the tube. As a rule, only one of the two ovaries ovulates. In the case of unilateral occlusion or absence of a tube, the tube of the opposite side can position itself over the follicle.

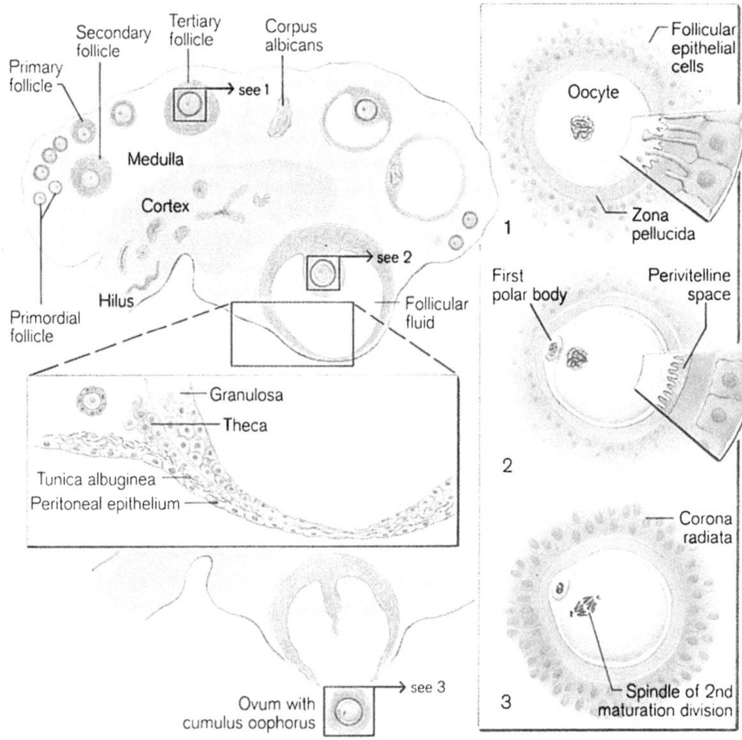

Primary follicle
Secondary follicle
Tertiary follicle
see 1
Corpus albicans
Medulla
Cortex
see 2
Hilus
Primordial follicle
Follicular fluid
Granulosa
Theca
Tunica albuginea
Peritoneal epithelium
see 3
Ovum with cumulus oophorus
Follicular epithelial cells
Oocyte
Zona pellucida
1
First polar body
Perivitelline space
2
Corona radiata
Spindle of 2nd maturation division
3


A. Ovary with preovulatory follicle

Suspensory ligament of ovary
Tube
Ampulla
Fimbria
Uterus
Ovarian ligament
Ovary with mature follicle
(after Martius)


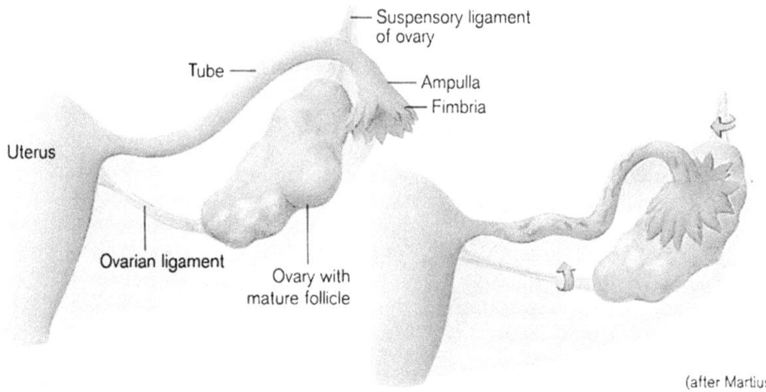

B. Movements of uterine tube and ovary

## 1.13 Menstrual Cycle

### A. Hormonal Regulation of the Menstrual Cycle

Ovulation occurs at day 14 of a 28-day cycle (**A3**). During the first half of the cycle (**follicular or proliferative phase**), the endometrium prepares for ovulation by intense proliferation (**A1**). In the second half of the cycle (**luteal or secretory phase**), the endometrium prepares for implantation of the fertilized ovum (*secretion* , **A1**).

In most mammals, the phase of receptivity around ovulation (estrus) determines the periodicity of the cycle. In humans, estrus is not as conspicuous as in other species. Instead, there is a sloughing off of the uterine mucosa (**menstruation**) so that one speaks of a **menstrual cycle**. By definition, the menstrual cycle begins with the first day of the last menstruation.

**Follicular Phase.** In the maturing *tertiary follicle* (**3a**), the *granulosa cells* produce progesterone (Pr) which remains in the follicular cavity and stimulates the maturation of the oocyte. The *theca interna* forms *estradiol* ($E_2$), which is released into the blood. Estradiol (**A2**) stimulates the proliferation (**A1**) of the endometrium and inhibits the pituitary-hypothalamic system (**4a**) so that a uniform level of FSH, LH, and estradiol is maintained (**A2**).

**Triggering of Ovulation.** Ovulation is induced by the *preovulatory follicle* itself. While the other tertiary follicles become atretic, $E_2$ from the theca interna of the dominant follicle stimulates its own granulosa cells to produce estradiol independently of the pituitary gland (→ 1.11). In the granulosa cells, androgens, which are formed in the theca, become aromatized into additional estradiol. This leads to a steep rise of estradiol in the blood. After 14 hours, the *estradiol peak* induces a surge of LH secretion (**4b**). The *LH peak* induces ovulation after 10 hours.

**Luteal Phase.** The ovulated follicle is transformed into the *corpus luteum*, which produces large amounts of estradiol and progesterone (**3c**). Progesterone induces the differentiation of the endometrium. Through feedback, a new equilibrium (**4c**) is created between the FSH and LH secretion in the pituitary and progesterone and estradiol production in the corpus luteum. The new equilibrium is at a higher level than in the follicular phase.

**Luteolysis.** If implantation does not occur and no human chorionic gonadotropin (HCG) is formed, oxytocin arises in the corpus luteum and brings about its degeneration (*luteolysis*). In other species the formation of oxytocin is elicited by *prostaglandins* from the endometrium (**A1**). The decline of progesterone and estradiol caused by the involution of the corpus luteum induces *menstruation* (withdrawal bleeding).

**Neuroendocrine Control.** The hypothalamus produces *gonadotropin releasing hormone* (GnRH), which leads to the secretion of follicular stimulating hormone (FSH) and luteinizing hormone (LH) from the *anterior lobe of the pituitary gland* (**4a**). The central endogenous rhythm is modified and overlapped by the ovary by feedback mechanisms

**Feedback Mechanisms.** The feedback between the ovary and the pituitary (**A4**) has two distinct effects: (1) The regulation of a **constant hormone level** by negative feedback (**4a** and **4c**) and (2) the induction of the **LH peak** that induces ovulation (positive feedback, **4b**). In the **follicular (proliferative) phase** (**4a**), an average estradiol level has an inhibitory effect on ovulation, whereas a low level of progesterone promotes the appearance of an LH peak. A surge *in estradiol* (**4b** and **A2**) induces the *LH peak* and ovulation. In the **luteal (secretory) phase** (**4c**), a high progesterone level reliably prevents further ovulations. The average estradiol level acts in the same way.

**Surge of $E_2$ (and low Pr):** positive feedback = induction of ovulation. **High Pr and/or average $E_2$:** negative feedback = suppression of ovulation.

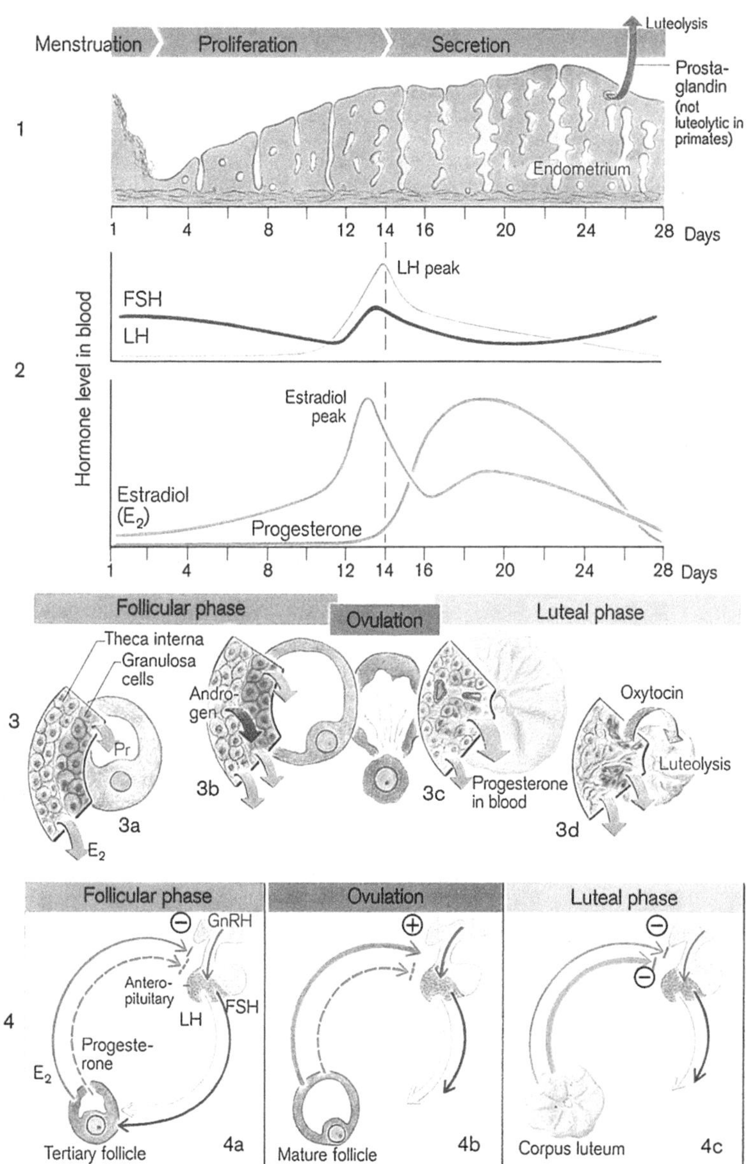


A. Menstrual cycle

## 1.14 Endometrium

### A. Preparation of the Endometrium for Implantation

**1. Cycle with Menstruation**

The endometrium prepares for implantation of the embryo in each cycle. When implantation fails to occur, the mucosa is sloughed at menstruation.

**2. Cycle with Implantation**

a. **Proliferative Phase**. After menstruation (or after a curettage), the endometrium regenerates from the remnants of the endometrial glands and the spiral arteries and veins between the trabeculae of smooth muscle at the border between the myometrium and endometrium. They regain their original height under the influence of estradiol. In the proliferative phase, histology of the sloughed material reveals slender, straight tubular glands with undifferentiated epithelium and abundant apical mitoses.

**b. Early Secretory Phase.** After ovulation on day 14, differentiation begins in the glandular tubes under the influence of progesterone. The glandular tubes become tortuous and the epithelial cells store glycogen. In histologic preparations, the dissolution of basally accumulated glycogen from the epithelial cells leads to the formation of typical pale vacuoles below the cell nuclei.

**c. Midsecretory Phase.** The glycogen vacuoles disappear.Dilated and tortuous, the glands assume a serrated leaf-like appearance in histologic sections. The cell fills apically with mucus, part of which is discharged into the lumen by apocrine secretion.

**d. Late Secretory Phase.** The three layers of the mucosa are complete: a cell-rich *zona basalis* with undifferentiated basal ends of glands that give rise to new formations after menstruation; a *zona spongiosa* with loose connective tissue and dilated tortuous glands; and a *zona compacta* below the superficial epithelium with densely lodged connective tissue cells, through which pass the straight excretory ducts of the glands with low cuboidal epithelium. The zona compacta and spongiosa together form the *zona functionalis*. *Granular cells* appear in the endometrium. They contain prolactin and relaxin. These local hormones assist the disintegration of the endometrium during menstruation and the decidual transformation during implantation.

In a cycle with menstruation, *no implantation* takes place (**A1**). The height of the endometrium decreases in the last week of the cycle. The corpus luteum regresses, and the sudden decline in estradiol and progesterone induces menstruation. Menstruation also commences if, because of genetic or other defects, the blastocyst cannot form sufficient HCG to maintain the corpus luteum (possible physiologic meaning of menstruation). In the case of the "**morning after pill**," a single high dose of estrogen produces a relative decline in hormone levels, which induces menstruation before the blastocyst has arrived in the uterine cavity.

If fertilization has occurred, the blastocyst arrives in the uterine cavity after about 5 days and implants in the zona compacta after 6 1/2 days (**implantation, 2d**). The trophoblast cells of the blastocyst penetrate into the mucosa and lyse and phagocytize the decidual cells.

**Decidual Reaction.** The endometrium reacts to implantation by transforming into a **decidua**. In the decidua, the connective tissue cells increase in size by the storing of glycogen and fat and form large polygonal cells. Blood becomes obstructed in the venous sinuses. The decidual transformation of the mucosa takes place under the influence of progesterone. A lesser degree of decidual transformation develops in a secretory phase without implantation.

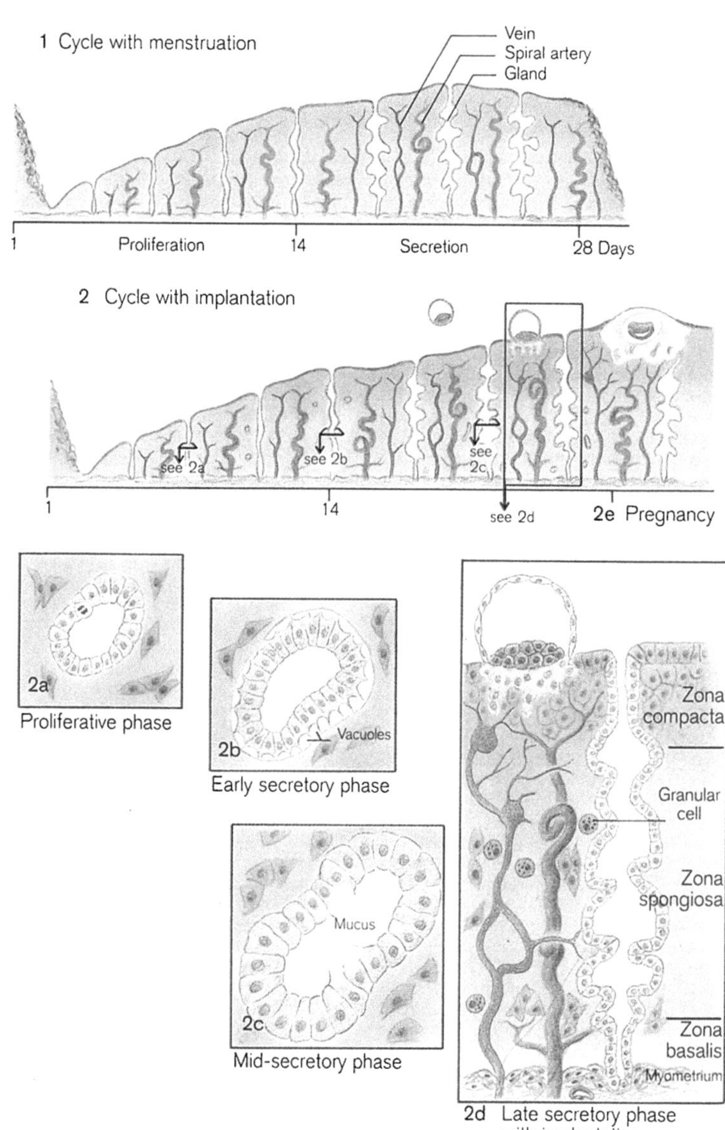


A. Preparation of endometrium for implantation

# Pregnancy and Delivery

## 1.15 Overview: Course of Pregnancy

### A. Early Development

**First Week: Oocyte Transport in the Tube.** *Fertilization* occurs within 6–12 hours of *ovulation*. During cleavage divisions, the *zygote* is transported into the uterus. Tubal transport lasts between 48 and 72 hours. The *morula* reaches the lumen of the uterus after 3 days and transforms into a *blastocyst*. On the 5th-6th day of its development, the blastocyst makes contact with the endometrium (*attachment*), which is now in the late secretory phase.

**Second Week: Implantation.** The blastocyst burrows into the endometrium and at the end of the 2nd week, makes contact with the maternal circulation. In so doing, *implantation bleeding*, which coincides with the time of menstruation, may occur.

*Pregnancy test*. From the 7th day, the trophoblast produces *human chorionic gonadotropic hormone* (HCG). The immunologic demonstration of HCG in the urine is already positive when menstruation fails to occur.

### B. Embryonic Period

**Third Week: Germinal Disc.** The extraembryonic nutritive organs are formed during the 3rd week *post ovulationem* (p.o.). The germinal disc is stretched out between yolk sac and amniotic cavity. The embryo is suspended in the wide chorionic cavity by the body stalk. Blood islands arise in the yolk sac mesoderm. The heart begins to beat.

**Fourth Week: Folding of Embryo.** The embryo develops its body form by folding off from the yolk sac and being enveloped by its amnion.

**Fifth to Eighth Weeks: Embryonic Period.** The placenta is delineated and the villi at the abembryonic pole recede ("chorionic baldness"). Organ systems differentiate (*organogenesis*). *Chorionic biopsy* can be done under ultrasound control between the 7th and 10th postovulatory week (9–12 weeks of gestation).

### C. Fetal Period

This period is characterized by fetal *growth and maturation*. Clinically, the pregnancy is dated from the first day of the last menstrual period or in *gestational weeks*.

**11th-14th Gestational Weeks** (3rd month). The decidua capsularis and the decidua parietalis fuse. The amnion and chorion fuse. *The chorionic cavity becomes obliterated.*

**15th-18th Gestational Weeks** (4th month). The fetus is freely mobile in the amniotic fluid. Its sex is recognizable. The uterus fundus rises above the symphysis (**C1**). *Amniocentesis* is possible after 15–16 weeks of gestation.

**19th-22nd Gestational Weeks** (5th month). First movements are recognized by the mother (quickening). Fetal heart sounds are audible.

**23rd-26th Gestational Weeks** (6th month). The uterine fundus is at the level of the umbilicus. The position of the fetus stabilizes. Dorsum left (left oblique) = position I. Dorsum right (right oblique) = position II. The limit of extrauterine viability begins.

**27th-40th Gestational Weeks** (7th - 10th month). The uterus inclines forward 3–4 weeks before birth. The fundus of the uterus lies deeper (lightening). *Lightening* (**C1**) can be used to confirm the date of delivery. Before engagement in the true pelvis, the head of the fetus is still freely movable during vaginal examination (**C2**). A **premature infant** is one born before 38 gestational weeks and < 2500 g.

**Expected Date of Delivery**

From day 1 of the last period (post menstruationem, p.m.): 280 days = 40 gestational weeks = 10 lunar months.

From conception (post ovulastionem): 266 days = 38 weeks p.o. = about 9 calendar months.

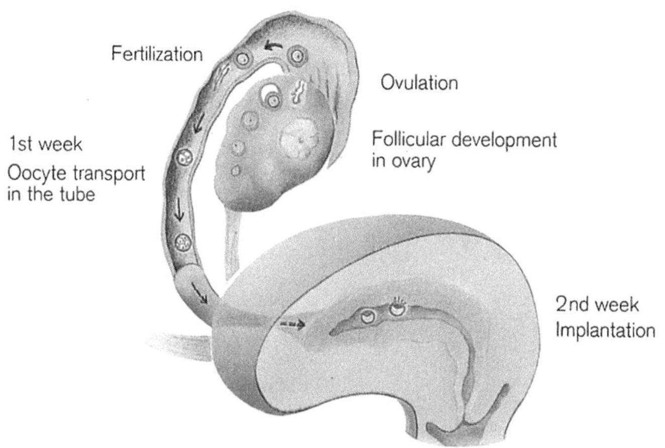


A. Early development

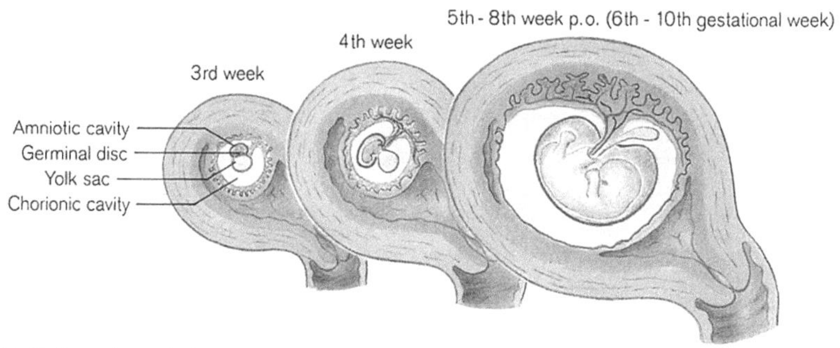


B. Embryonic period

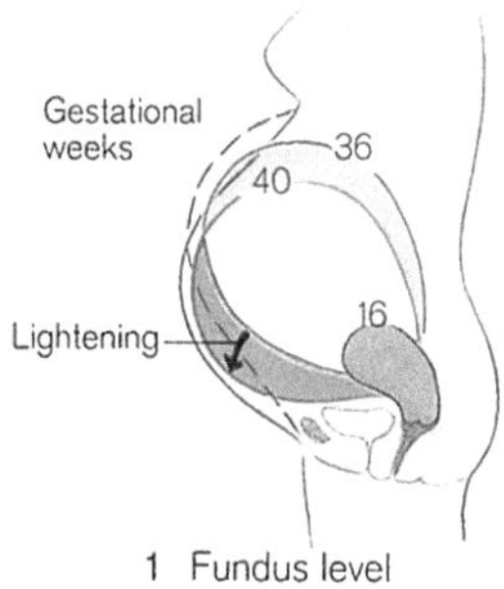


1 Fundus level

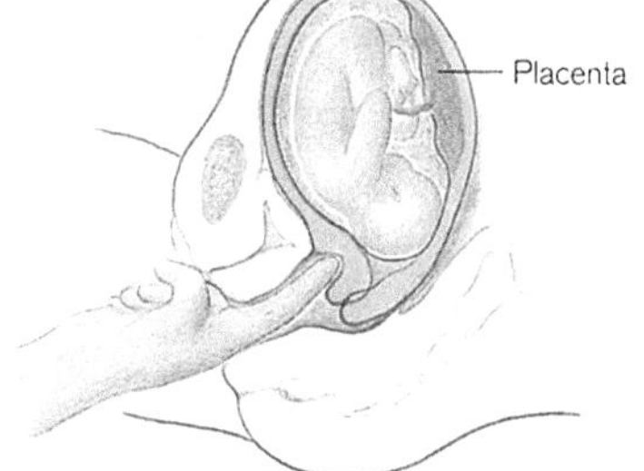


2 Antenatal examination (indication after Pinard)

C. Fetal period

## 1.16 Gravidarium

### A. Pregnancy Calculator Wheel for Calculating the Expected Date of Delivery

The estimated date of delivery, as well as the expected fetal size at the day of antenatal examination, can be obtained by consulting a pregnancy calculator wheel. It consists of two discs sitting on a common axis. The external disc shows 12 months and the days of the calendar year. The internal disc shows the *postmenstrual gestational period* (10 lunar months of 28 days or 40 weeks). The empty segment on the inner disc corresponds to the difference between the calendar year and the gestational period (minus 3 months plus 7 days, Nägele's rule). The portrayed pregnancy calculator wheel is set for the first day of the last menstrual period on June 1st. The setting shows the time of ovulation at June 15 and an expected date of delivery on March 5th of the following year. The antenatal examination is on January 5th, the pregnancy is in the 32nd gestational week, 8 weeks before the estimated date of delivery.

**Duration of Pregnancy**

**1. Post Menstruation.** Absence of menstrual bleeding is an early sign of pregnancy. For practical reasons, a pregnancy is dated in weeks or months from the first day of the last menstrual period in obstetrics. The figure insert shows the variation of gestational age in the normal course of pregnancy, in days calculated from the first day of the last menstrual period: The large variations are due to mistakes in estimating the last period, irregularities in the cycle, a variable time span between ovulation and fertilization and the natural variation of the gestational period itself. Nevertheless, experience shows that little error is introduced when pregnancy is considered to last 280 days, starting from the first day of the last menstrual period.

Duration of pregnancy post menstruation: 280 days = 40 weeks = 10 lunar months.

**2. Post Ovulation.** Ovulation marks the true beginning of pregnancy, since the activation of the oocyte by fertilization occurs within 24 hours of ovulation.

*Ovulation age = Fertilization age*

The age of an embryo is calculated from the moment of ovulation. The figure inset shows that the variation of gestational age is less when calculated from the date of ovulation (indicated by the increase in basal body temperature) than from the first day of the last menstrual period. Formally, ovulation age is 14 days (2 weeks) less than menstrual age.

*Ovulation age = menstrual age minus two weeks*

Duration of pregnancy post ovulation: 280 days - 14 days = 266 days = 38 weeks. 266 days are approximately equal to 9 calendar months of 30 days.

**Estimated Date of Delivery**

On the basis of menstrual age, the date of delivery can be estimated according to the following formula (**Nägele's law**):

First day of last menstrual period + 1 year - 3 calendar months + 7 days ± X days.

X indicates the number of days that the cycle deviates from the assumed 28 days. This adjustment is made because of the observation by Knaus and Ogino that the first part of the cycle (proliferative phase) varies widely, whereas the number of days (14) between ovulation and the onset of menstruation is relatively constant.

**Ultrasonography**

Ultrasonography is carried out to evaluate the fetus and to check the gestational age. The size of the fetus and the biparietal diameter of the head are measured and compared with normal values.

Pregnancy calculator wheel from Hansmann, photograph: Vaclav Reischl, Stuttgart. Ultrasound image from: Martius, Geburtshilfe. Data from G.K. Döring (1962).

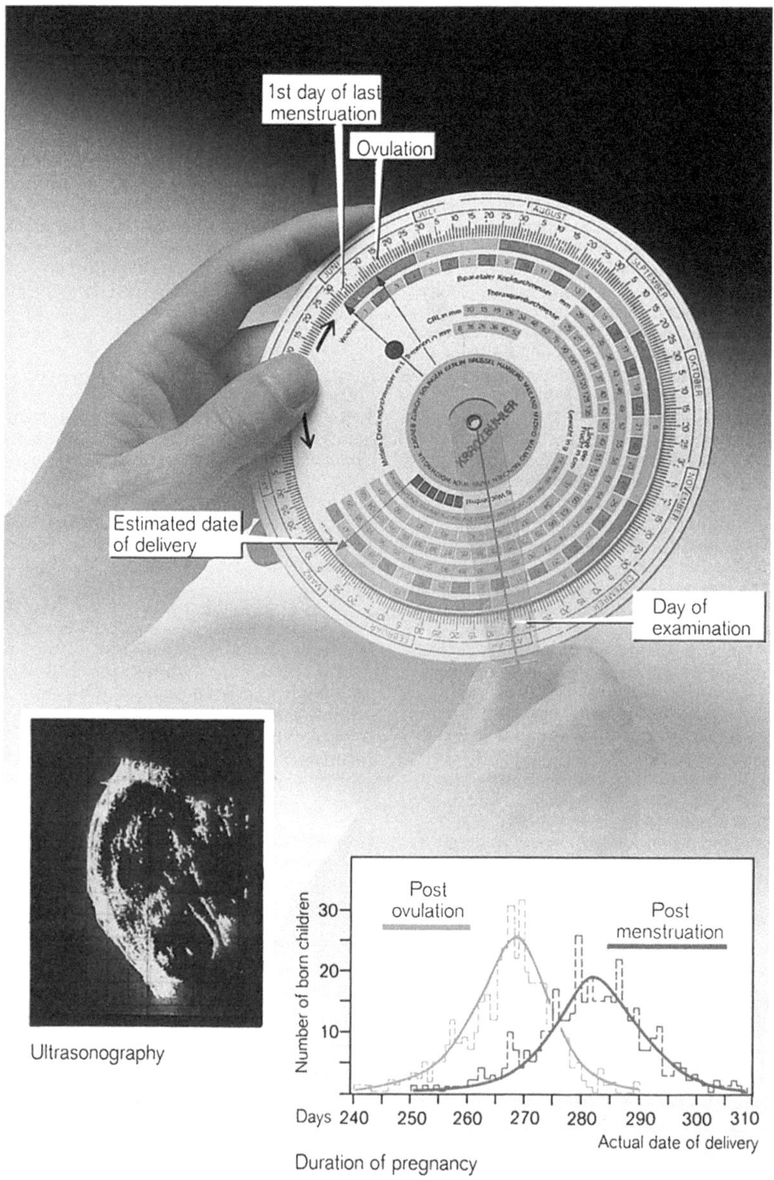


A. Gravidarium for calculating the expected date of delivery

## 1.17 Hormone Levels

### A. Hormone Levels during Pregnancy

**1. Human Chorionic Gonadotropin (HCG).** After implantation, the trophoblast begins to produce the hormone HCG. HCG is similar to LH from the pituitary gland and binds to LH receptors of the corpus luteum. The *corpus luteum* becomes the *corpus luteum of pregnancy,* which prevents the sloughing of the uterine decidua and is initally necessary to maintain pregnancy. From the 8th day of gestation, the trophoblast itself produces so much progesterone that the pregnancy is no longer influenced by the removal of the ovaries.

**2. Progesterone.** Toward the end of pregnancy, the placenta produces about 10 times as much progesterone as the corpus luteum in the second half of the cycle. The high blood levels of progesterone are partly due to the increase of transcortin (corticosteroid-binding globulin), which also binds progesterone. Interaction between progesterone and aldosterone receptors in the kidney leads to an increase of aldosterone and angiotensinogen, which in turn are responsible for sodium and water retention in the second half of the cycle and during pregnancy.

**3. Estrogen.** Free estrogen also increases markedly during pregnancy. The largest part of estrogen, however, consists of the biologically less active *estriol* and *estrone*, the precursors of which originate from the fetal adrenal cortex.

**4. Human Placental Lactogen (HPL).** Parallel with the formation of prolactin in the maternal pituitary gland, the placenta produces HPL, which is similar to prolactin. Both hormones stimulate growth and differentiation of the mammary glands.

### B. Fetoplacental Unit

Not only the *placenta*, but also the fetal *adrenal cortex* and the *fetal liver* synthesize steroid hormones. The steroid hormones are *conjugated* in the fetal adrenal cortex and the liver so that they exist in an inactive form in the fetus and do not disturb development. They are *deconjugated* by the placenta when passed into the maternal circulation and thus become active. Forty percent of the estrone and estriol synthesized in the placenta are formed from dihydroepiandrosterone sulfate (DHEA sulfate) from the fetal adrenal gland. A decrease in the estriol-estrone levels in the case of constant estradiol, therefore indicates a defect in the early pregnancy (*hydatiform mole, chorionic epithelioma*) or indicates fetal distress (indication for induction of labor).

### C. Endocrine Control of Parturition

**1. Relaxation of the Cervix.** During pregnancy, the fetus is secured in the uterus by the closed cervical canal. The cervix consists of dense collagenous connective tissue that must be loosened for the passage of the fetus. The hormone, *relaxin,* which is formed in the corpus luteum and endometrium, contributes to this relaxation.

**2. Onset of Labor.** Labor can only be effective if the cervix is prepared for birth. Locally, contraction of the uterine musculature is elicited by *prostaglandins,* which are formed in the endometrium and in the musculature itself at the beginning of parturition. Systemically, labor is controlled by *oxytocin,* secreted by the posterior lobe of the maternal pituitary gland. Oxytocin intensifies the local formation of prostaglandins. The secretion of oxytocin is stimulated by a neuronal reflex, the afferent arm of which reports irritations of the cervix via *sensory nerve tracts* to the hypothalamus (*Ferguson reflex*). How the fetus contributes to the onset of labor is still unclear in humans. A possible mechanism is via steroid hormones from the *fetal adrenal gland,* which are aromatized in the *placenta* into *estrogen* and stimulate the formation of prostaglandins.

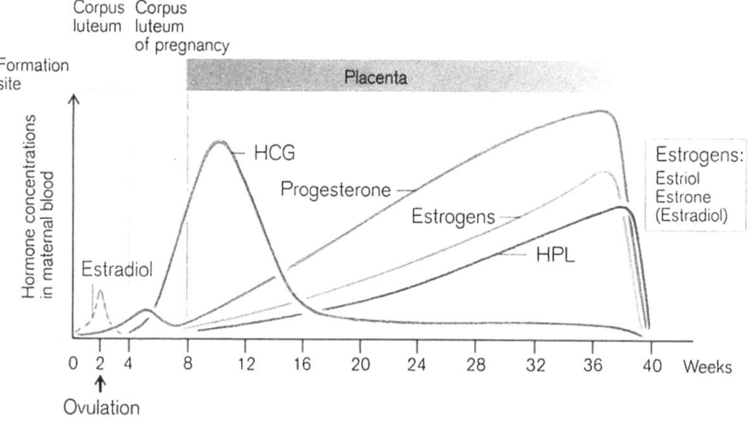


A. Hormone levels during pregnancy

Activation by deconjugation in placenta

Inactivation by conjugation in fetal adrenal gland and liver

DHEA sulfate

Estriol
Estrone
Estradiol
in blood

Precursors from mother (cholesterol, pregnenolone)

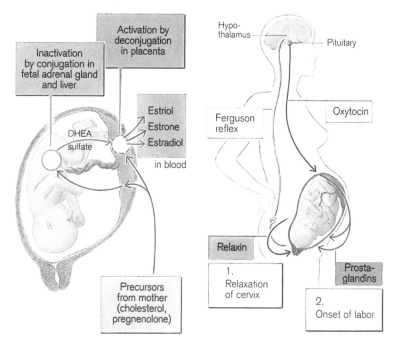

B. Fetoplacental unit

Hypothalamus

Pituitary

Ferguson reflex

Oxytocin

Relaxin

1. Relaxation of cervix

Prostaglandins

2. Onset of labor

C. Endocrine control of parturition

## 1.18 Parturition

### A. Passage through the Birth Canal: The Stages of Labor

**1. First Stage, Stage of Dilation.** The birth process begins after relaxation of the cervix, with the establishment of regular, strong labor pains at intervals of about 3 minutes. In this first stage of labor, the cervix is dilatated for passage of the fetal head. Initially, the fetal head is protected by the cushion of the intact amniotic sac. Rupture of the membranes and the loss of the amniotic fluid accelerate the process of parturition. The cervix and the external os of the uterus are drawn out into a thin edge. At entry into the oval true pelvis, the fetal head fits in the transverse diameter, as indicated by the position of the sagittal suture (dorsum left = I, or left occiput anterior position; Dorsum right = II or right occiput anterior position).

**2. Second Stage, Stage of Delivery.** After the complete delation of the uterine os, *expulsive contractions* set in. Labor is now carried out not only by uterine contractions,but additionally by the striated abdominal musculature. A disparity exists in humans between the size of the fetal head and the diameter of the pelvis (development of a large head and the upright gait produced by evolution). This causes the relative narrowness of the birth canal and determines the progress of childbirth.

**a Rotation of the Head in the Birth Canal.** During the expulsive contractions, the head of the fetus is guided by the physiological landmarks of the birth canal. At the level of the linea terminalis, the head rotates into the first or second *oblique diameter.* It avoids the *promontory,* which protrudes into the birth canal dorsally.

**b Crowning of the Head.** By continuing internal rotation, the head lies on the floor of the pelvis in the *sagittal diameter*. In exiting, the head must overcome the curvature of the birth canal. It thereby distends the *maternal pelvic floor* into a broad tube formed by the vaginal wall and vulva, and exteriorly by the muscles of the pelvic floor. For protection against overdistension and uncontrolled lacerations, a decompressive incision of the perineum (episiotomy) may be performed at the height of an expulsive contraction.

**3. Delivery of the Head.** The fetal head is pressed against the symphysis with the nape of the neck. It then undergoes extension. By this means, the face is developed above the perineum.

**4. Delivery of the Shoulders.** The shoulders follow the path of the sagittal suture and rotate from the transverse into the oblique and then into the sagittal diameter. The obstetrician guides the head further toward the side (external rotation of the head) and, amidst a flood of amniotic fluid, lifts the newborn and reaches it toward the mother before cutting the umbilical cord. During a labor of about 8–14 hours, 1–1.5 hours are involved with the delivery period.

**5. Third Stage (Placental Stage).** After delivery of the fetus, the placenta is detached by the formation of a *retroplacental hematome* and is expelled by further uterine contractions.

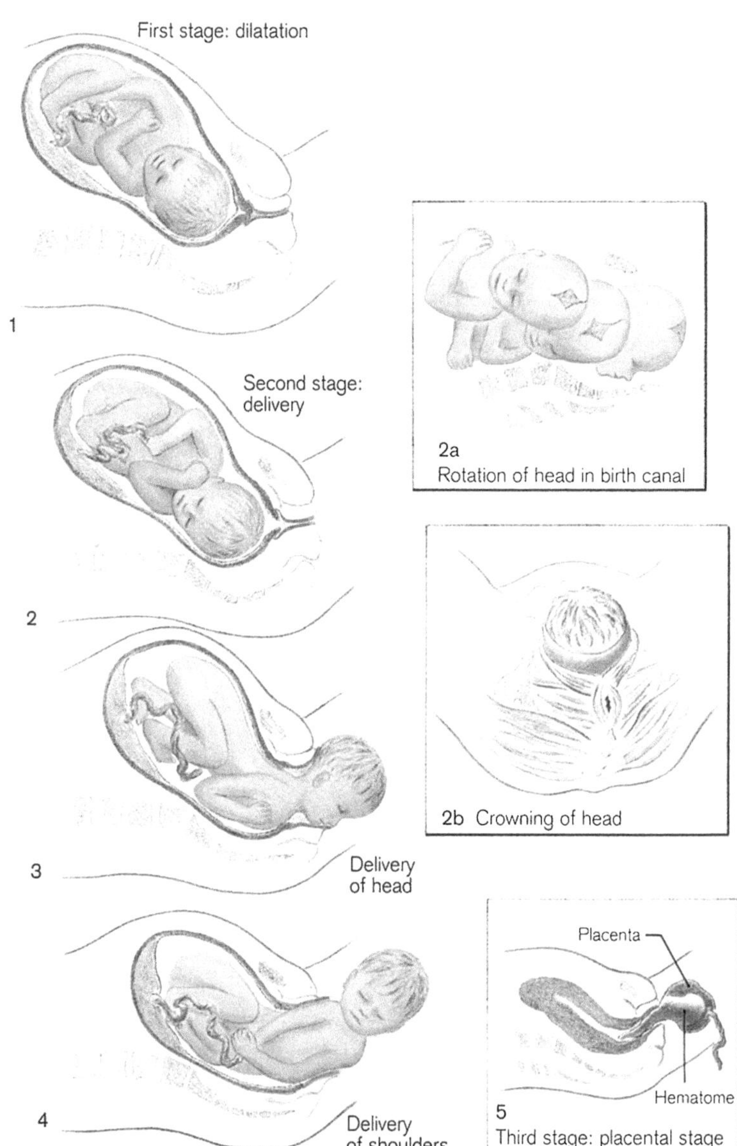
First stage: dilatation
1
Second stage:
delivery
2
2a
Rotation of head in birth canal
2b Crowning of head
3
Delivery
of head
4
Delivery
of shoulders
Placenta
Hematome
5
Third stage: placental stage

A. The stages of labor

# Chapter 2: Human Development

## Introduction

Chapter 2 covers the development of the human embryo from the fertilized egg to birth. The chapter concentrates on medically relevant knowledge ("Human Embryology," "Medical Embryology").

**Classification into Stages (2.1 and 2.2).** An embryo can be characterized by its *age*, its *size* or its *developmental stage*.

**Age Data.** In the embryonic period, age data is given in days or weeks after fertilization, or equivalently, after ovulation (*fertilization age, ovulation age*). The ages of human embryos that are studied histologically after abortion, or for other medical reasons, are very imprecise, since the date of conception is rarely known. In these specimens, the age is usually calculated on the basis of the last menstrual period obtained from the case history or on the basis of the developmental stage of the embryo.

**Size Data.** In young embryos, size data are based on the *greatest length* (GL). After formation of the cephalic flexure, the greatest length is equivalent to the crown-rump length (CRL). A slight variation between the two measurements appears only in Carnegie stages 13–17, as in these stages, the curvature of the cervical flexure is transiently higher than the crown (mesencephalic region, → 2.4). Tissue shrinkage due to fixation, or varying degree of curvature of the embryo, can give rise to discrepancies between length data and true developmental stage.

**Carnegie Stages.** Streeter (1942) and O'Rahilly and Müller (1987) have classified human embryonic development into 23 stages based on specimens from the Carnegie collection. These *Carnegie stages* are used in this pocket atlas. Plate 2.1 contains definitions of the Carnegie stages according to O'Rahilly and Müller and a graph relating length, age, and stage data to one another.

The first "Normentafel" of human development was published by Keibel and Elze in 1908, and by Keibel and Mall in 1910. It was an attempt to organize the individual specimens of human embryos available at the time into a developmental series. In 1914, Franklin P. Mall, a student of Keibel, founded the "Department of Embryology of the Carnegie Institution of Washington," named after the industrialist and philanthropist, Carnegie. In 1942, his successor, G.L. Streeter ordered the embryos of the Carnegie Collection into defined stages and named his classification "Developmental Horizons (I-XXIII)." Since early human specimens were not available, co-workers at the Carnegie Laboratory studied the early development of rhesus the monkey and extrapolated the observations to humans. The early implantation stages of the human embryo were first described between 1942 and 1956 in the landmark publications of the pathologist A.T. Hertig and the gynecologist J. Rock. Since an implantation only becomes perceptible after the 2nd week (absence of menstruation), Hertig and Rock searched carefully for implantation sites in the endometrium of uteri removed for surgical indications. In 210 uterine extirpations from women of childbearing age, they found 34 implantation sites. Specimens were photographically documented, histologically prepared, and reconstructed in the Embryological Laboratory of the Carnegie Institution where they, like all other specimens of the Carnegie collection, are available to every researcher. This pocket atlas is based on the embryos of the *Blechschmidt collection*, which were classified by Blechschmidt himself according to the Carnegie stages and were incorporated into the Carnegie collection.

**Chorionic Sac (→ 2.2).** The *chorion* grows much more rapidly than the embryo until the end of the 4th week. From the 5th week onward, both growth curves are parallel. Embryologic data on the size of the chorion are based on the outer diameter including the villi, since after an abortion, the chorion is covered with villi (→ 2.41) and the chorionic cavity is usually collapsed. The chorionic cavity is readily discerned by ultrasonography, whereas the border between the villi and the uterine decidua is not so clear. The inner diameter of the chorionic cavity is thus determined in ultrasonographic examinations.

Modern **ultrasonography** now permits the examination of the embryo in the first three weeks of development and in the embryonic period. The medical significance lies in the early diagnosis of disturbances in implantation and of embryo deformities. Until recently, descriptive embryology was useful only for the understanding of developmental processes and had no clinical relevance. This explains why obstetricians calculate the weeks of pregnancy from the last menstruation. From the embryologic perspective, the embryo, at the point of ovulation and fertilization, has already reached the end of the 2nd week of pregnancy!

For *endosonographic examination* of early pregnancy a transducer is positioned in the vagina in front of the vaginal portion of the cervix (→ 2.2). In *abdominal sonography*, ultrasound is transmitted through the abdominal wall. Interpretation of ultrasound images requires considerable knowledge of the position and the proportions of the fetal organs. Plates 2.2, 2.32 and 2.37 provide examples of transvaginal sonograms and schematic representations of the corresponding embryos.

**Embryonic Period (2.3–2.32).** In the *overview of early development* (→ 2.3), weeks 1–3 are illustrated. The total 21 days are divided into three developmental periods. These subperiods may be summarized as "*first week*": tubal migration, "*second week*": implantation, and "*third week*": trilaminar embryonic disc. The term "week" is used, although the first two developmental subperiods last only 6 days and the third 9 days.

In the overview of the *embryonic period: 4–8 weeks* (→ 2.4), the early development of the first 3 weeks is included in condensed form on the same axis in order to illustrate the exponential growth of the embryo. The 4th week is expanded separately from the 8-week time axis. In the 4th week, the embryonic disc is transformed into an embryo (*folding*). The 4th week is also the central period of embryonic development in which the organ systems are established. The developmental period from the 5th to the 8th week is the time of *organogenesis* . The embryo assumes a human shape and the large organ systems of the body – bones and muscles, gastrointestinal canal, liver, heart, and lungs, as well as kidneys – are established.

Embryos in the overview plates are drawn to the same scale in each developmental period. The scale is indicated in each case. In the 4th week, the drawing scale is 1:10.

**Fetal Period (2.33–2.38).** The fetal period is much longer than the embryonic period. In relation to the total time of pregnancy, therefore, the difference in age determinations based on the last menstruation, or based on ovulation is relatively insignificant. The representations of fetuses under the *growth curve* (→ 2.33), which are true to scale, illustrate the enormous growth up to the 20th week of gestation. Until birth, all growth parameters continue to increase at high rates.

**Placenta and Fetal Membranes (2.39–2.45).** The extraembryonic organs are developed in the human before the embryo itself is formed. Purely morphological consideration of early human development has led to complicated interpretations of the development of the amniotic cavity, chorionic mesoderm, and "primary" and "secondary" yolk sacs that appear to substantiate a special position for humans. Implantation and formation of the placenta are species-specific processes in the reproduction strategy. Homology to the fetal membranes of the chick embryo (→ 3.11) and comparisons with the yolk sac placenta and allantoic placenta of other mammals (→ 3.14) facilitate an understanding of human placental development.

# Embryonic Period

## 2.1 Carnegie Stages

### A. Definition of the Carnegie Stages

The plate contains the criteria for the Carnegie stages according to O'Rahilly and Müller (1987). In the graph, greatest lengths (GL) are correlated with age and Carnegie stages.

**"First Week": Migration through the Fallopian tube**

**Stage 1:** Fertilized oocyte.

**Stage 2:** 2–3 days. Cleavage. Differentiation into outer and inner cells.

**Stage 3:** 4–5 days. Free blastocyst. Trophoblast and inner cell mass. Blastocyst cavity. Separation from zona pellucida ("hatching").

**"Second Week": Implantation**

**Stage 4: 5–6 days.** Attaching Blastocyst (no human specimens described).

**Stage 5:** 0.1–0.2 mm. 7–12 days. Implantation. 5a: Solid trophoblast. 5b: Trophoblastic lacunae. 5c: Lacunar vascular circle. Bilaminar embryonic disc. Amniotic cavity and primary yolk sac.

**"Third Week": Trilaminar Embryonic Disc**

**Stage 6:** 0.2 mm. 13–15 days. Proliferation of extraembryonic mesoderm. Chorionic cavity and chorionic villi. Transformation of primary yolk sac into secondary yolk sac. Primitive streak and embryonic mesoderm.

**Stage 7:** 0.4 mm. 15–17 days. Notochordal process. Body stalk and allantoic diverticulum. Extraembryonic blood vessels.

**Stage 8:** 1.0–1.5 mm.17–19 days. Primitive pit. Notochordal canal. Axial (neurenteric) canal.

**Stage 9:** 1.5–2.5 mm. 19–21 days. 1–3 somites. Neural folds. Cardiac primordium. Head fold.

**"Fourth Week": Folding**

**Stage 10:** 2–3.5 mm. 22–23 days. 4–12 somites. Neural folds fuse. Two pharyngeal arches. Optic sulcus.

**Stage 11:** 2.5–4.5 mm. 23–26 days. 13–20 somites. Rostral neuropore closes. Optic vesicle.

**Stage 12:** 3–5 mm. 26–30 days. 21–29 somites. Caudal neuropore closes. Three pharyngeal arches. Arm buds appear.

**Stage 13:** 4–6 mm. 28–32 days. 30 somites. Leg buds. Lens placode. Otic vesicle.

**5–8 Weeks: Organogenesis**

**Stage 14:** 5–7 mm. 31–35 days. Lens pit and optic cup. Endolymphatic duct.

**Stage 15:** 7–9 mm. 35–38 days. Cerebral vesicles. Lens vesicle. Nasal pit. Facial swellings. Hand plate.

**Stage 16:** 8–11 mm. 37–42 days. Nasal pits are directed ventrally. In the unfixed embryo, the eye is pigmented. Auricular hillocks are visible. Foot plate.

**Stage 17:** 11–14 mm. 42–44 days. Relative enlargement of head and elongation of trunk. Nasolacrimal groove and auricular hillocks are distinct. Finger rays.

**Stage 18:** 13–17 mm. 44–48 days. Cuboidal body form. Elbows and toe rays are defined. Eyelids are discernable. Apex of nose is distinct. Appearance of nipples. Onset of ossification.

**Stage 19:** 16–18 mm. 48–51 days. Elongating and straightening of trunk.

**Stage 20:** 18–22 mm. 51–53 days. Upper limbs are longer and bend at the elbows.

**Stage 21:** 22–24 mm. 53–54 days. Hands and feet are turned inward.

**Stage 22:** 23–28 mm. 54–56 days. Eyelids and external ears develop.

**Stage 23:** 27–31 mm. 56–60 days. Rounded head. Body and limbs developed.

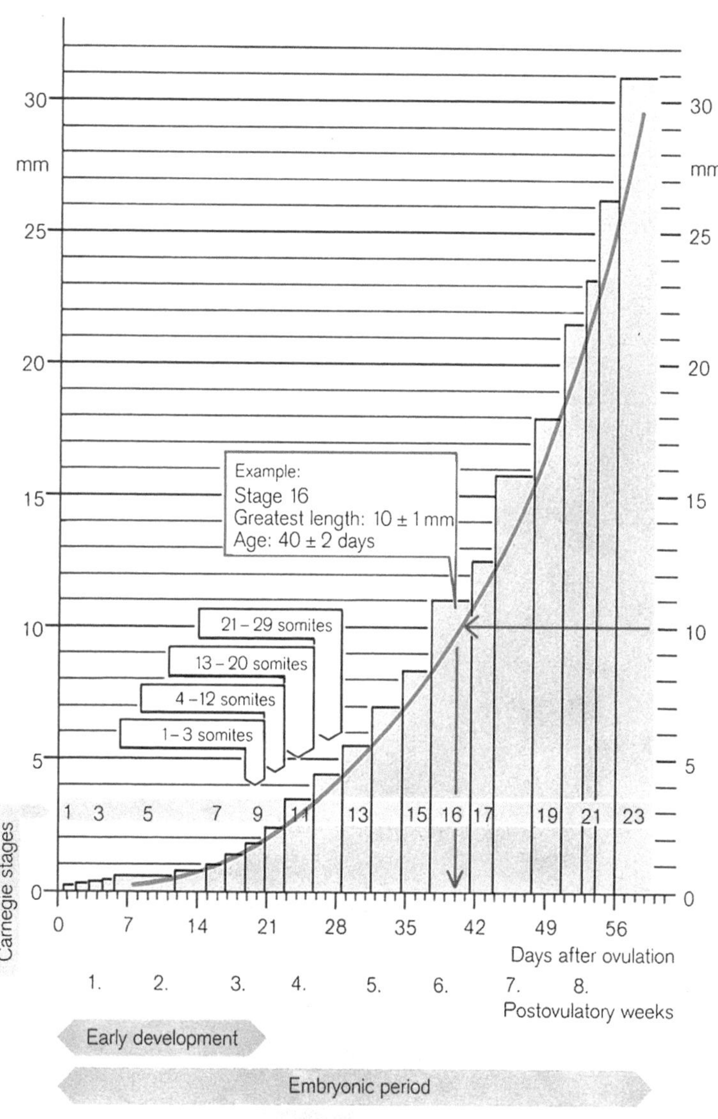


A. Carnegie stages

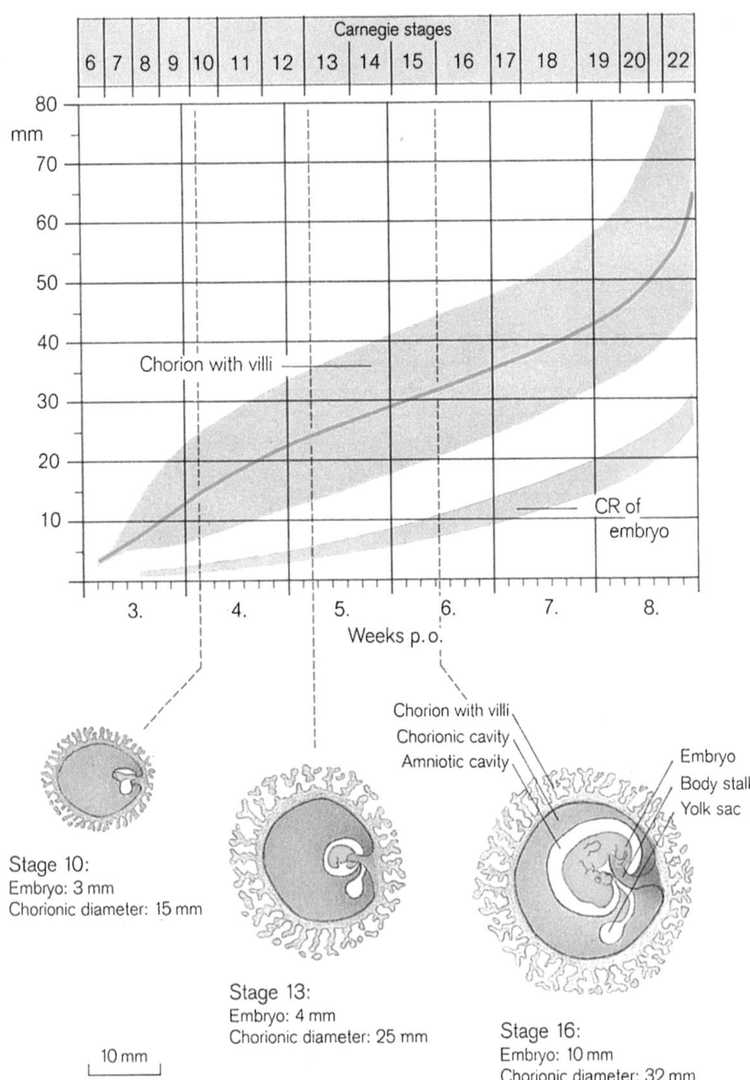


A. Chorionic diameter in the embryonic period

Data after O'Rahilly

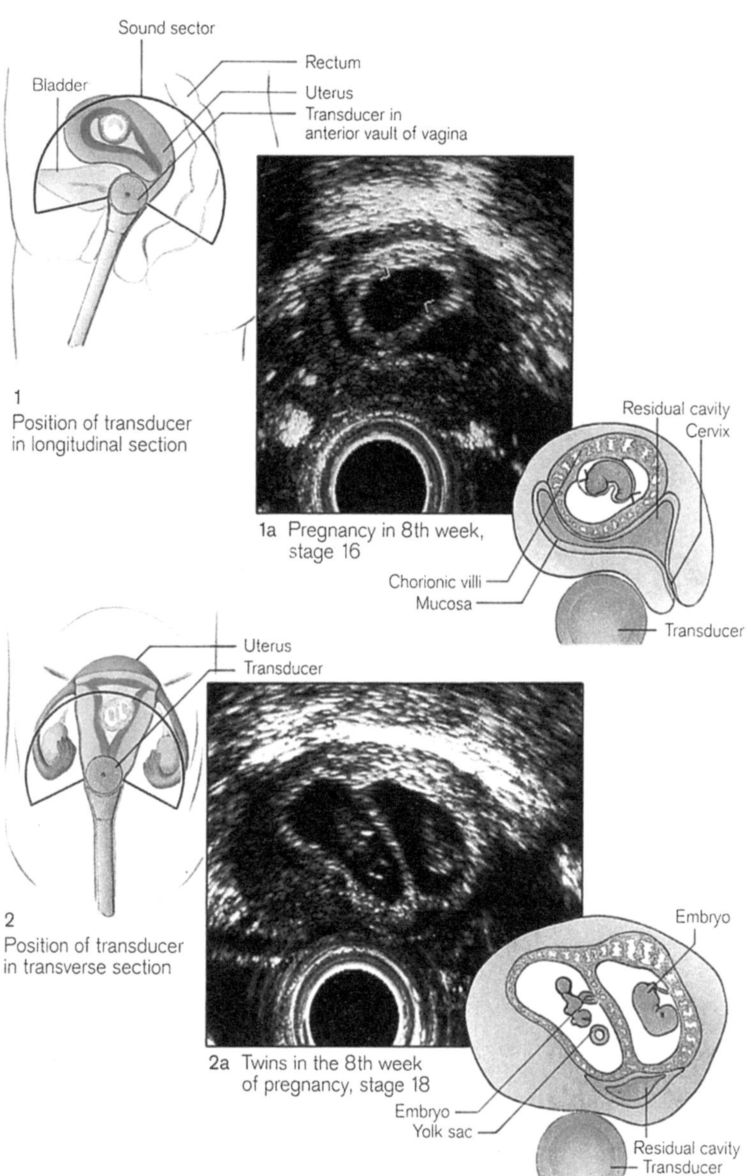


1
Position of transducer in longitudinal section

1a Pregnancy in 8th week, stage 16

2
Position of transducer in transverse section

2a Twins in the 8th week of pregnancy, stage 18

B. Endosonographic examination in the 8th week of pregnancy
The ultrasound photographs were kindly made available by F. Degenhard, Hannover

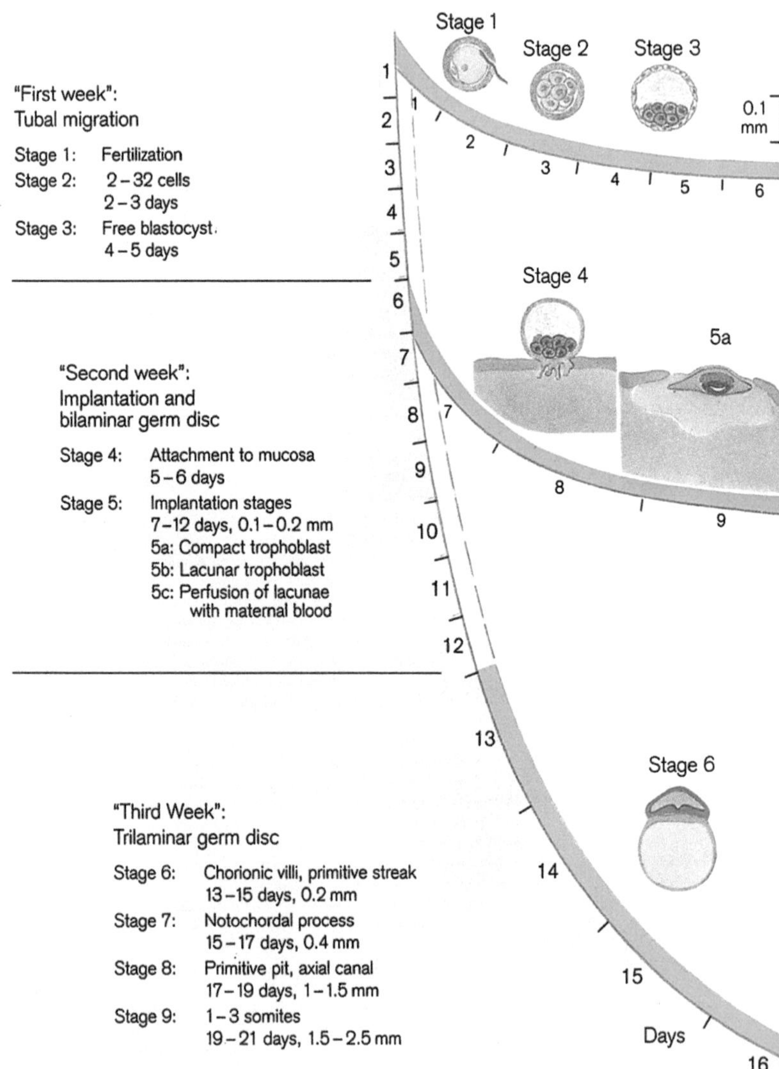
"First week":
Tubal migration
Stage 1: Fertilization
Stage 2: 2–32 cells
2–3 days
Stage 3: Free blastocyst
4–5 days
"Second week":
Implantation and
bilaminar germ disc
Stage 4: Attachment to mucosa
5–6 days
Stage 5: Implantation stages
7–12 days, 0.1–0.2 mm
5a: Compact trophoblast
5b: Lacunar trophoblast
5c: Perfusion of lacunae
with maternal blood
"Third Week":
Trilaminar germ disc
Stage 6: Chorionic villi, primitive streak
13–15 days, 0.2 mm
Stage 7: Notochordal process
15–17 days, 0.4 mm
Stage 8: Primitive pit, axial canal
17–19 days, 1–1.5 mm
Stage 9: 1–3 somites
19–21 days, 1.5–2.5 mm
Stage 1
Stage 2
Stage 3
0.1 mm
Stage 4
5a
Stage 6
Days

C. Early development: 1–3 weeks

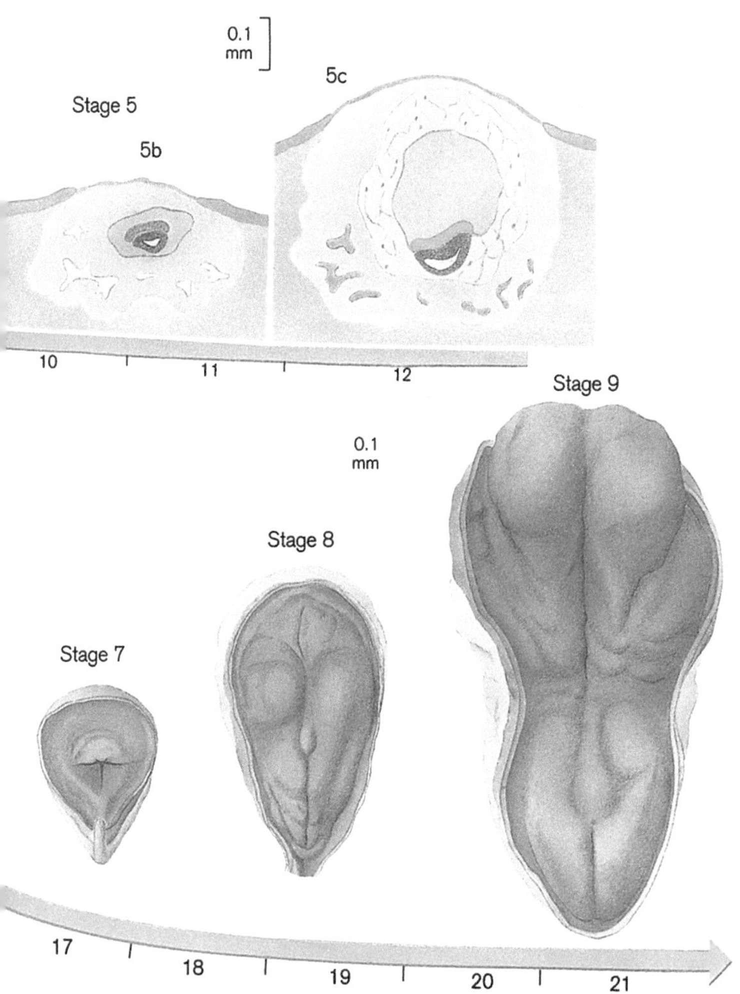
0.1
mm
Stage 5
5b
5c
10
11
12
Stage 9
0.1
mm
Stage 8
Stage 7
17
18
19
20
21

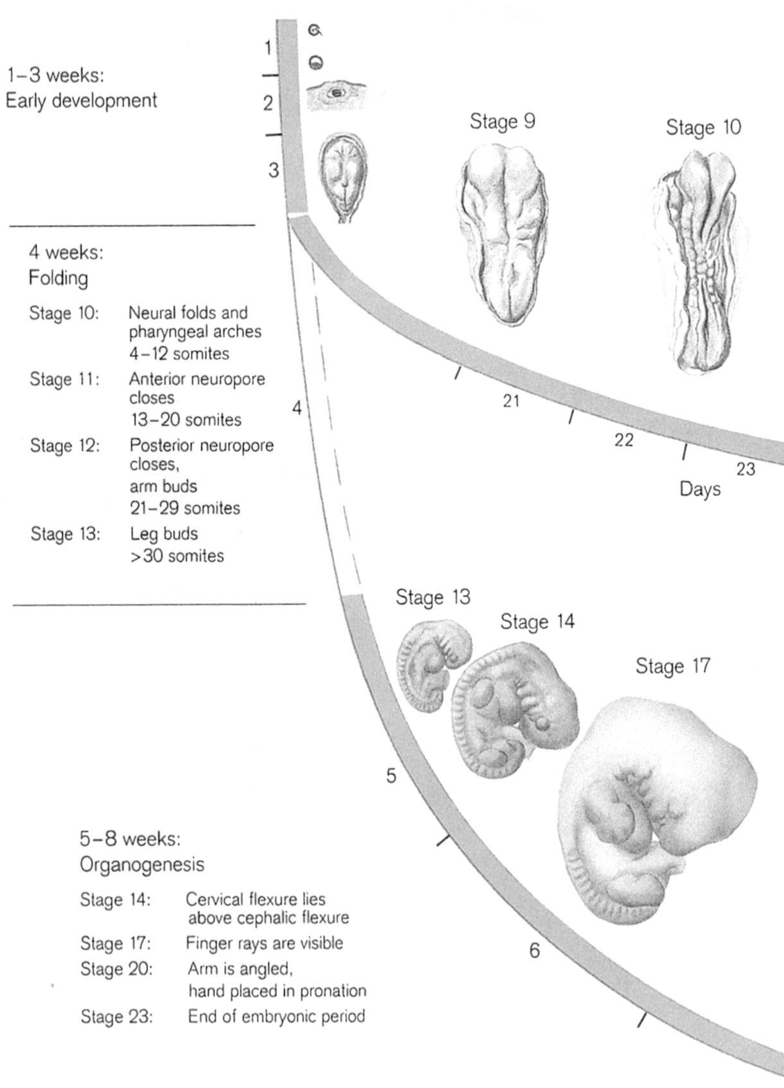
1–3 weeks:
Early development
1
2
3
Stage 9
Stage 10
4 weeks:
Folding
Stage 10: Neural folds and pharyngeal arches 4–12 somites
Stage 11: Anterior neuropore closes 13–20 somites
Stage 12: Posterior neuropore closes, arm buds 21–29 somites
Stage 13: Leg buds >30 somites
4
21
22
23
Days
Stage 13
Stage 14
Stage 17
5
6
5–8 weeks:
Organogenesis
Stage 14: Cervical flexure lies above cephalic flexure
Stage 17: Finger rays are visible
Stage 20: Arm is angled, hand placed in pronation
Stage 23: End of embryonic period

D. Embryonic period: 4–8 weeks

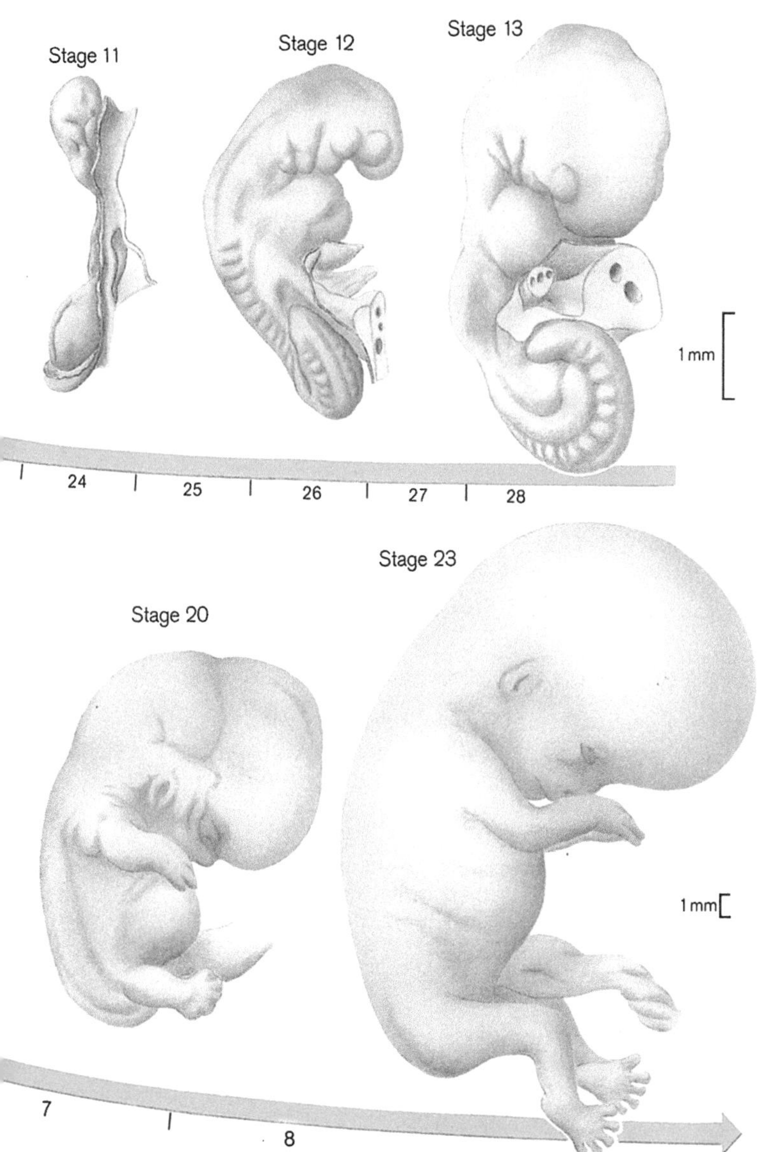
Stage 11
Stage 12
Stage 13
1 mm
24
25
26
27
28
Stage 23
Stage 20
1 mm
7
8

# "First Week": Migration through Tube

## 2.5 Overview: "First Week"

*Background*

The first developmental period **from ovulation to implantation,** lasting 6 days, is slightly less than a week. The embryo goes through the cleavage stage during migration through the Fallopian tube, reaches the uterus as a morula on the 3rd or 4th day after ovulation, and remains in the uterine cavity until about the 6th day as a free blastocyst.

### A. From Ovulation to Implantation

**1. Migration through the Fallopian Tube.** After ovulation, the oocyte is fertilized in the ampulla of the Fallopian tube and is activated. Unfertilized oocytes remain in a state of reduced metabolic activity and die after 12–24 hours. The fertilized oocyte is transported to the uterus by ciliary action and contractions of the Fallopian tube.

**2. Free Blastocyst in Uterine Lumen.** On the 4th day after ovulation, the endometrium is already in the secretory phase and is about 5 mm thick. The endometrial glands produce mucus that carries the morula into the lumen of the uterus. While in the lumen, the 0.1–0.2 mm size morula develops into a blastocyst.

### B. Development of the Oocyte into a Blastocyst

Shortly before ovulation, the oocyte completes the first meiotic (maturation) division and expels the first polar body, which comes to lie beneath the zona pellucida (→ 1.12). The second meiotic division, which follows immediately, is arrested in metaphase. The block in metaphase II is released only by fertilization. The first polar body may undergo a division corresponding to the second meiotic division, giving rise to a fertilized oocyte with three polar bodies.

**Stage 1: Fertilized Oocyte.** Fertilization activates the oocyte (→ 1.5). Metabolic activity increases. The haploid egg nucleus and the haploid sperm nucleus are transformed into *female* and *male pronuclei.* Both pronuclei go through a phase of DNA synthesis and their replicated chromosomes are arranged on a common spindle.

**Stage 2: Cleavage.** The *2-cell stage* arises directly from the first cell division. During transport through the Fallopian tube, cell divisions continue within the zona pellucida. A *4* and an *8-cell stage* are formed. Since furrows (clefts) appear as the cytoplasm is divided, this process is called cleavage. The daughter cells are called blastomeres. The fact that specimens with 3, 12, or 20 blastomeres have been described, indicates that the divisions proceed asynchronously. At this point the *morula* is still surrounded by the zona pellucida and therefore is no larger than the original oocyte. As the blastomeres form junctional complexes, the morula gains an epithelial character ("**compaction**" in the mouse in the 8- cell stage).

**Stage 3: Free Blastocyst.** The blastocyst cavity begins to form when the cell number reaches between 32 and 58. The blastomeres segregate into an internally situated *inner cell mass* and surrounding *outer trophoblast cells*. The trophoblast cells form an epithelial arrangement with tight junctions and secrete fluid that accumulates in the blastocyst cavity between the trophoblastic layer and the inner cell mass. Before attaching to the uterine epithelium, the blastocyst actively slips from the zona pellucida ("hatches") and swells to a diameter of about 0.25 mm by the absorption of fluid.

Morula
Fertilized oocyte
Implantation
Free blastocyst
Fertilization
Endometrium
Myometrium
Oocyte
Developing follicles
Ovulation

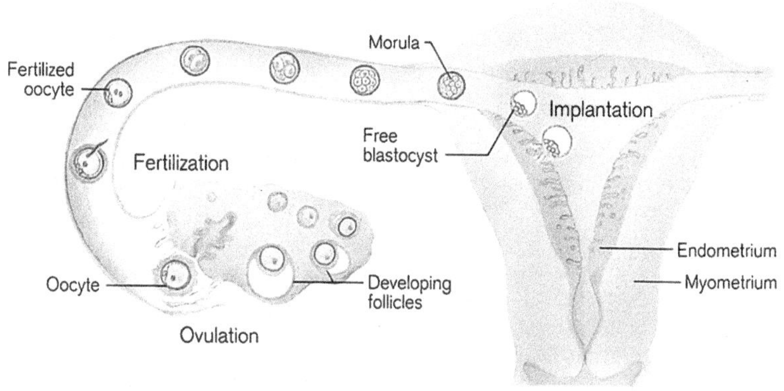

A. From ovulation to implantation

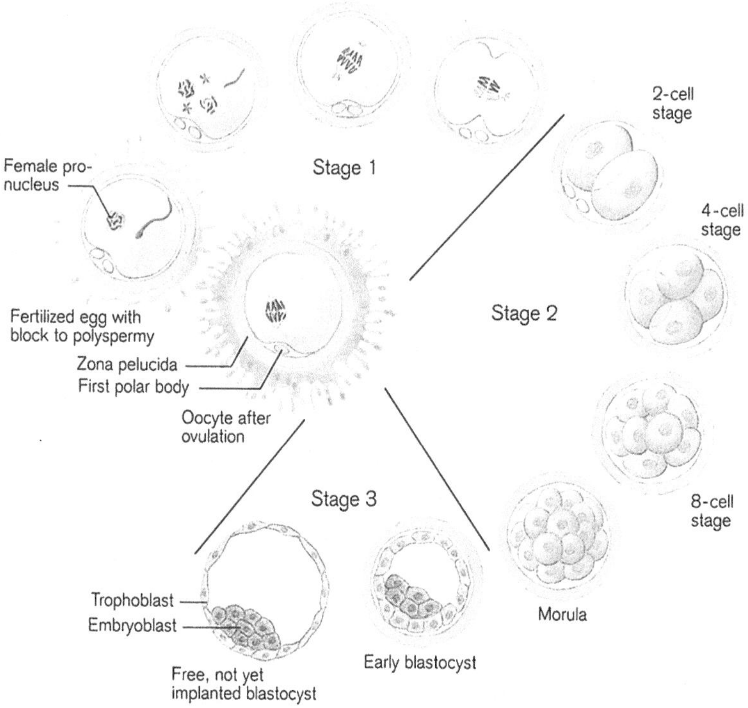

2-cell stage
Female pro-nucleus
Stage 1
4-cell stage
Fertilized egg with block to polyspermy
Stage 2
Zona pelucida
First polar body
Oocyte after ovulation
Stage 3
8-cell stage
Trophoblast
Embryoblast
Morula
Early blastocyst
Free, not yet implanted blastocyst

B. Development of oocyte to blastocyst

## 2.6 Stage 4: Attachment

*Background*

The human blastocyst attaches to the endometrial epithelium between the 5th and 6th day after ovulation. To date, no human embryos in **stage 4** have been described. However, no essential differences exist from the attachment of the blastocysts of rhesus monkeys, which was studied in detail by Heuser and Streeter in 1941 in order to compensate for the absence of human material for this stage.

### A. Attachment of the Blastocyst to the Endometrium

During stage 3 the zona pellucida of the free-swimming blastocyst is enzymatically loosened. The blastocyst then slips ("hatches") from the zona pellucida (**A1**) and settles on the epithelial surface. Attachment can only take place when the endometrium has entered the secretory phase. At the point of contact, the *trophoblast cells* are transformed into a syncytium and penetrate into the endometrial epithelium (**A2**). The *inner cell mass* migrates along the inner wall of the trophoblastic cavity to the attachment site, so that the blastocyst penetrates the endometrium "head first." The embryological stage in which the first contact is made with the maternal epithelium is defined as **Stage 4**.

### B. Human Morula and Free Blastocyst

After in vitro fertilization, the human oocyte can be directly observed under the microscope up to the blastocyst stage. The **32-cell morula (B1)** is one of the first living human cleavage stages and was described by Shettles (1968). A fissure has formed between the zona pellucida and the blastomeres.

The blastocysts shown (**B2** and **B3**) are classic specimens that were found in the uterine lumen after surgery and were prepared histologically by Hertig and Rock (1954). The **blastocyst (B2)** consists of 58 cells. Its age is estimated to be 96 hours. The *cells* of the inner cell mass (epiblast) have begun to separate from the trophoblast. The trophoblast cells already form an epithelial structure. Remains of the *zona pellucida* and the *polar bodies* are still present.

The **blastocyst (B3)** consists of 107 cells. Its age is approximately 103 hours. The blastocyst has "hatched" from the zona pellucida and has become pumped up with fluid. The cells of the epiblast are larger and less differentiated than the trophoblast cells.

### C. Attachment of the Rhesus Monkey Blastocyst

The blastocyst has emerged from the zona pellucida and swims in the fluid film secreted by the endometrial glands (**C1**). It settles on the epithelium like a balloon (**C2**). The trophoblast cells make active contact with the superficial epithelium of the uterus. They form pseudopodia, which penetrate into the intercellular spaces between the epithelial cells (**C3**).

In the further course of implantation, differences exist between the two species. Whereas the human blastocyst penetrates entirely into the mucosa (interstitial implantation), the blastocyst of the rhesus monkey at first also forms a hemochorial placenta at the attachment site, but then instead of penetrating further, spreads out in the uterine lumen (central implantation) and forms a second attachment site on the opposite wall of the uterus, where a second placenta develops (bidiscoidal placenta, → 3.15).

Photograph B1 from Shettles (1968), B2 and B3 from Hertig and Rock (1954), and photograph C1-C3 from Streeter (1941).

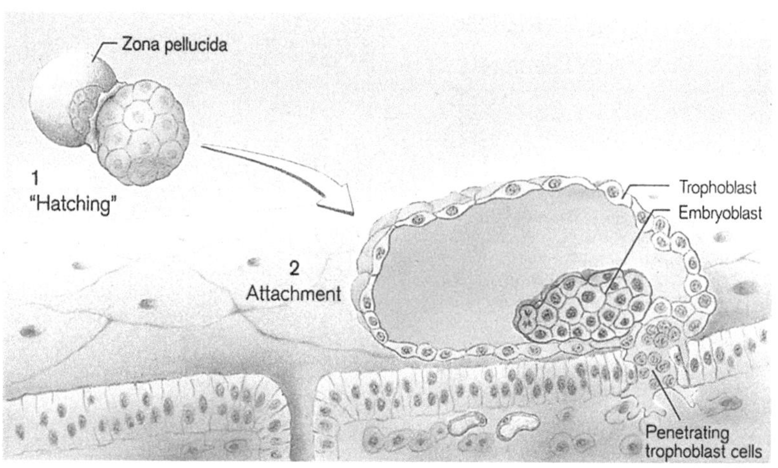


A. Attachment of blastocyst to mucosa

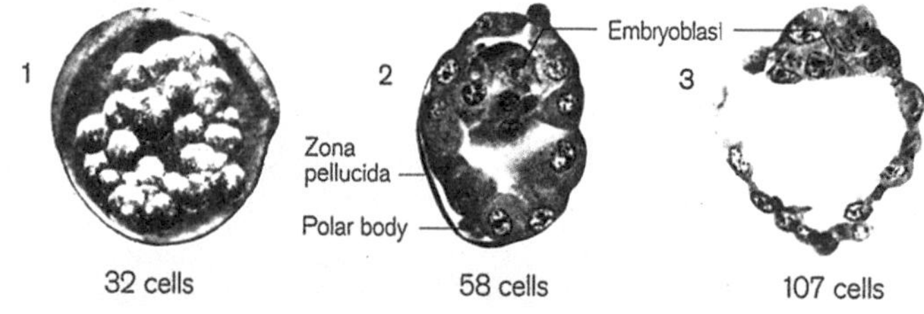


B. Human morula and free blastocyst (stage 3)

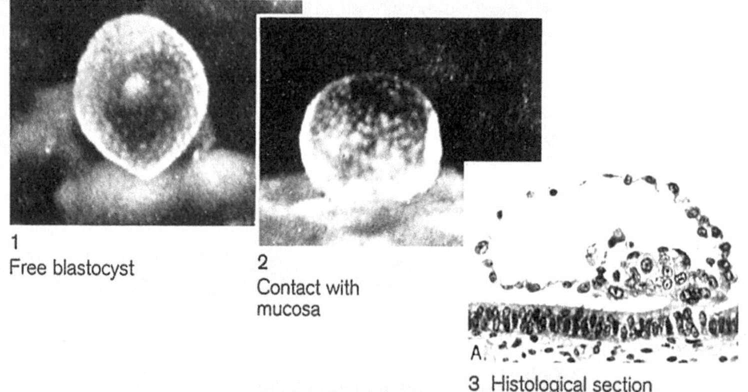


C. Attachment of Rhesus monkey blastocyst

## "Second Week": Implantation

## 2.7 Overview: "Second Week"

*Background*

In the 2nd week, the blastocyst becomes embedded in the maternal mucosa (implantation). **Implantation** begins around the 6th day with the attachment of the blastocyst to the endometrial epithelium and ends with the beginning of the utero-placental circulation on about the 12th day after ovulation. The developmental period "second week" is therefore somewhat shorter than a calendar week.

### A. Implantation of the Blastocyst

**1. Early Phase.** The fluid filled cavity of the free blastocyst collapses during penetration of the endometrial epithelium (**implantation collapse**). The trophoblast layer thickens and moves deeper into the endometrium. Trophoblastic cells lyse the decidual cells of the endometrium, resorb released proteins, sugars, and lipids, phagocytize cell residues, and erode the glandular tubules. This **invasive growth** stops in the *zona compacta* of the endometrium, which lies between the epithelium and the zone with dilated glands (*zona spongiosa*) (→ 1.14). The blastocyst becomes implanted in the connective tissue (interstitium) of the endometrium (**interstitial implantation**). The connective tissue cells of the zona compacta have differentiated into decidual cells in the secretory phase of the cycle.

**2. Final Phase.** After penetration into the endometrium, the blastocyst cavity (trophoblast cavity) expands again. Its lumen becomes filled by the *primary yolk sac* and by the *endodermal reticulum* , which try to keep up with the **expansion of the blastocyst.** The blastocyst becomes spherical and increases its diameter more than twofold. A labyrinth of interconnected fluid-filled lacunae is formed in the trophoblast. The trophoblast cells finally penetrate the maternal arterioles and venules. Maternal blood streams from the arteries into the lacunae and leaves them again through the venules. This perfusion of the lacunae is the beginning of the **uteroplacental circulation**.

A mushroom-shaped fibrin clot (**closing-plug**) is formed over the penetrating implant, and the defect is healed by mucosal epithelium growing in from the margins.

The changes in the mucous membrane in the region of the implantation site go beyond the general decidual transformation in the secretory phase of the cycle and are therefore considered a reaction to implantation. This so-called **"decidual reaction"** involves an edematous swelling of the tissue induced by the trophoblast, as well as an increased blood flow in the adjacent maternal sinusoids and a further swelling of the decidual cells.

### B. Implantation Cone in the Uterine Epithelium

The expansion of the blastocyst leads to a cone-shaped bulge at the mucosal surface. After the mucosal defect is healed with the closing-plug, the implantation site can only be recognized externally by this bulge.

Judging by the position of the normal discoid placenta, 55.5% of implantations take place at the posterior wall and 44.5% at the anterior wall of the uterus.

The perfusion of maternal blood into the lacunae of the trophoblast on the 12th or 13th day may cause minor hemorrhages (**implantation bleeding,** → 1.15), which can be confused with menstrual bleeding (on the 28th day of the cycle), leading to an incorrect calculation of the estimated date of delivery.

2.7B is a macro-photograph of the implantation cone of 'the 12-day-old Barnes embryo (about 12X) (From Boyd, Hamilton: The Human Placenta).

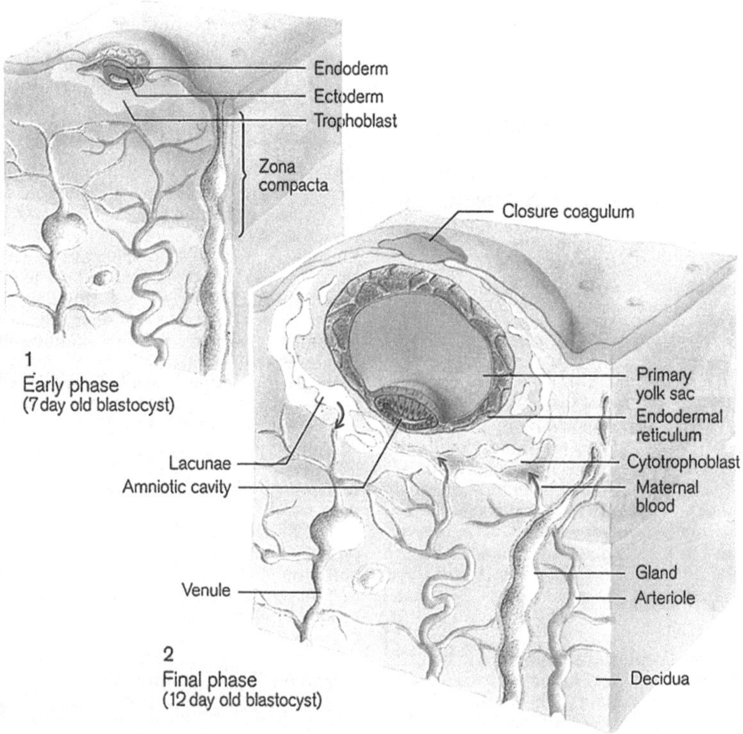

Endoderm
Ectoderm
Trophoblast
Zona compacta
1
Early phase
(7 day old blastocyst)
Closure coagulum
Primary yolk sac
Endodermal reticulum
Cytotrophoblast
Maternal blood
Lacunae
Amniotic cavity
Gland
Arteriole
Venule
2
Final phase
(12 day old blastocyst)
Decidua

A. Implantation of blastocyst

Mucosa
Implantation cone

Macro-photo

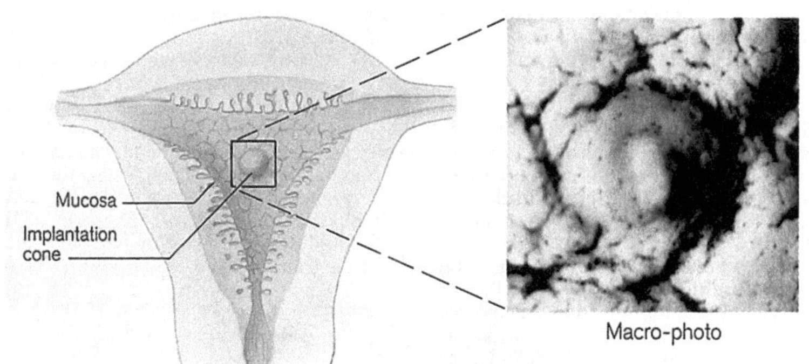

B. Implantation cone in the uterine mucosa

## 2.8 Stage 5: Bilaminar Embryonic Disc

*Background*

Stage 5 encompasses the penetration of the blastocyst into the endometrium up to the beginning of the uteroplacental circulation. It is subdivided according to the **differentiation of the trophoblast,** since until the nutrition of the embryo is secured, the trophoblast grows rapidly. The embryonic disc, however, remains relatively behind in its development.

### A. Development of the Bilaminar Embryonic Disc and Trophoblast

**1. Implantation collapse.** While penetrating the uterine endothelium, the inflated blastocyst collapses. Contact with the uterine mucosa induces strong mitotic activity in the trophoblastic cells. The newly formed trophoblastic cells coalesce into **multinucleated giant cells**. The trophoblastic cells that have no contact with the mucosa still have the characteristic flat epithelial morphology of the free blastocyst.

**2. Solid Trophoblast** (stage 5a). Initially, giant cells with one or more nuclei are irregularly distributed. The multinucleated areas finally form a continuous external layer, which is called the **syncytiotrophoblast** or syncytium (**A4**). The inner, cellular layer is called the **cytotrophoblast**. Cell divisions occur only in the cytotrophoblast. The newly formed cells are continuously taken up into the syncytium by fusion.

**3. Lacunar Trophoblast** (stage 5b). The syncytium spreads out radially into the mucosa and intercommunicating, labyrinthine cavities (lacunae) appear in the syncytium.

**4. Final Phase: Perfusion of Lacunae with Maternal Blood** (stage 5c). The syncytium invades the decidua of the endometrial zona compacta. In the deeper layers, it penetrates maternal capillaries. The syncytial lacunae fill with maternal blood. When small arterioles and venules with a pressure difference are finally reached, the uteroplacental circulation begins. The **embryoblast (inner cell mass)** develops into a bilaminar embryonic disc of *ectoderm* and *endoderm* (A2),which is bordered ventrally by the *primary yolk sac* and dorsally by the *amniotic cavity* (4A).

**1a Primary Cavity Formation.** In the formation of the ectoderm, the cells of the embryoblast become connected into a pseudostratified, columnar epithelium, thereby becoming concavo-convex. During this reorganization of cells to the embryonic disc, a cleft is formed in the embryoblast (**A1**) that later opens into the trophoblast (arrows in **A1a**), enabling the trophoblast to form the roof of this primary cavity.

**2a Formation of the Amniotic Cavity.** The newly formed cavity is then lined by *amnioblasts* that grow inward from the margins of the ectodermal disc (arrow in **A2a**, *modified fissure amnion* according to Luckett [1975]). The amnion is an ectodermal structure that arises from the embryonic disc (epiblast) and not by delamination from the trophoblast, as postulated by Hertig and Rock (→ 3.13).

**3a Formation of the Primary Yolk Sac.** Endodermal cells migrate inward from the margins of the ectoderm of the bilaminar embryonic disc and line the blastocyst cavity (arrow in **A3a**), thus forming the primary yolk sac in the blastocyst cavity (**A4**).

**4a Spreading of the Trophoblasts.** In the final phase of implantation, the blastocyst cavity expands enormously. The radial growth of the trophoblast (arrow in **A4a**) leads to the formation of a cleft between the trophoblast and the newly formed primary yolk sac, which is filled by a network of spread out endodermal cells, the *endodermal reticulum*. According to Luckett (1978), the reticulum is of endodermal origin and does not arise by delamination from the trophoblast.

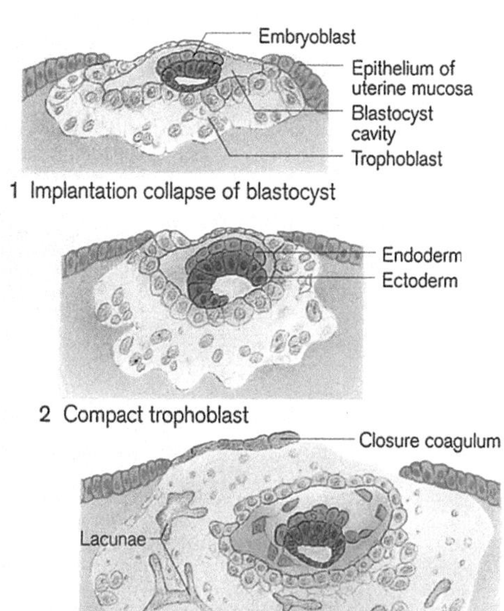


1 Implantation collapse of blastocyst

2 Compact trophoblast

3 Lacunar trophoblast

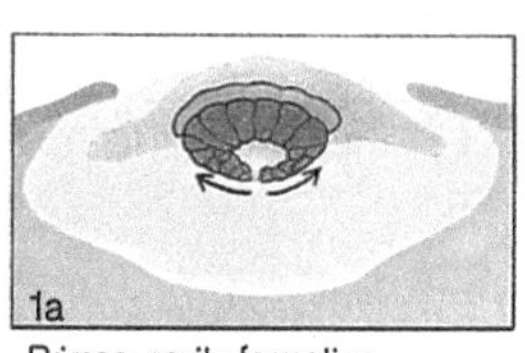


Primary cavity formation

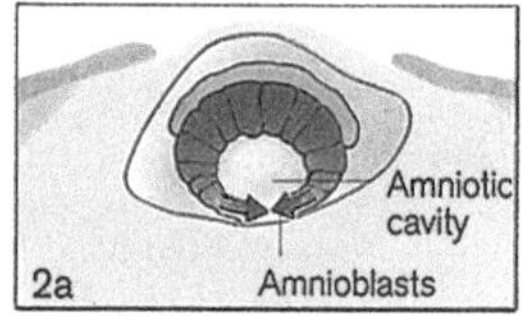


Formation of amniotic cavity

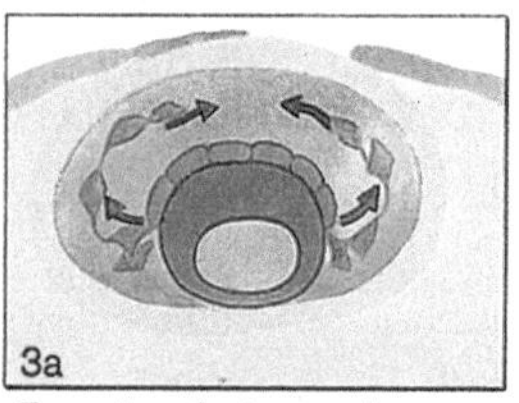


Formation of primary yolk sac

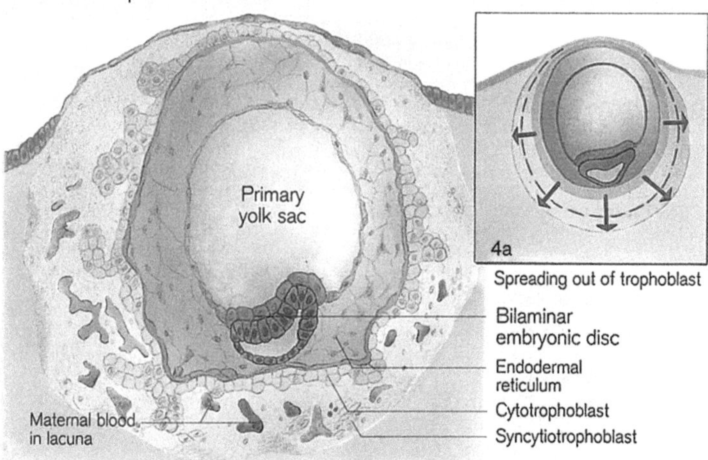


Spreading out of trophoblast

4 Closure phase of implantation

A. Development of bilaminar embryonic disc and trophoblast

# "Third Week": Trilaminar Embryonic Disc

## 2.9 Overview: "Third Week"

*Background*

This developmental phase begins in stage 6a with the formation of extraembryonic mesoderm and the reorganization of the embryonic cavities (rupture of the primary yolk sac). The primitive streak arises in stage 6b, the notochordal process in stage 7 and the axial (neurentric) canal in stage 8. In stage 9 the head folds appear, the heart begins to beat, and the chorionic villi float in maternal blood.

### A. Reorganization of the Embryonic Cavities by Rupture of the Primary Yolk Sac

In the 3rd week the expansion of the trophoblast continues rapidly, whereas the relative growth of the embryonic disc lags further behind (note the separation of the growth curves of chorion and embryo in 2.1 B). The primary yolk sac cannot keep pace with the widening of the trophoblastic cavity and is therefore reduced to the definitive (secondary) yolk sac. A wide *chorionic cavity* arises, in which a small *two chambered embryo* is suspended by a body stalk made up of extraembryonic mesoderm. In the reorganization of the early embryonic cavities, the yolk sac cavity is reduced and is replaced by a large chorionic cavity.

**1. The Embryo before Reorganization.** The expanding trophoblastic cavity is filled by the *primary yolk sac* and by loose *endodermal reticulum* (same embryo as 2.7, A2).

**2. The Embryo after Reorganization.** At the beginning of the 3rd week, the primary yolk sac has been replaced by a smaller *secondary yolk sac* beneath the embryonic disc. The diameter of the chorionic cavity enlarges to more than double its size, whereas the embryonic disc hardly grows. **A1** and **A2** are shown on the same scale. The reorganization of the cavities proceeds with the spread of extraembryonic mesoderm, which arises before the intraembryonic mesoderm at the thickened caudal pole of the embryonic disc. The extraembryonic mesoderm lines the trophoblastic cavity, forming *chorionic mesoderm*, and also covers the *amniotic cavity* and the *yolk sac* with a layer of investment mesoderm. Cytotrophoblastic cells move through the trophoblastic trabeculae to the exterior and form the *cytotrophoblastic shell*. The chorionic mesoderm penetrates into the trabeculae of the trophoblast, which thereby become the *chorionic villi*.

### B. Direction of Growth of the Embryonic disc

After the reorganization of the cavities at the beginning of the 3rd week, the bilaminar embryonic disc is transformed into a **trilaminar embryonic disc** by the formation of a mesodermal layer. The intraembryonic primitive streak mesoderm arises just after the extraembryonic mesoderm. Until folding begins in the 4th week, the embryonic disc remains stretched out above the yolk sac.

**1. The Chorionic Sac in stage 8**. The section illustrated in B passes in the longitudinal direction of the embryonic disc and is rotated 90 degrees with respect to **A2**.

**2. Embryo.** With the forward growth of the primitive streak, the embryonic disc is stretched and is elongated cranially. The body stalk, originally attaching over the entire top of the amnion, is shifted posteriorly. The embryonic disc adjusts itself to the contour of the fluid-filled yolk sac. The strong craniocaudal and lateral curvature of the human embryonic disc in the 3rd week is due to this adjustment to the yolk sac.

**Orientation of the Embryo.** In the illustration of the embryo becoming implanted in the endometrium during the 2nd week (see 2.7, A1), by convention, the epithelial lining of the endometrium is on top and the ectoderm and amniotic cavity of the embryo are below. From the 3rd week onward, the embryo is oriented with the ectoderm and the amniotic cavity upward; whereas the endometrium (decidua) lies below.

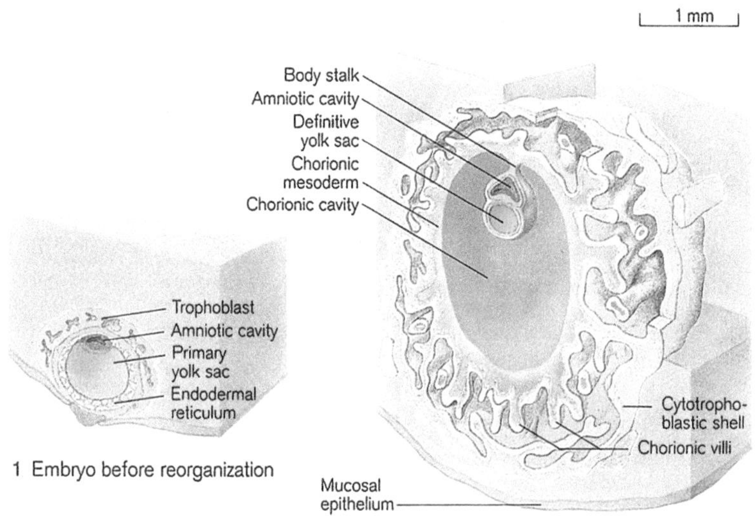


1 Embryo before reorganization

2 Embryo after reorganization

A. Reorganization of the embryonic cavities

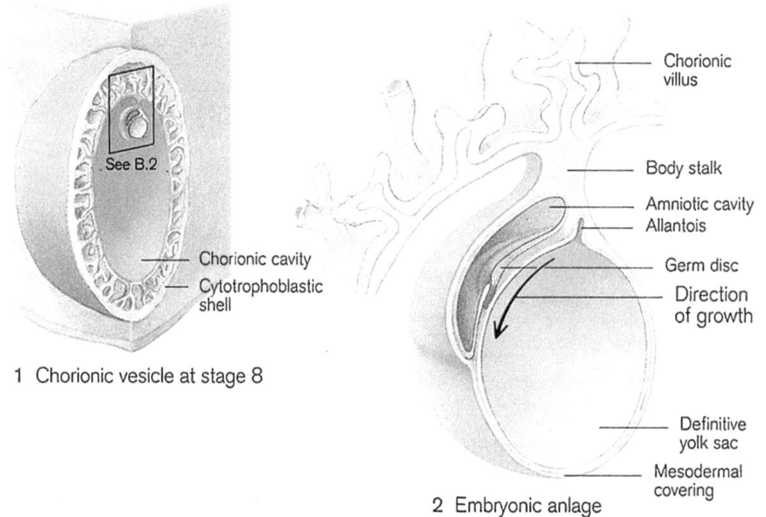


1 Chorionic vesicle at stage 8

2 Embryonic anlage

B. Direction of growth of germ disc

## 2.10 Stage 6: Transformation of Yolk Sac

*Background*

**Stage 6:** The primary yolk sac ruptures and its remnants give rise to a smaller, *definitive (secondary) yolk sac* in the region of the embryonic disc. Extraembryonic mesoderm lines the trophoblastic cavity, converting it to the *chorionic cavity. Chorionic villi* arise by the invasion of mesoderm into the trabeculae of the trophoblast. Stage 6 is defined by the first appearance of chorionic villi. Measurements of the external diameter of the chorion vary from 1 mm to 4.5 mm, while those of the embryonic disc range from 0.15 mm to 0.5 mm. The age is approximately 13 days. In younger stage 6 specimens, no axial structures can yet be recognized (*stage 6a*); in older specimens, a primitive streak is present (*stage 6b*).

### A. Extraembryonic mesoderm and Transformation of the Yolk Sac

**1. Onset of Mesoderm Formation.** In a 12-day-old embryo at *stage 5c* (longitudinal section), the *extraembryonic mesoderm* arises in a thickening at the caudal pole of the embryonic disc, which at the same time, is the point of origin of the primitive streak that grows craniad somewhat later. Individual mesodermal cells migrate outward from the thickened epithelial region. The formation of the extraembryonic mesoderm precedes the development of the primitive streak mesoderm in the embryo.

The derivation of extraembryonic mesoderm from the embryonic disc advocated by Luckett (1978), is in accordance with experimental results in the mouse. Earlier authors assumed a delamination of mesodermal cells from the trophoblast.

**2. Spreading of Mesoderm and Rupture of the Primary Yolk sac.** In a 13-day-old embryo at *stage 6* (longitudinal section), the mesodermal cells spread out on the yolk sac and amnion of the embryonic anlage, as well as on the inner side of the trophoblast below the endodermal reticulum. At the same time, the primary yolk sac ruptures. Individual epithelial remnants form irregular, isolated cysts ("exocoelomic cysts"). The cells of the endodermal reticulum disappear in the extraembryonic mesoderm.

**3. Formation of the Secondary Yolk sac, Chorionic Cavitys and Body Stalk.** In a 14-day-old embryo at *stage 6* (transverse section), the remnants of the ruptured primary yolk sac are united beneath the embryonic disc into a small secondary yolk sac. Extraembryonic mesoderm covers the two-chambered embryonic anlage and lines the trophoblastic cavity. The wall of the trophoblast, lined by mesoderm, is now designated as the *chorion*. The *chorionic cavity,* a cell-free, fluid-filled space, arises between the chorion and the embryonic disc. Mesoderm invades the trophoblastic trabeculae giving rise to villi (*chorionic villi*). The bridge of extraembryonic mesoderm between the chorion and the embryo is the *body stalk*.

**4. Differential Growth of Embryoblast and Trophoblast.** The transformation of the primary into the secondary yolk sac is only observed in primate development. It is explained functionally by the interstitial mode of implantation, in which the trophoblast expands enormously, while the embryo barely increases in size.

The transformation of the yolk sac is induced by the extraembryonic mesoderm that lines the chorionic cavity and initiates the development of blood vessels in the villi. The extraembryonic mesoderm arises before the intraembryonic mesoderm because the trophoblast must differentiate and villi must form, securing nutrition before the development of the embryo can set in.

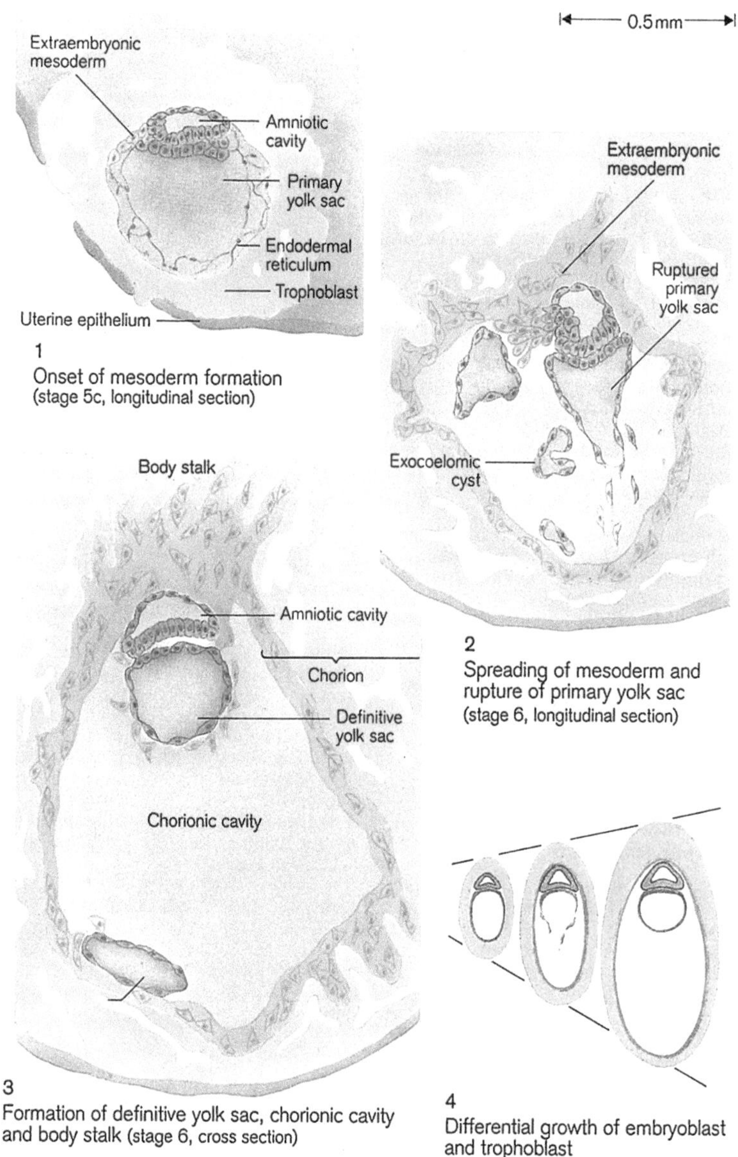


1
Onset of mesoderm formation (stage 5c, longitudinal section)

2
Spreading of mesoderm and rupture of primary yolk sac (stage 6, longitudinal section)

3
Formation of definitive yolk sac, chorionic cavity and body stalk (stage 6, cross section)

4
Differential growth of embryoblast and trophoblast

A. Extraembryonic mesoderm and transformation of yolk sac

## 2.11 Stage 6b and 7: Primitive Streak

*Background*

**Stage 6b and 7:** The embryonic disc, comprised of ectoderm and endoderm, is stretched out between the amniotic cavity and the yolk sac. After cells for the extraembryonic mesoderm have migrated from the thickened ectoderm at the caudal pole, the ectodermal thickening grows craniad as the **primitive streak.** Through the **primitive groove** arising on the streak, cells invaginate, migrate laterally, and insert themselves between the ectoderm and endoderm, forming **intraembryonic mesoderm.** When the primitive streak has reached its endpoint between the middle and the anterior third of the embryonic disc, its apex thickens into the **primitive node,** through which material invaginates to form the **notochordal process**. The primitive streak defines the anteroposterior axis and the bilateral symmetry of the embryo. The structure of the primitive streak can be interpreted as an elongated **blastopore** (→ 3.18). The invagination of mesodermal material through the streak was deduced from labelling experiments using chick embryos. **Invagination** probably does not exclusively involve the movement of a continuous tissue sheet, but also the separation and migration of individual cells from the ectoderm (→ 3.7).

### A. Development of the Primitive Streak (Stage 6b)

In the graphic reconstruction of a 14-day-old embryo (**A1**), the extraembryonic mesoderm covering the yolk sac and amnion, as well as the *body stalk*, have been removed on the left side up to the midline, so that the amniotic cavity and the yolk sac become visible. The amniotic cavity is opened, exposing the ectoderm of the embryonic disc with the advancing primitive streak. The *arrows* indicate the spread of **extraembryonic mesoderm** ,originating at the posterior pole of the embryonic disc.

The *cross sections* (**A2**) show the development of **intraembryonic mesoderm**. In the region of the *primitive streak* (**A2a**), a layer of intraembryonic mesoderm already lies between the ectoderm and endoderm and is laterally continuous with the extraembryonic mesoderm. At the tip of the *primitive streak* (**A2b**), the migration of individual mesodermal cells from the ectoderm is schematically represented (→ 3.7). *In front of the primitive streak* (**A2c**), the endodermal layer is closely apposed to the ectoderm. At the lateral margins of the embryonic disc, extraembryonic mesoderm is already present.

### B. Development of the Notochordal Process (Stage 7)

In the reconstruction of a 16-day-old embryo (**B1**), the *notochordal process* (situated in the mesodermal layer in front of the primitive node) is visible through the ectoderm. The cranial growth of the embryonic disc results in the ectoderm and amniotic cavity projecting out over the yolk sac. In the **sagittal section** (**B2**), the arrow indicates the invagination of cellular material through the primitive node to form the notochordal process.

**Allantoic Diverticulum.** At the caudal pole of the embryonic disc, a dead-ended duct extends into the body stalk from the endodermal yolk sac. This duct represents the rudimentary allantoic primordium (**B1**). The allantoic diverticulum exhibits great variability. As a rudimentary component of body stalk and chorion, it points to the fact that chorion and placenta of the human are derived from a chorioallantois (→ 3.11 and 3.13).

**Amniotic Duct.** The amniotic cavity possesses a diverticulum projecting into the body stalk that is referred to as the amniotic duct (**B1**). The development of such a duct is very variable in human embryos.

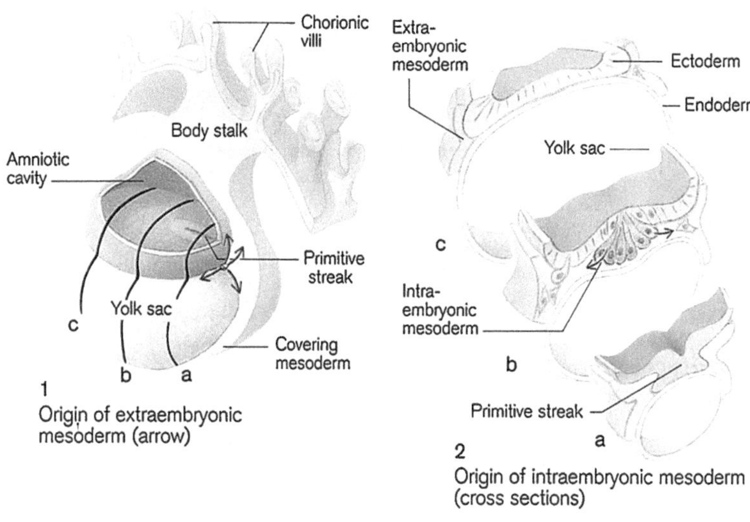


1
Origin of extraembryonic mesoderm (arrow)

2
Origin of intraembryonic mesoderm (cross sections)

A. Development of primitive streak (stage 6 b)

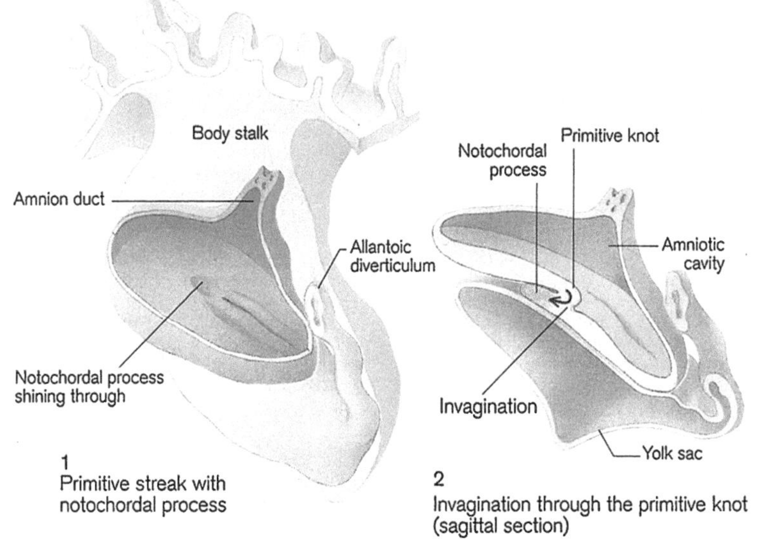


1
Primitive streak with notochordal process

2
Invagination through the primitive knot (sagittal section)

B. Development of notochordal process (stage 7)

## 2.12 Stage 8: Axial Canal

*Background*

In **stage 8,** embryos are characterized by a deep primitive pit that extends into the notochordal process and later opens ventrally into the yolk sac. The formation of the axial canal (neurenteric canal) and the intercalation of the notochord into the roof of the gut exhibit great variability. This suggests that the formation of these structures is phylogenetically in a state of transition.

### A. Axial canal and Intercalation of the Notochord into the Roof of the Gut

The primitive pit arises by the invagination of material for the notochordal process. The pit deepens and extends into the notochordal process as an initially still dead-ended canal, known as the notochordal canal. The hollow notochordal process fuses with the underlying endoderm. The fused epithelial regions then disintegrate, so that the canal of the notochordal process opens into the yolk sac. The cellular material of the notochordal process is intercalated into the roof of the gut, forming the epithelial *notochordal plate*. The resulting canal, which extends from the primitive pit into the notochordal process and opens into the yolk sac, is termed the **axial canal** (after Blechschmidt). In stage 10 and 11 the notochord again becomes delimited from the roof of the gut and the axial canal disappears.

The axial canal is also known as the neurenteric canal, since it unites the future neural canal and the future intestinal canal. Formation of an axial canal and intercalation of the notochord into the endoderm are observed in the human, guinea pig, and hedgehog. The primitive pit in the primitive node is reminiscent of a blastopore, through which the mesodermal cells of the notochordal process invaginate. The position of the notochordal plate on top of the yolk sac corresponds to the position of the chordamesoderm complex in the roof of the archenteron of the amphibian embryo (→ 3.4). The axial canal may play a functional role in the maintenance or the adjustment of pressure equilibrium between the amniotic cavity and the yolk sac.

**1. Embryonic Disc with Axial Canal.** In the wax plate reconstruction of an 18-day-old embryo (**A1**), the body stalk is oriented downward, together with a piece of the chorionic plate and two sectioned *chorionic villi.* The *primitive streak* lies in the caudal half of the embryonic disc. The primitive groove ends in the narrow *primitive pit.* The club-shaped protrusion (attached cranially) corresponds to the notochordal process, which bulges through the ectoderm at the floor of the still flat neural groove. The neural folds are raised laterally as flat domes.

**2. Median Section.** In front of the primitive node, the floor of the axial canal fuses with the endoderm and disintegrates. The material of the *notochordal process* is intercalated into the endoderm and at this site forms the roof of the yolk sac. The primitive pit now opens into the yolk sac via the axial canal (arrow). Cranially, a thickened region of endoderm known as the *prechordal plate* lies in front the notochordal process. At the caudal end of the primitive streak, in front of the allantois, ectoderm and endoderm are tightly adherent and represent the site of the future *cloacal membrane.*

**3. Transverse Sections.** In the region of the *primitive streak* (**a**), ectoderm and mesoderm are continuous with one another. The flat endodermal layer is slightly detached. The *primitive pit* (**b**) in the primitive node continues anteriorly into the axial canal. The *axial canal* (**c**) passes into the *notochordal process* as a small epithelial canal. The floor of the axial canal in the notochordal process disintegrates. The notochordal process is thus intercalated into the endoderm as the *notochordal plate* (**d**). The *prechordal plate* (**e**) subsequently gives rise to head mesoderm.

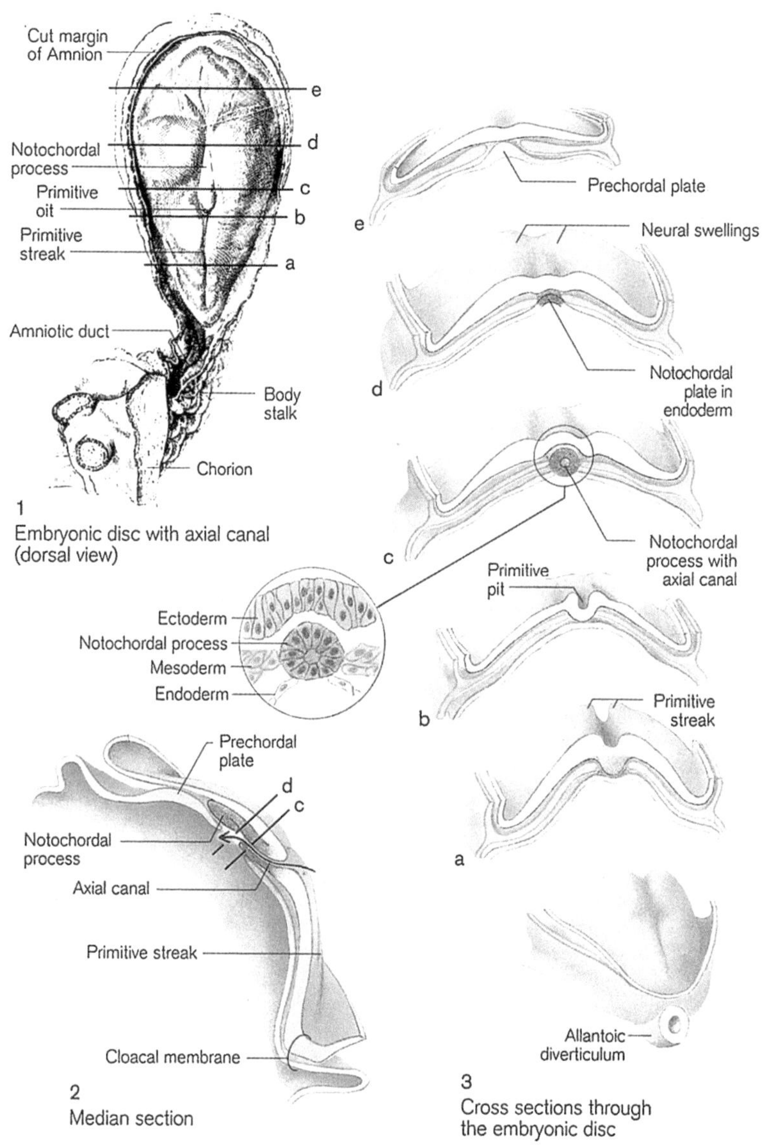


1
Embryonic disc with axial canal (dorsal view)

2
Median section

3
Cross sections through the embryonic disc

A. Axial canal and intercalation of notochord into roof of gut

## 2.13 Stage 9: First Somites

*Background*

**Stage 9:** One to three pairs of somites can be observed. The embryonic disc is shaped like a shoe-sole, with broad neural plates above the head folds and a constriction in the region of the first somite. The **lordotic flexure** of most specimens in stage 8 to 10 is probably caused by the rupture of the yolk sac, e.g., during curettage. The decrease in pressure releases the inner tension of the embryonic disc, causing it to bend in the lumbar region between the head fold and the tail fold.

### A. Head Fold, Somites, and Lateral Plates

**1. Reconstruction of the "Embryo Ludwig"** (Wax plate reconstruction. Dorsal view; length of embryo: 1.8 mm; age: about 21 days). The embryo was described by Ludwig in 1928 as a specimen with one pair of somites. The countour of the somites is visible in the narrow region of the embryonic disc between the *head fold* and the *tail fold* (**A1**). The *primitive node*, with the still open axial canal, lies on the *tail fold*.

**2. Foregut and Hindgut in Median Section.** The foregut and hindgut invaginate from the yolk sac into the head and tail folds, respectively (**A2**). With the active elevation of the head fold above the level of the embryonic disc, the delimitation of the embryonic body begins. The tail fold, on the other hand, arises rather passively by the lordotic bending of the embryonic disc. In the midline, the roof of the yolk sac is formed by the *notochordal plate*. The *axial canal* connects the amniotic cavity and the yolk sac. It can be imagined that a decrease in pressure due to the collapse of the yolk sac has caused the bending (dorsal flexure) of the embryonic disc.

**3. Differentiation of the Germ Layers.** The caudally retreating primitive node is an organization center that induces the formation of axial organs in the germ layers (→ 3.8). By invagination through the primitive pit, cellular material in the primitive streak is deposited in front of the primitive node as the notochord. The somites are induced laterally and the neural groove is induced dorsally.

**a** At the level of the *primitive streak*, the mesoderm is still unsegmented.

**b** In front of the *primitive node* with the still open axial canal, the notochordal process is intercalated into the endoderm as the *notochordal plate*, which extends cranially into the head fold.

**c** The ectoderm above the notochordal plate forms the *neural groove*, bringing the notochordal plate into direct apposition with the neural ectoderm. The paraxial mesoderm situated laterally to the notochord aggregates to form the epithelial somites. The lateral plate mesoderm forms two epithelial plates (visceral and parietal), between which the cleft of the *intraembryonic coelom* appears.

**d** At the level of the *anterior intestinal portal*, the coelomic cleft widens into the caudal, paired segments of the *pericardial cavity*. The visceral mesodermal layer at the base of the pericardial cavity contains the cardiac primordium. The *neural plate* blends laterally, without a sharp boundary into the surface ectoderm, which in turn is connected to the amniotic epithelium at the *amnioectodermal fold* (**A1**).

**e** The *head fold* arises by the bulging of the *neural plate*, which is divided into two lobes by the deep neural groove. The endoderm below the neural plate is curved inward into the *foregut*, forming a cylindrical, pseudostratified epithelium, out of which cells for the *head mesenchyme* later migrate. The thickened *endoderm* of the anterior intestinal portal is at least partially identical with the endoderm of the prechordal plate (→ 3.8).

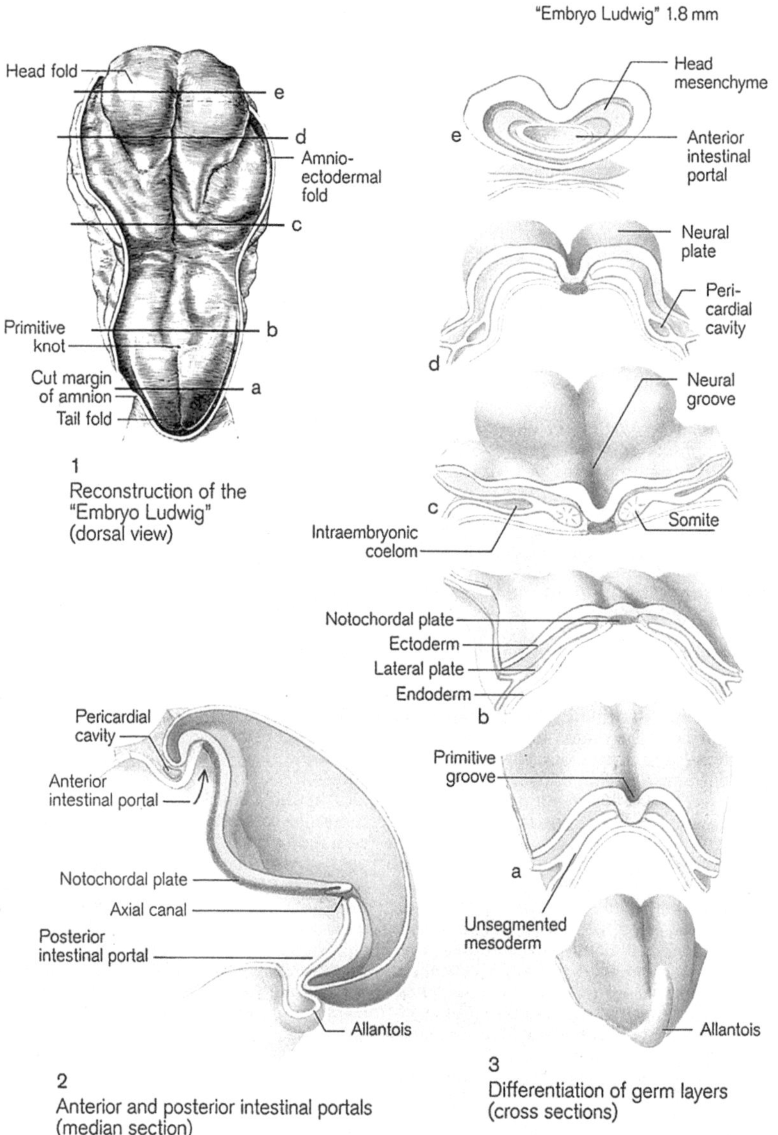


1
Reconstruction of the "Embryo Ludwig" (dorsal view)

2
Anterior and posterior intestinal portals (median section)

3
Differentiation of germ layers (cross sections)

A. Headfold, somites, and lateral plates (stage 9)

# "Fourth Week": Folding of Embryo

## 2.14 Overview: "Fourth Week"

*Background*

The developmental period of the **"fourth week"** comprises stages 10–13. At the beginning of the 4th week, the heart begins to beat (stage 9 or 10) and the embryonic circulation sets in. The neural tube closes. The embryo folds off from the yolk sac. The somites arise, so that subsequent developmental stages can be designated by the number of somites. At the end of the 4th week, over 30 somites are present and the first somites begin to disintegrate. The differential growth between the small embryo and the chorion reaches its maximum. At the beginning of the 4th week, the length of the embryo is about 2 mm and toward the end, about 5 mm. The diameter of the chorion increases from 2 to 3.5 cm.

### A. Implantation Site in the Fourth Week

In the uterus (**A1**) opened from the ventral aspect, the implantation site in the posterior wall is visible on the surface of the endometrium (decidua). The implantation site consists of a round bulge, flattened on top, with a diameter of about 2 cm. The decidua above the implant (*decidua capsularis*) is smooth and stained brownish-red, whereas the remaining decidua (*decidua parietalis*) is lined by deep folds.

The height of the endometrium is 68 mm. Directly underneath the epithelium lies the *zona compacta* with many decidual cells, followed by the *zona spongiosa* with broadened glandular ducts. The chorion is embedded in the zona compacta and is covered by a thin layer of decidual cells with mucosal epithelium, the *decidua capsularis.* The widened glands in the *zona spongiosa* and the secretory ducts in the zona compacta are compressed toward the surface (displacement growth of the blastocyst). The *spiral arteries* lose their muscle layer as they pass through the cytotrophoblastic shell. Basally, the blood drains into a wide venous sinus, into which some villi extend. The *chorionic villi* and the cytotrophoblastic shell are larger and further developed at the basal than at the lumenal side of the uterus.

The *embryo* with the *amniotic cavity* and the *yolk sac* is suspended in the wide *chorionic cavity* by the *body stalk* . The embryo initially spreads out between the two cavities as the embryonic disc (**B1**). In the course of the 4th week, the embryo folds off from the yolc sac and becomes enclosed by the amnion, so that it lies in the amniotic cavity (**B2**).

### B. Enlargement of Amniotic Cavity and Development of Umbilical Cord

During the folding off of the yolk sac and the closure of the ventral body wall, the amniotic cavity enlarges and the border between ectoderm and amnion (amnio-ectodermal fold) is shifted ventrally, forming the *umbilical ring* (**B1**). The amnion, which now completely envelops the embryo, becomes constricted at the umbilical ring until only the umbilical cord remains to suspend the embryo in the amniotic fluid (**B2**). The connection between the intraembryonic coelom and the chorionic cavity is reduced to the narrow umbilical coelom surrounding the *vitelline duct.* The yolc sac, which has been almost completely ligated, comes to lie in the chorionic cavity between amnion and chorion.

In the *umbilical ring,* the amnioectodermal fold ensheaths the *body stalk,* containing the *allantois* and the umbilical vessels, the *umbilical stalk*, and the rudimentary vitelline vessels, forming the *umbilical cord* (**B2**). At the end of the 4th week, the embryo floats in the amniotic cavity and is connected with the *chorionic plate* only by the umbilical cord, which subsequently is covered by amnion (→ 2.42).

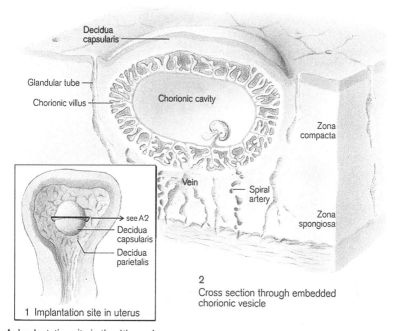

Decidua capsularis
Glandular tube
Chorionic villus
Chorionic cavity
Zona compacta
Vein
Spiral artery
Zona spongiosa

see A2
Decidua capsularis
Decidua parietalis

1 Implantation site in uterus

2
Cross section through embedded chorionic vesicle

A. Implantation site in the 4th week

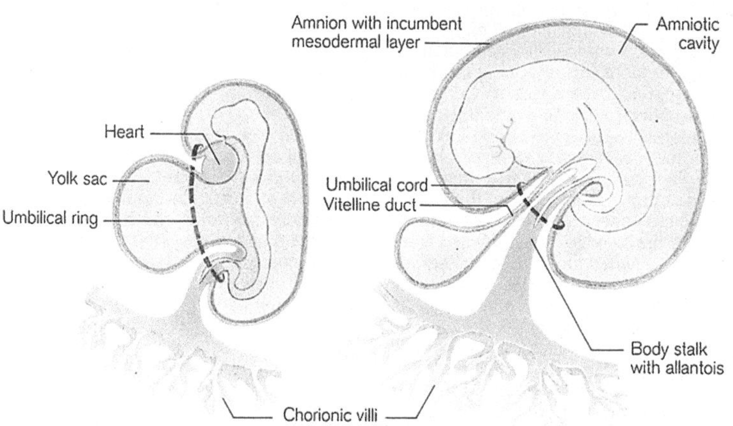


1 Beginning of 4th week

2 End of 4th week

B. Enlargement of amniotic cavity and development of umbilical cord

## 2.15 Overview: Folding

*Background*

**Mechanism of Folding.** The transformation of the embryonic disc into the embryonic body is driven by thick epithelial plates derived from epithelial layers of ectoderm and endoderm or from mesodermal tissue (→ 3.25). After actively carrying out morphogenetic movements, the epithelial plates disintegrate and the cells subsequently differentiate according to their determined fate and position.

### A. Folding and Development of Body Form

**1. Formation of the Axial Organs.** In stage 10 the head and tail folds of the embryo are raised above the level of the yolk sac. Subsequently, the axial organs rise and delimit the embryonic body by folding movements. In a **cross section (1a)** through the anterior intestinal portal, the developmental movements are designated by numbered arrows: (1) The neural epithelium rises to form the *neural groove* and then the neural tube. The cells in the paraxial mesoderm become arranged into the epithelial *somites*. (2) The notochordal plate forms a small ventrally opened groove, which closes to become the compact *notochord* and simultaneously detaches from the endoderm. (3) The *intestinal tube* closes. The anterior intestinal portal migrates caudally. The foregut elongates. (4) The driving force for these latter processes comes from the *visceral mesoderm* (→ 3.9). The mesodermal cells in the visceral layer of the lateral plate become organized into a compact epithelium that wedges itself inward from both sides, closing the foregut in zipper fashion, and thus separating it from the yolk sac. (5) The ventral body wall is formed by the turning in of the *lateral folds* (ectoderm and parietal mesoderm) and by the constriction of the anmioectodermal fold around the umbilical ring enveloping the body stalk, vitelline duct, and the umbilical coelom (See A3 and 2.14B).

**2. Craniocaudal Curvature.** By the enlargement and elongation of the neural tube in stage 11, the dorsally situated axial organs become arched above the ventrally situated viscera and yolk sac. The head fold, containing the cerebral vesicles, overgrows the stomodeum and the *cardiac primordium*. The tail fold becomes curved, shifting the cloacal membrane and the allantoic duct ventrally with a turning movement. The *anterior* and *posterior neuropore* close (**A3**). The primitive node has disappeared into the blastema of the *tail bud*. Caudal segments of the neural tube, notochord, and somites directly emerge from the tail bud (→ 3.10).

**3. Closure of Intestinal Tube.** In stage 13 the anterior and posterior intestinal portals migrate toward each other,further constricting the opening of the yolk sac . In the anterior fusion zone of the endoderm, the *thyroid gland, lungs* , and *liver* arise successively. The wedge-shaped apices of the visceral mesoderm (wall of the coelomic canal, arrow 4 in 1a) fuse below the digestive tube. After the closure of the digestive tube, the epithelial structure disintegrates and forms loose mesoderm. The upper sides of the wedges give rise to the mesoderm that will form the wall of the esophagus and stomach. The lower sides fuse below the digestive tube, lengthening the cardiac loop (→ 6.2). Further caudally, the mesenchyme for the liver is formed (transverse septum).

The liver primordium arises at the anterior-intestinal portal, at the boundary of the yolk sac. **Cross section 3a** shows how (by closure of the digestive tube) the endoderm of the *hepatic diverticulum* is separated ventrally from the foregut. A connection remains only in the lower segment (hepatic bile duct). The hepatic cell cords sprout into the mesoderm of the *transverse septum*, which arises earlier from the fused visceral mesoderm. The *vitelline veins* extend into the developing liver; by fusing with one another, they form the network of the hepatic sinusoids (→ 7.9).

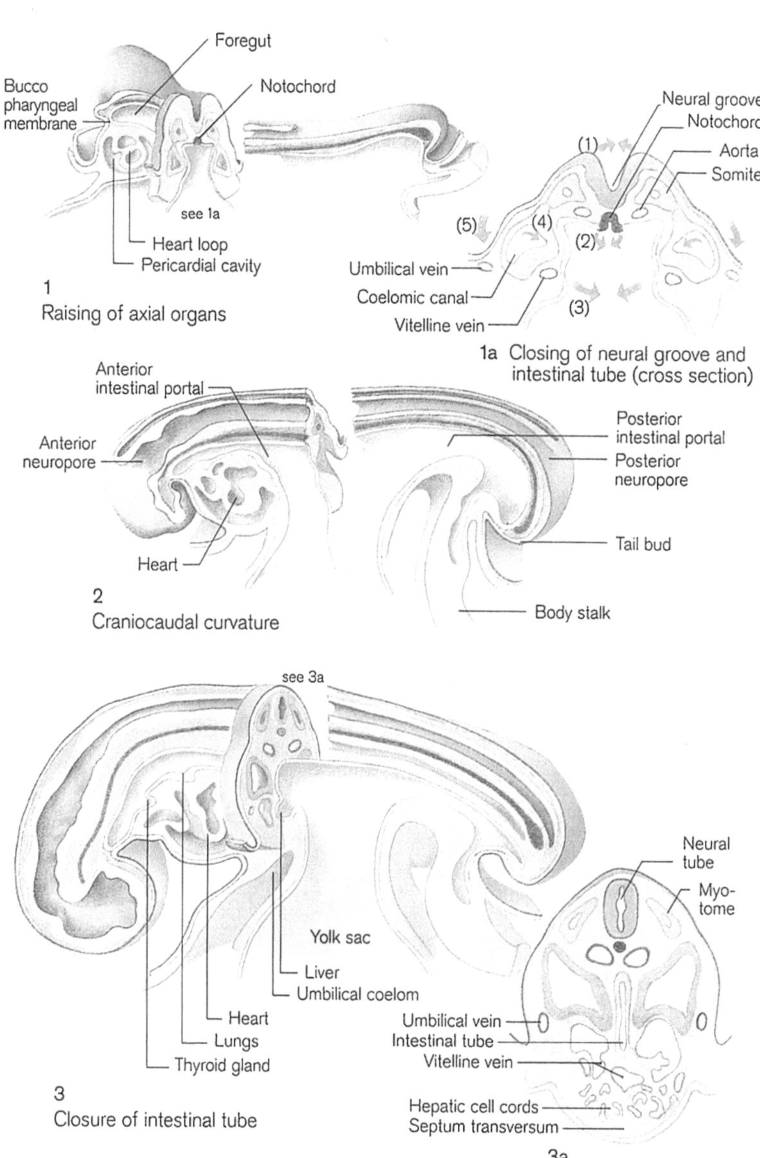
Foregut
Bucco pharyngeal membrane
Notochord
see 1a
Heart loop
Pericardial cavity
1
Raising of axial organs
Neural groove
Notochord
Aorta
Somite
(1)
(2)
(3)
(4)
(5)
Umbilical vein
Coelomic canal
Vitelline vein
1a Closing of neural groove and intestinal tube (cross section)
Anterior intestinal portal
Anterior neuropore
Heart
2
Craniocaudal curvature
Posterior intestinal portal
Posterior neuropore
Tail bud
Body stalk
see 3a
Yolk sac
Liver
Umbilical coelom
Heart
Lungs
Thyroid gland
3
Closure of intestinal tube
Neural tube
Myo-tome
Umbilical vein
Intestinal tube
Vitelline vein
Hepatic cell cords
Septum transversum
3a

A. Folding from yolk sac and development of body form

## 2.16 Stage 10: Circulation

*Background*

**Stage 10: Beginning of the Embryonic Circulation.** The cardiovascular system is the first functional organ system. The embryo is dependent on the placental circulation, as it is not supplied with yolk and nourishment via diffusion is not sufficient. The heart develops in the pericardial cavity below the foregut. In stages 8 and 9, capillary networks are formed along the path of the aorta, as well as in the body stalk, the chorion, and the villi. The endothelium-lined capillaries are not yet completely linked. Only when the heart begins to beat in stage 9 or 10 does a continuous vascular circuit arise. The main blood stream flows through the placental circulation. The vessels of the yolk sac (vitelline circulation) and those of the remaining organs (systemic circulation) lag behind in development (→ 6.1).

### A. Blood Vessels at Stage 10

**1. Blood Islands and Capillary Plexus in the "Embryo Ingalls" with 7 Somites.** In the reconstruction of the endothelium-lined vessels on the right side of the body, the direction of the vascular flow is marked by arrows. The endothelial lining of the *heart* still consists of a capillary plexus. Blood flows via the aortic arches into the dorsal aorta and from there directly into the *umbilical arteries*, which pass through the body stalk into the chorionic villi (placental circulation). The exits of the vitelline arteries are indicated. Blood returns to the heart via the umbilical and vitelline veins. The umbilical vessels in the body stalk are unusally wide.

**2. Course of Vitelline and Umbilical Veins.** The vitelline veins arise in the wall of the yolk sac and course along the endoderm through the splanchnic mesodermal layer to the heart. The umbilical veins lie in the lateral body wall and course in the somatic mesoderm.

### B. Vessels in the "Embryo Payne" with 7 Somites

**1. Dorsal View.** The neural tube is closed between somites 4 and 6.

1 Optic sulcus
2 Region of first pharyngeal cleft
3 Bulge of pericardial cavity
4 Otic plate
5 Neural crest
6 Somite 1
7 Section of yolk sac
8 Entrance into neural canal
9 Cut edge of amnion

**2. Dorsal View of Vessels. Isolated Presentation after Removal of Ectoderm.** The somites are presented on the right side (**10**). On the left side they are removed. At the anterior intestinal portal, the vitelline and umbilical veins form a common stem (**4**).

1 Pharyngeal pouch 1
2 Foregut
3 Dorsal aorta
4 Common stem of vitelline and umbilical veins
5 Vitelline vessels
6 Left umbilical vein
7 Left umbilical artery
8 Primitive groove
9 Primitive pit
10 Somite 4

**3. Position of the Heart below the Foregut in Sagittal Section.** The endocardial tube (**7**) is separated from the myocardial layer (**6** ) by cardiac jelly traversed by fine fibers.

1 Pharyngeal membrane
2 Thyroid primordium
3 Cut edge of amnion
4 Cut edge of yolk sac
5 Pericardial cavity
6 Myocardium
7 Endocardial tube
8 Anterior intestinal portal
9 Level of somite 2
10 Neural tube
11 Endoderm of yolk sac
12 Allantois
13 Primitive node with discontinuous (closed) neurenteric canal (axial canal)
14 Amnioectodermal fold

Umbilical arteries
Exit of vitelline arteries
Dorsal aorta
Umbilical vein
Neural plate
Pharynx
Cardiac plexus
Body stalk
Allantois
Sinus venosus
Vitelline vein
Yolk sac
Blood islands

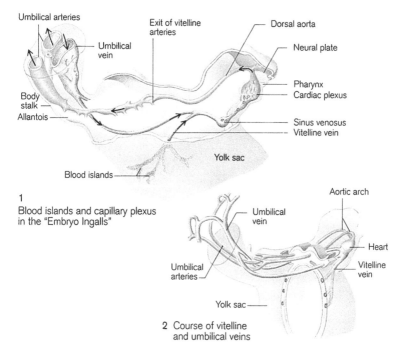

1
Blood islands and capillary plexus in the "Embryo Ingalls"

Aortic arch
Umbilical vein
Heart
Vitelline vein
Umbilical arteries
Yolk sac

2 Course of vitelline and umbilical veins

A. Blood vessels (stage 10)

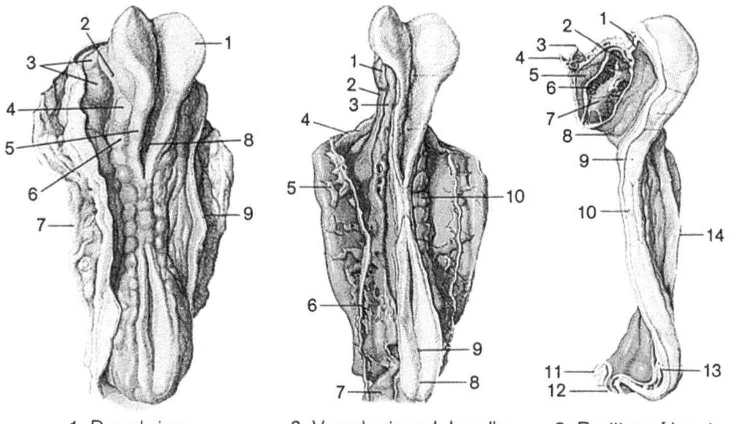


1 Dorsal view

2 Vessels viewed dorsally

3 Position of heart

B. Vessels in the "Embryo Payne" with 7 somites (originals)

## 2.17 Stage 10: Embryo Corner

*Background*

**Source of the Embryo.** The embryo with 10 somites was removed from the body cavity, together with a large blood clot, in 1925 during the operation of a perforated tubal pregnancy. The chorionic sac was not damaged. After the chorion was opened, the intact embryo was visible. It could be fixed in its natural position and was prepared histologically in the Carnegie Laboratories in Baltimore, Maryland. A wax plate reconstruction was made. The description of the embryo was published in the series, "Contributions to Embryology" by the embryologist G. W. Corner in 1929. The Corner embryo shows the natural body form at stage 10, in contrast to the embryos of Ingalls and Payne (→ 2.16) and Blechschmidt 3,1 mm, which have a lordotic curvature that is probably due to damage of the yolk sac with subsequent decrease in pressure prior to fixation.

The artist of the Embryological Laboratories of the Carnegie Institution, James Didusch, drew the embryo immediately after fixation. The present illustration in a colored steel engraving is based on the original drawing of the specimen, which was corrected in detail by the artist after reconstruction of the embryo from serial sections.

### A. Stage 10: "Embryo Corner"

**1. Left View of the Embryo.** Magnification: 60 times. The *amniotic cavity* (**1**) is open, revealing the *somites* (**2**), neural tube (**3**), cerebral vesicles with the *prosencephalon* (**4**), *mesencephalon* (**5**) and *rhombencephalon* (**6**), the bulge of the *first pharyngeal arch* (**7**), and the indentation of the *first pharyngeal cleft* (**8**), as well as the *cardiac prominence* (**9**). Under the swelling caused by the *umbilical vein* (**10**), the intraembryonic coelom and the left *coelomic canal* (**11**) open slit-like into the chorionic cavity. The *yolk sac* (**12**) exhibits *blood islands* (**13**). The *body stalk* (**14**) is distended by the coiled and enlarged *umbilical arteries* (**15**) (fenestrated in the drawing).

**2. View into the Anterior Neuropore.** The neural tube is closed in the region of the *mesencephalon* (**1**) and still wide open in the *prosencephalon* (**2**). Therefore, one has an inside view of the beginning evagination of the optic vesicles (optic sulcus, **3**) that progresses laterally toward the ectoderm, where the lens placodes are later induced.

**3. Median Section.** The "embryo Corner" possesses a *dorsal mesocardium* (**1**), which suspends the cardiac loop in the *pericardial cavity* (**6**). As a sign of the beginning involution, a hole (**2**) is already present in the dorsal mesocardium. A ventral mesocardium is not established in the human. Between the *myocardial mantle* (**3**) and the *endocardial tube* (**4**) there is a wide cleft (**5**) that (in other embryos) contains *cardiac jelly*. In the "embryo Corner," this space contained only serous fluid (a, b, and c = position of sections of 2.18).

1 Dorsal mesocardium
2 Hole in dorsal mesocardium
3 Myocardium
4 Endocardial tube
5 Cleft (cardiac jelly)
6 Pericardial cavity
7 Oropharyngeal membrane (or: Oral membrane)
8 Thyroid primordium
9 Pharyngeal pouch 1
10 Anterior intestinal portal
11 Allantois
12 Cloacal membrane
13 Tail bud
14 Notochord

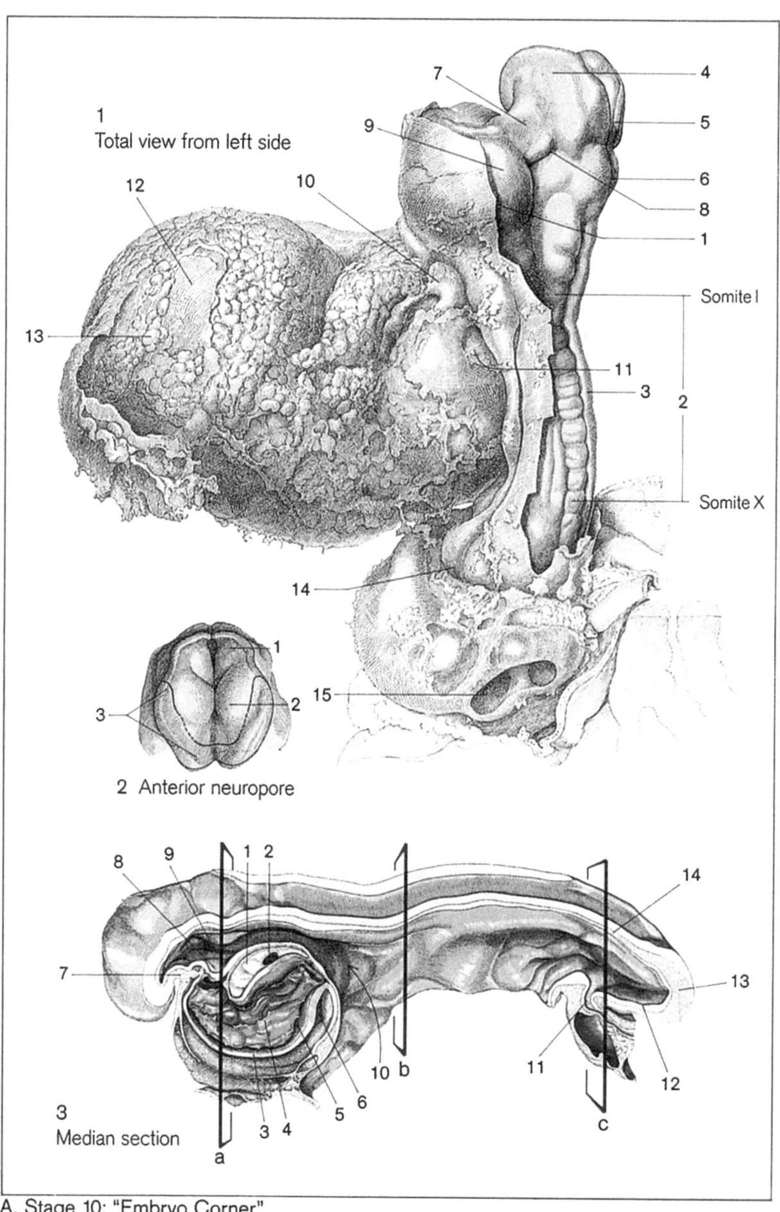


A. Stage 10: "Embryo Corner"

## 2.18 Stage 10: Histology

*Background*

**Histology of the "Embryo Corner."** In front of the primitive node the embryonic body is organized into notochord, neural tube, somites, and lateral plates. The caudally migrating primitve node represents the organization center for the development of these basic elements from the germ layers. The basic body plan is most distinctly recognized in the middle, segmented region of the embryo. The anterior body segment arises from the head fold and is thus independent of the primitive node. Here, the basic design is altered by the absence of somites and by the formation of mesoderm from the prechordal plate, neural crest, and the placodes. The primitive node is transformed in the tail fold into the blastema of the tail bud, from which the neural tube and the caudal somites emerge directly.

### A. Basic Structure of the Embryonic Body

#### 1. Organization of the Germ Layers

**Ectoderm.** The ectoderm gives rise to the *neural tube* and the *surface ectoderm,*which is continuous laterally with the *amniotic epithelium*. After closure of the neural tube, the *neural crest cells* migrate from the neural crest.

**Mesoderm.** Beneath the neural tube, the *notochord* is detached from the roof of the intestine. The *somites* lie laterally. Between the somites and the lateral plates lies the *intermediate mesoderm*, which will give rise to nephrons. The lateral plate mesoderm separates and splits off into a *parietal* and a *visceral mesodermal layer*; intraembryonic coelom fills the space between the two. The parietal mesodermal layer is associated with the ectoderm and is continuous laterally with the extraembryonic *amniotic mesoderm*. The visceral mesodermal layer is associated with the endoderm and is continuous laterally with the *mesoderm* of the yolk sac. The intraembryonic coelom opens at the sides into the extraembryonic coelom (*chorionic cavity*).

**Endoderm**. Above the yolk sac, the endoderm forms an intestinal groove that later closes to form the digestive tube.

#### 2. Histological Sections of the "Embryo Corner"

**a Section at the Level of the Pericardium.** The embryonic body has already folded off at this site (→ 2.15 A2). Laterally from the neural tube, the ectoderm thickens to form placodes. The *otic placode* gives rise to the inner ear. Further placodes give rise to cells that migrate outward and form the sensory ganglia of the pharyngeal nerves (→ 5.2). The pharynx has a triangular form in cross section. In the "Embryo Corner," the *notochord* is attached to the roof of the gut for its entire length. The *pharyngeal pouches* are situated at the lateral ends of the pharynx. The medial groove (*hypobranchial groove*) contains, in sequence, the primordia of the thyroid gland, the lungs and finally the liver (→ 2.15).

The *pericardium* consists of a thin, drawn out visceral mesodermal layer; it is covered in the upper segment by ectoderm that merges laterally with the amnion. The two layers of the visceral mesoderm unite, forming first the *dorsal mesocardium* and then the *myocardial mantle*, which surrounds the *endocardial tube*. The space between the endocardium and myocardium contains cardiac jelly. In the "Embryo Corner," no fibrous or gelatinous components were present.

**b Section through Somite 5 above the Yolk Sac.** The intestinal groove is still open (→ 2.15 A2). The course of the paired *aorta* and *umbilical vein* in the *parietal mesoderm* were described previously (→ 2.16 A2).

**c Section through the Tail Fold and Body Stalk.** In the tail fold in front of the primitive node, the *paraxial mesoderm* is not yet organized into somites. The caudally dead-ended *coelomic sacs* (→ 2.19) lie beside the hindgut diverticulum. The *body stalk* is distended by the umbilical vessels.

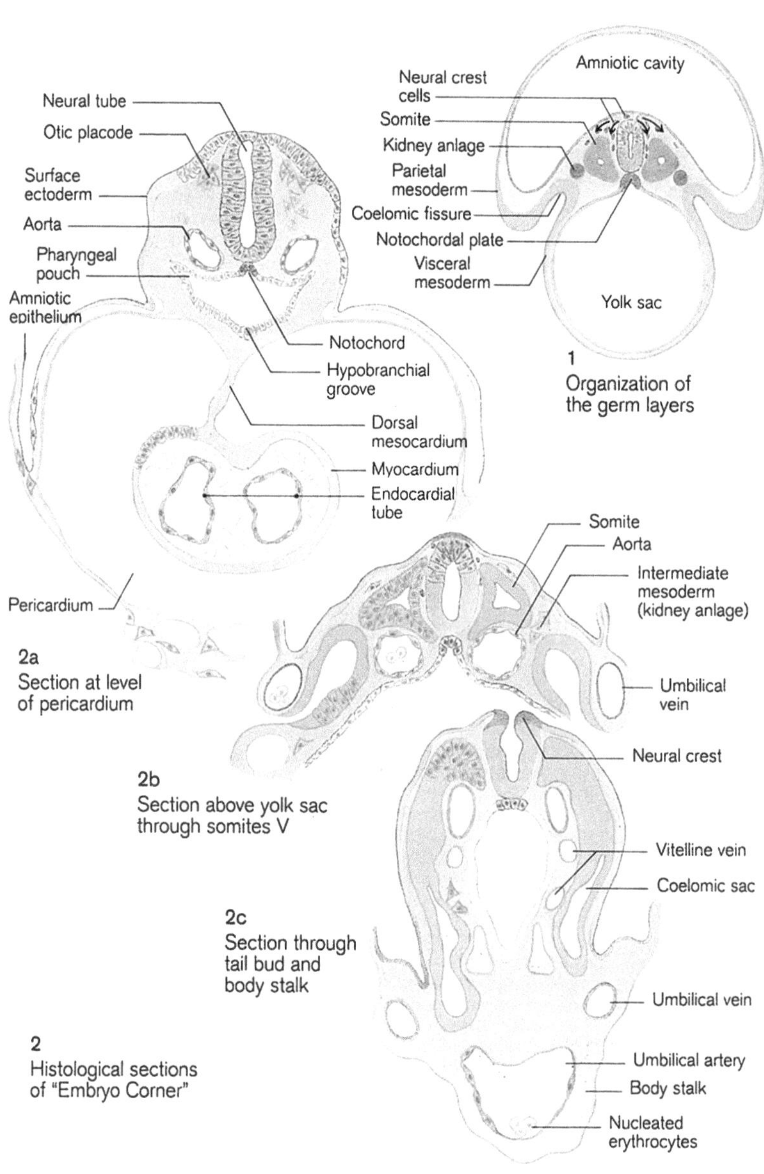
Amniotic cavity
Neural crest cells
Somite
Kidney anlage
Parietal mesoderm
Coelomic fissure
Notochordal plate
Visceral mesoderm
Yolk sac
1
Organization of the germ layers
Neural tube
Otic placode
Surface ectoderm
Aorta
Pharyngeal pouch
Amniotic epithelium
Notochord
Hypobranchial groove
Dorsal mesocardium
Myocardium
Endocardial tube
Pericardium
2a
Section at level of pericardium
Somite
Aorta
Intermediate mesoderm (kidney anlage)
Umbilical vein
Neural crest
2b
Section above yolk sac through somites V
Vitelline vein
Coelomic sac
2c
Section through tail bud and body stalk
Umbilical vein
Umbilical artery
Body stalk
Nucleated erythrocytes
2
Histological sections of "Embryo Corner"

A. Basic structure of the embryonic body

# 2.19 Stage 10: Coelomic Ring

## A. Coelomic Ring at the Beginning of the 4th Week

The definitive body cavities, the pericardial, pleural, and peritoneal cavities, are derived from the **intraembryonic coelom.** The intraembryonic coelom arises as a cleft between the splanchnic (visceral) and somatic (parietal) layers of the lateral plate mesoderm. At the beginning of the 4th week, the cranial body segments including the head region and pericardium, as well as the caudal body segments including the exit of the umbilical vessels and the allantois, are raised from the yolk sac (**A1**). The digestive tube and yolk sac still form a single unit in the middle body region. Intraembryonic coelom surrounds the opening of the yolk sac like a ring (coelomic ring according to Blechschmidt). The **coelomic ring** is indicated in **A2** and **A3** by a black line that passes anteriorly through the coelomic canal and the pericardial cavity. In the region of the future peritoneal cavity (body cavity proper), the intraembryonic coelom is not yet closed off from the chorionic cavity (extraembryonic coelom).

**Pericardial Cavity.** The coelomic cleft first appears in the human in the region of the pericardial cavity. This is associated with the precocious development of the heart. The pericardial cavity begins as a horseshoe-shaped fissure that encompasses the head fold and foregut diverticulum at the base (→ stage 9, 2.13 A2). As folding takes place, the limbs of the "horseshoe" become united below the foregut, enlarging the pericardial cavity caudally (→ 2.15 A1).

**Coelomic Canals.** The coelomic cleft continues on both sides as a closed coelomic canal travelling caudally from the pericardial cavity into the ventrally open peritoneal cavity (**2a**). Later, the lung buds grow into the coelomic canals, forming pleural cavities, which are then separated from the pericardial and peritoneal cavity.

**Peritoneal Cavity.** In the region of the peritoneal cavity, the embryo is spread out flat on the yolk sac before folding off begins. The coelomic cleft opens laterally into the chorionic cavity (extraembryonic coelom). Only with the closure of the body wall does the body cavity separate from the chorionic cavity. At the *anterior intestinal portal* (**A3**), the *septum transversum* and liver develop in the ventral mesentery between the heart and the base of the yolk sac. The development of the liver primordium in the ventral foregut causes the right and left body cavities to separate from each other. At the *posterior intestinal portal,* on the other hand, no ventral mesentery develops. Thus, the right and left body cavity communicate with one another below the hindgut (unpaired body cavity).

### 1. and 2. The Coelom in the "Embryo Corner"

The planes of section a, b, and c correspond to the histological sections in the preceding plate.

**a** The *pericardial cavity* below the foregut is represented without the heart and vessels.

**b** The *coelomic canals* unite the pericardial cavity with the right and left peritoneal cavity, which in some regions open laterally into the *chorionic cavity*.

**c** In the region of the hindgut the coelom ends blindly (*coelomic sacs* ).

### 3. The Coelom in the Contour of the "Embryo Davis"

The reconstruction of the lining of the coelom in the "Embryo Davis" (20 somites, stage 12), seen from the ventral side, has been fitted into the body outline. The embryonic coelom surrounds the base of the yolk sac in the form of a ventrally open ring. As folding proceeds, the base of the yolk sac constricts to form the vitelline duct (→ 2.14B). The opening of the embryonic coelom is simultaneously constricted into the umbilical coelom. The umbilical coelom surrounds the vitelline duct on the caudal side in a ring fashion. On the rostral side, the opening of the coelom is interrupted by the septum transversum with the liver primordium.

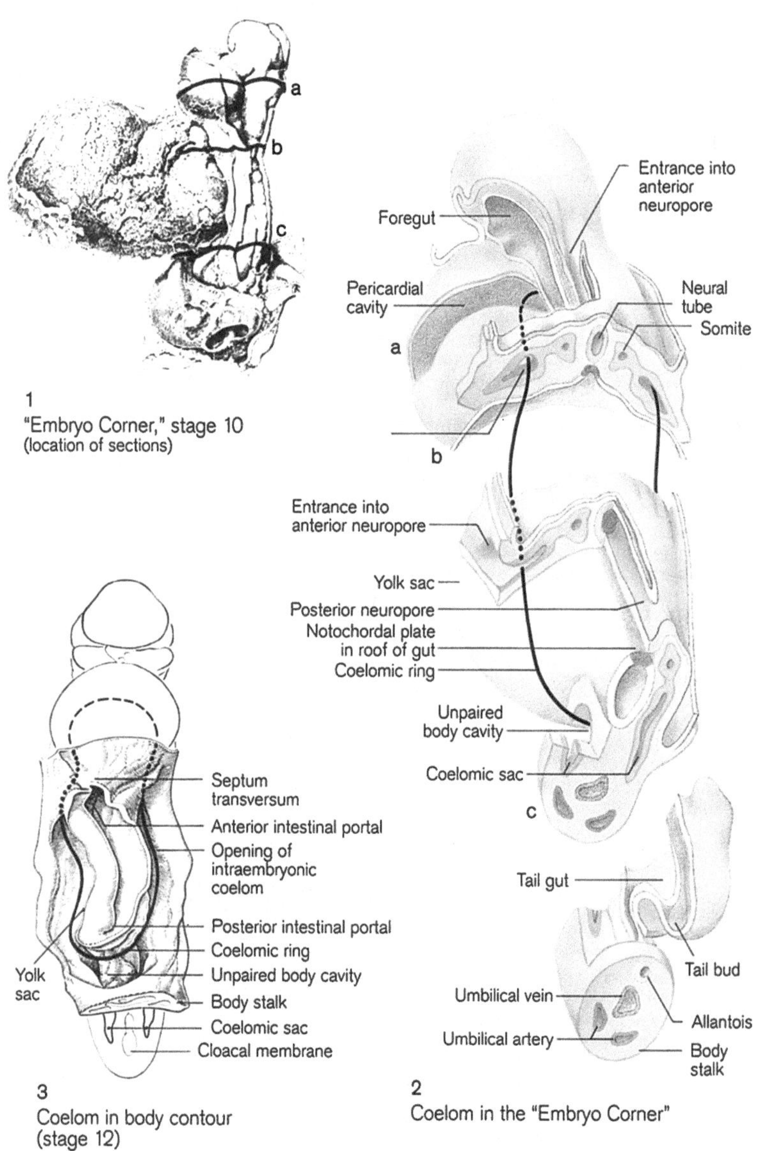


1
"Embryo Corner," stage 10
(location of sections)

2
Coelom in the "Embryo Corner"

3
Coelom in body contour
(stage 12)

A. Coelomic ring at beginning of 4th week

## 2.20 Stage 11: Anterior and Posterior Neuropore

*Background*

**Stage 11:** 2.5–4.5 mm, 23–26 days, 13–20 somites. The optic sulci are visible in the neuropore. In the course of stage 11 the anterior neuropore closes.

### A. "Embryo Blechschmidt," 3.1 mm

**1. Photograph of the Original Specimen.** The embryo possesses 13 pairs of somites and is about 24 days old. It was photographed in oblique light after fixation and opening of the chorionic sac. It is connected to the chorion by the body stalk. The embryonic body lies in the amniotic cavity. The anterior and posterior ends of the body are elevated and extend into the amniotic cavity, whereas the middle portion of the body containing the somites is stretched out flat above the yolk sac. The yolk sac itself is torn and its outline is indistinct. The pronounced dorsal flexure (lordosis) of the embryo appears also in this case to be caused by the tearing of the yolk sac during the preparation. Of the 13 pairs of somites, only the posterior ones can be recognized as bulges on the surface.

1 Cut edge of chorion
2 Chorionic villi
3 Chorionic cavity
4 Body stalk
5 Translucent Amnion
6 Posterior neuropore
7 Somites
8 Optic primordium
9 Cardiac bulge
10 Yolk sac
11 Entrance into intraembryonic coelom

**2. Reconstruction of the Same Embryo**

**a View from the Right Side.** Yolk sac (**4**) and amnion ( **5**) have been removed. At the interface between amniotic and umbilical mesoderm (**3**), the extraembryonic coelom (chorionic cavity) borders on the embryo. The arrow (**2**) shows the transition from extraembryonic to intraembryonic coelom. At this stage the intraembryonic coelom consists of the unpaired, U-shaped pericardial cavity that opens caudally on both sides.

**b Dorsal View.** The neural tube has not yet closed caudally (**1**) or cranially (**6**). The optic sulci are visible within the still open prosencephalon (**10**).

**c View from the Left Side.** The pericardial cavity is open (**18**) and the mesoderm at the boundary between amnion and yolk sac is removed so that the large vessels are visible. The unpaired aorta (**9**) lies between the roof of the yolk sac (endoderm) and the axial organs; and the umbilical vein lies (**13**) in the mesoderm of the future body wall.

**d Ventral View.** Below the cardiac bulge (**15**), one looks into the anterior intestinal portal (**14**, arrow). Somites and the notochord are visible through the roof of the yolk sac (endoderm).

1 Posterior neuropore
2 Entrance into intraembryonic coelom. The arrow leads via the coelomic canals into the pericardial cavity
3 Transition between amniotic and umbilical mesoderm
4 Cut margin of yolk sac
5 Cut margin of amnion
6 Anterior neuropore
7 Cardiac bulge
8 Segmental border between two somites
9 Endothelial tube of aorta with intestinal and vitelline vessels
10 Optic primordium
11 Pharyngeal arch 1 (mandibular arch)
12 Pharyngeal arch 2 (hyoid arch)
13 Left umbilical vein
14 Anterior intestinal portal
15 Umbilical endoderm above cardiac bulge
16 Optic sulcus in still-open prosencephalon
17 Maxillary process
18 Cardiac loop exposed by opening the pericardial cavity
19 Amnion from below
20 Unpaired umbilical vein in body stalk

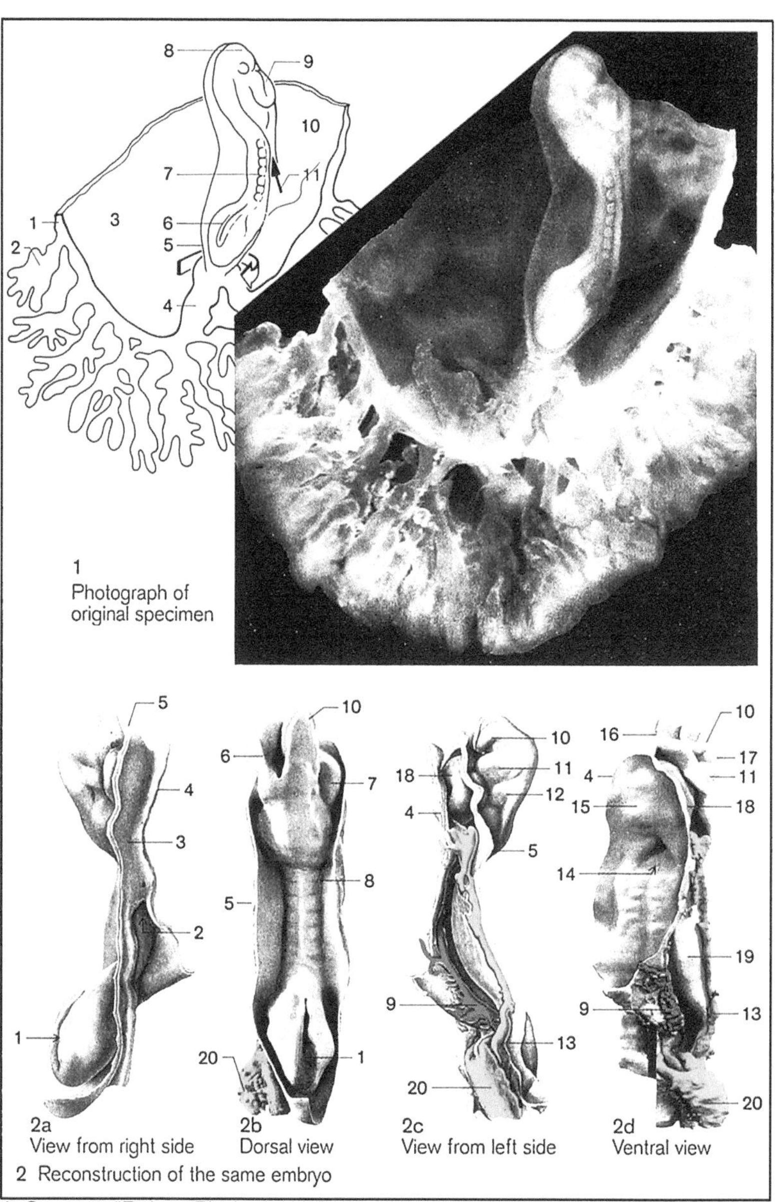


A. Stage 11: "Embryo Blechschmidt," 3.1 mm

## 2.21 Stage 12: Cranio-Caudal Curvature

*Background*

**Stage 12:** 3–5 mm, 26–30 days p.o., 21–29 somites. The caudal neuropore is closed. Three pharyngeal arches are present. The arm buds are distinct. During the folding off from the yolk sac and the formation of the umbilical ring, the embryo bends and rotates so that the yolk sac comes to lie on the right side.

### A. "Embryo Blechschmidt," 2.57 mm

**1. Surgical Specimen of Tubal Pregnancy.** The embryo possesses 23 pairs of somites and is about 26 days old. It has become implanted in the ampulla of the Fallopian tube. The chorionic villi infiltrate the wall of the tube. (Because of the penetration of maternal vessels, bleeding occurred in the body cavity of the mother, an absolute indication for operation). The embryo lies in the opened chorionic cavity. The amniotic cavity is opened above the head and the tail end. As a result of the folding off from the yolk sac and the convex dorsal curvature, the axis of the embryo has rotated so that the yolk sac comes to lie on the right side.

**2. Embryo before Fixation.** The isolated embryo is illustrated from the dorsal aspect. It is covered by the transparent amnion. Comparison with the 3.1 mm embryo (stage 11) shows that folding off from the yolk sac is accompanied by a transition from the dorsally concave to the dorsally convex shape and also by constriction of the amnion in the umbilical ring. The dorsal convex curvature accounts for the smaller size of 2.57 mm.

**3. Reconstruction.** Neural tube, endoderm, vascular system, and urinary system were reconstructed from serial sections and drawn after the reconstruction.

1 Optic vesicle
2 Trigeminal nerve (V)
3 Facial nerve (VII)
4 Glossopharyngeal nerve (IX)
5 Anterior cardinal vein. Its continuation into the head can be recognized by the capillary sprouts in front of and behind the otic vesicle
6 Left sinal horn of sinus venosus at the inflow tract of the heart
7 Inferior cardinal vein
8 Notochord
9 Intersegmental artery
10 Mesonephric duct

**4. Organization of the Coelomic Cavities**

**a. Reconstruction of the Intraembryonic Coelom on the Left Side with the Digestive Tract and Large Vessels.** The visceral and parietal lining of the coelom is reconstructed as a surface (brown). The endocardial tube of the cardiac loop is shown; whereas the space of the myocardium is empty.

1 Pericardial cavity between epicardium and endocardium
2 Endocardium of cardiac tube
3 Arterial outflow tract
4 Pharynx with pharyngeal pouches
5 Dorsal aorta
6 Left sinus horn in the inflow tract of the heart
7 Inferior cardinal vein
8 Right umbilical vein
9 Intestinal tube
10 Allantois
11 Umbilical vein
12 Umbilical coelom

**b Isolated Coelom of Left Side**

1 Pericardial cavity with view of the epicard from the myocardial side
2 Left coelomic canal (future pleural cavity)
3 Visceral peritoneum of left body cavity with contour of removed mesonephros (dorsally) and digestive tract (ventrally)
4 Entrance into umbilical coelom

**c The Entire Intraembryonic Coelom.** The right coelomic canal is removed and the umbilical coelom is opened from the right side.

1 Pericardial cavity
2 Passage of esophagus through the coelomic ring (arrow)
3 Peritoneal cavity

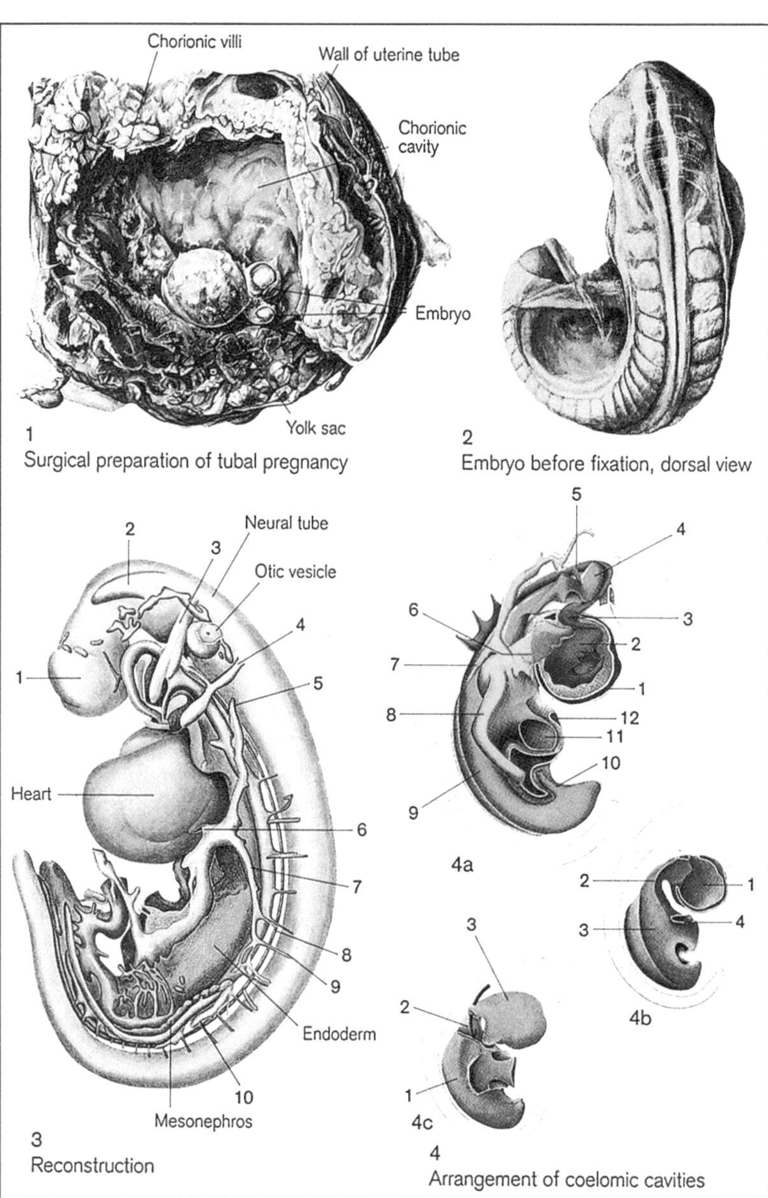


A. Stage 12: "Embryo Blechschmidt," 2.57mm

## 2.22 Stage 13: Primary Brain Vesicles

*Background*

**Stage 13:** 4–6 mm, 28–32 days, more than 30 somites. Arm and leg buds are present. The bulge of the optic vesicle can be recognized at the surface. The optic vesicle induces the lens placode in the overlying ectoderm; the otic vesicle has sunk inward.

### A. "Embryo Blechschmidt," 4.2 mm, 30 Pairs of Somites, about 28 Days

**1. Development of the Umbilical Cord.** At the end of the 4th week, the structures in the umbilical ring are gathered into the umbilical cord (→ 2.14 B). The stalk of the yolk sac (**10**) containing the vitelline vessels and the body stalk (containing the umbilical vessels) (**6**) are enveloped by a layer of amnion (**12**). The amnion is continuous with the ectoderm. The umbilical coelom (**9**) is the only remaining connection between the body cavity and the chorionic cavity. It is closed at the end of the embryonic period with the obliteration of the chorionic cavity. Until then, the yolk sac remains in the chorionic cavity (→ 2.32).

1 Optic vesicle
2 Maxillary process
3 Pharyngeal arches 1 and 2
4 Arm bud
5 Bulge of mesonephros
6 Body stalk with umbilical vessels (allantois no longer found)
7 Umbilical artery (normally paired)
8 Umbilical vein
9 Entrance into umbilical coelom
10 Vitelline duct (omphalomesenteric duct) with vitelline vessels
11 Cardiac bulge
12 Cut margin of amnion
13 Tail bud
14 Somites

**2. Reconstruction of Internal Organs**

**Nervous System.** The anlage of the brain is divided into the prosencephalon with the optic vesicles (**1**), the mesencephalon (**2**),and the rhombencephalon (**3**). The pharyngeal arch nerves (**4**, **5**, **7**, and **8**) grow out from the neural tube in the region of the rhombencephalon, followed by the spinal nerves, which are indicated by the thickening of the spinal ganglia (**9**).

**Heart and Vessels.** The illustration shows the myocardial surface of the cardial loop. The atrial segment (**a**), ventricle (**b**), and bulbus (**c**) are delimited from each other by furrows.

**Intestinal Tube.** The lung buds (**20**) are visible below the pharyngeal pouches, and beneath the heart, the network of liver cell cords can be seen (**21**) sprouting into the vascular bed of the vitelline and umbilical veins (**22**).

**Mesonephros.** The apex of the mesonephros (**14**) still lies above the umbilicus. The mesonephric duct opens into the cloaca (**16**) from behind.

1 Optic vesicle
2 Mesencephalon
3 Rhombencephalon
4 Trigeminal nerve
5 Facial nerve
6 Otic vesicle
7 Glossopharyngeal nerve
8 Vagus nerve
9 Spinal ganglion
10 Superior cardinal vein
11 Common cardinal vein
12 Inferior cardinal vein
13 Aorta with intersegmental arteries
14 Mesonephric duct with glomeruli
15 Notochord below the neural tube
16 Cloaca
17 Umbilical vein
18 Umbilical artery
19 Allantoic diverticulum
20 Lung bud
21 Liver cell cords
22 Plexus of vitelline veins

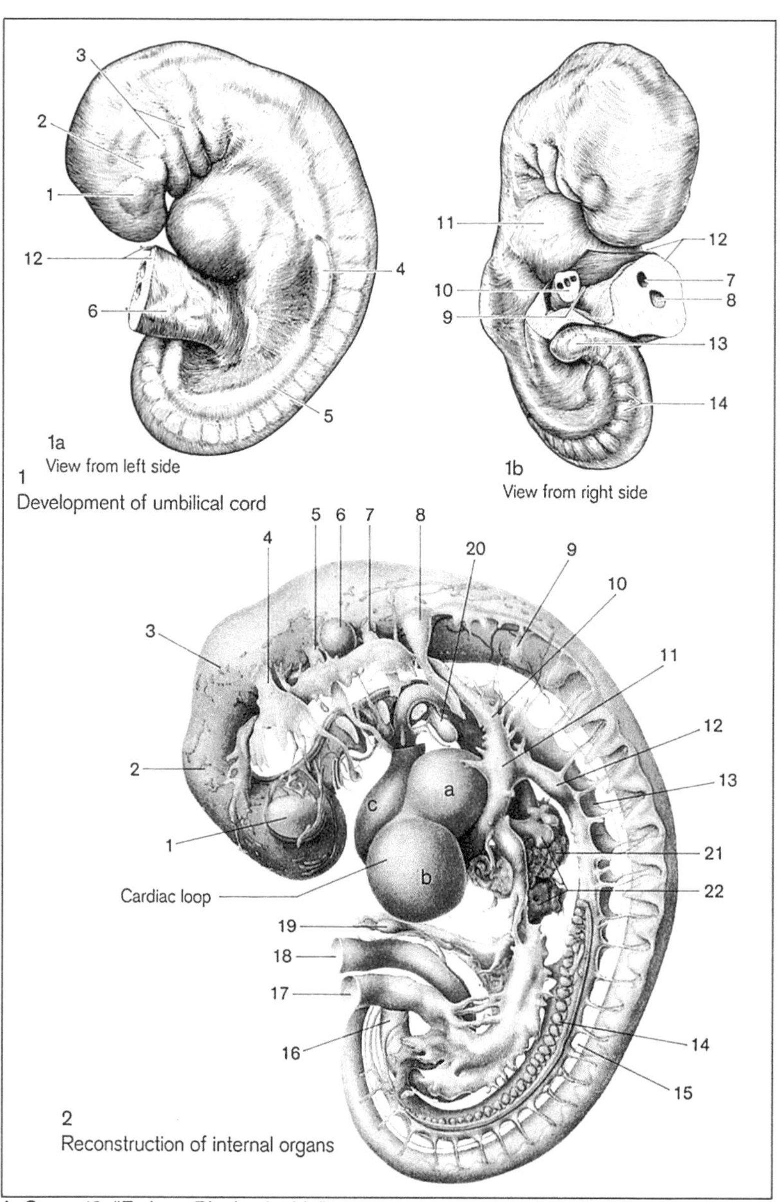


A. Stage 13: "Embryo Blechschmidt," 4.2 mm

# 5th–8th Weeks: Organogenesis
## 2.23 Stage 14: Myotomes

*Background*

**Stage 14:** 5–7 mm, 31–35 days. The lens pit invaginates into the optic cup. The endolymphatic duct emerges from the otic vesicle. Cephalic flexure and cervical flexure are pronounced.

### A. "Embryo Blechschmidt," 6.3 mm, 33 Pairs of Somites, about 30 Days

**1. External Morphology.** The number of definable somite pairs has reached its maximum. The cranial somitic borders have already disintegrated. Arms and legs are established as paddle-shaped buds. There are four pharyngeal arches, of which the second (hyoid arch) starts to cover the third and fourth as operculum (→ 7.3).

1 Optic primordium
2 Maxillary process
3 Nasal plate
4 Bulge of liver
5 Roof of 4th ventricle

**2. Illustration of Intestinal Tract, Heart,and Kidneys**

**Intestinal Tract.** The stomodeum (**1**) is opened from the left side. Its roof gives rise to an outpocketing, Rathke's pouch (primordium of the anterior lobe of the pituitary) (**2**), which becomes closely associated with the diencephalon. The first pharyngeal pouch (primordium of the middle ear) is followed by the second to fourth pharyngeal pouches and the trachea with two lung buds (**5**). The fourth pharyngeal pouch is associated with the vagus nerve (indicated only in outline) (**4**). Below the elongated stomach, the dorsal pancreatic bud (**6**) evaginates dorsally and the hepatic duct, together with the ventral pancreatic bud and the gallbladder primordium, evaginates ventrally (**7**). The umbilical loop (with the remains of the vitelline duct) and the allantois (**8**), extend into the umbilical ring. The large intestine (**9**) already exhibits the bulge of the caecum in its upper segment.

**Heart.** The embryonic ventricle is opened from the left, making the internal trabecular network visible. The arrow shows the entry of the blood stream from the atrium through the atrioventricular canal. The third and fourth aortic arches (**13**) represent the outflow tract of the heart, while the venous ring (**14**) in the region of the sinus venosus represents the venous inflow tract.

**Kidney.** The mesonephric (Wolffian) (**11**) duct opens into the not yet divided cloaca (**10**). Dorsally, the ureteric bud (**12** ) grows out. The glomeruli of the mesonephros extend cranially past the stomach. The segment of the mesonephric duct between the cloaca and the ureteric bud is later incorporated into the bladder.

**3. Representation of Myotomes and Body Cavities**

The myotome plates of the somites (**2**) are fused with one another. Ventrally, the myoblasts migrate out to form the striated musculature of the extremities and the ventral body wall. The remaining material becomes the "autochthonous" back musculature. The intraembryonic coelom is divided into the pericardial cavity (**3**, cut open) and the peritoneal cavity (**5**, also opened). The two cavities are connected by coelomic canals, into which the lung buds invaginate (**4**, covered by visceral peritoneum). The liver (**6**), stomach (**7**), and mesonephros (**8**) project into the body cavity. They are covered by visceral peritoneum.

1 Crest of spinal ganglia
2 Myotomes fusing with one another (origin of striated muscle)
3 Cut edge of pericardium
4 Lung bud covered by visceral pleura
5 Cut edge of peritoneum
6 Bulge of liver
7 Bulge of stomach covered by visceral peritoneum
8 Bulge of mesonephros (Wolffian body)
9 Umbilical veins situated in body wall
10 Exit of left umbilical artery from the aorta
11 Ureteric bud
12 Cloaca
13 Umbilical coelom

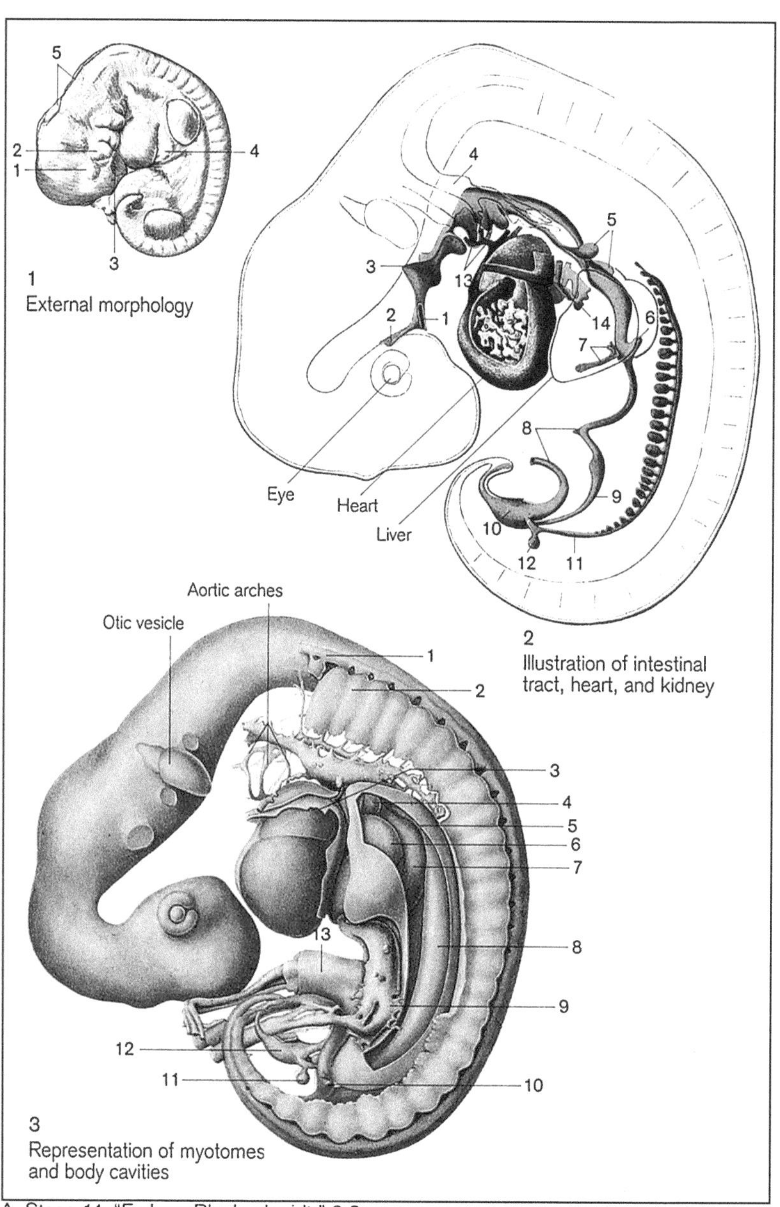


A. Stage 14: "Embryo Blechschmidt," 6.3 mm

## 2.24 Stage 15: Topography of Blood Vessels

*Background*

**Stage 15:** 7–9 mm, 35–38 days. The ectoderm closes over the lens vesicle. The nasal plate invaginates to form a pit. The auricular hillocks arise.

### A. "Embryo Blechschmidt," 7 mm and 7.5 mm

**1. "Embryo Blechschmidt," 7 mm Original Photograph.** The embryo is about 34 days old and was photographed before histological preparation. The nasal plate (**1**) is depressed into a pit that still borders on the telencephalon (**2**). In the optic primordium (**3**), lens closure is almost complete and only the narrow opening of the lens pit can be recognized. The furrow running towards the eye is the nasolacrimal groove between the frontal and maxillary processes. The maxillary process (**4**) is a part of the first pharyngeal arch (**5**). On the first (**5**) and second (**6**) pharyngeal arches arise the auricular hillocks. The second pharyngeal arch (**6**) forms an **operculum** over the third and fourth pharyngeal arches (**7**), which recede into the cervical sinus. The fourth ventricle of the rhombencephalon (**8**) is visible through the ectoderm. As the first myotome disintegrates, the somite borders in the cervical region disappear. The arm buds are angled off ventrally, whereas the leg buds still project paddle shaped from the trunk.

**2. "Embryo Blechschmidt," 7.5 mm. Topography of Blood Vessels (→ 6.7).** The aortic arches (**a13**) arise from the outflow tract of the heart. The first aortic arch between the first and second pharyngeal pouches has already receded. In the head, an arterial loop is formed by the carotid artery (**c29**) ascending behind the pharyngeal gut and by the stem of the vertebral and basilar arteries (**c27**). The vertebral artery arises from anastomosing intersegmental arteries of the neck (**c26**) that later recede cranially except for the well-developed exit of the subclavian artery (**14**). The **venous plexus** (→ 9.4) over the cerebral vesicles forms three large venous stems (**aI-III**) that empty into the superior cardinal vein (**a15**). In the trunk, the intersegmental arteries (**a7**) exit from the descending aorta at regular intervals. Blood returns via the parallel branches of the inferior cardinal vein.

**a Lateral View**
1 Telencephalon
2 Mesencephalon with cephalic flexure
3 Rhombencephalon
4 Cervical flexure
5 Ventral and dorsal roots of spinal nerve (cut margin)
6 Lung bud
7 Intersegmental vessels
8 Mesonephric duct with glomeruli
9 Cloaca with ventrally growing urorectal septum
10 Umbilical vessels
11 Umbilical loop
12 Remains of vitelline duct with vitelline vessels
13 Aortic arches
14 Vertebral artery
15 Superior cardinal vein with the three venous stems for the brain (I-III)
16 Pterygoid plexus

**b Anterior View.** The arrows show the blood flow in the cardiac loop.
17 Optic cup
18 Atrium
19 Descending limb of cardiac loop
20 Ascending limb
21 Liver
22 Marginal sinus of leg bud
23 Leg arteries
24 Allantoic diverticulum

**c Arteries of the Head.** The **arterial loop** between the **carotid** (**29**) and **basilar arteries** (**27**) shown in the reconstruction (**2a**, lateral view) is illustrated schematically.
25 Descending aorta
26 Intersegmental arteries of the neck
27 Basilar artery
28 Arteries of the mesencephalon
29 Internal carotid artery
30 Ophthalmic artery
31 Middle cerebral artery

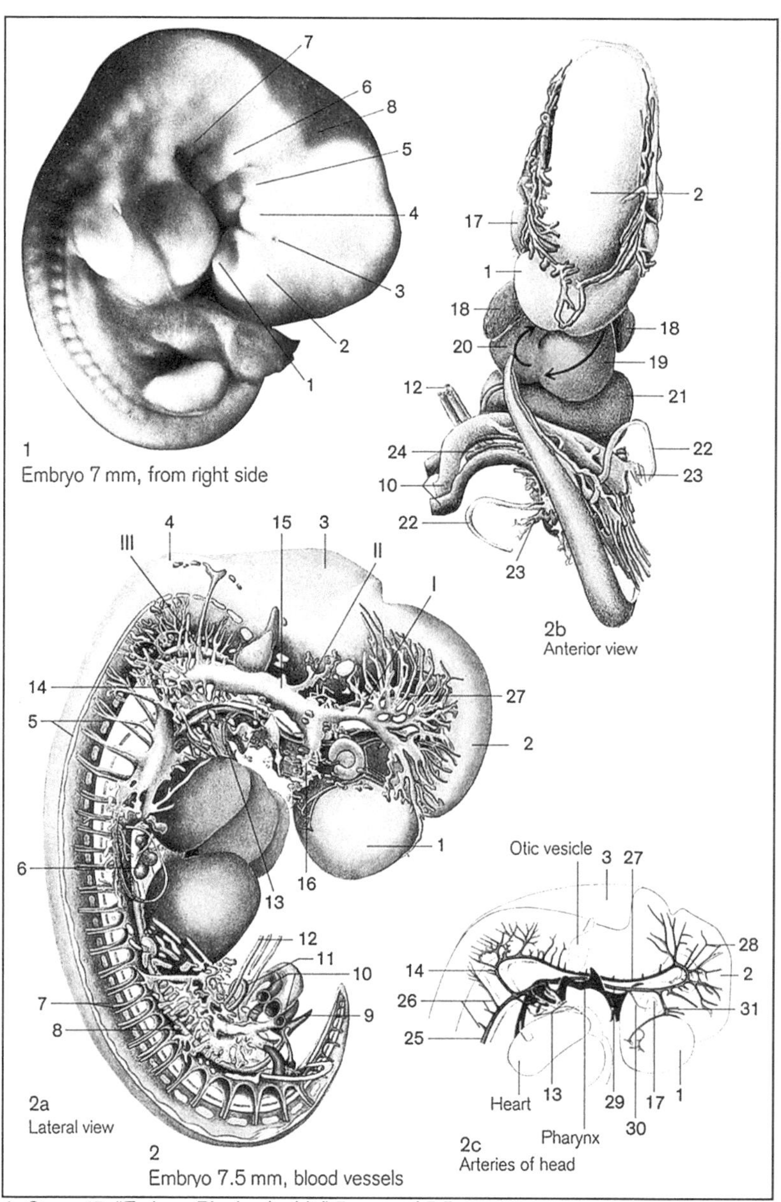


A. Stage 15: "Embryo Blechschmidt," 7 mm and 7.5 mm

## 2.25 Stage 16: Facial Swellings

*Background*

**Stage 16:** 8–11 mm, 37–42 days. Deep nasal pits. In unfixed embryos, the eyes are already pigmented. The auricular hillocks are distinguishable. The cervical sinus is closed. The hand plate is distinct; the foot plate is emerging.

### A "Embryo Blechschmidt," 8.8 mm, 9.6 mm and 10 mm

In the 5th and 6th week, the cerebral vesicles are situated anteriorly and inferiorly relative to the body axis. The cervical flexure is more elevated than the cephalic flexure (**A2**, → 2.4). The face lies on the heart-liver bulge. The front side of the face (**A1**) is only visible when the head is raised from the heart-liver bulge.

**1. Frontal View of Face in the 8.8 mm Embryo.** The stomodeum is bordered below by the mandibular swelling (**1**, first pharyngeal arch) and above by the frontal process (**2**). The **lateral** (**3**) and **medial nasal processes** (**4**) lie laterally below the frontal process and border the nasal pit, which later invaginates to form the primary choana. From behind, the **maxillary process**, a part of the first pharyngeal arch, grows forward. Between the lateral nasal process (**3**) and the maxillary process (**5**) arises the nasolacrimal groove, which is directed toward the eye.

**2. 9.6 mm Embryo. Original Photograph.** In the view from the right side, the nasolacrimal groove between the lateral nasal swelling (**4**) and the maxillary process (**5**) appears as a wide furrow (same numbers as in A1). The first pharyngeal cleft is surrounded by six **auricular hillocks,** three of which reside on the first (mandibular) pharyngeal arch (**1**) and the other three on the following second (hyoid) arch. The second pharyngeal arch forms a ventral segment (operculum) that covers the third and fourth arches, causing them to recede into the cervical sinus (→ 7.3). The arm bud exhibits a broad, flat hand plate that develops earlier than the foot plate.

**3. Partial Reconstruction of the 10 mm Embryo**

**Intestinal Tract and Body cavities.** The invaginating epithelium of the nasal pit (**1**) meets the roof of the stomodeum (**2**). The adenohypophysis (Rathke's pouch) evaginates from the roof of the stomodeum (**3**) and makes contact with the floor of the diencephalon. The first pharyngeal pouch (**4**) grows laterally toward the otic vesicle. The digestive tube, lying behind the pericardial cavity (**5**), enters the peritoneal cavity (**6**) from behind. The peritoneal cavity is almost entirely filled by the liver. The tip of the umbilical coelom is removed, making the umbilical loop (**7**) visible. The digestive tube enters the cloaca as the rectum (**8**). The bladder and the urethra arise from the ventral segment of the cloaca (**9**, urogenital sinus). The apex of the bladder merges with the allantoic duct (**10**), which joins the umbilical coelom in the umbilical cord.

**Locomotor System.** The striated musculature derived from the myotomes aggregates into the longitudinal fiber tracts of the back musculature (**11**), which are cranially inserted into the cartilaginous anlage of the occipital bone (**12**). The anlage of the scapula, humerus, radius, and ulna, as well as the five rays of the hand skeleton, are visible in the cartilaginous skeleton of the arm (**13**). In the leg bud, only the femur (**14**) is laid down as a cartilaginous model (→ 3.32B).

1 Ectodermal invagination of olfactory pit with nasal placode.
2 Oral cavity
3 Rathke's pouch
4 Pharynx
5 Pericardial cavity
6 Peritoneal cavity
7 Umbilical loop in the tip of the (opened) umbilical coelom
8 Rectum
9 Urogenital sinus
10 Allantois
11 Back musculature
12 Occipital bone
13 Arm skeleton
14 cartilage anlage of femur
15 Metanephros (covered by femur)

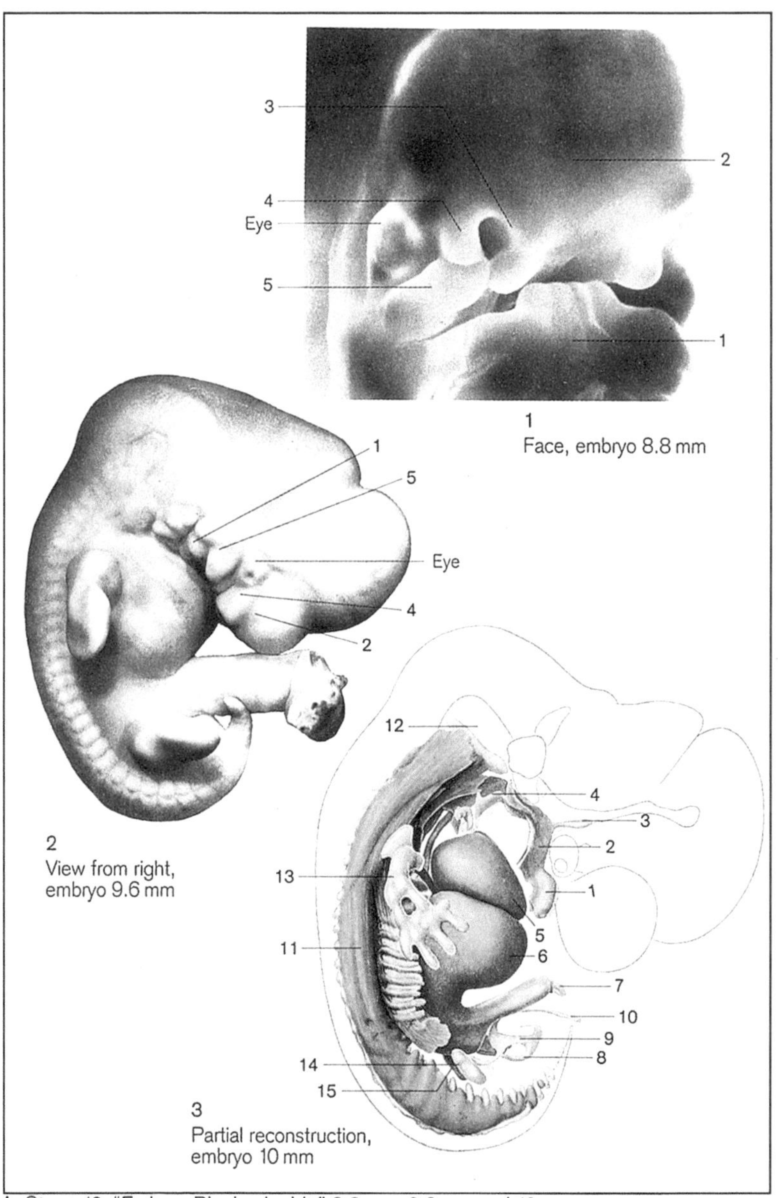


1
Face, embryo 8.8 mm

2
View from right, embryo 9.6 mm

3
Partial reconstruction, embryo 10 mm

A. Stage 16: "Embryo Blechschmidt," 8.8 mm, 9.6 mm and 10 mm

## 2.26 Stage 17: Telencephalon Vesicles

*Background*

**Stage 17:** 11–14 mm, 42–44 days. Relative enlargement of the head and extension of the trunk. Nasolacrimal groove and auricular hillocks are distinct. Arm buds are angled off. Finger rays are well defined.

### A. "Embryo Blechschmidt," 9.8 mm and 11.7 mm

**1. 9.8 mm Embryo, Dorsal View.** The ectodermal and mesenchymal layers are translucent. The zone of fusion is thus visible between the alar plates of the neural tube (**1**). Laterally, the contour of the spinal ganglia (**2**) is apparent; below it are the contours of the myotomes (**3**) and the segmental musculature that will form the ventral trunk wall. This contour image is intensified by dehydration and shrinkage of the loose mesenchyme. The arm buds are already angled off at the prospective elbow joint (**4**), whereas the leg buds (**5**) still project at right angles from the body.

**2. Cleared Preparation of 11.7 mm Embryo.** The specimen was cleared in xylol or methyl benzoate and the inner structures made visible by transillumination. In the clearing process, however, the tissue hardens and becomes fragile (x, fracture sites). In the head, the cerebral vesicles can be recognized (**1 telencephalon, 2** diencephalon, **3** mesencephalon). They are surrounded by loose mesenchyme. The abdomen is almost completely filled by the liver. The liver is strongly enlarged due to blood formation and appears dark. The heart (**4** right atrium, **5** right ventricle, **6** left atrium, **7** left ventricle) lies at the base of the liver (**8**). The thin-walled atria appear as empty spaces. In the right ventricle, the trabecular network shines through. The umbilical cord is distended by the displacement of the umbilical loop into the umbilical coelom (**9**).

**3. Dissection of the 11.7 mm Embryo**

**a. After Removal of the Head.** By removal of the head, the cartilaginous anlage of the cervical vertebral bodies were also removed from the loose mesenchyme in front of the neural tube. The intact elastic notochord (**6**) slipped out from the vertebral bodies and remained behind as isolated structure in the preparation. The cut surfaces of the second and first pharyngeal arches (**9, 11**) and the tongue on the floor of the mouth (**12**) are visible. The thin body wall above the heart (**14**) and liver (**3**) was also removed.

1 Neural tube
2 Trunk wall with mesonephros shining through medially
3 Liver
4 Right atrium
5 Pharyngeal cleft 1
6 Notochord
7 Neural tube
8 Spinal ganglion with dorsal and ventral branch of spinal nerve
9 Hyoid arch
10 Pharyngeal pouch 1 (future auditory tube)
11 Nerve of pharyngeal arch 1 (V.3)
12 Tongue
13 Left atrium
14 Left ventricle
15 Umbilical vein
16 Umbilical loop of small intestine
17 Future heel
18 Genital tubercle

**b Organs after Removal of Heart and Liver**

19 Mesonephros
20 Gonad
21 Lower lobe of right lung
22 Outline of peritoneum
23 Visceral pleura of right upper lobe
24 Posterior body wall
25 Entrance into larynx
26 Trachea
27 Outline of common cardinal vein
28 Upper lobe of left lung
29 Lower lobe of left lung
30 Stomach
31 Spleen
32 Vitelline vein
33 Superior mesenteric artery
34 Umbilical loop
35 Rectum

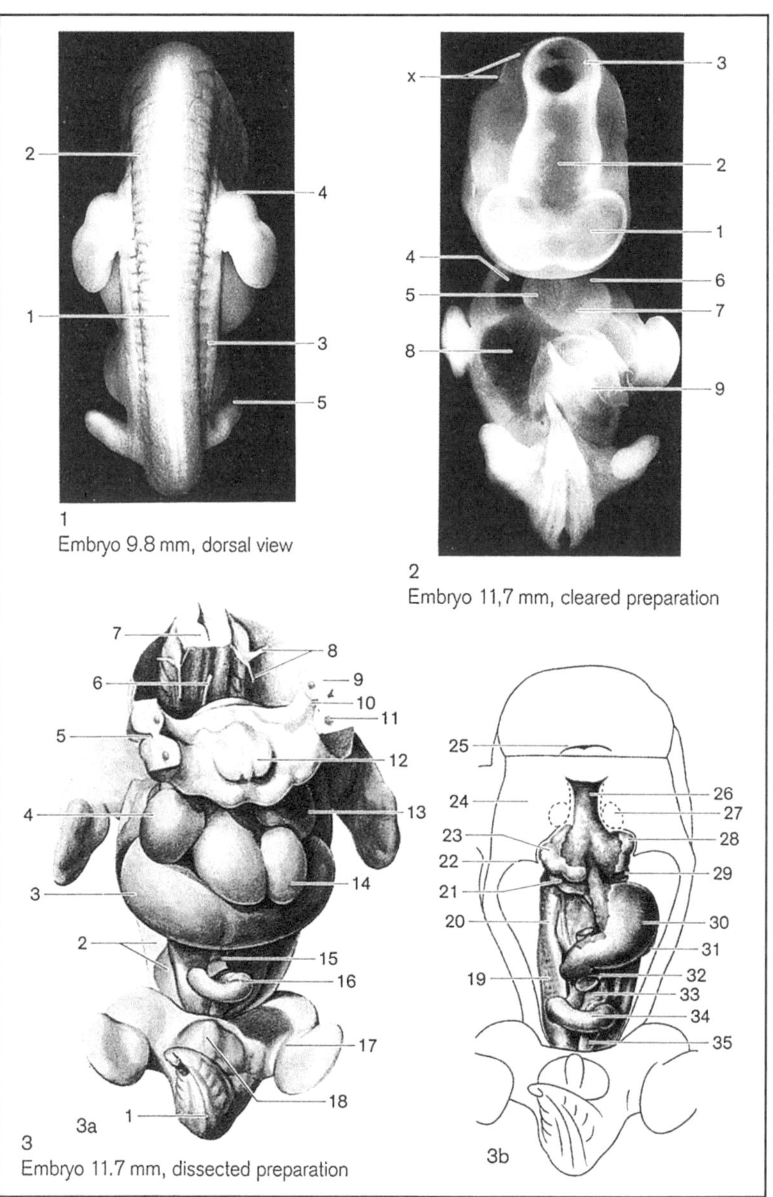


1
Embryo 9.8 mm, dorsal view

2
Embryo 11,7 mm, cleared preparation

3
Embryo 11.7 mm, dissected preparation

A. Stage 17: "Embryo Blechschmidt," 9.8 mm and 11.7 mm

## 2.27 Stage 18 and 19: Cuboid Body Shape

*Background*

**Stage 18:** 13–17 mm, 44–48 days, cuboid body form. Toe rays are delimited. Eyelid folds appear. Tip of nose is distinct. Nipples form. Ossification may begin.
**Stage 19:** 16–18 mm, 48–51 days. Eyes and external ears gain definite shape. Finger rays are distinctly differentiated.

### A. Stage 18 and 19

**1. "Embryo Blechschmidt," 13 mm, in Situ with Yolk Sac.** The chorionic sac has been opened and the transparent amnion (**1**) cut at the umbilical cord. The vitelline vessels (**2**) travel from the umbilical stalk to the yolk sac (**3**), which lies in the narrow space between the amnion and the inner surface of the chorion (**4**) (→ 2.42).

**2. "Embryo Blechschmidt," 13.5 mm, Partial Reconstruction.** Isolated presentation of the nervous system, arteries, and digestive tract. The veins (blue) are concealed by arteries or not shown.

**Central Nervous System (yellow)**

1 Telencephalon
2 Diencephalon
3 Mesencephalon with oculomotor nerve projecting at the ventral surface
4 Rhombencephalon with trigeminal and vestibulocochlear nerves
5 Neural tube
6 Ventral root
7 Dorsal root of spinal nerves

**Arteries (red) (→ 6.7)**

8 Right aortic arch. The two aortic arches embrace the esophagus and trachea
9 Vertebral artery. It originates from anastomoses between the cranial intersegmental arteries, the proximal roots of which disappear
10 Right subclavian artery. It arises from the 7th intersegmental artery of the neck
11 Carotid artery. It is a continuation of the paired ventral aorta
12 Ophthalmic artery
13 Middle cerebral artery
14 Dorsal aorta with intersegmental arteries
15 Umbilical artery

**Digestive Tract (green) (→ 7.1)**

16 Primary choanae
17 Stomodeum
18 Pharynx
19 Epithelial branching out of the lung bud
20 Stomach
21 Duodenum with the ventrally directed exit of the hepatic duct and the dorsally directed dorsal and ventral pancreas
22 Umbilical loop
23 Allantoic diverticulum
24 Remains of the mesonephros
25 Epithelial ramification of the ureteric bud in the metanephros

**3. "Embryo Blechschmidt," 16.2 mm, Isolated Embryo after Fixation**
**a View from Right Side.** The development of the upper and lower eyelid is indicated by deep furrows above and below the optic primordium. The auricular hillocks have merged to form the external ear. In the hand plate, notches are visible between the finger rays, whereas the foot plate still has a smooth border. The **nipple** (**1**) is evident beneath the hand.

**b Dorsal View.** The border between the future vertebral column and future ribs appears as a groove. The leg buds are now angled off at the knee joint. The **tail** has receded by physiological necrosis.

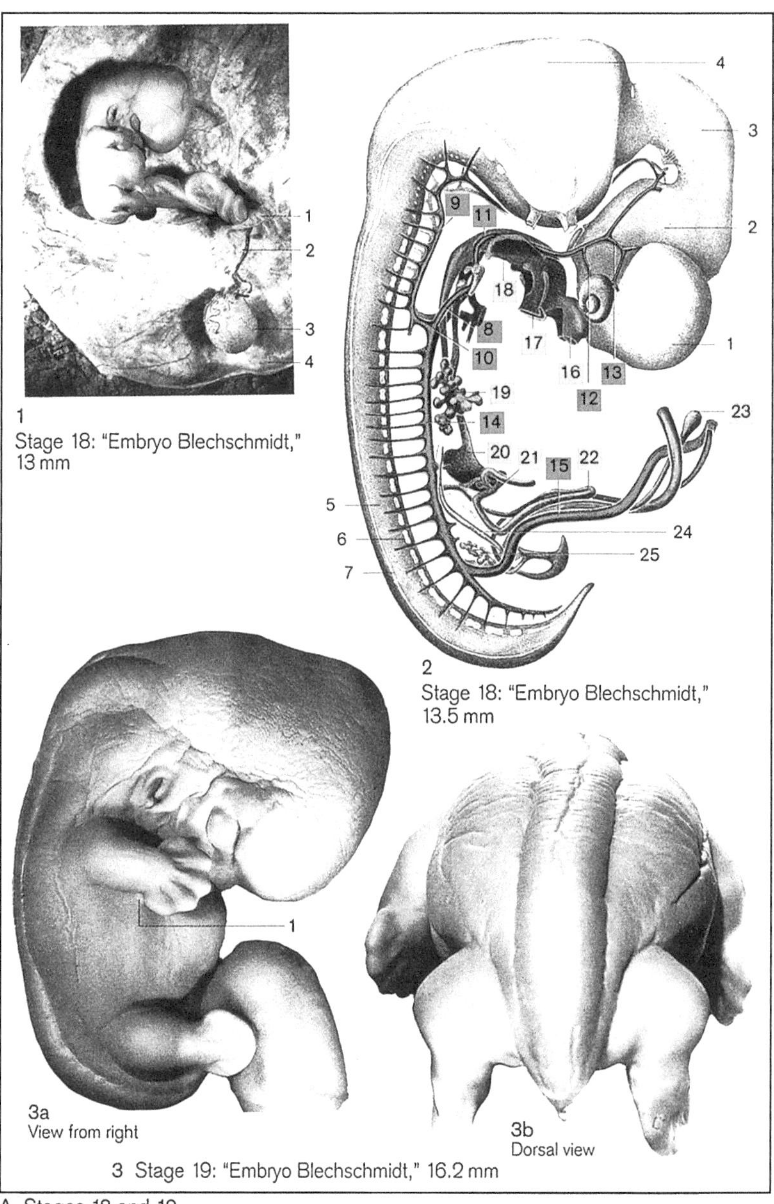


1
Stage 18: "Embryo Blechschmidt," 13 mm

2
Stage 18: "Embryo Blechschmidt," 13.5 mm

3a
View from right

3b
Dorsal view

3 Stage 19: "Embryo Blechschmidt," 16.2 mm

A. Stages 18 and 19

## 2.28 Stage 20: Hand in Pronation

*Background*

**Stage 20:** 18–22 mm, 51–53 days. Arms angled and hands curved (pronate). Fingers are separated. Toe rays are defined.

### A. "Embryo Blechschmidt," 17.5 mm

**1. External Morphology.** As the base of the nose is delineated from the forehead and the nose forms a snount (preceding the snub nose), the embryonic face becomes childlike. The finger rays are separated from one another. The hands are curving medially over the cardiac region (pronate). The foot plate exhibits notches between the toe rays.

**2. Digestive Tract and Body Cavities**

**a Isolated Intestinal Canal in Relation to the Neural Tube.** The external shape of the embryo is determined by the dorsally convex curvature of the neural tube, into which the digestive tract is fitted.

The primordia of the salivary glands (**4**) sprout downward from the epithelium of the oral cavity (**2**). The tongue bulges upward. The hypophysial diverticulum (**3**) becomes associated with the infundibulum of the diencephalon. A thin epithelial connection still exists between the hypophysis and the roof of the oral cavity. The thyroid gland and thymus lie below the larynx. The stomach (**10** ) has rotated and shifted in such a way that it covers the duodenum, the exit of the bile duct, and the gallbladder. The small intestine and the large intestine (including the caecum) form an intestinal loop (**12**) outside of the body cavity, in the umbilical cord (physiological umbilical herniation). The rectum (**15**) has separated from the urogenital sinus (**18**) and the urethra (**17**). At the posterior wall of the bladder (**19**), the genital ducts (**22**) open between the two ureters (**20**).

**b View into the Body Cavities.** The parts of the digestive tract shown in **2b** are numbered as in **2a**.

The trachea and esophagus (**6**) extend downward behind the pericardial cavity (**7**). The coelomic canals between the pericardial and body cavities have broadened into the pleural cavities (**8**). All three cavities are opened so that one can look into the pericardial cavity (**7**) at the apex of the heart, into the left pleural cavity (**8**) at the lung with its covering of visceral pleura, and into the peritoneal cavity (**9**) at the stomach (**10**), and (behind) the bulge of the mesonephros with the genital ducts (**22**). The body cavity extends into the umbilical cord; this extension has been removed (**14**) to make the umbilical loop (**12**) visible. A peritoneal duplication (**16**) extends down over the rectum (**15**) as the anlage of the rectovesical or rectouterine pouch. The ureters (**20**) extend in a dorsal direction to the retroperitoneally situated metanephros (**21**).

1 Epithelial lining of the primary choana
2 Endoderm of oral cavity
3 Hypophysial diverticulum
4 Duct of salivary glands
5 External auditory canal with external ear
6 Trachea and esophagus
7 Pericardial cavity, opened at apex
8 Left pleural cavity, opened
9 Lining of peritoneal cavity
10 Stomach
11 Lesser omentum
12 Umbilical loop
13 Vessels of umbilical stalk (future superior mesenteric artery and vein)
14 Umbilical coelom
15 Rectum
16 Leg (cut margin)
17 Urethra
18 Urogenital sinus
19 Bladder
20 Ureter
21 Metanephros
22 Genital ducts
23 Allantois

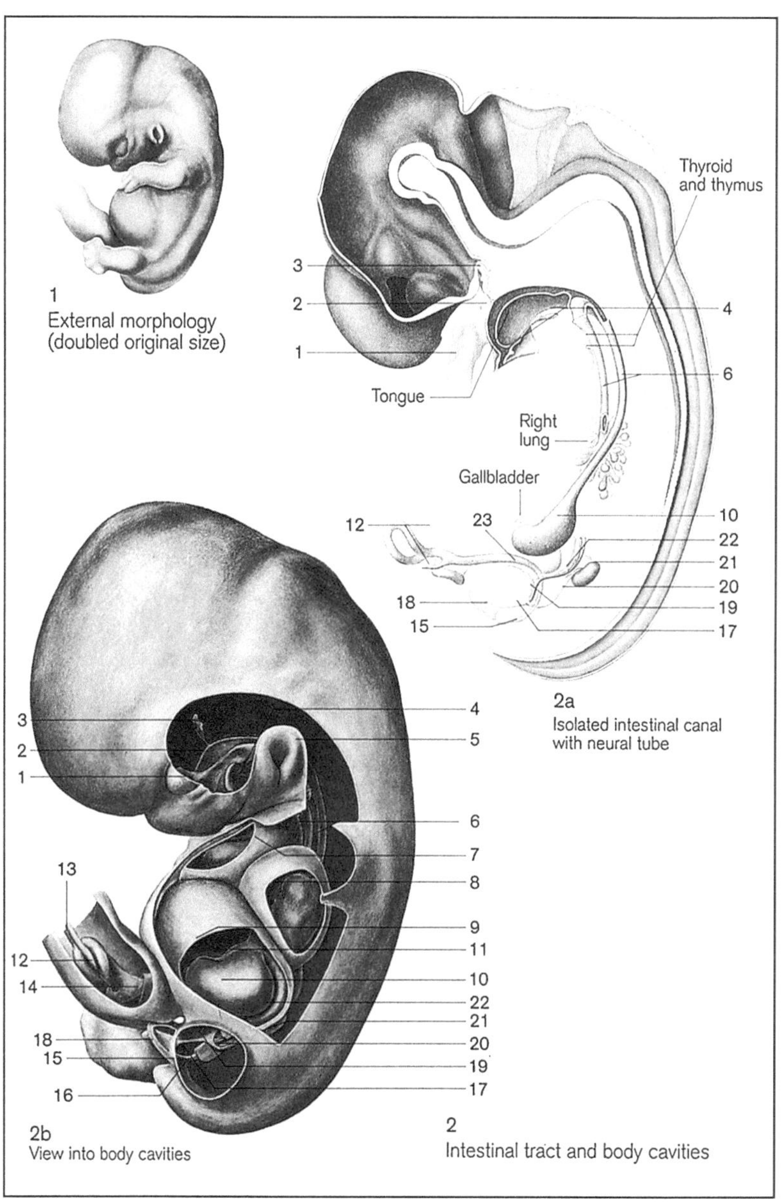


A. Stage 20: "Embryo Blechschmidt," 17.5 mm

## 2.29 Stage 20: Cartilage Skeleton

### B. "Embryo Blechschmidt," 17.5 mm. Reconstruction of Organ Systems

#### 1. Cartilaginous Skeleton and Venous System of Head

**Skeleton.** The vertebral column, ribs, limb skeleton, and base of the skull develop as hyaline cartilage, which later undergoes endochondral ossification and forms bone. At this stage the members of the cartilaginous skeleton are still continuous and not separated from each other. Joints develop from the richly vascularized, loose connective tissue that grows in between the cartilaginous primordia.

1 Cartilaginous nasal capsule
2 Greater wing of sphenoid
3 Anlage of auditory ossicles
4 Otic capsule (future petrous bone)
5 Occipital bone
6 Vertebral body with attachments of vertebral arches
7 Hand skeleton with dorsal venous arch
8 Foot skeleton with marginal venous sinus

**Venous System of Head (→ 9.4).** The otic capsule interrupts the course of the anterior *cardinal vein* (**9**), which in the young embryo, drains blood from the anterior half of the body and from the head. The venous drainage is now shifted upward via the *sigmoid sinus* (**15**) and the *superior* (**11**) and *inferior petrosal sinus* (**12**), which arise from local venous plexuses. The anterior segment of the cardinal vein forms the *cavernous sinus* (**13**), retaining its original connections to the veins of the face via the *ophthalmic vein* (14), the angular vein, and the *pterygoid plexus* ( **15**).

#### 2. Base of Skull and Skeletal Musculature

**Base of Skull (→ 9.2).** The base of the skull is composed of central elements that represent a continuation of the vertebral column, and of elements that form cartilaginous capsules for the central sense organs. Central elements include the *occipital bone* with cartilagenous primordium of the proximal part of the occipital squama (**1**), the *basilar bone* (**3**), and the *hypophysial cartilages* (**4**).

The most prominent capsular structure is the *otic capsule* (**2**), which completely encloses the inner ear (containing the cochlea and the semicircular canals) and later ossifies into the petrous bone. The *orbit*, the anteriorly open capsule of the eye, arises from the cartilaginous anlage of the *greater* and *lesser wings* (**5**) of the *sphenoid*. The *nasal capsule* (**6**) contains the invagination of the nasal pit and is the cartilaginous primordium of the nasal skeleton.

Below the otic capsule lies the chain of auditory ossicles (**7**), linked to *Meckel's cartilage* (**8**), the cartilage of the first pharyngeal arch (mandibular). Above Meckel's cartilage is a lamella of *membrane bone* (**9**), the anlage of the definitive mandible. The mandible arises by membraneous ossification, while Meckel's cartilage regresses. The bony lamella in the mandible is the first ossification center in this stage.

**Skeletal Musculature.** The *ocular musculature* (**11**), the *masticatory musculature* (**10**), and the muscles of the neck (**12**) appear at the underside of the base of the skull. The *trapezius* (**13**) and *latissimus dorsi* (**14**) muscles (shoulder girdle musculature) extend over the entire trunk and cover the deeper back musculature. The liver bulges through a wide open gap in the *rectal musculature* (**15**) (diastasis of rectus abdominis). The extensors in the lower arm (**16**) and the extensors in the lower leg (**17**) are completely muscular right up into the hand and foot plate, respectively; the tendons form later. The hand lies on the liver bulge in a curved (pronate) position. The leg is similarly held in a curved (pronate) position until pronation is fixed as the definitive foot position.

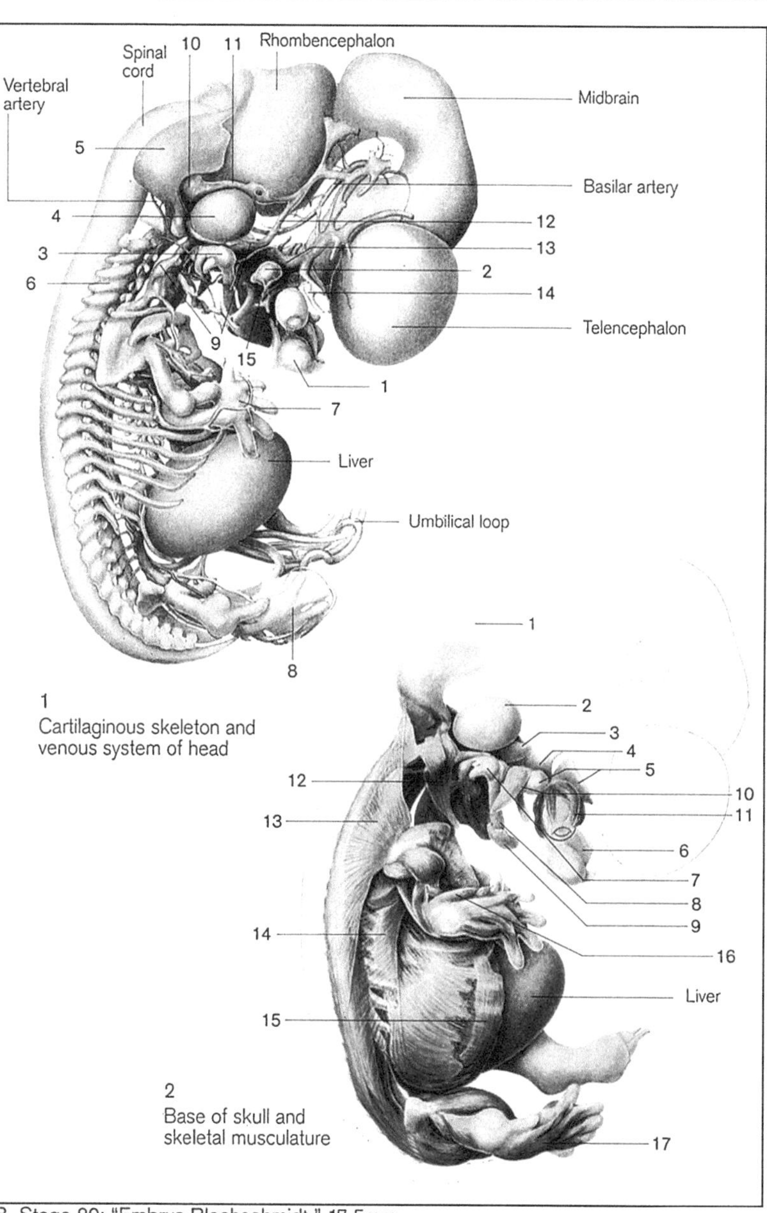


1
Cartilaginous skeleton and venous system of head

2
Base of skull and skeletal musculature

B. Stage 20: "Embryo Blechschmidt," 17.5mm

## 2.30 Stage 23: Histology

### A. Stage 23: Embryo, 30 mm, Sagittal Sections

The embryo corresponds in its development to the 29 mm "Embryo Blechschmidt" (→ 2.31 A2) and to the third phase of the dissection of the head (2.31 A1c). It is less developed than the 30 mm fetus of Blechschmidt (→ 2.34), but this fetus can be used to localize the sections. Section A1 lies slightly to the right of the midline. In the sagittal section A2, the left ovary has been cut.

**Central Nervous System.** The brain comprises more than a third of the entire embryo (**A1**). The choroid plexus (**4**) can be seen in the lateral ventricle (**1**) and the fourth ventricle (**3**). The mesencephalon still possesses a wide ventricle (**2**) that later narrows to form the cerebral aqueduct. The brain and spinal cord are surrounded by richly vascularized, loose mesenchyme (**5**), which differentiates into the meninges.

**Vertebral Column and Base of Skull.** The vertebral column consists of dense connective tissue zones, corresponding to the intervertebral discs, and paler cartilaginous zones, corresponding to the vertebral bodies. It extends horizontally into the base of the skull. The adenohypophysis is located in the cartilaginous primordium of the sella turcica (**7**). It has now separated from the roof of the oral cavity.

**Gastrointestinal Tract.** The oral cavity is filled by the large tongue (**8**). Below the larynx (**9**), the thymus (**10**) descends into the mediastinum. Behind the pericardial cavity, the right main bronchus (**11**) is cut transversely. Further down, the esophagus (**12**) passes through the diaphragm into the body cavity. The stomach, lying further left, is cut in section 2 (**A2**, 24). The transverse antrum portion of the stomach (**13**) lies below the liver. In A1 the attachment of the dorsal mesogastrium (**14**) at the large curvature of the stomach is visible. In A2 this thin tissue layer separates the stomach from the mesonephros and the ovary (**15**), which lie at the dorsal body wall; it also ensheaths the pancreas (**16**). The unpaired umbilical vein (**17**) passes from the umbilical cord directly into the liver. Phallus and labioscrotal folds (**19**) consist of undifferentiated, dense mesoderm.

**Ovary and Mesonephros.** The section (**A2**) is situated further laterally. The ovary (**15**) is seen to connect with the mesonephros (**20**) through a broad mesenteric root. The mesonephros lies at the lower pole of the metanephros (**21**) and has well-developed glomeruli and renal tubules. Below, the mesonephric duct (**22**) and the paramesonephric duct (**23**), of the mesonephric body appear in cross section. Above the ovary and behind the fundus of the stomach, the apex of the pancreas (**16**) can be seen, lying in the dorsal mesogastrium (**14**). The mesogastrium forms a separate tissue layer lying parallel to the dorsal body wall and covering the descending ovary and the mesonephros.

1 Telencephalon
2 Mesencephalon
3 Rhombencephalon
4 Choroid plexus
5 Meninges
6 Defect in section
7 Sella turcica with hypophysis (pituitary gland)
8 Tongue
9 Larynx
10 Thymus
11 Right main bronchus
12 Esophagus
13 Antrum portion of stomach
14 Dorsal mesogastrium
15 Ovary
16 Pancreas
17 Umbilical vein
18 Umbilical artery
19 Phallus and labioscrotal folds
20 Mesonephros
21 Metanephros
22 Mesonephric duct
23 Paramesonephric duct
24 Fundus of stomach

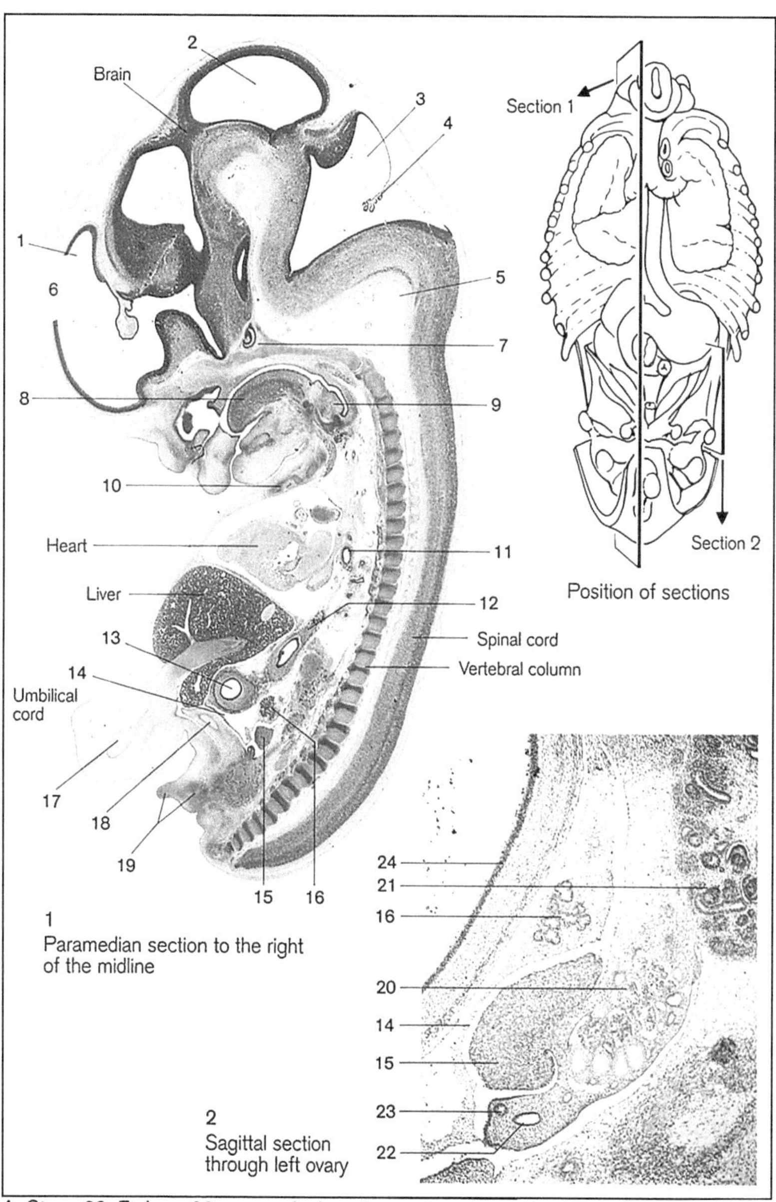


A. Stage 23: Embryo 30 mm, sagittal sections

## 2.31 Stage 23: Dissected Preparation of Head

### A. "Blechschmidt Embryo," 29 mm, Dissected Preparation

**1. Dissection of Head.** The dissected preparation has been drawn directly from the specimen instead of being reconstructed from histological sections.

**a. Brain and Visceral Skeleton.** The skull cap is removed. In the *telencephalon* (**1**), the rotation of the hemispheres begins. The *insular region* (**2**) is retarded in growth. In the dorsal rhomboid lip of the rhombencephalon, the *cerebellar bulge* (**11**) develops. The cerebellum is divided into an intraventricular and an extraventricular portion by the *ruptured margin* (**12**) of the thinly drawn-out roof of the 4th ventricle. The cartilaginous elements of the pharyngeal arches are visible below the base of the skull. The cartilage of the *first pharyngeal arch* (**8**) articulates with the cartilage of the *second pharyngeal arch* (**9**); the auditory ossicles form from the articulation between the two.

1 Telencephalon
2 Insula
3 Diencephalon
4 Optic nerve
5 Hypophysis (Pituitary gland)
6 Wing of sphenoid
7 Nasal capsule
8 Cartilage of first pharyngeal arch
9 Cartilage of second pharyngeal arch
10 Mesencephalon
11 Cerebellar bulge
12 Ruptured margin of roof of fourth ventricle
13 Occipital squama
14 Otic capsule

**b. Opening of Lateral Ventricle and Fourth Ventricle**. Below the *insula*, (**a,2**) the *ganglionic prominence* (**16**), which will give rise to the basal ganglia, is visible. The *otic capsule* (**a,14**) and the visceral skeleton are removed from the right side.

15 Tenia choroidea
16 Ganglionic prominence
17 Nasal septum
18 Olfactory fibers of rudimentary vomeronasal organ (→ 5.5)
19 Palate
20 Primary choana
21 Semicircular canal
22 Cochlea

**c. Median Section through the Diencephalon, Mesencephalon, and Rhomboid Fossa**. The lateral ventricle of the opposite side is opened medially so that the left choroid plexus (**25**) becomes visible. In sagittal section the *thalamus* (**24**) bulges into the upper half of the diencephalon. The exit into the left *lateral ventricle* (**26**) is visible above the *lamina terminalis* (**27**). The *mesencephalon* (**31**) still possesses a wide lumen that later narrows down to form the cerebral aqueduct. The *nasal septum* (**b,17**) is removed. In the median section through the nasopharyngeal space, the *cochlea* (**33**) remains in place and projects out from the preparation.

23 Epiphysis (Pineal gland)
24 Thalamus
25 Choroid plexus in left ventricle
26 Interventricular foramen
27 Lamina terminalis
28 Olfactory bulb and olfactory fibers
29 Nasal concha of left side
30 Quadrigeminal plate
31 Mesencephalic vesicle
32 Mamillary body
33 Cochlea
34 Basilar bone
35 Dens of axis

**2. Thorax and Pelvic Position.** The thoracic wall is opened on the right side, allowing the attachments of the ribs and the thoracic and abdominal musculature to be seen.

1 Ribs
2 Rectal musculature
3 Physiological umbilical hernia
4 Phallus
5 Tip of pericardium
6 Lung
7 Diaphragm above liver
8 Cartilaginous pelvis

**Subcutaneous Vascular Plexus of Head.** (→ 2.32, A1). From stage 20 to 23, the subcutaneous vascular plexus spreads throughout the skull. Vascularization proceeds from the base of the skull to the vertex. A sharp V-shaped boundary arises between vascularized and not yet vascularized mesoderm.

Illustration 2.32 A2 from Boyd, Hamilton: The Human Placenta.

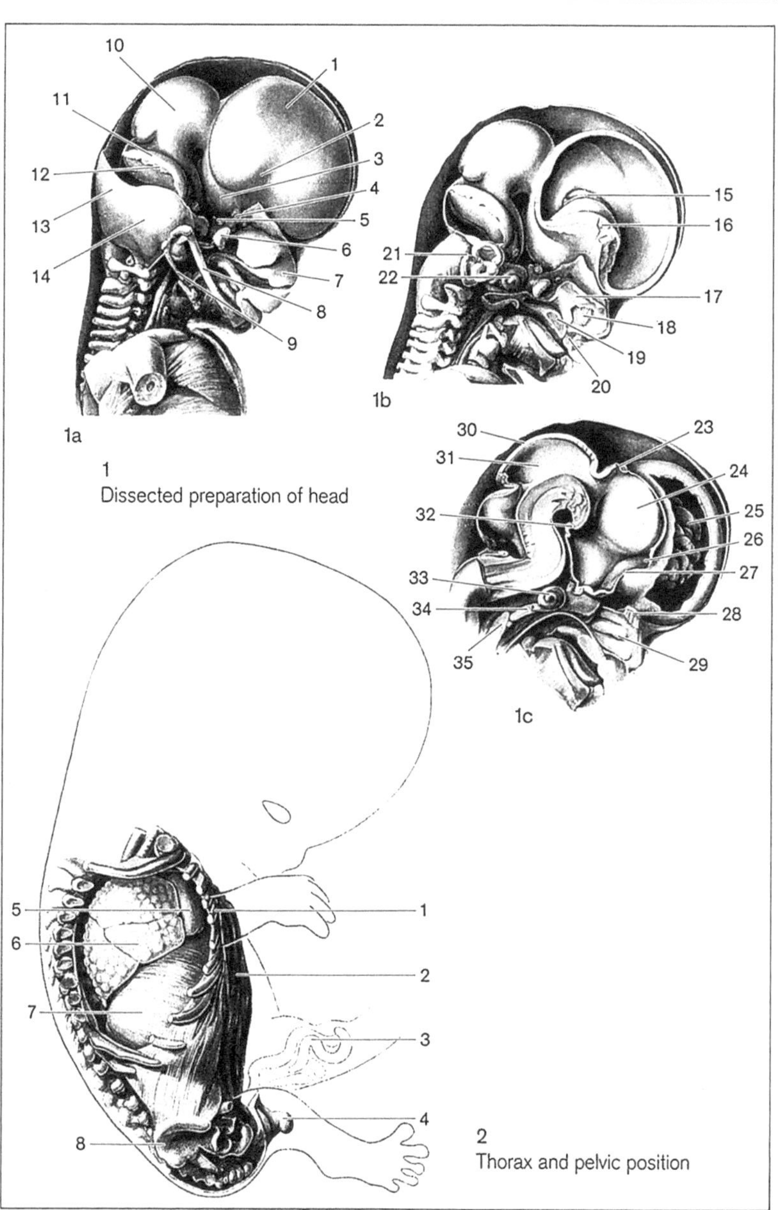


1
Dissected preparation of head

2
Thorax and pelvic position

A. Stage 23: "Embryo Blechschmidt," 29 mm

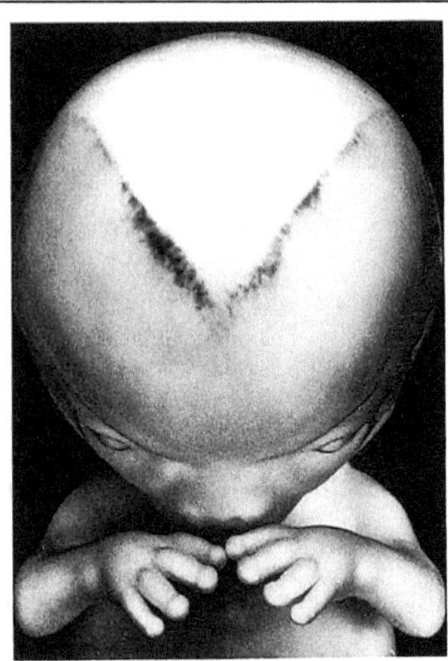

1
Face at stage 2
"Embryo Blechschmidt," 29 mm

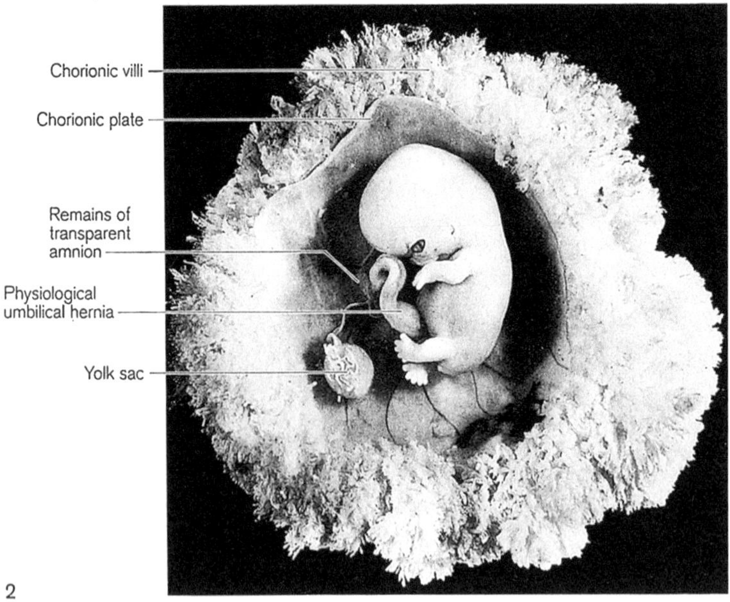

Chorionic villi
Chorionic plate
Remains of transparent amnion
Physiological umbilical hernia
Yolk sac

2
Embryo at stage 22

A. Body form and fetal membranes at the end of the embryonic period

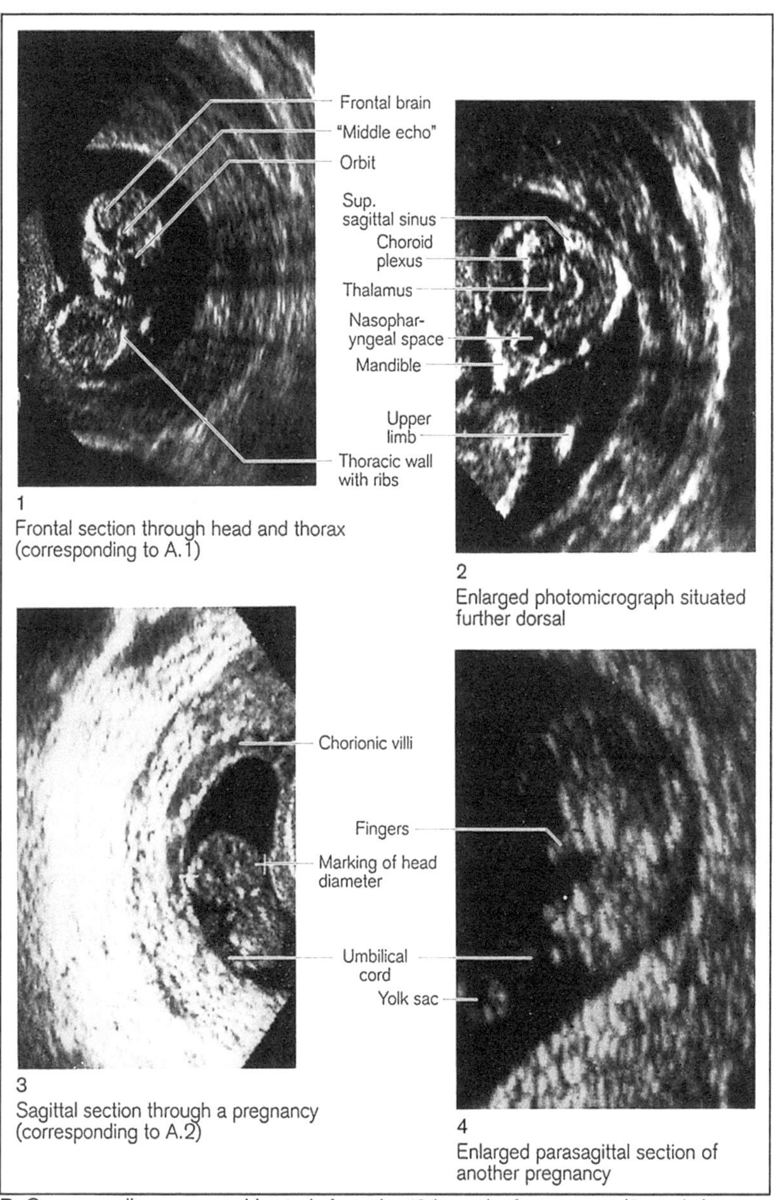


1
Frontal section through head and thorax (corresponding to A.1)

2
Enlarged photomicrograph situated further dorsal

3
Sagittal section through a pregnancy (corresponding to A.2)

4
Enlarged parasagittal section of another pregnancy

B. Corresponding sonographic study from the 10th week of pregnancy (8 weeks)

The pictures were kindly placed at my disposal by F. Degenhardt, Hannover

# Fetal Period

## 2.33 Overview

*Background*

The embryonic period ends in the 10th week of pregnancy (stage 23; 8th postovulatory week). During the **fetal period**, growth of the embryo and maturation of the organ systems take place. In the first half of the fetal period (up to the 20th week of pregnancy), the embryo grows mainly in length, whereas toward the end of pregnancy it gains weight.

### A. Growth Curve in the Fetal Period

**Characterization of the Fetal Period.** In the **third month**, the physiological umbilical hernia recedes (11th week of pregnancy) and the chorionic cavity is obliterated. In the **4th month**, sex can be determined by inspection of external genital organs. Beginning in the **5th month**, the mother can perceive fetal movements. At this time, the fetus is covered by lanugo hair. In the **6th month** the fetus is characterized by a wrinkled skin, as subcutaneous adipose tissue is still absent. Subcutaneous fat appears in the **7th month**. Toward the end of pregnancy, the skin is covered by a whitish, fatty substance, the vernix caseosa, which is formed by sebaceous glands.

The viability of a premature infant during the 6th or beginning of the 7th month depends on the maturation of the lungs and brain. After the 28th week of pregnancy, the fetus is, in principle, capable of living.

**Weeks of Pregnancy.** In the fetal period, the age of the fetus is given in weeks of pregnancy, which are counted from the first day of the last menstrual bleeding (menstrual age). The calculation of the duration of a pregnancy after the last menstruation corresponds to the usage in obstetrics in which the last menstruation can always be ascertained, whereas the moment of ovulation, which has led to a pregnancy and to an implantation, is generally not known. *Menstrual age* given in weeks of pregnancy, therefore, is always around two weeks longer than the *ovulation* or *fertilization age* specified in days or weeks.

**Lunar months.** The time between the first day of the last menstruation and the day of birth is a total of 40 weeks. This period can be divided into 10 lunar months of 4 weeks each. In this calculation, a month has 28 days.

**Trimester.** The designation trimester comprises 3 lunar months. The first trimester extends to the 12th week of pregnancy and is, therefore, 2 weeks longer than the embryonic period.

**Crown–Rump Length (C.R.).** In the embryonic period, the C.R. length of an embryo is equivalent to its greatest length,since the extremities are perpendicular to the body axis. During further development in the fetal period, the C.R. length is still used as a measure, since it can be determined reliably by sonography. In the middle of the pregnancy (20 weeks), the fetus is 15–20 cm C.R., which is about half its birth size.

**Crown–Heel Length (C.H.)**. The size of a newborn infant is measured with extended legs and denoted as C.H. length. In the second half of pregnancy, the crown-heel length increases about 5 cm per month (rule of thumb: 5th month 5 x 5 cm; 6th month 6 x 5; 7th month 7 x 5; 8th month 8 x 5; 9th month 9 x 5 and 10th month 10 x 5 cm).

**Weight Development.** Weight gain is minimal during the first half of pregnancy and increases sharply only in the second half. The weight increase in the last third of pregnancy is accompanied by the development of subcutaneous fat and amounts to about 700 g per month.

**Development of Body Form (Inset).** At the end of the embryonic period, the C.R. length is 3 cm. It then increases steeply, reaching a length of 15 cm in the 20th week. The head straightens, the cervical flexure is adjusted, and the body loses its cuboid form. The differentiation of the brain is apparent from the size of the head. The head is as large as the trunk and in the 20th week of pregnancy, still comprises 50% of the C.R. length.

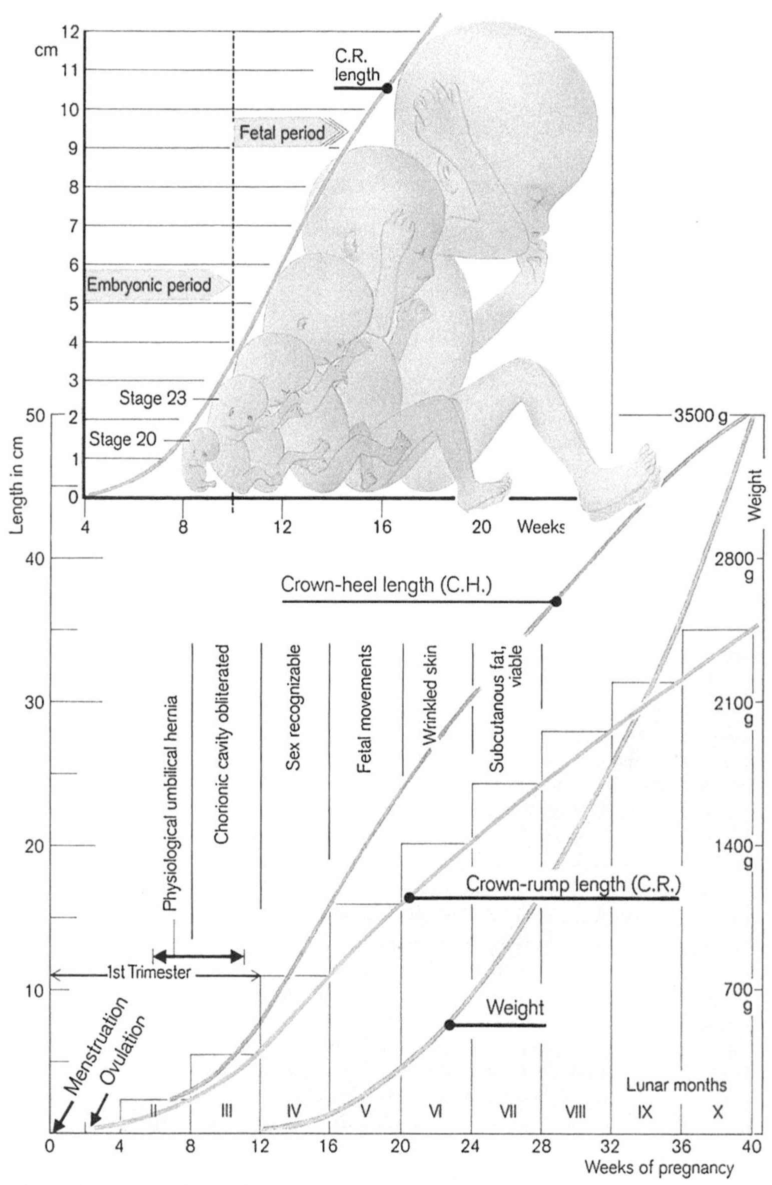


A. Growth curves in the fetal period

## 2.34 10th Week of Pregnancy: Situs

### A. 30 mm Fetus, Dissected Preparation (Blechschmidt)

#### 1. View into Lateral Ventricles and of the Body Wall

**Brain.** The lateral ventricles of the brain are opened horizontally. On account of the still pronounced bending of the head, the section lies in the frontal plane relative to the body axis. In the anterior horn of the ventricle, the lumen of the *olfactory bulb* (**1**) can be seen exiting from the ventricle. The *corpus callosum* (**2**) arises in the U shaped border between the two hemispheres. Beneath it lies the *interventricular foramen* (**3** ). The ventricular lumen is almost completely filled by the *choroid plexus* (**4**). The thinly streched roof of the *diencephalon* (**5**) is shown as a transparent lamella; at the posterior end lies the *pineal gland* (epiphysis) (**6**). The *mesencephalon* (**7**) still extends further past the cephalic flexure than the cerebral vesicles. The bulges of the quadrigeminal bodies are not yet visible. The choroid plexus has been removed on the left side so that the *fusion zone* (**8**) between the medial wall of the lateral ventricle and the wall of the diencephalon is visible. The bulge of the basal ganglia is prominent at the floor of the lateral ventricle. The *caudate nucleus* (**9**) passes into the temporal, following the rotation of the hemispheres. The medial wall of the hemisphere sinks inward to become the *insula* (**10**).

**Body Wall.** The ribs are shown on the right side, the musculature of the thoracic wall on the left (**11**). The rectal musculature with its *tendinous intersections* has contracted above the liver. The dilatated *umbilical cord* (**12**) contains the convoluted small intestine, which is still outside the body cavity in the *physiological umbilical hernia*.

#### 2. View of Thorax and Abdomen

**Thoracic View.** The thoracic wall is removed, as well as the thymus, heart, liver,and diaphragm, revealing the *trachea* (**2**) and lobed *lungs* (**1**). The *vagus nerve* (**3**) descends into the mediastinum lateral to the trachea and the esophagus. On the left side, the recurrent nerve loops around the *arch of the aorta* (**4**) and the *ductus arteriosus* (**5**), so that after the obliteration of the ductus, the nerve lies lateral to the ligamentum arteriosum. Because of the rotation of the stomach, the left main stem of the vagus is shifted to the ventral side of the *esophagus* and the right stem to the dorsal side.

**Abdominal View.** The umbilical loop was removed together with the liver so that only the stumps of the *duodenojejunal flexure* (**9** ) and the *rectum* (**15**) are visible. Except for the *stomach* (**7**), all depicted organs, including the duodenum and *pancreas* (**8**), later lie retroperitoneally. The bulges of the *ovary* (**10**), *mesonephros* (**11**), and the *genital ducts* (**12**) occupy the V-shaped folds that meet in front of the rectum. The *caudal mesonephric band* (**13**), originating from the lower end of the mesonephric swelling, extends ventrally into the inguinal canal (which was removed with the body wall). In the female, as in this case, it becomes the ligamentum teres of the uterus; in the male it forms the gubernaculum testis ( 8.7). At this stage, the *phallus* (**14**) in the female fetus is also relatively large. On the right side, above the ovary and mesonephros, the peritoneal covering of the dorsal body wall has been removed, exposing the right *metanephros* (**16**) and the large *adrenal gland* (**17**). The large size of the fetal adrenal gland is related to the involvement of the adrenal cortex in the metabolism of steroid hormones, which is greatly increased during pregnancy (→ 1.17).

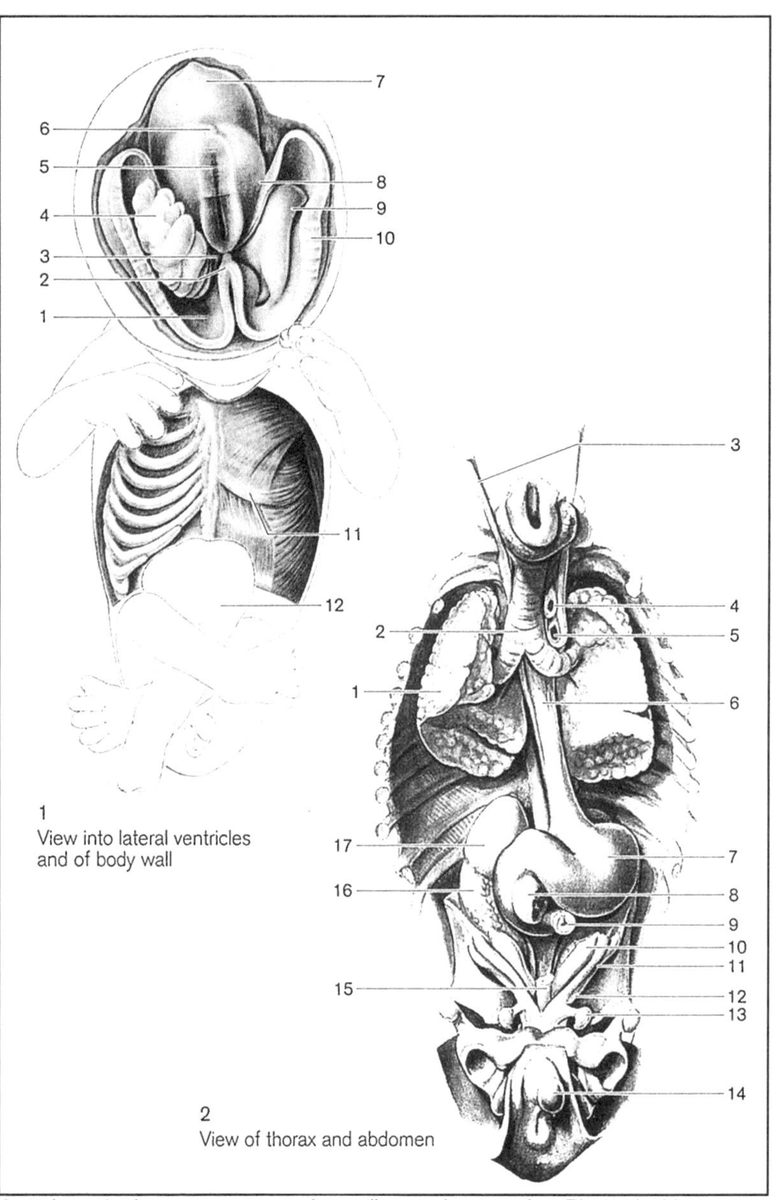


A. 10th week of pregnancy: 30 mm fetus, dissected preparation, Blechschmidt

# 2.35 12th Week of Pregnancy: Ossification Centers

## A. Cartilage Skeleton and Ossification Centers

### 1. Cartilage skeleton of a 40 mm C.R. Fetus (Blechschmidt)

**Skull.** The base of the skull consists of the primordia of the *occipital bone* (**1**), *otic capsule* (**2**), *sphenoid bone* (**3**), and *nasal capsule* (**4**). According to Blechschmidt, mechanical tension zones (dural belts, **5**) that develop in the connective tissue covering of the brain determine the growth of the membrane bones. Venous plexuses between the dural belts fuse to form the *sagittal sinus* (**6**) and the *confluence of the sinuses* (**7**). The visceral skeleton consists of the cartilage of the lower jaw (*Meckel's cartilage* , **8**); its upper end is attached to the *hammer* (**9**), which in turn articulates with the *anvil* (**10**) in the primary temporomandibular joint.

**Trunk.** The funnel-shaped thorax is filled by the *lungs* (**11**) and the *dome of the diaphragm* (**12**), below which lies the large *liver* (**13**). The *intestinal loops* (**14**) have returned into the body cavity. Below them lie the *urogenital sinus* (**15**) and the *rectum* (**16**).

The cartilage models of the *vertebral arches* (**17**), *ribs*, and *vertebral bodies* (**19**) are still continuous with each other and lack joints. The vertebral arches of the cervical vertebral column are still open (**1b**).

### 2. Ossification Centers

In translucent (cleared) embryos, bony trabeculae can be stained with alizarin red. In the illustrations, the hyaline cartilage models are indicated by white outlines and the ossification zones are filled in with black.

**Cranium.** The finely ramified bony trabeculae in the cranium indicate **intramembranous ossification** of the membrane bones. The membranous cranium is composed of the *frontal bone* (**1**), *parietal bones* (**2**) and the *occipital squama* (**3**) (an extension of the cartilaginous skull base), and the squamous portion of the *temporal bone* (**4**).

**Visceral Skeleton.** The phylogenetically recent membranous portions of the facial skeleton (*nasal bone*, **5**; *maxilla*, **6**) are inserted as a wedge-like zone between the base of the skull and the original cartilaginous visceral skeleton formed by the pharyngeal arches (→9.3). As the *mandible* (**7**) ossifies, a bony lamella of membrane bone is formed over Meckel's cartilage. Only the tip of Meckel's cartilage, in the region of the future chin, develops an endochondral ossification center; the remaining cartilaginous rod desintegrates. The *secondary jaw articulation* (**8**) develops between intramembranously ossified bones. An endochondral ossification center appears in the cartilage model of the *hammer* (**9**).

**Vertebral Column and Ribs.** The elements of the axial skeleton develop as hyaline cartilage models, which secondarily ossify by endochondral ossification (→3.32). **Endochondral ossification** is characterized by the sprouting of blood vessels into the cartilage models and the formation of ossification centers. Sharply defined ossification centers are formed in the spinous processes of *vertebrae* (**10**), *ribs*, (**11**) and the *vertebral bodies* (**12**).

**Appendicular Skeleton.** Ossification of the long tubular bones begins in the 8th week of pregnancy, when compact perichondral bone is deposited around the cartilage models and centers of ossification form within the diaphysis (**2a** , **13**).

The ossification centers in the epiphyses of long tubular bones do not appear until the 32nd week of pregnancy. In the short tubular bones, they first appear only after birth. The hyaline cartilage of the cartilage models between the *central ossification centers* (**2b**, **13**) and the *ossification center in the epiphysis* (**2b**, **14**) gives rise to a growth zone known as the *epiphysial plate* (**2b**, **15**). Longitudinal growth ends with the ossification of the epiphysial plate at puberty.

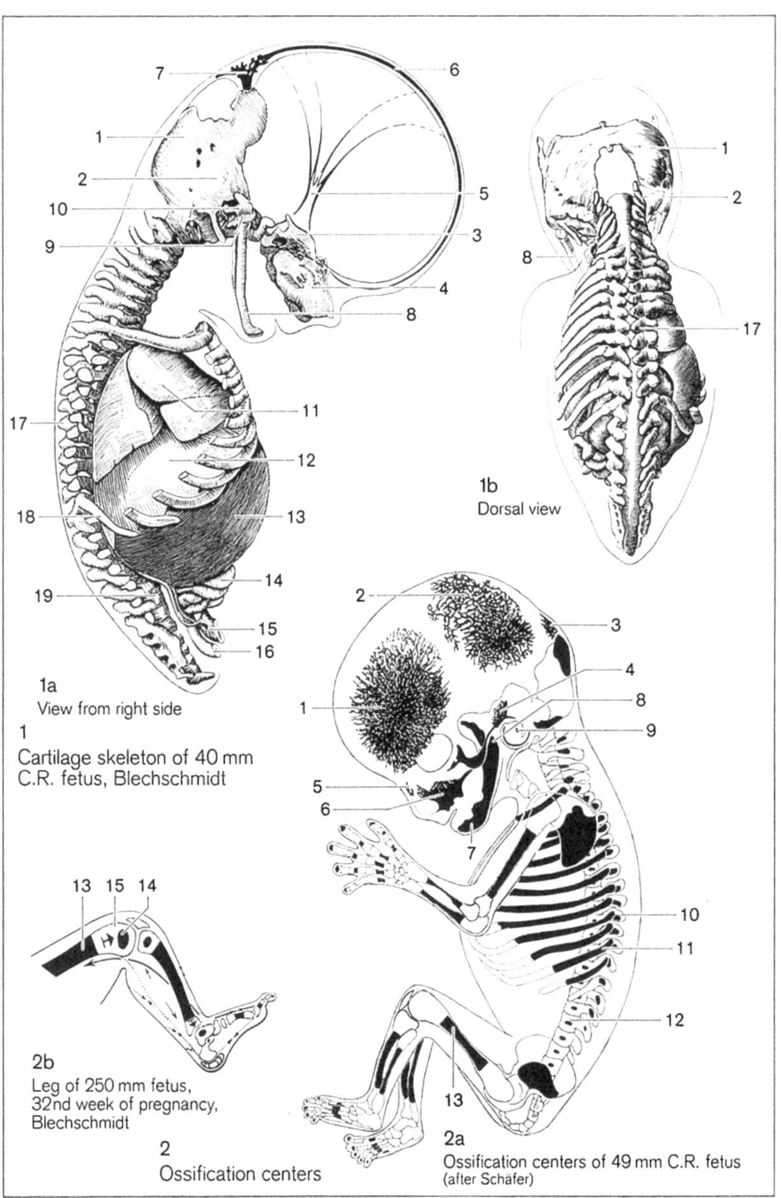


A. 12th week of pregnancy: Cartilage skeleton and ossification centers

## 2.36 14th Week of Pregnancy: Sagittal Section

### A. Sagittal section of 60 mm Fetus, Tonutti Collection

The sagittal section through the right half of the body (part of a histological series) was stained with HOPA (hematoxylin, orange G, phosphomolybdic acid, and aniline blue, after Tonutti).

**Head.** In the right lateral ventricle the *matrix zone* (**1**) of the neuroepithelium, is still thick and can be distinguished from the delicate *cortical plate* (**2**) (→4.17). Beneath the anterior horn of the ventricle, one can see an outpocketing of the ventricle into the exit of the *olfactory bulb* (**6**). Basally, the hillock of the *basal ganglia* (**4**) and the *thalamus* (**5**) form bulges. The *choroid plexus* (**3**) spreads cloud-shaped into the interior of the ventricle. Below the primitive *tentorium* (**28**) lie the *cerebellar swelling* (**31**) and the *rhomboid fossa* (**32**) and the 4th ventricle, into which the choroid plexus invaginates. The brainstem is surrounded by a wide, empty looking *arachnoid space* (**30**), in which several blood-filled vessels can be seen. This area is bounded by the more highly condensed tissue of the *dura mater* (**29**), which becomes compressed into the *tentorium cerebelli* (**28**), between the telencephalon and cerebellum. In the triangular, looser tissue region of the tentorium, the venous plexuses merge to form the transverse sinus. The tentorium cerebelli extends to the otic capsule as a thin layer of tissue. The base of the skull is formed by the endochondrally ossifying part of the *occipital bone* (**33**), by the *otic capsule* (**34**) (in which the semicircular canals are sectioned), by the cartilage model of the *sphenoid bone* (**8**), and by the *trabeculae cranii* (**7**) (sectioned in front). Between the primordia of the wings of the sphenoid, the *optic nerve* (**9**) and the *ocular musculature* appear in cross-section (**10**). Membranous ossification of the cranium begins at the apex of the occipital squama and in the frontal bone. In the visceral skeleton, membranous ossification is visible in the *maxillary process* (**11**) and in the tip of the *mandible* (**12**). The musculature of the floor mouth is between the cartilaginous *hyoid bone* (**13**) and the mandible.

**Neck.** Between the laterally sectioned cartilaginous vertebral elements, the *spinal ganglia* (**35**) and the *vertebral artery* can be seen. In front of the prevertebral musculature lie the vagus (**16**), the *carotid artery* (**15**), the *jugular vein* (**17**), the right lobe of the *thyroid gland* (**14**), and the pretracheal musculature.

**Thoracic Space.** In the right *lung* (**21**), one can recognize the branchings of the bronchial tree and the divisions of the lung segments. In front of the lung is the *right atrium* (**22**) and above it the stem of the *superior vena cava* (**20**) and a tip of the left lung. The ribs and *sternum* (**19**) are still cartilaginous. Endochondral ossification begins in the head of the *clavicle* (**18**).

Above the clavicle and in front of the heart lie conspicuously dilated lymphatic spaces. The spontaneous abortion of this fetus may be linked to the striking hyperplasia of the lymph vessels.

**Abdominal Space.** Over half of the body cavity is filled by the large liver. Dorsally below the liver, lies the *kidney* (**37**) with sectioned *renal pelvis* (**38**) and the strikingly large fetal *adrenal gland* (**36**). The lower *lobe of the liver (caudate lobe)* (**25**) is delimited by the *gallbladder* (**24**) and by the bile duct, which is situated above it. Below it, the *duodenum* (**26**) and a series of *duodenal loops* (**27**) appear in cross section. At the level of the pelvis , the remains of the right *mesonephros* (**39**) and the right *ovary* (**40**), with its broad cortical zone, can be distinguished under higher magnification. On the hyaline cartilage model of the os ilium, ossification begins at the exterior (osseous shell). The still cartilaginous, round *head of the hip joint* (**41**) is inserted into the primordium of the pelvis.

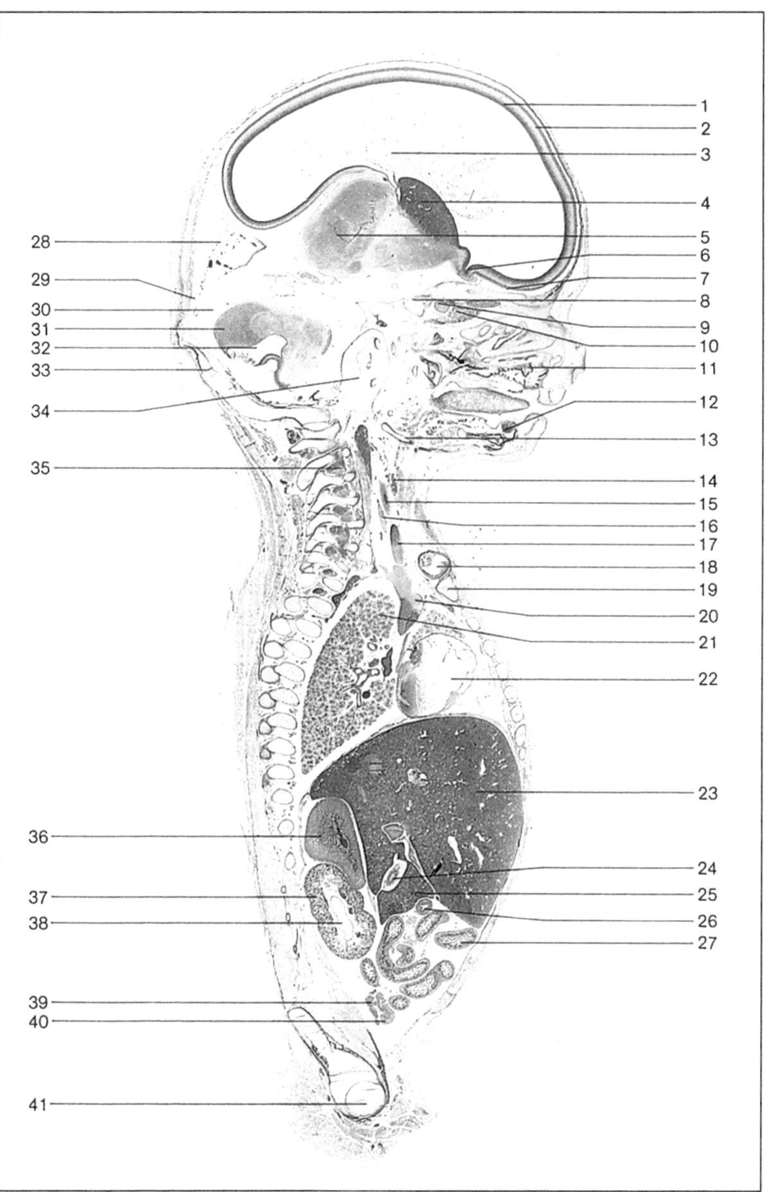


A. 14th week of pregnancy: sagittal section through right half of body, Tonutti collection

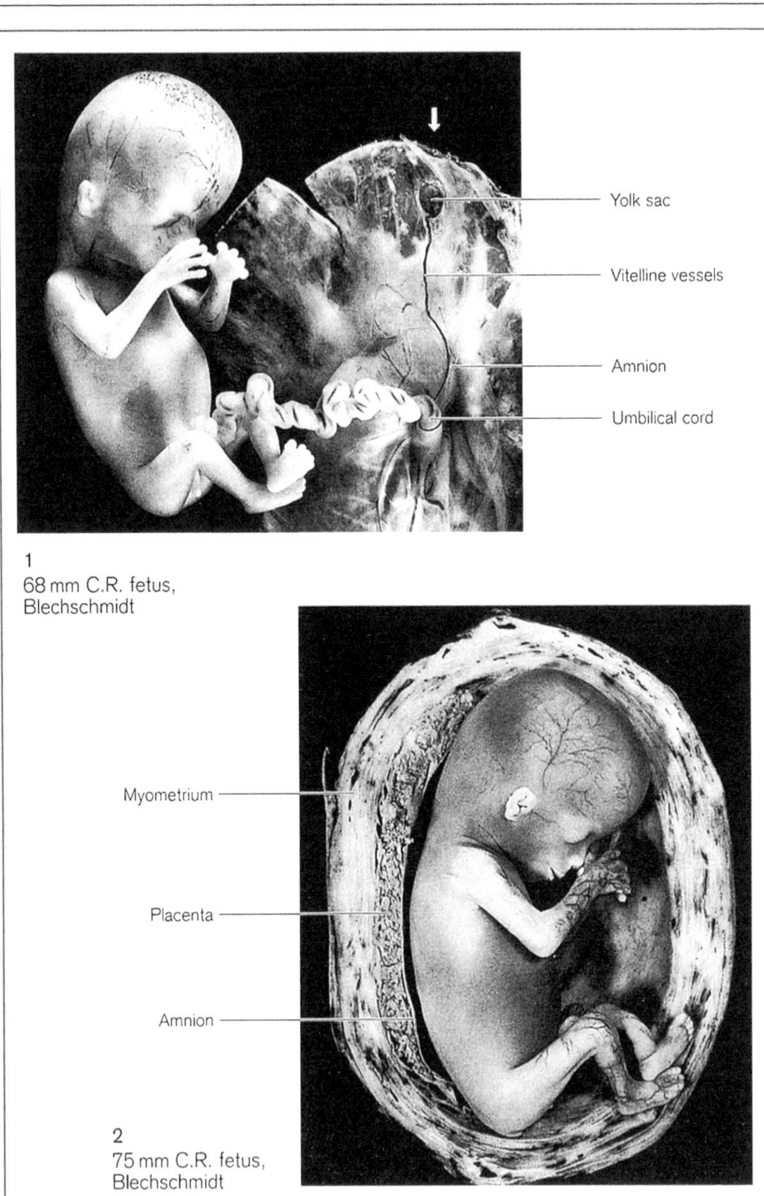


1
68 mm C.R. fetus,
Blechschmidt

2
75 mm C.R. fetus,
Blechschmidt

A. 16th week of pregnancy

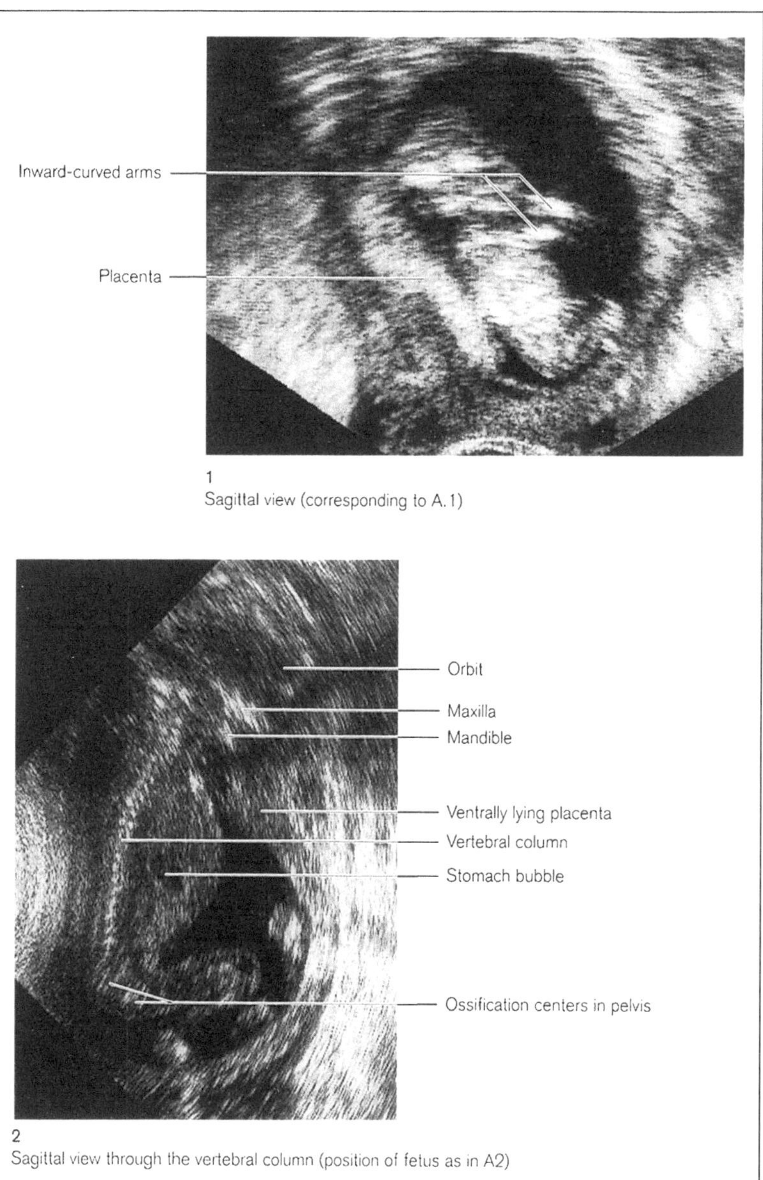


1
Sagittal view (corresponding to A.1)

2
Sagittal view through the vertebral column (position of fetus as in A2)

B. Endosonography at 16th weeks of pregnancy
Pictures were kindly provided by F. Degenhardt, Hannover

## 2.38 Newborn

### A. Skull of the Newborn Infant

In the human, the diameter of the skull at the time of birth is significantly larger than that of the remaining body, making the skull (**A2**) a physiological obstacle to birth. The enlargement of the skull is a consequence of the enlargement of the telencephalon. To facilitate the birth process, the cranial sutures and the fontanelles between the covering bones of the skull are not ossified (**A11**). During birth, these bones (particularly the parietal bones) can be pushed over one another, adjusting the head size to the birth canal.

**1. Fontanelles and Cranial Sutures.** The sagittal suture (**4**) lies between the *parietal bones* (**5**). Anteriorly, it merges into the *large fontanelle* (**6**), a rhomboid-shaped structure situated between the right and left primordia of the *frontal bone* (**8**). Laterally, the *coronal suture* (**7**) between the frontal and parietal bones also merges with the large fontanelle. Posteriorly, the sagittal suture ends in a *small fontanelle* (**3**) that extends into the *lambdoid suture* (**2**) between the parietal bones and the *occipital squama* (**1**). Between the parietal and frontal bones on the one side and the squama of the *temporal bone* (**12**) and the *greater wing of the sphenoid* (**10**) on the other side, lies the *anterolateral fontanelle* (**9**), and between the temporal bone and the occipital bone, the *posterolateral fontanelle* (**15**).

**2. Proportions of the Skeleton.** Because of the strongly bent condition of the head, the occiput and the sagittal suture (**4**) emerge first during parturition. The sagittal suture connecting the small and large fontanelle (**6**) assists the obstetrician in judging the position of the head in the birth canal. The facial skeleton is relatively small; the paranasal sinuses have not yet developed. Since the bulge of the mastoid process is still absent, the exit of the facial nerve (**A1**, **14**, *stylomastoid foramen*) lies close to the surface. The *facial nerve* can therefore be easily damaged by a forceps delivery.

The *external acoustic meatus* (**13**) is formed by an intramembranously ossifying ring (tympanic bone) that initially serves to suspend the eardrum (→ 5.10, D2). After birth, the tympanic ring becomes incorporated into the tube of the external acoustic meatus.

1 Occipital bone
2 Lambdoid suture
3 Small fontanelle
4 Direction of sagittal suture
5 Parietal bone
6 Large fontanelle
7 Coronal suture
8 Frontal bone
9 Anterolateral fontanelle
10 Greater wing of sphenoid
11 Zygomatic bone
12 Temporal bone
13 External acoustic meatus
14 Stylomastoid foramen
15 Posterolateral fontanelle

### B. Development of Body Proportions up to Birth

At the beginning of the fetal period (*10th gestational week*), the head takes up about half of the total C.R. length. The relative proportions do not change in the first half of pregnancy, although the legs grow longer. In the crown-heel (C.H.) measurement, the head, trunk, and legs take up a third of the total length.

During the second half of pregnancy (*24th gestational week*), the trunk and the legs increase more in length than the head. *At birth* the head thus accounts for a fourth of the total length (C.H.). The change in body proportions continues during childhood. In the adult, the head represents about one-seventh of the total body height.

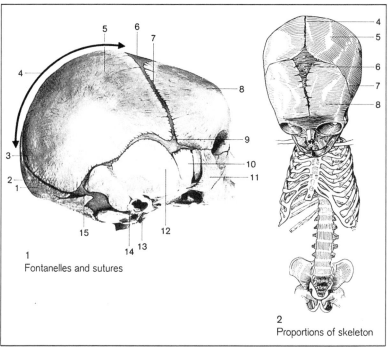

1
Fontanelles and sutures

2
Proportions of skeleton

A. Newborn skull

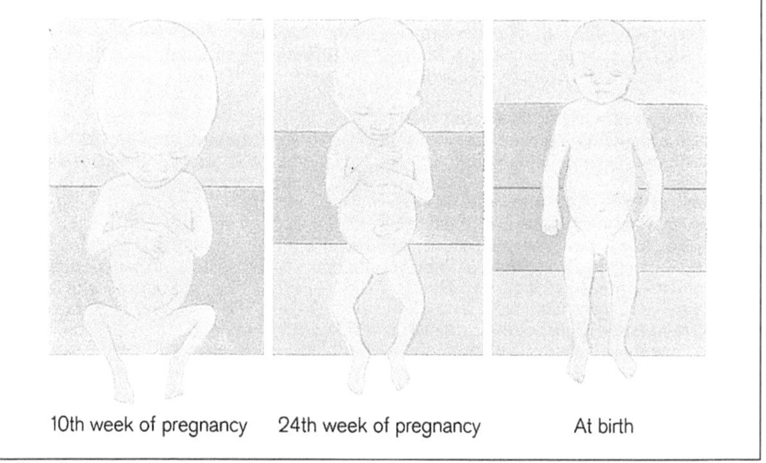


B. Development of body proportions up to birth

# Fetal Membranes and Placenta

## 2.39 Overview: Chorion and Chorionic Villi

*Background*

During **implantation** in the second week, the blastocyst initially secures the nourishment of the embryo with precocious differentiation of the chorion and the chorionic villi. During the **embryonic period,** the chorionic sac is completely covered by villi. In the **fetal period** (starting at 10 weeks of pregnancy), only the villi at the embryonic pole undergo further development and become part of the placenta. The remaining chorion loses its villi and, together with the amnion, forms the transparent fetal membranes (→ 2.42).

### A. Development of Chorionic Villi

**1. Compact Trophoblast.** During implantation in the second week, the trophoblastic cells actively invade the maternal mucosa. After the initial phase of rapid invasion and growth of the trophoblast cells in the inner zone form an epithelial structure, the *cytotrophoblast*. In the outer zone, the trophoblast cells fuse to multinucleated giant cells that unite into a *syncytium* (→ 2.6 A1 and 2.7 A1). Cell proliferation takes place only in the cytotrophoblast, with the cells becoming incorporated into the syncytium by cell fusion.

**2. Lacunae in the Syncytium.** Intercommunicating, irregular lacunae arise in the syncytium and become filled with fluid.

**3. Inflow of Maternal Blood and Formation of Trabeculae.** Maternal blood enters the lacunae from eroded branches of the spiral arteries and exits via opened venules. The blood-filled lacunae dilate, allowing the syncytial segments lying between them to be transformed into septa or, as seen in cross section, into *trabeculae* . The trabeculae are aligned radially, forming a spoke-like structure in cross sections of the trophoblast.

**4. Ingrowth of Cytotrophoblast.** The cytotrophoblast grows with cone-shaped extensions into the trabeculae of the syncytium. Simultaneously, the trophoblastic cavity is covered by chorionic mesoderm that arises as extraembryonic mesoderm at the posterior pole of the embryonic disc (→ 2.10) and spreads on the inner side of the cytotrophoblast. After the mesodermal lining has formed, the trophoblast is by definition transformed into the *chorion*. The trophoblast cavity becomes the *chorionic cavity*.

**5. Cytotrophoblastic Shell.** The cones from the cytotrophoblast advance forward to the decidual side and grow rapidly around the blastocyst inside of the *external syncytial layer*. The peripheral portions of the syncytium remain behind in the decidua as *syncytial residue*. The development of the *cytotrophoblastic shell* is essential for the anchorage of the embryo to the decidua. An incomplete cytotrophoblastic shell leads to defects in the formation of villi and can cause fetal loss.

**6. Penetration by Mesoderm and Blood Vessels.** Chorionic mesoderm grows from the chorionic cavity into the cytotrophoblastic core of the trophoblastic trabeculae, giving rise to *chorionic villi*. Only the external third of the trabeculae is preserved as a compact core of cytotrophoblast (*cytotrophoblastic column*). Beginning at stage 7, blood vessels appear in the mesoderm of the villi. Fetal blood circulates through these vessels when the embryonic circulation is established in stages 9 and 10, at the transition from the third to the fourth week (→ 2.10).

**7. Villous Tree and Anchor Villi**. Further chorionic villi sprout from the radial trabeculae (primary villi) and from the chorionic plate, branching out into the lacunae. The primary villi anchored between the chorionic plate and cytotrophoblastic shell are now termed *anchor villi* (stem villi). The branching villi (*villous trees*) float freely in the maternal blood that fills the lacunar spaces. If the fetus is lost (abortion), the anchor villi detach and the cytotrophoblastic shell remains behind in the mucosa (→ 2.41).

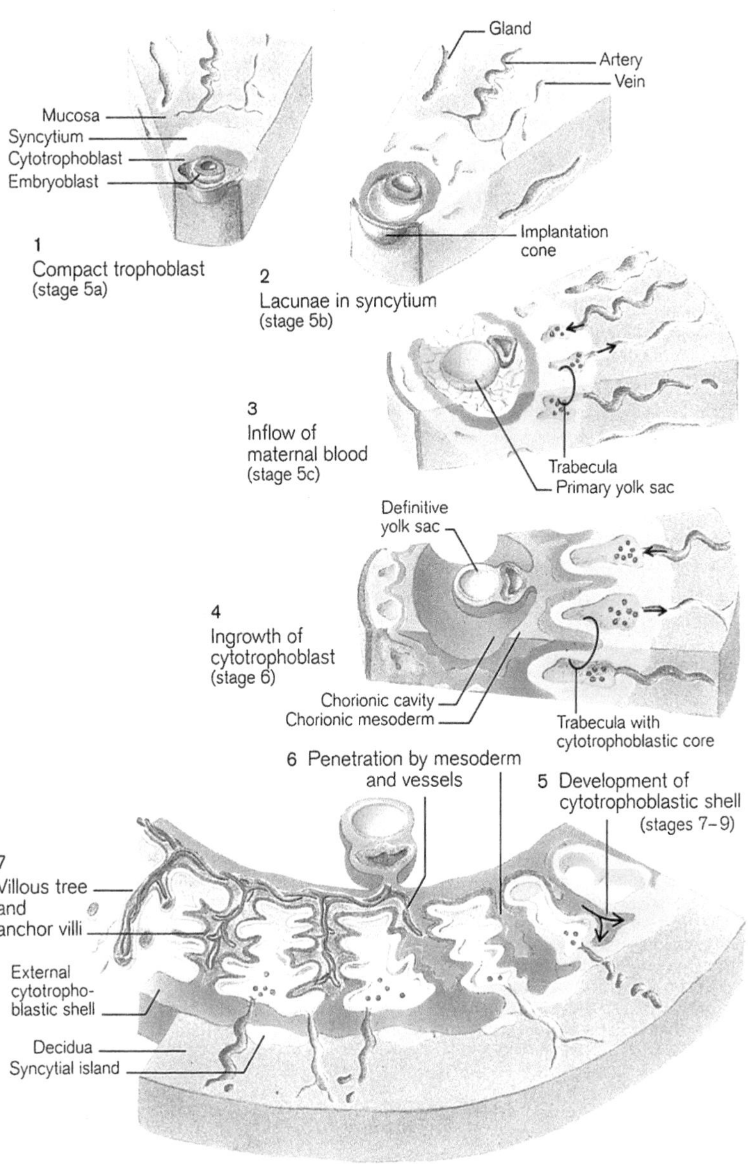
Mucosa
Syncytium
Cytotrophoblast
Embryoblast
1
Compact trophoblast
(stage 5a)
Gland
Artery
Vein
Implantation
cone
2
Lacunae in syncytium
(stage 5b)
3
Inflow of
maternal blood
(stage 5c)
Trabecula
Primary yolk sac
Definitive
yolk sac
4
Ingrowth of
cytotrophoblast
(stage 6)
Chorionic cavity
Chorionic mesoderm
Trabecula with
cytotrophoblastic core
6 Penetration by mesoderm
and vessels
5 Development of
cytotrophoblastic shell
(stages 7–9)
7
Villous tree
and
anchor villi
External
cytotropho-
blastic shell
Decidua
Syncytial island

A. Development of chorionic villi

## 2.40 Cytotrophoblastic Shell

*Background*

In stages 6 and 7, at the beginning of the "3rd week," the cytotrophoblast layer of the trophoblast grows outward through the syncytium, delimiting the blastocyst from the decidua. With the development of the **cytotrophoblastic shell**, implantation is complete. The invasive growth of the trophoblast is arrested by the outer cytotrophoblastic shell. The implant remains confined to the zona compacta of the endomentrium and grows only by displacement (→ 3.15).

### A. Development of Cytotrophoblastic Shell

**1. Segment of the Wall of the Chorionic Sac.**

**Chorionic Plate.** The chorionic plate consists of *extraembryonic mesoderm*, a *cytotrophoblastic layer*, and a *syncytial layer* that lines the *lacunae*, filled with *maternal blood*. The mesoderm of the *chorionic plate* lines the *chorionic cavity* without an epithelial covering.

**Basal Plate.** The basal plate is formed by the *syncytium*, the *cytotrophoblastic shell*, and the surrounding *decidua*. The stem villi are anchored in the basal plate on the maternal side via compact *cytotrophoblastic columns*. Fetal mesoderm does not penetrate further into these columns, which are preserved into the fetal period.

The cytotrophoblastic cells of the columns connect to each other laterally, forming the *cytotrophoblastic shell*, which borders the maternal tissue. As the cytotrophoblastic cells grow into the syncytium, they divide the external syncytial layer into a continuous inner layer that lines the lacunae and into an external portion consisting of individual *syncytial remnants*. These fragments extend from the syncytium further into the decidua as islands, cords, and fingers.

The *decidua* is edematously swollen at the implantation site. The interstitial spaces are large (→ decidual reaction, 2.6 implantation). Many decidual cells die, giving rise to tissue regions filled with disintegrating cells. Parts of the decidua are enveloped and subsequently resorbed by the syncytium and by the advancing cytotrophoblastic cells. Many of the tissue gaps in the decidua communicate with dilated maternal vessels and with the lacunae. In some gaps, fibrin deposits exist, which are preserved during later stages (**Nitabuch's membrane**).

Alarge number of multinucleated syncytial cells advance by amoeboid movement far into the decidua, up to the venules of the uterine musculature. This infiltration of maternal tissue with fetal *giant cells* is thought to play a role in the inactivation of the maternal immune system, by which the rejection of the fetus is prevented. After the trophoblastic shell has developed, this infiltration process continues with syncytial giant cells that detach from the villi and are washed into the maternal circulation (syncytial knots → 2.41).

**2. Section through the Implantation Site.** To indicate the direction of penetration of the blastocyst, the uterine epithelium is oriented upward and the developing *embryo* (with the *yolk sac* and *amniotic cavity*) downward. Extraembryonic mesoderm has lined the blastocyst cavity, completing the formation of the chorion and the conversion of the blastocyst cavity into the chorionic cavity. The mesoderm penetrates the villi, which are still devoid of capillaries. After the cytotrophoblastic shell has formed, the invasive growth of the blastocyst ceases and the further embryonic growth occurs by expansion of the chorion. As the chorion enlarges, it displaces the maternal *glands* ascending from the *zona spongiosa*.

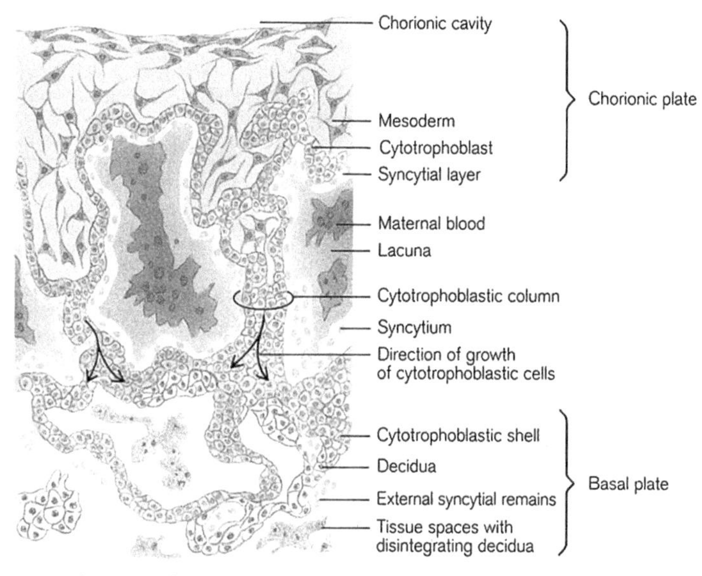


1
Segment of the wall of the chorionic sac of the "Nissen embryo"

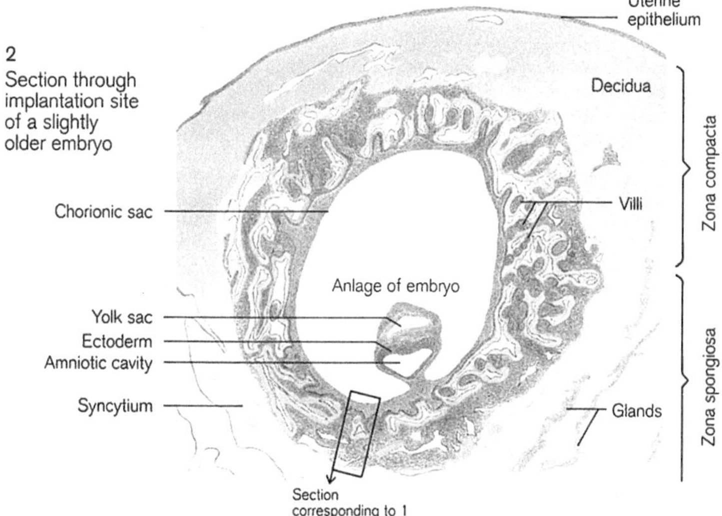


2
Section through implantation site of a slightly older embryo

A. Development of the cytotrophoblastic shell at stage 7

## 2.41 Differentiation of Chorionic Villi

*Background*

Until the villi differentiate and the placental circulation begins, the trophoblast takes up nutrients from the decidua by enzymatic digestion of tissue and by **phagocytosis**.

The fully differentiated villi function in **resorption** of nutrients (later taken over by villi in the small intestine), in **excretion** of metabolic end products (later taken over by the kidneys), and in **respiration** (later taken over by the lungs).

During **differentiation,** the villi increase in number and branch extensively. The syncytial layer forms a brush border at the surface. The cytotrophoblastic layer (Langhans cells) disintergrates, thus improving the diffusion path in the terminal ramifications of the villi.

### A. Differentiation of Chorionic Villi in the 4th Week

**1. Isolated Chorionic Sac.** Aborted specimen, beginning of the 4th week. With the detachment of the embryo, the stem villi were released from the cytotrophoblastic shell in the uterine mucosa. The chorionic sac is covered by free villi and would have been filled with fluid in the undamaged condition. The 8-somite embryo (stage 11) is visible through a hole in the chorion.

**2. Chorionic Villi in the 4th Week.** Villi with many delicate branchlets sprout from the *stem villi* and the chorionic plate, representing the functioning villous tissue. The stem villi are anchored via the *cytotrophoblastic columns* to the *cytotrophoblastic shell*, which has grown into a compact epithelial structure with up to 10 cell layers. It is now increasingly difficult to distinguish between fetal cytotrophoblastic cells and maternal decidual cells with histological stains. Fetal vessels coursing in the stem villi supply the villous capillaries in the villous branchlets.

**Syncytial Knots.** In some areas, the syncytium exhibits undifferentiated, multinucleated segments that bulge into the intervillous spaces. These sites give rise to new *villous sprouts*, or represent *syncytial bridges* that link adjacent villi with one another. The protruding areas of the syncytium (syncytial knots) may also detach and become washed out into the maternal circulation as *giant cells* . Such cells can be found, for example, in the pulmonary capillaries of the mother. They disintegrate without adverse immune reaction.

**Primary, Secondary, and Tertiary Villi.** On the basis of their histological structure in transverse sections, three stages can be distinguished in the development of villi.

**a Primary Villus.** The villus consists of a compact cytotrophoblastic core with a syncytial covering.

**b Secondary Villus.** Extraembryonic mesoderm has penetrated into the cytotrophoblastic core.

**c Tertiary Villus.** Capillaries have developed within the mesoderm.

**Section Detail: Differentiation of the Trophoblastic Layer.** The syncytium and cytotrophoblast, the epithelial components of the villus, share a common basement membrane (**2c**). The **cytotrophoblastic cells** form a single layer of cuboidal cells (Langhans cell layer), connected to each other and to the syncytium by desmosomes. The cytoplasm of the cytotrophoblastic cells is only slightly differentiated and resembles that of basal cells in stratified epithelia. In the terminal branchings of the villi, the Langhans cell layer recedes, and fetal capillaries are directly apposed to the syncytium. The **syncytium** is the differentiated cell layer. It is stretched into a thin, homogeneous surface with individual cell nuclei lying far apart. The syncytium possesses a brush border and is densely filled with dilated endoplasmic reticulum and vesicles.

Photograph A1 from Boyd, Hamilton: The Human Placenta

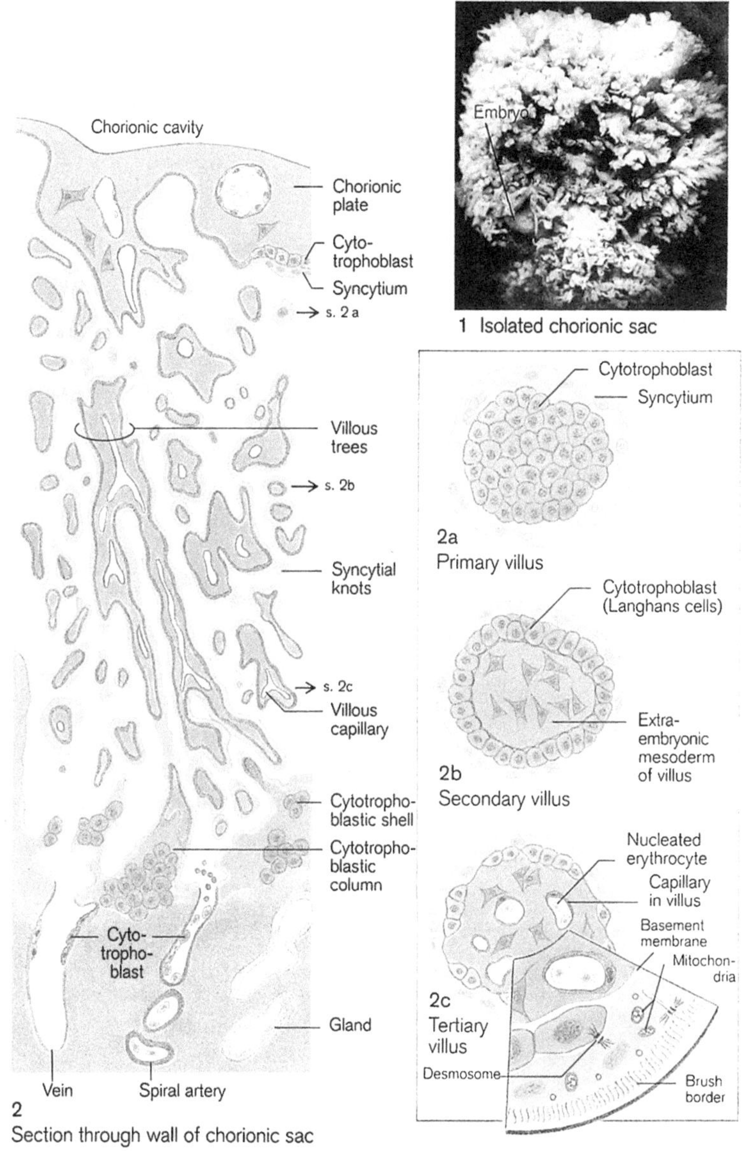


1 Isolated chorionic sac

2a
Primary villus

2b
Secondary villus

2c
Tertiary villus

2
Section through wall of chorionic sac

A. Differentiation of chorionic villi in the 4th week

## 2.42 Overview: Placenta and Fetal Membranes

*Background*

**Formation of the Placenta.** In the fetal period, the chorionic villi enlarge and condense at the embryonic pole of the chorionic sac, i.e., the pole at which the umbilical cord inserts into the chorionic plate. Due to the mode of implantation (→ 2.40) the embryonic pole is directed toward the uterine wall. At the abembryonic pole, which is directed toward the uterine lumen, the villi disappear. This region gives rise to the transparent fetal membranes (amnion and the smooth chorion).

### A. Development of Placenta and Fetal Membranes

**1. Chorionic Baldness.** Up to the end of the embryonic period, the chorionic sac is completely covered by villi. The villi at the embryonic pole of the chorion undergo further growth and branching (*chorion frondosum*, bushy chorion), whereas the villi at the abembryonic pole beneath the decidua capsularis thin out (bald chorion) and disappear completely by about the 10th week of pregnancy, giving rise to the smooth chorion (*chorion laeve*).

**2. Uterus and Placenta**

**a In the 10th Week of Pregnancy.**

**Obliteration of Chorionic Cavity.** At the end of the embryonic period, the amniotic cavity expands at the expense of the chorionic cavity (**2a**). The amnion then fuses with the chorion, and the chorionic cavity is obliterated. The yolk sac, squeezed between the chorion and amnion, is dissolved.

**Obliteration of Uterine Cavity.** The chorionic sac is embedded in the zona compacta of the endometrium. The implantation site bulges into the uterine lumen. The mucosal layer above the implant (*decidua capsularis*) ultimately fuses with the mucosa of the opposite uterine wall (*decidua parietalis*), so that the uterine cavity is obliterated.

**b In the 13th Week of Pregnancy.**

**Placenta.** The placenta is formed by the *chorionic plate*, to which the chorionic villi are attached, and by the *basal plate* bordering the *material tissue* (**2c**). The basal plate consists of the fetal cytotrophoblastic shell and the remaining decidua of the zona compacta of the endometrium. The thickness of the endometrium decreases and the glands recede. The maternal vessels multiply and enlarge beneath the placenta. At its margin the chorionic plate merges with the villus-free *chorion laeve*. The chorionic plate and the umbilical cord are covered by the amnion.

**Fetal Membranes.** The *amnion* and *chorion (laeve)* form a delicate transparent covering around the fetus floating in the amniotic fluid.

**Section detail:** The *amnion* consists of a single layer of flat amniotic epithelial cells and a thin layer of extraembryonic *amniotic mesoderm* (investing mesoderm, → 2.16). As the chorionic cavity is obliterated, the amniotic mesoderm fuses with the *chorionic mesoderm* bordering the chorionic cavity. (The chorionic cavity has no epithelial covering.) Surrounding the chorionic mesoderm are *fragments of the syncytium and trophoblast* derived from the degenerated intervillous spaces of the chorion laeve. These remnants in turn are surrounded by the *decidua capsularis*, which fuses with the decidua parietalis after degeneration of the *uterine epithelium*.

**c Toward the End of Pregnancy.**

The **placenta** grows in proportion to the growth of the fetus and the uterus. During the entire fetal period, it occupies about 25–30% of the inner surface of the uterus. Its increase in thickness occurs by ramification and multiplication of existing villi and not by further penetration into the maternal tissue.

**Fetal Membranes.** The trophoblast of the chorion laeve regresses completely, causing the chorionic mesoderm to directly appose the maternal decidua. The amnion possesses no blood vessels. The vessels radiating into the fetal membranes lie in the chorionic mesoderm.

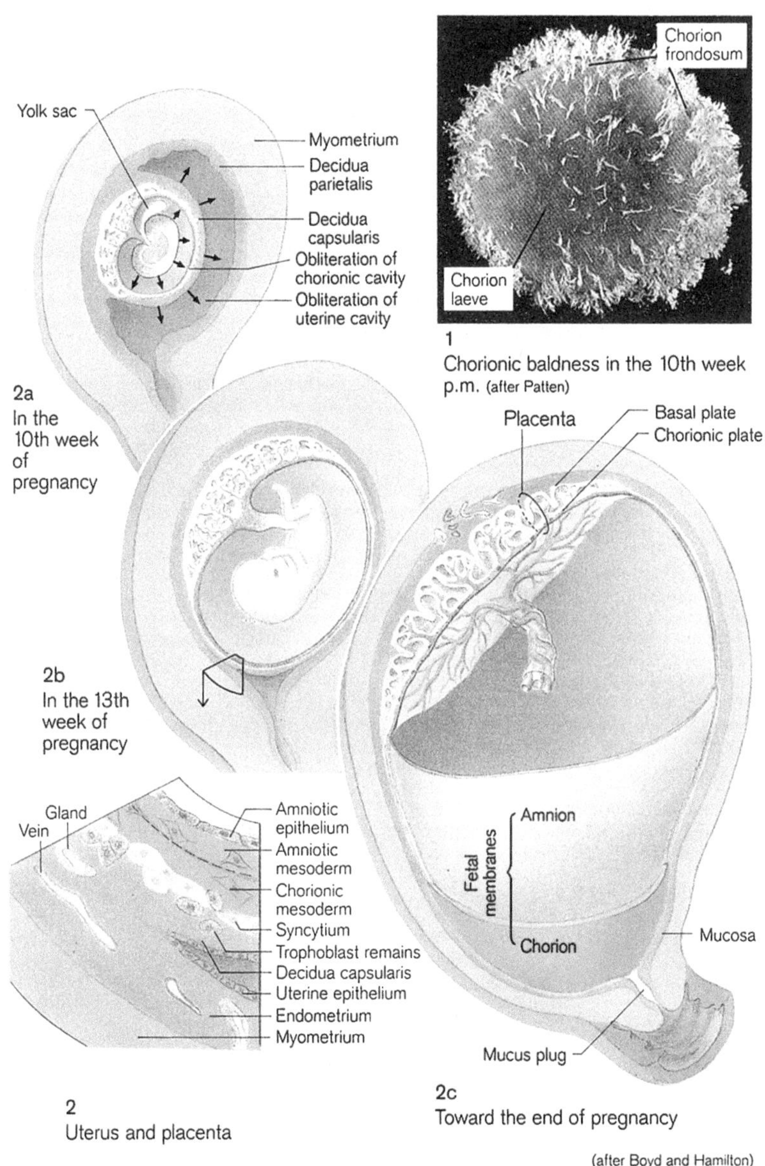


1
Chorionic baldness in the 10th week p.m. (after Patten)

2a
In the 10th week of pregnancy

2b
In the 13th week of pregnancy

2
Uterus and placenta

2c
Toward the end of pregnancy

(after Boyd and Hamilton)

A. Development of placenta and fetal membranes

# 2.43 Structure of the Placenta

## A. Functional Structure of the Placenta

### 1. Placental Villi

The villus is composed of a connective tissue core with blood vessels. It is surrounded by a single cytotrophoblastic layer, which in turn is covered by the syncytium. The surface of the syncytium possesses microvilli (brush border). The stem villi are attached to the basal plate via cytotrophoblastic columns that are also covered by syncytium. The basal plate consists of the cytotrophoblastic shell and the decidual cells of the zona compacta.

**a Cross Sections of Villi after the 4th Month.** In the second half of pregnancy, the *cytotrophoblastic layer* beneath the *syncytium* of the villi disappears, thus eliminating one of the diffusion barriers between fetal capillaries and maternal blood. Many of the capillaries of the villi are in direct contact with the syncytium so that at these sites, the fetal connective tissue is also eliminated as a diffusion barrier. At the same time, the villous branchlets undergo further branching and ramification and thus increase the exchange surfaces. The syncytium is transformed into an epithelial layer with a brush border (→ 2.15) and becomes specialized for resorption and secretion. Only few undifferentiated, multinucleated nodes remain; these project into the intervillous spaces and can be washed out into the maternal circulation as *syncytial knots.*

**b Involution of Cytotrophoblastic Columns.** The cytotrophoblastic columns in the *stem villi* finally undergo involution, so that *fetal connective tissue* of the villi directly contacts the basal plate. Cytotrophoblastic cells and decidual cells intermingle and are very difficult to distinguish histologically.

### 2. Cotyledon Structure

The placenta possesses a fetal and a maternal portion. The **fetal portion** consists of the chorionic plate and the chorionic villi projecting into the intervillous spaces filled with maternal blood, as well as the trophoblastic portion of the basal plate. The **maternal portion** consists of the decidua of the basal plate and the decidual septa, which divide the intervillous space into pot-shaped regions. The placental septa from the maternal decidua are covered by a layer of cytotrophoblastic cells and syncytium. The villous areas between the septa are called *cotyledons* and represent the functional unit of the placenta. Since the placental septa do not extend to the chorionic plate, connections exist between the intervillous spaces of adjacent cotyledons.

**a Vessels of the Villi.** On the fetal side, the oxygen-poor blood is pumped by the fetal heart through the two *umbilical arteries.* It passes through the capillaries of the villous branchlets and returns to the embryo through the *umbilical vein.* Because of the diffusion gradient relative to the maternal blood in the intervillous space, oxygen can be taken up, and soluble waste materials can be excreted.

**b Villous Trees.** The ramifications of the villous trees and stem villi are highly developed over the exit of the maternal spiral arteries and sparse in the region of the septa. From this observation it can be deduced that the outflow of oxygen-rich blood from the spiral arteries stimulates growth of the villi and thus has led to the organization of the placenta into cotyledons.

**c Spiral Arteries.** A *spiral artery* exits at the base of each cotyledon and discharges a stream of oxygen-rich arterial blood into the intervillous space of the cotyledon. The blood is squeezed laterally through the dense network of villi and flows back to the basal plate in the periphery of the cotyledon through the capillary spaces formed by the meshwork of villous branchlets. There it is taken up by irregularly distributed *venous openings* and returns into the maternal circulation.

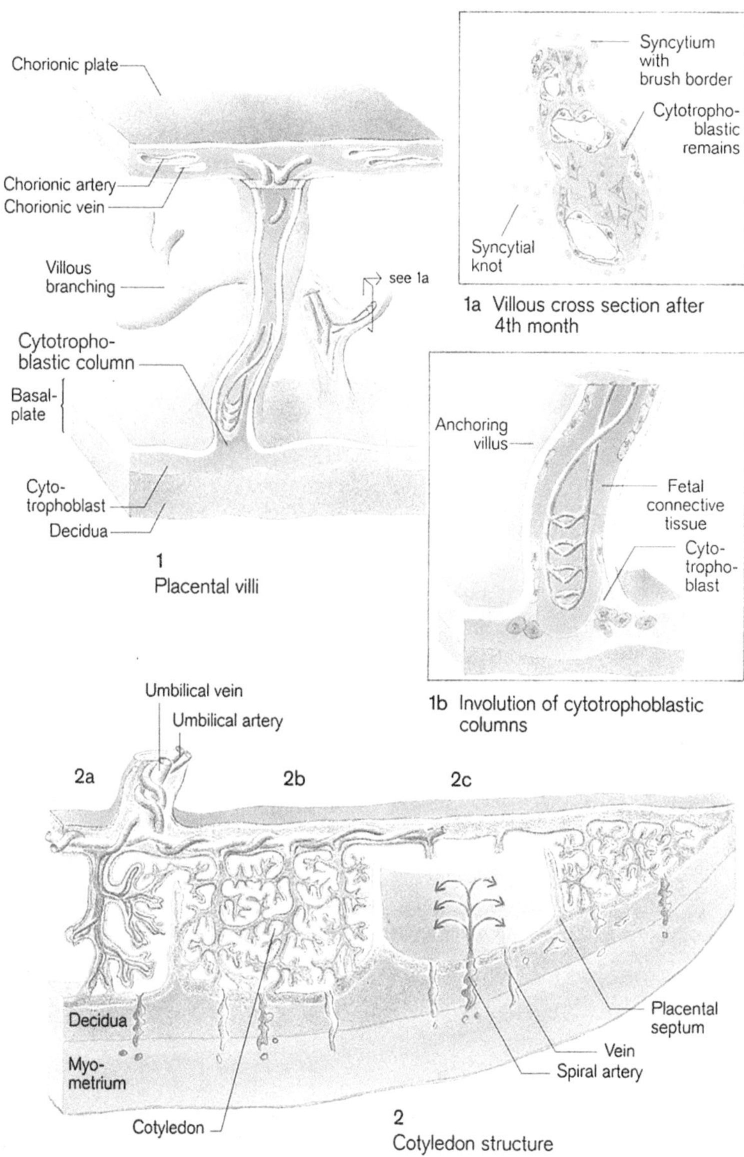
Chorionic plate
Chorionic artery
Chorionic vein
Villous branching
see 1a
Cytotropho-blastic column
Basal-plate
Cyto-trophoblast
Decidua
1
Placental villi
Syncytium with brush border
Cytotropho-blastic remains
Syncytial knot
1a Villous cross section after 4th month
Anchoring villus
Fetal connective tissue
Cyto-tropho-blast
1b Involution of cytotrophoblastic columns
Umbilical vein
Umbilical artery
2a
2b
2c
Decidua
Myo-metrium
Cotyledon
Placental septum
Vein
Spiral artery
2
Cotyledon structure

A. Functional structure of the placenta

## 2.44 Mature Placenta

*Background*

In the **mature placenta**, the villous trees are maximally extended and well supplied with blood. The fetal capillaries are separated from maternal blood only by the syncytial layer. Small hemorrhages, in which passage of fetal erythrocytes pass into the maternal circulation, are frequent. In the case of **Rh incompatibility**, such hemorrhages lead to sensitization of the mother, which in subsequent pregnancies can lead to hemolysis in the fetus.

### A. Section through the Mature Placenta with a Placental Septum

The *chorionic plate* of the fetal side consists of dense embryonic mesoderm and is covered by a thin layer of *amniotic epithelium*. A stem villus emerges from the chorionic plate and contacts the upper margin of the *placental septum* (decidual septum). The stem villus and the fine villous ramifications in the intervillous space are covered by the syncytium. The syncytium is continuous between the stem villus and the surface of the placental septum. The core of the placental septum consists of maternal *decidua* and still contains several dilated *glands*. Most of the septum consists of *fibrin deposits*. The cytotrophoblastic cells resemble the decidual cells in histological preparations and are difficult to distinguish. The situation is similar at the base of the anchor villi: dense fetal connective tissue merges into the cytotrophoblast and maternal decidua without a clear boundary.

Toward the end of pregnancy, the intervillous spaces contain approximately 150 mL of blood, which is renewed about 3–4 times per minute.

### B. Placental Detachment

About 30 minutes after childbirth, the placenta detaches and is expelled from the uterus as the **afterbirth.** The interruption of fetal circulation, and the decline in pressure on the fetal side lead to a hemorrhage below the basal plate, which induces the detachment of the placenta (→ 1.18). The illustration indicates the layer in which the detachment takes place. A part of the maternal decidua is expelled, together with the maternal portion of the *basal plate.*

### C. The Placenta after Birth

**1. Maternal side**

The expelled placenta is covered on the maternal side by the violet-colored decidua, through which the organization into cotyledons can be seen. The basal plate is opened in the drawing, providing a view of the villous branchlets and the placental septa that give the colyledons their structure.

**2. Fetal side**

On the fetal side, the placenta is covered by the amnion. The fetal blood vessels in the chorionic plate converge at the insertion site of the umbilical cord, which is generally inserted centrally.

After expulsion, the placenta and the fetal membranes (afterbirth) must be examined to ensure that they are complete. Defects in the cotyledon structure indicate that villous tissue has remained behind in the uterus. This can lead to prolonged postpartum hemorrhage.

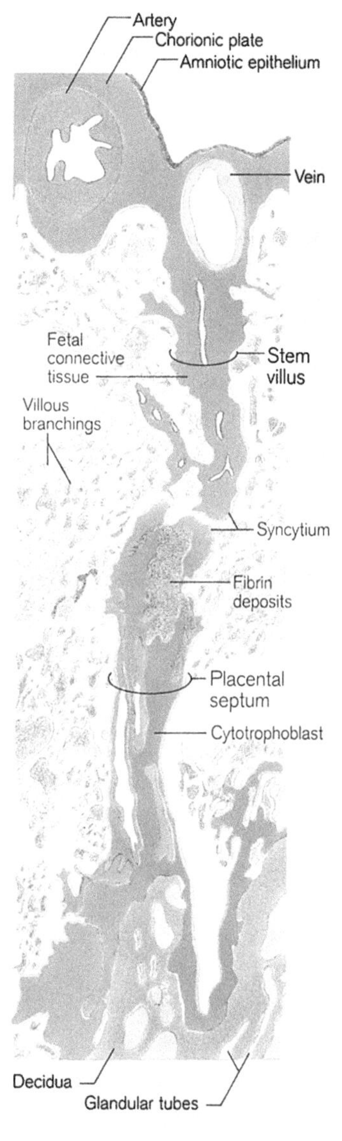


A. Section through the mature placenta

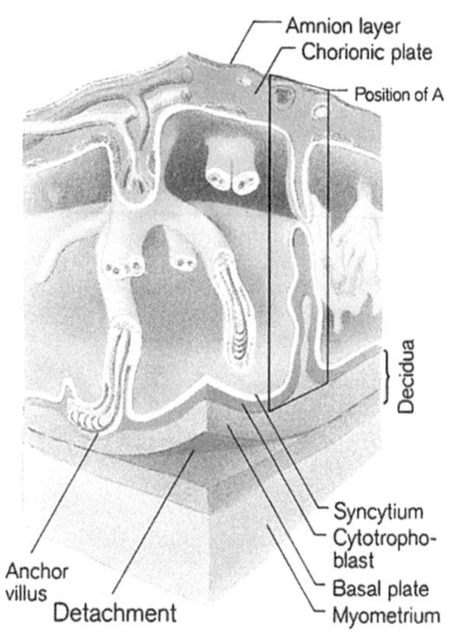


(after Tuchmann-Duplessis)

B. Placental detachment

1 Maternal side

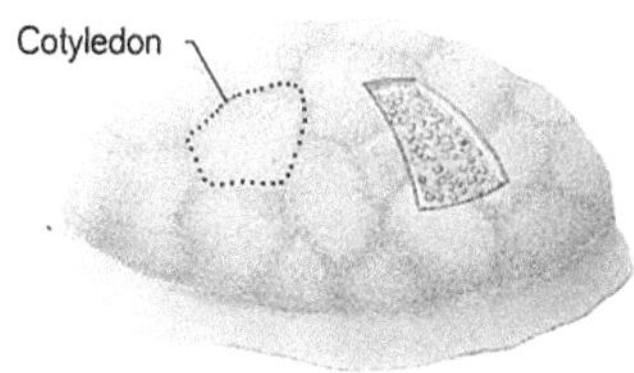


2 Fetal side

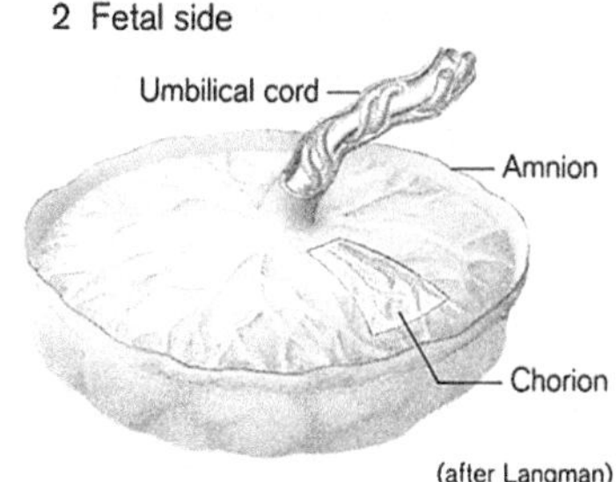


(after Langman)

C. Placenta after birth

## 2.45 Fetal Membranes in Twins

*Background*

**Fetal Membranes in Twins.** Inspection of the fetal membranes after birth allows monozygotic (identical) twins to be diagnosed by the presence of a common chorion or a common amnion and chorion.

Slightly more than 1% of all births are twins. Of these, about 70% are dizygotic and about 30% are monozygotic.

### A. Dizygotic Twins

If several oocytes are released at ovulation, they can be simultaneously fertilized and implanted in the uterus. In the case of twins or triplets, two or more equivalent follicles develop during the ovarian cycle instead of only one dominant follicle. The age and genetic constitution of the mother are important factors influencing multiple pregnancies.

**Fusion of Placentas.** Dizygotic twins are implanted separately in the uterus. Thus, each embryo forms its own amnion, its own chorionic coverings, and its own placenta. The placentas can, however, fuse with one another. When chorionic vessels thereby fuse in this process, fetal blood cells can be exchanged between the twins (erythrocyte mosaicism). In all other respects, dizygotic twins are not different from normal brothers and sisters.

**Multiple Artificially Induced Ovulations.** Hormone administration used to induce ovulation during treatment for infertility can induce ovulation, not only of the dominant follicles, but also of all other maturing tertiary follicles (→ 1.11). In this way, a multiple pregnancy can arise.

### B. Monozygotic Twins

Monozygotic (genetically identical) twins develop from a single fertilized oocyte. During early development, the cells of the zygote or the inner cell mass divide into two embryonic anlagen from which separate embryos are formed. The development of fetal membranes depends on the time at which the two embryos separate. The mechanism of twin formation can be determined at birth by analysis of the fused fetal membranes.

**1. Separation in the Morula.** If separation takes place at the morula stage, two completely separated embryos arise, the fetal membranes of which are similar to those of dizygotic twins.

**2. Separation in the Blastocyst Stage.** A division of the inner cell mass in the blastocyst stage gives rise to twins with separate amniotic cavities, but with a common chorionic cavity and a common placenta.

**3. Separation after Formation of the Amniotic Cavity.** If the separation of the two embryos takes place in the germ layer stage after development of the amniotic cavity, two embryos arise with a common amniotic cavity, a common chorionic cavity, and a common placenta.

**Conjoined Twins.** If the division of the embryonic anlage is not complete, the twins may be fused with one another at different body regions (Siamese twins) or may possess unpaired, common body segments.

**Blood Supply of Twins.** Fusion of the placenta can lead to an unequal blood supply and thus to the development of a very small and a very large twin.

Separated
placentae
Embryoblast
Zygote
Morula
Blastocyst
Amniotic cavity
Chorionic cavity
Fused placentae

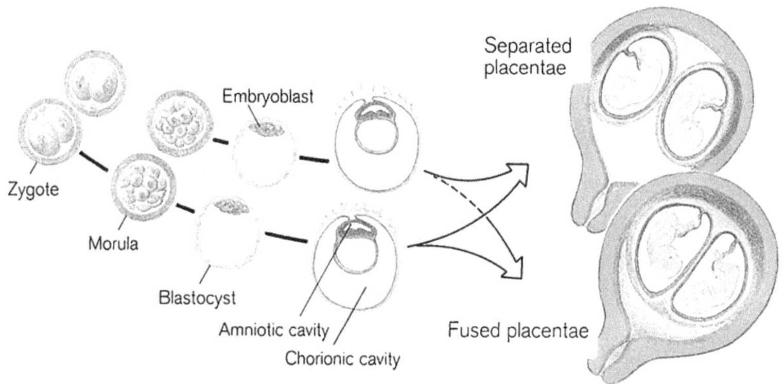

A. Dizygotic twins

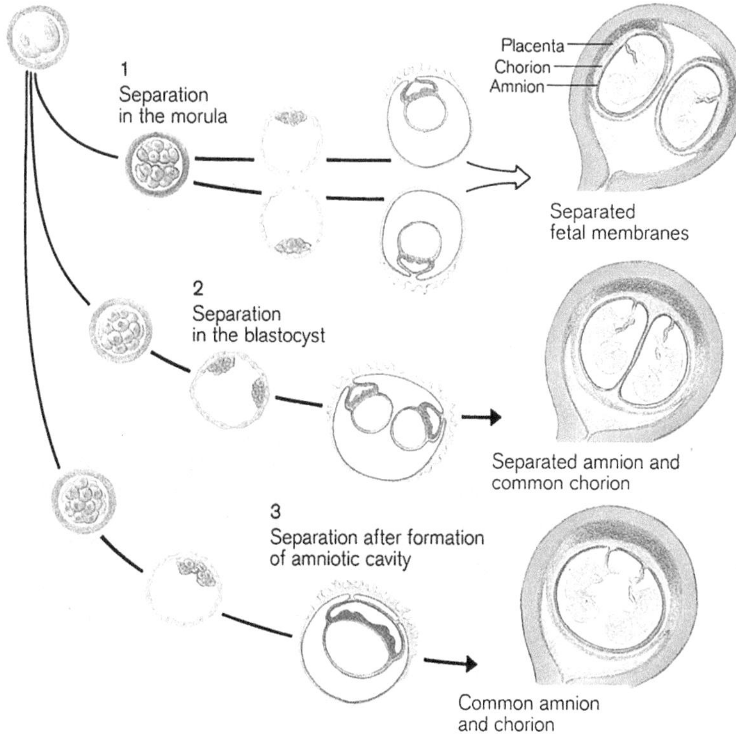

Placenta
Chorion
Amnion
1
Separation
in the morula
Separated
fetal membranes
2
Separation
in the blastocyst
Separated amnion and
common chorion
3
Separation after formation
of amniotic cavity
Common amnion
and chorion

B. Monozygotic twins

# Chapter 3: General Embryology

## Introduction

A morphological description of embryonic development cannot provide insight into the stepwise expression of the genome and the molecular-biological aspects of development. This insight can be obtained through experimental embryology, using sea urchins, Drosophila, or mouse embryos as model systems. The chapter "General Embryology" introduces important results from the field of experimental embryology and shows how experimentation provides a basis for generalizations (and for extrapolation to human development).

**Comparative Embryology.** In the overview on the relation between phylogeny and ontogeny (→ 3.1), the stages of embryonic development (ontogeny) are related to the development of species (phylogeny). In the second *overview* (→ 3.2), the development of the body form in the vertebrate embryo is correlated with the amount of yolk in the egg. In the following plates, the developmental stages summarized in 3.2—from the blastula via the germinal disc to the folding stage—are described in more detail, together with relevant experiments. In the *sea urchin* (→ 3.3), cell movements in fertilization and gastrulation can be observed directly under the microscope. The *amphibian embryo* (→ 3.4–3.6) is the classic model for Spemann's induction experiment. The long unknown and sought after primary inductor belongs to the large family of growth factors of the TGF-β (beta)-type ("transforming growth factor"). This unexpectedly suggests a common denominator for embryogenesis and tumorigenesis. The *chick* (→ 3.7–3.12) is the most easily accessible object for study of the embryonic disc, the primitive node, the folding process, and the development of fetal membranes. Grafting of quail tissue into the chick is the method of choice for analysis of cell movements in the embryo. The study of early development and comparative placenta formation in *mammals* (→ 3.13–3.16) is the key to understanding human implantation and placental development. The technique of gene transfer is exemplified by transfection experiments with the sex-determining DNA sequence of the mouse Y chromosome. Homeotic genes, discovered in *Drosophila* (→ 3.17), regulate the determination of body segments in all species investigated to date, including humans. The study of these genes provides key insights into the fundamental mechanisms of gene regulation during development. A single plate is perhaps too short to cover normal development of insects and the molecular biology of homeotic genes. This should be considered a stimulus for further reading.

**Basic Body Plan.** Analysis of the *basic body plan* (→ 3.18–3.24) of vertebrates by comparative embryology is fundamental for an understanding not only of the embryonic body, but also of definitive anatomy. This analysis includes the system of *pharyngeal arches* and *somites*, as well as general principles in the differentiation of the *germ layers*. The *limb bud*, a small region of homogeneous mesoderm with an ectodermal covering, gives rise to a complex system of bones and muscles. Experiments aimed at revealing how the axes are determined and how tissues differentiate in the limb bud illustrate the spectrum of questions that remain and the approaches used to answer them.

**Regulation of Development.** What is the mechanism of "morphogenesis" and what is meant by "induction?" Experiments have revealed *cell adhesion molecules* (CAMs), *growth factors*, and *homeotic genes* (→ 3.25–3.29) as the molecular mechanisms responsible for cell determination and differentiation. Regulation of growth is equivalent to regulation of the *cell cycle*. During the last two decades in the war against cancer, researchers have investigated cell growth regulation, using and inventing a large array of modern molecular biological techniques. The hypothesis that viruses cause cancer ultimately led back to the question of how cell determination and proliferation are regulated during embryonic development. "Oncogenes" turned out to play a central part in regulating the cell cycle. Thus, they determine whether cells proliferate or terminally differentiate in the embryo and in cancer.

**Differentiation of Tissues.** Some aspects of embryology will be covered that will facilitate an understanding of the organism from the histological perspective (→ 3.30–3.35). *Teeth* are homologous to scales. Intramembranous ossification has its origins in the exoskeleton of early vertebrates. The susceptibility of the *mammary glands* to cancer can be explained (in part) by their delicate hormonal control and by the steady presence of embryonic stem cells that reform the glandular tissue in each successive pregnancy. The differentiation of *striated muscle cells* is an example of how primitive systems that are expressed during embryonic development are transformed into differentiated tissues by the expression of optimized variants from the same gene family. The development of the *immunoglobulin family* by gene duplication and the function of some of the gene products in cell determination and proliferation are typical for *cell adhesion molecules*. A unique aspect of immunoglobulin formation is the generation of an individual antibody diversity by somatic mutations in the variable regions of immunoglobulin genes, which exceeds the coding capacity of the transmitted genome. It can be speculated that the number of CAMs involved in processes such as axonal "pathfinding" or synapse formation in the CNS is just as high as the number of antibodies in the immune system and may rely on similar mechanisms.

**Gastraea Theory and Germ Layer Theory.** Influenced by Darwin's theory on the evolutionary origin of species, Haeckel developed the gastraea theory at the beginning of the last century. The gastraea theory is the foundation for the germ layer theory. Haeckel postulated that in the origin of multicellular organisms (metazoa) from single cells (protozoa), a hollow sphere, similar in organization to the spherical alga Volvox, was first formed. He called the hollow sphere a blastaea. This form corresponds to the blastula stage in the ontogeny of higher animal species. A gastraea is formed by the development of a primitive gut (archenteron). The gastraea corresponds to the gastrula stage in the ontogeny of higher animal species and is the definitive body form in polyps (Hydra). At Haeckels time the germ layer theory was supported by the concomitantly developing modern microscopic and histological techniques. It became the foundation for a scientifically based biology. The homology between embryological stages in ontogeny and stages of evolution in phylogeny received the significance of a law of nature known as the *"fundamental biogenetic law."* It includes the concept that the germ layers in the embryo give rise to tissues. The differentiated functions of these are predetermined according to the functions assigned to ectoderm, endoderm, and mesoderm by evolution.

**Molecular Biological Approach.** The fundamental biochemical processes of transcription, translation, and protein synthesis use the same mechanisms and the same basic components in bacterial cells and eukaryotic cells. However, the cell nuclei of eukaryotic cells contain more DNA than is necessary to handle specific (acute) life situations. Gene duplications and gene transfers (via phages and viruses) produced multiple copies of genes for a large array of additional cellular proteins. Only a single copy of each gene is active. The gene duplications represent a genetic reservoir for metazoan evolution. Activation and inactivation of specific genes, expressing different sets of proteins and glycoproteins, give rise to the specialized cells of different organs. On the basis of homologies in the DNA sequences, gene families can be traced back to an "ancestral gene." Thus, the molecular biological approach is also based on evolutionary theory. The germ layer theory, founded on studies of morphology and comparative anatomy, is being refined and partially replaced on the basis of new insights into the structural organization and genomic regulation of the cell as derived from the fields of biochemistry and cell biology.

# Comparative Embryology

## 3.1 Ontogeny and Phylogeny

### A. Relation between Ontogeny and Phylogeny of Vertebrates

In the study of *phylogeny*, relationships between species are deduced by common features in body structure. Thus, animal species existing today can be organized into phylogenetic trees. Similarities in body structure are more apparent in embryonic development than in the adult organisms, which are specifically adapted to their different habitats.

In *ontogeny*, the embryo passes through a series of embryonic stages characterized by different body forms. Each of these forms represents the basic body plan of some species in the animal kingdom. This observation suggests that an embryo and an animal species at the corresponding level of organization have a common ancestor with the same body plan. However, organ structures such as somites or pharyngeal arches do not have the same functions in the embryo as in the corresponding animal species (in this example, movement or respiration). In the embryo, such functions are fulfilled by embryonic nutritive organs such as the yolk sac, the fetal membranes, and the placenta. In the embryo, somites and pharyngeal arches do not consist of terminally differentiated cells. They can thus develop into the next organizational stage.

The different stages in *phylogeny* and *ontogeny* are each characterized by the appearance of a new structural principle. This new design enables the species to expand its habitat and to multiply, often at the expense of the original species. The new development is not reversible. Mammals living in the sea cannot develop gills from the embryonic pharyngeal arches; their lungs must be adapted to life in the water.

**1. Spermatozoon and Oocyte.** In the haploid phase of the life cycle, the gametes are at the same level of organization as the protozoans. Multicellular organisms have emerged from unicellular ones. By analogy, embryonic development begins in the single-cell stage, the fertilized oocyte (egg). The oocyte, of course, is not the (abstract) primordial cell; like the sperm cell or the unicellular *Paramecium*, it is highly differentiated.

**2. Blastula Stage.** The development of a hollow sphere is a basic principle for *multicellular organisms*. The spherical form is found in the *spherical alga* Volvox and in the embryo at the blastula stage. The underlying principles are the development of epithelial polarity with an inner (basal) and an outer (apical) surface, and the formation of junctional complexes between cells.

**3. Gastrula Stage.** The gastrula arises from the blastula by involution of the primitive gut. The inner cells become specialized in the uptake of nutrients (endoderm) and the outer cells become specialized for protection and perception (ectoderm). The primordial gastrula-type animal can be envisaged as functioning like a suction cup that creeps along the ground and grazes on a bacterial lawn. The structural principle of the *gastrula* is exemplified by the *coelenterates*, which consist of an ectodermal and an endodermal layer. A fringe of tentacles serves to whirl food through the primitive mouth and into the blind-ending primitive gut. The coelenterates propagate by germ cells and by budding. Colonies of coelenterates give rise to coral reefs by depositing calcium on their undersides. The small freshwater Hydra serves as an experimental model for regeneration: cut pieces of the body can regenerate head and tail segments.

**4. Formation of Mesoderm.** During gastrulation of the sea urchin, i.e., during the involution of the archenteron, mesenchymal cells segregate to become the third germ layer, the *mesoderm*. The ciliated larvae of the echinoderms (*sea urchins, starfish, sea cucumber*), which have an asymmetrical opening of the intestinal tube at the animal pole, possess bilateral symmetry. This disappears again in the adult forms.

The nematode, *Caenorhabditis elegans*, is also at this level of organization. It consists of about 1000 somatic cells, each of which can be traced back to the zygote by cell lineage analysis. C. elegans represents a typical organism in which the fate of each cell seemed to be solely genetically determined (**mosaicism**) and not influenced (induced) by interactions with neighboring cells (**regulation**). Careful analysis has shown that a cell experimentally "knocked out" can be replaced by a neighboring cell due to specific cellular interactions. Caenorhabditis elegans, therefore, has become a model for perfect developmental regulation by cell interactions, thus outdating the concept of mosaicism.

**5. Metamerism.** Metamerism is based on an initial subdivision of the embryonic body into an ordered series of equal *segments*. Segmentation is the basis for the development of the two large animal classes on the earth, the *vertebrates* and the *insects*. In the phylum Annelida (roundworms), segmentation persists into the adult form. The genes responsible for segmentation were first identified in *Drosophila*. These *homeotic genes* possess a consensus sequence called a homeobox. The homeobox was used as a probe to demonstrate that homeotic genes are expressed in all classes of vertebrate embryos.

In the larva of a primitive *tunicate* (Crustacea), two segmentally organized regions can be distinguished: the head gut region, formed from pharyngeal arch elements alternating with gill slits and the trunk segment, which possesses a segmental musculature. During development, the trunk segment (including the notochord and the segmental musculature) regresses, giving rise to the adult tunicate—a sessile filter feeder that filters seawater through its branchial gut. In the evolution of vertebrates, the principle of the motile embryonic larva is developed further. The adult form of the lancetfish, another filter feeder, possesses a branchial gut, a notochord, and a segmental musculature. The muscle segments extend cranially over the branchial gut, indicating the position in which the *prootic myotomes* (external eye muscles) develop in vertebrate embryos. In fish, cartilaginous or bony vertebral elements arise around the notochord. Gills represent a specialized differentiation of the branchial gut (respiratory organs of fish → 3.19).

**6. Yolk Sac and Embryonic Disc.** Increased amounts of yolk in the egg lead to the development of an embryonic disc and the formation of an extraembryonic yolk sac supplied with its own vessels. This development already occurs in fish.

Amphibian eggs can be cleaved completely despite their relatively large yolk content. During development, the yolk is shifted into the intestinal tube, so that no extraembryonic yolk sac is formed. After hatching, the amphibian larva lives in the water and breathes through gills. During metamorphosis, the gills disappear and lungs develop, enabling the adult form to live on land.

**7. Amniotic Cavity.** Embryos of terrestrial *reptiles* and of *birds* that arose from them develop within a hard eggshell. They are enclosed in the fluid-filled *amniotic cavity* and respire initially by means of the extraembryonic yolk sac and later by the chorioallantois. The successful transition from water to land and into the air can be ultimately attributed not to the amphibian invasion of the terrestrial environment, but rather to the invention of the yolk sac and the amniotic cavity.

**8. Placenta.** Mammals with a well-developed *placenta* (euplacentalia) are distinguished from the *egg-laying mammals* (*duckbill platypus*) and the marsupials. For embryos growing within an eggshell, the placenta develops from the yolk sac and the chorioallantois. With the disappearance of the eggshell, the chorioallantoic vessels connect to the maternal vessels, forming the placenta, a nutritive and respiratory organ. Although the yolk content of the oocyte is markedly reduced, the formation of an embryonic disc and the mechanism of gastrulation (by means of a primitive streak), are retained, as is the secondary development of body form (by folding processes).

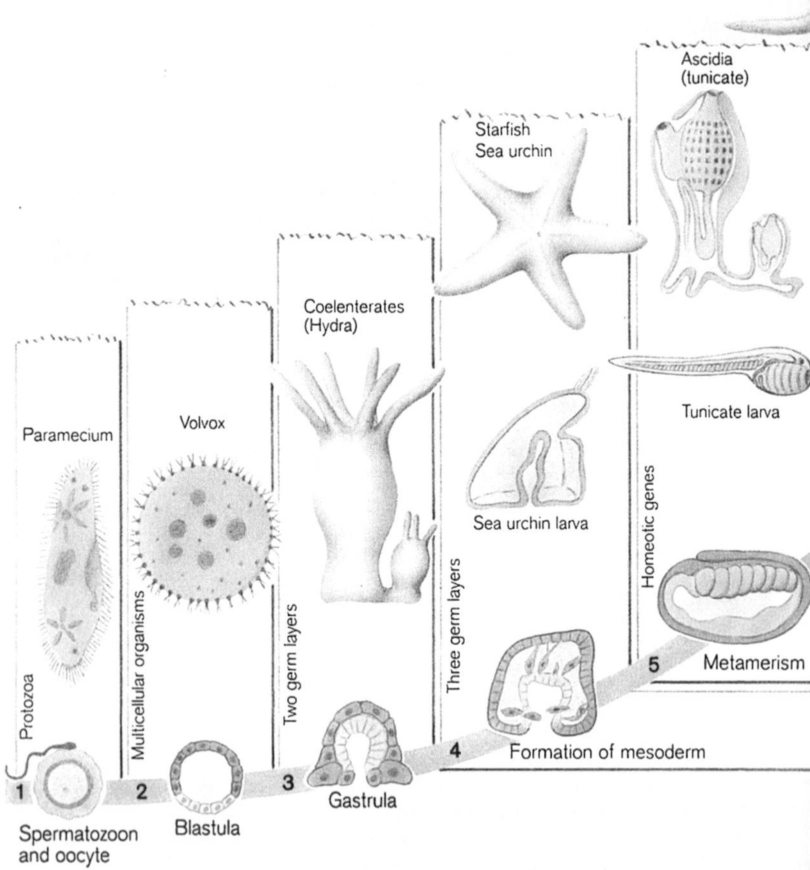


A. Relation between ontogenesis and phylogenesis in the vertebrate series

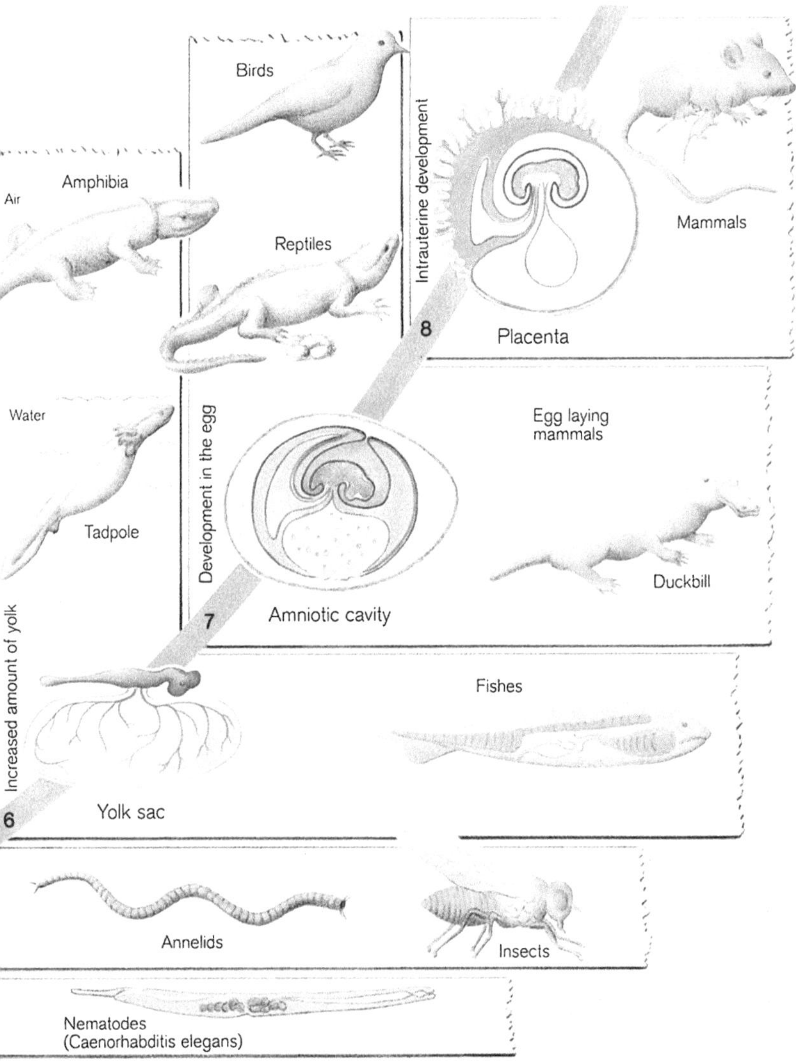
Birds
Amphibia
Air
Reptiles
Intrauterine development
Mammals
8
Placenta
Water
Egg laying mammals
Development in the egg
Tadpole
Duckbill
Increased amount of yolk
7
Amniotic cavity
Fishes
6
Yolk sac
Annelids
Insects
Nematodes
(Caenorhabditis elegans)

## 3.2 Overview: Early Development

*Background*

**Influence of Yolk Content of the Oocyte on Embryonic Development.** In the series from sea urchins via amphibians to birds, the eggs become larger and the amount of yolk increases. The plate compares the development of sea urchins, amphibians, birds, and mammals in relation to yolk content and size of the egg. In the *sea urchin*, the yolk is distributed equally between the blastomeres. In *amphibia*, the cells at the vegetal pole contain more yolk. After gastrulation, this yolk comes to lie in the digestive tube of the embryo. Increased yolk size enables the embryo to attain a higher degree of organization prior to hatching. In *birds*, the yolk is so large that it can no longer be divided during cleavage, and it does not fit into the primitive gut at gastrulation. The embryo therefore forms an embryonic disc and separates (folds off) from the yolk. The yolk lies in the extraembryonic yolk sac as a food reservoir and is transported to the embryo by vitelline vessels. Up to the time of hatching from the calcareous shell, the excretions of the embryo accumulate in an extraembryonic outpocketing of the cloaca (allantois). In *mammals*, embryonic development occurs in the mother. The female oviduct is expanded to form the uterus. The embryo is connected to the maternal circulation by the formation of a placenta derived from the yolk sac or the allantois. Although the oocytes are secondarily poor in yolk, the formation of an embryonic disc is retained.

### A. Comparison of Early Development

Sea urchins and amphibians develop in water and possess no amniotic cavity (**anamniotes**). Birds and mammals, inhabiting dry land, create an aqueous environment for the embryo by the development of an amniotic cavity (**amniotes**).

**1. Sea Urchins.** The eggs contain very little yolk. At *cleavage*, almost equal-sized blastomeres are formed. They form a *blastula* with a single-layered wall. The blastula hatches from the zona pellucida and swims freely in the seawater by means of cilia. During *gastrulation*, the first mesodermal cells separate (primary mesoderm). Most of the mesoderm segregates from the roof of the primitive gut and forms secondary mesoderm. The primitive gut becomes apposed to the ectoderm and breaks through to form the definitive mouth opening. The blastopore becomes the anus.

**2. Amphibians.** The eggs contain much yolk. Cleavage is still complete, but unequal: Large *yolk-rich blastomeres* are formed at the vegetal pole. The *blastula* is compact at the vegetal pole and possesses a stratified wall. During *gastrulation*, a yolk plug forms in the blastopore; this plug ultimately comes to lie in the intestinal canal of the larva. The *mesoderm* segregates from the roof of the primitive gut as a plate. The *body form* arises directly by segmentation of the mesoderm and elongation of the embryo.

**3. Birds.** Cleavage takes place only in the germinal region, giving rise to a *germinal disc* that grows on top of the yolk. A *primitive streak* develops in place of an invagination of the archenteron. *Mesoderm* arises by invagination through the streak. The *body form* arises secondarily by folding off from the yolk. In this process, the embryo sinks into the yolk, becoming enfolded and ultimately enclosed by the amnion (amniotic cavity).

**4. Higher Mammals (Human).** The oocyte is secondarily poor in yolk. *Cleavage* is complete (i.e., the egg is divided completely) and equal (i.e., equal-sized blastomers are produced). The blastomeres segregate into an inner cell mass and a trophoblast and form a *blastocyst*. The trophoblast gives rise to the extraembryonic organs before the embryo itself develops. The inner cell mass forms a *germinal disc* between the amniotic cavity and the yolk sac. Mesoderm arises via the primitive streak. The *embryonic body* folds off from the yolk sac as in yolk-rich eggs.

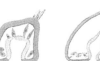

| | Cleavage | Blastula | Gastrula | Mesoderm | Body form |
|---|---|---|---|---|---|
| Anamniotes: Sea urchin, Egg type: less yolk | Total, almost equal | Round, single layered | Invagination by blastopore | Emigration from archenteron | Elongation of embryo |
| Anamniotes: Amphibians, Egg type: much yolk | Total unequal | Round, multilayered | Involution around blastopore lip | Segregation from roof of archenteron | Elongation of embryo |
| Amniotes: Birds, Egg type: very much yolk | Partial discoidal | Germ disc | Delamination of endoderm | Involution through primitive streak | Folding off from yolk |
| Amniotes: Higher mammals (man), Egg type: little yolk | Total, equal | Blastocyst of trophoblast and embryoblast | Delamination of endoderm | Involution through primitive streak | Folding off between yolk sac and amniotic cavity |

A. Comparison of early development

Sea Urchin

## 3.3 Sea Urchin and Amphioxus

*Background*

**Sea urchins** release their gametes into the seawater. The development from fertilization to a larva (Pluteus) capable of feeding lasts about 40 hours. The short period of embryonic development corresponds to a small amount of yolk in the egg.

### A. Development of the Sea Urchin

**1. Fertilization.** Upon sperm entry, the oocyte forms a *fertilization cone*. From this center, the secretion of cortical granules, development of the perivitelline space, and formation of a fertilization membrane from the jelly coat (Zona pellucida) spread over the entire egg surface within 20 seconds. The fertilization membrane is impermeable to sperm (→ 1.5).

**2. Cleavage.** After activation of the egg by fertilization, the first cell divisions occur in rhythmic succession. Under the microscope, the cell divisions are visible by the appearance of clefts in the surface of the zygote (cleavage). The daughter cells are the *blastomeres*. Since no nourishment can be taken up from the exterior, cleavage progresses without increase in size of the total embryo. At the 16, 32, and 64 cell stages, the embryo resembles a mulberry (morula). In the sea urchin, eight medium-sized blastomeres (mesomeres) arise at the animal pole, while four large blastomeres (macromeres) and four small ones (micromeres) arise at the vegetal pole. The macromeres contain the material for the endoderm, the micromeres, the material for the mesoderm.

**3. Blastula.** The cells of the morula form a hollow sphere, the blastula. The cavity of the blastula is the *blastocoel*. The blastula possesses an animal and a vegetal pole. The *animal pole* of the sea urchin blastula is characterized by a tuft of cilia. In general, it contains the material for the surface ectoderm and the nervous system. The *vegetal pole* contains prospective endoderm and mesoderm. About 10 hours after fertilization, the blastula of the sea urchin hatches from the gelatinous envelope (*jelly coat, zona pellucida*), which surrounds the egg and begins to move by ciliary motion.

**4. Early Gastrula.** The cells at the vegetal pole of the blastula send out pseudopodia into the interior of the blastula. At the animal pole, the pseudopodia form solid contact points, so that they bridge over the blastocoel as cytoplasmic cords. The pseudopodia then contract, pulling the primitive intestinal pouch (archenteron) into the blastocoel.

**5. Gastrulation and Mesoderm Formation.** During gastrulation, some of the epithelial cells migrate into the blastocoel and form *primary mesoderm* (**A4**). The remaining mesoderm arises by migration of cells from the roof of the archenteron (*secondary mesoderm*).

**6. Larval Stage.** The bilateral symmetry of the sea urchin larva results from the development of the *mouth (stomodeum)*. The diverticulum of the archenteron curves forward and touches the ectoderm. The ectoderm invaginates to form the stomodeum. Ectoderm and endoderm become closely apposed, forming a *pharyngeal membrane* that subsequently ruptures. The blastopore becomes the anus. After metamorphosis, the bilateral symmetry of the sea urchin, starfish, and sea cucumber is lost. A five-rayed, radially symmetric body arises. It possesses a skeleton of calcareous plates and a “hydraulic” movement apparatus.

### B. Formation of Mesoderm in Amphioxus

In lancelets (Amphioxus), the notochord is retained in the adult animal as a stout, elastic, axial rod (**B1**). Amphioxus has neither vertebrae nor head. **B2** illustrates the archetypic fashion in which mesoderm segregates from the *roof of the archenteron* (**2a**) in the Amphioxus embryo. Segmented *coelomic sacs* evaginate laterally (**2b**) and separate into *somitic musculature and body cavities* (coelom) (**2c**). The *notochord* arises from the medial region of the roof of the archenteron.

Fertilization cone
Jelly coat
1
Fertilization
2
Cleavage
64 cells
Macromeres
Micromeres
3
Blastula
Animal pole
Blastocoel
Vegetal pole
4
Early gastrula
Primary mesodermal cells
Secondary mesoderm
Primitive gut
Primary mesoderm
Blastopore
5
Gastrula
Definitive opening of mouth
Skeletal element
6
Larval stage

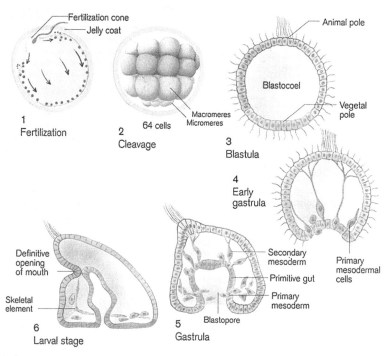

A. Development of the sea urchin embryo

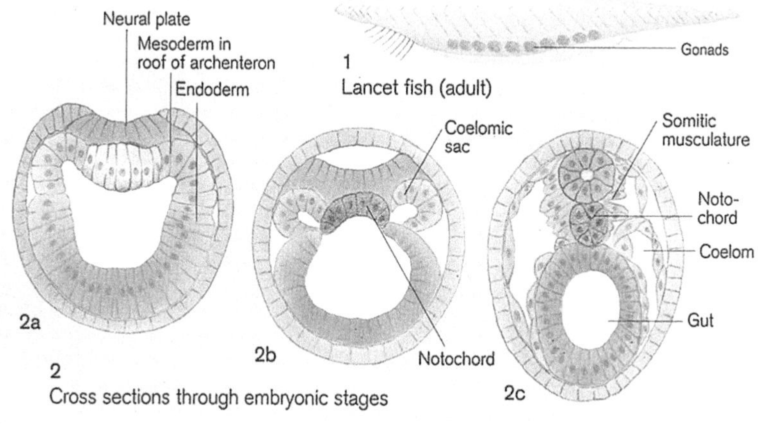


B. Mesoderm formation in Amphioxus (lancet fish)

# Amphibia
# 3.4 Normal Development

*Background*

**Amphibians** (newt, salamander, frog) lay their eggs (spawn) on grasses and reeds in shallow water. The eggs develop within a protective gelatinous envelope until they become swimming larvae. The hatched larvae live in the water and breathe through gills. After metamorphosis, the adult animals adapt to life on land and breathe through lungs.

## A. Early Development of Amphibians

### 1. Cleavage and Gastrulation

The pinhead-sized eggs contain a large mass of yolk that is concentrated at the vegetal pole. Despite the large amount of yolk, the egg divides completely. The blastomeres at the *vegetal pole* are larger than those at the *animal pole* (**1a**). The wall of the *blastula* is stratified (**1b**). At the vegetal pole, the yolk-rich blastomeres bulge into the *blastocoel*. The blastopore arises in a zone with lighter pigmentation (*gray crescent*) opposite the sperm penetration site. Here, the epithelial structure loosens and cells migrate by amoeboid movements into the blastocoel. With their slender posterior poles, they pull the lip of the blastopore inward (*bottle cells*) (**1c**).

### 2. Cell Movement and Induction in the Gastrula

The peculiarities of **gastrulation** in amphibians are due to the sluggishness of yolk-rich cells at the vegetal pole. Gastrulation begins with the involution of prospective mesodermal material into the sickle-shaped dorsal lip of the *blastopore* ( **2a**). As the archenteron invaginates, the continuity of the epithelium is interrupted at the ventral lip of the blastopore. The large yolk-rich cells remain as a *yolk plug* (**2b**) in the opening of the blastopore. Toward the end of gastrulation, some mesoderm also involutes into the ventral lip of the blastopore and pushes forward between the yolk plug and the ectoderm.

The prospective mesoderm invaginates around the dorsal lip of the blastopore and comes to lie in the region of the *roof of the archenteron* (**2a**). Mesoderm in the roof of the archenteron induces the ectoderm lying above to form the *neural plate* (**2b**).

In *frogs* (*Anurans*), mesoderm and endoderm are united in the archenteron during gastrulation (**1b**); the mesodermal plate separates later. In *salamanders* (*Urodeles*), mesoderm and endoderm separate at the beginning of gastrulation. After separation from the endoderm, the mesoderm forms a ventrally open "shell" that inserts between the ectoderm and endoderm at its edges (**2c**).

### 3. Differentiation of Germ Layers

In the **neurula** (**3a**), the *mesoderm* becomes organized into the *notochord* (situated in the median plane), the material for the *somites*, and the *lateral plates*.

In the **tail-bud stage** (**3b**), the edges of the *neural plate* rise and form neural folds that subsequently fuse in the region of the *neural crest*. This process gives rise to a *neural tube* with a central canal that is detached from the surface ectoderm. In the trunk region, the neural tube becomes the spinal cord; in the head region, it forms the brain vesicles. After fusion of the neural folds, outward migration of neural crest cells begins. The *notochord* differentiates into a stout, elastic axial rod with a tough collagenous sheath and swollen vacuolated cells. The paraxial mesoderm becomes organized into *somites*, laying a foundation for the metameric arrangement of the body into vertebral segments and muscle plates. The *lateral plate mesoderm* grows around the digestive tube as a continuous plate; the coelomic space is formed secondarily. As the *notochord-mesoderm complex* (**2a**) separates from the roof of the archenteron, the margins of the endoderm close to form the definitive intestinal tract.

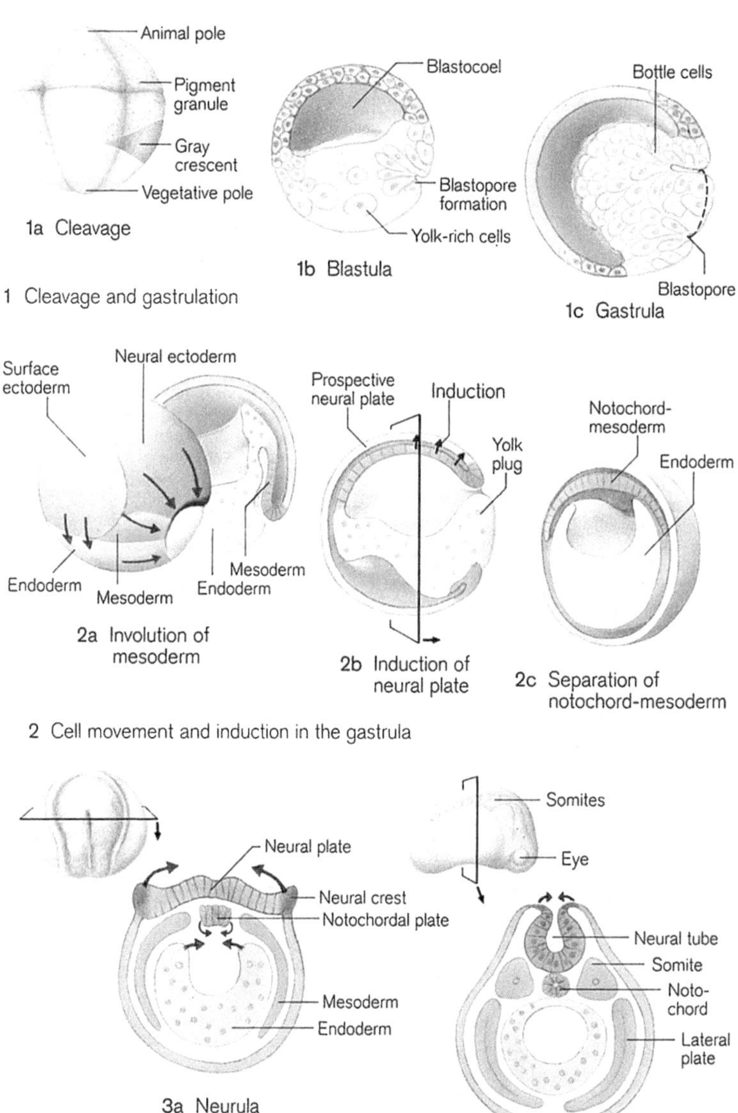


A. Early development of amphibians

## 3.5 Amphibia: Classic Experiments

### A. Constriction Experiments

If a gastrula is severed with a fine loop of hair into a dorsal and ventral half (**A1**), the dorsal half develops into a smaller, complete embryo. The ventral half, however, develops only into a clump of endoderm with a covering of epidermal ectoderm. On the other hand, severance of the gastrula in the median plane (**A2**) produces two complete embryos that can develop as twins in a common jelly coat (zona pellucida). This experiment shows that the animal pole can give rise to all body tissues, whereas the vegetal pole can form only endoderm.

### B. Prospective Significance and Prospective Potency

Using vital dyes, Vogt (1929) charted the migration of cells during gastrulation. In this technique, pieces of agar soaked with Nile blue sulfate or neutral red are applied to specific regions of the blastula. The cells in these regions take up the dye, allowing their migration to be followed into the neural tube, somites, notochord, intestine, etc. In this way, the organ primordia, which in normal development originate from the cells of the blastula, can be traced (projected) back to the blastula. From such a fate map, the **prospective significance** (**B1**) of cells can be deduced.

"Prospective significance" specifies into which tissue the cells *normally* develop. The term **prospective potency** (**B2**), on the other hand, represents *all* possible developmental fates that occur experimentally in a given region. The projection of prospective potency into the early gastrula shows that the prospective potency of cells is greater than their prospective significance.

During development, the prospective potency of embryonic cells is further restricted. The irreversible fixation of cells on a developmental path is called **determination** (→ 3.28). Determination precedes the visible differentiation of cells.

If the cells of a blastula are isolated and further grown in culture, they exhibit a certain **self-differentiation capacity** (**B3**), which is less than their prospective significance. For example, the dorsal ectoderm, which normally differentiates into the neural tube, forms only epidermal ectoderm.

### C. Spemann's Organizer Experiment

**1. Transplantation of the Dorsal Lip of the Blastopore.** A piece of tissue from the dorsal lip of the blastopore is removed just before the beginning of gastrulation and inserted into another blastula. In the blastocoel of the host embryo, the transplant comes to lie in the region of the future ventral body wall, where it induces the formation of a second neural plate. The transplanted tissue becomes integrated into the corresponding notochord-mesoderm complex (→ 3.4 A2). The result is an embryo with two complete embryonic axial systems.

**2. Induction of Archencephalic and Spinocaudal Structures.** Chemical isolation of the primary induction factor has shown that the factor is neither species- nor organ-specific and can be isolated from different tissues (chick embryos, guinea pig bone marrow). To assay the inducing activity, the isolated fractions were placed in a blastula (see **C1**). Two protein factors were isolated, one inducing head structures (*archencephalic inductor*), and the other, tail structures (*spinocaudal inductor*). The total body axis is believed to be induced by opposing gradients of both factors.

The biochemical substrates for Spemann's organizer are probably ubiquitous growth factors, the specificity of which depends on their temporal and spatial patterns of expression (phase specificity).

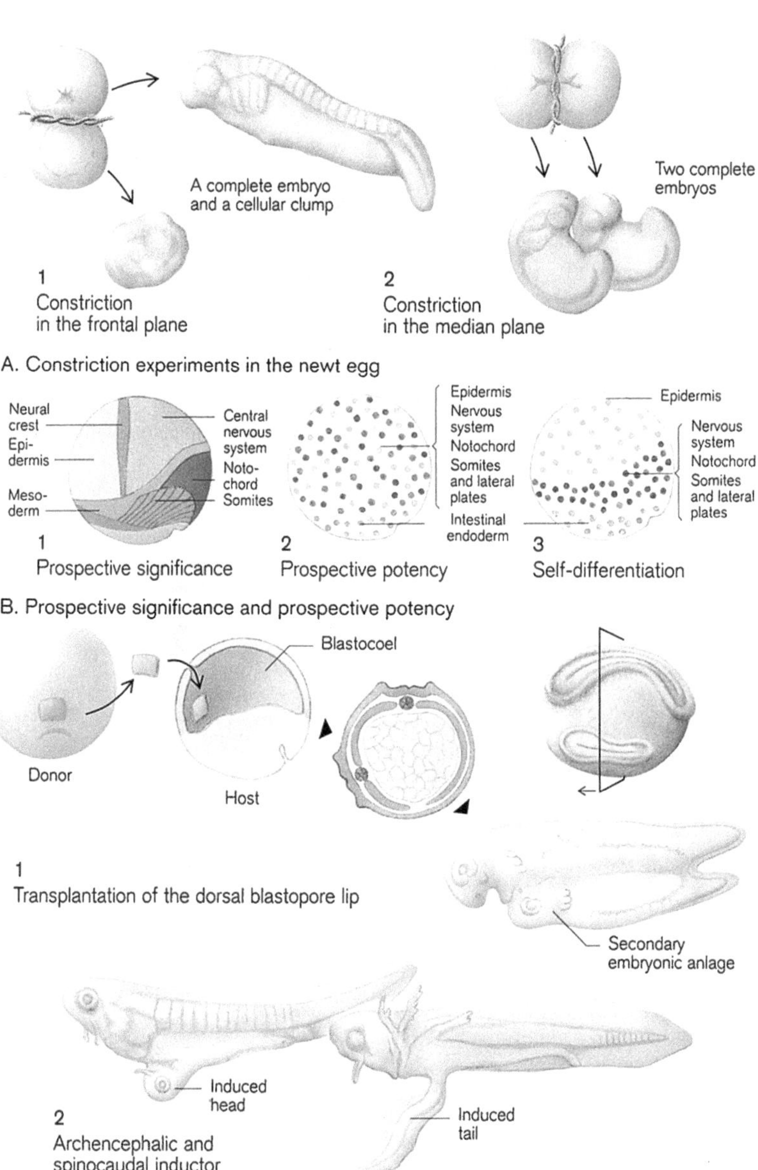
A complete embryo and a cellular clump
1
Constriction in the frontal plane
Two complete embryos
2
Constriction in the median plane
A. Constriction experiments in the newt egg
Neural crest
Epi-dermis
Meso-derm
Central nervous system
Noto-chord
Somites
1
Prospective significance
Epidermis
Nervous system
Notochord
Somites and lateral plates
Intestinal endoderm
2
Prospective potency
Epidermis
Nervous system
Notochord
Somites and lateral plates
3
Self-differentiation
B. Prospective significance and prospective potency
Blastocoel
Donor
Host
1
Transplantation of the dorsal blastopore lip
Secondary embryonic anlage
Induced head
Induced tail
2
Archencephalic and spinocaudal inductor

C. Spemann's organizer experiment

## 3.6 Amphibia: Embryonic Induction

*Background*

Inductive relations between tissues can be studied in amphibian embryos with a simple **induction experiment:** The reacting tissue (here the ectoderm) is cultured together with the *inductor* in question. Up to the blastula stage, development is determined by *maternal factors* that are already present in the oocyte before fertilization. During cleavage, these factors determine the dorsoventral polarity. The *animal cap* of the blastula contains the *prospective ectoderm*. The yolk-rich cells of the *prospective endoderm* lie at the vegetal pole. The first step in the induction cascade is the *induction of mesoderm*.

### A. Induction Cascade in the Amphibian Embryo

**1. Induction of Mesoderm.** In a now classic experiment, Nieuwkoop (1969) demonstrated that culture of an isolated ectodermal cap of the blastula in contact with cell material from the vegetal pole causes the ectoderm to differentiate into mesodermal tissue such as *notochord*, *musculature*, and *connective tissue*. If, on the other hand, the ectodermal cap is cultured without inducing tissue, the ectoderm gives rise only to an epidermal-type epithelium. This induction experiment shows that vegetal cells of the equatorial zone of the blastula induce the formation of mesodermal tissues in the ectoderm.

**2. Induction of Neural Plate.** Culture of the ectoderm of the gastrula, together with tissue from the archenteron roof (notochordomesodermal plate), gives rise to tissues corresponding to the *neural tube* and the *cerebral vesicles*. Without an inductor, the ectoderm again forms only epidermis. This in vitro induction experiment corresponds to the organizer experiment (→ 3.5 C1) by Spemann and Hilde Mangold (1938). This investigation showed that the prospective mesoderm that invaginates through the dorsal lip of the blastopore and forms the roof of the archenteron induces the neural plate.

**3. Induction of the Lens Placode.** The optic vesicle evaginates from the cranial portion of the neural tube. The neural epithelium of the *optic vesicle* contacts the surface ectoderm and induces the *lens placode,* which in turn invaginates to form the lens vesicle, the cells of which differentiate to lens fibers (→ 5.6). If one explants the optic cup or optic cup extract together with ectoderm of the neurula, a lens placode is formed. In the absence of contact with the optic vesicle, the prospective epithelium of the lens placode again forms only epidermis.

The induction experiments show that differentiation of the germ layers is determined by interaction of tissues via inductive factors, and that the primary induction in the gastrula is followed by a cascade of secondary induction steps.

### B. Identification of Growth Factors in the Induction of Mesoderm

The mesoderm-inducing factor is present not only in the vegetal cells of the blastula but is also secreted by a cell line derived from embryonic *Xenopus cells* (XTC cells) into their culture medium. When cultured in medium conditioned by XTC cells, suspensions of animal cap cells of the blastula form aggregates of mesodermal tissues. If the cells are cultured in a normal control medium, aggregates of epidermis arise. With this assay system, the mesoderm-inducing factor could be isolated biochemically from the conditioned medium of XTC cells (Smith et al. 1990). The factor is identical to *activin*, a peptide hormone responsible for the secretion of FSH from the pituitary gland (its antagonist is called inhibin). Activin belongs to a family of *peptide growth factors* that also include the TGF-βs (transforming growth factor-β). In appropriate concentrations, these factors also possess mesoderm-inducing activity. Different mesodermal tissues arise depending on the concentration of the inducing factor used.

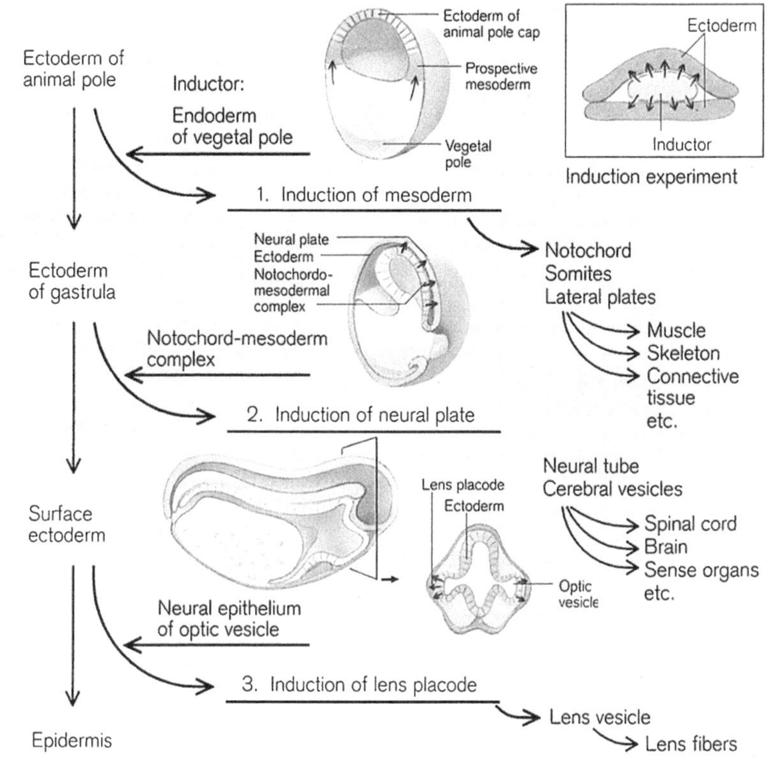

Ectoderm of animal pole cap
Prospective mesoderm
Vegetal pole
Ectoderm
Inductor
Induction experiment
Ectoderm of animal pole
Inductor:
Endoderm of vegetal pole
1. Induction of mesoderm
Notochord
Somites
Lateral plates
Muscle
Skeleton
Connective tissue
etc.
Neural plate
Ectoderm
Notochordo-mesodermal complex
Ectoderm of gastrula
Notochord-mesoderm complex
2. Induction of neural plate
Neural tube
Cerebral vesicles
Spinal cord
Brain
Sense organs
etc.
Lens placode
Ectoderm
Optic vesicle
Surface ectoderm
Neural epithelium of optic vesicle
3. Induction of lens placode
Lens vesicle
Lens fibers
Epidermis


A. Induction cascade in amphibian embryos (experimental)

Animal pole of blastula
Cell suspension
Control medium
Aggregates
Cartilage
Muscle
Epidermis
Mesodermal tissue
XTC–cells
280 nm absorption
Conditioned medium with mesoderm inducing factor
"Activin-like activity"
Isolation of activin


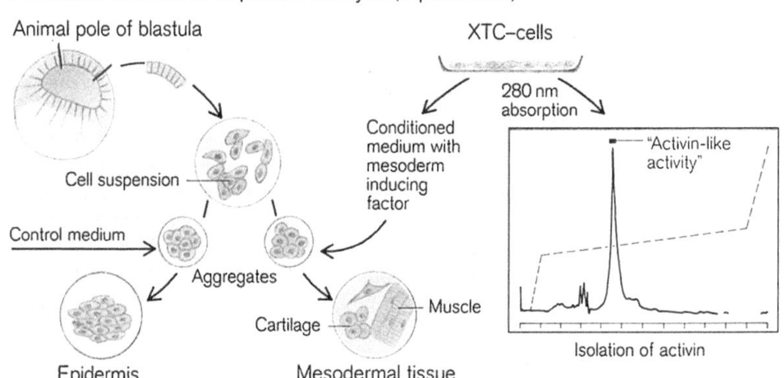

B. Identification of growth factors in the induction of mesoderm

# Chick Embryo
# 3.7 Embryonic Disc

*Background*

**Development of the Chick Embryo.** As an adaptation to the size of the egg, only the left ovary is active in birds; the right ovary already recedes during embryonic life. Fertilization of the egg occurs in the uterine tube after ovulation. Albumen and a calcareous shell are deposited during migration through the oviduct. The egg yolk is the oocyte. It is surrounded by the vitelline membrane, which corresponds to a zona pellucida. The incubation time is 21 days.

## A. Development of the Embryonic Disc

**1. Cleavage.** In the giant oocyte, the clear cytoplasm that contains the pronuclei separates from the yolk-filled cytoplasm and becomes recognizable as a *germinal spot* below the vitelline membrane (**1a**). Cleavage is restricted to this central cytoplasmic region; at the periphery, the furrows disappear into the large yolk mass (**1b**). The peripheral cell nuclei get lost in the yolk. Cleavage proceeds during migration through the uterine tube (**1c**). When the egg is laid, an embryonic disc with about 60 000 cells is already present (**A2**).

**2. Epiblast and Hypoblast of the Embryonic Disc.** Below the vitelline membrane, the cells form a stratified epithelium. On the underside of this epithelium, cells detach and penetrate into the yolk, causing it to liquefy. A *subgerminal cavity* arises beneath the embryonic disc. Epithelial cells transport fluid into the space between the embryonic disc and the vitelline membrane, causing the central cells to detach from the membrane. At the margins of the embryonic disc, the cells adhere firmly to the underside of the vitelline membrane and migrate outward with amoeboid movements. This active pulling by the *blastoderm edge cells* stretches and enlarges the embryonic disc. In surface view, the embryonic disc, lying above the subgerminal cavity, is translucent and is centrally separated from the vitelline membrane by fluid (*area pellucida*). Peripherally, it is opaque and firmly attached to the vitelline membrane (*area opaca*). At the border between the area pellucida and area opaca, lies a ridge of large, yolk-rich cells known as the "*germ wall*."

The embryonic disc of an unincubated chicken egg already consists of two cell layers that have arisen during migration through the oviduct. Since they are not identical with the definitive germ layers, the upper epithelial layer is called the *epiblast* and the lower the *hypoblast*. Individual cells migrate from the epiblast and integrate into the loose hypoblastic layer (*droplet cells*). This process corresponds to the formation of the primary mesoderm in the sea urchin embryo (→ 3.3) or the appearance of bottle cells at the beginning of gastrulation in amphibians (→ 3.4). The hypoblast is separated from the subgerminal cavity and the yolk by a flat layer of cells known as *primary endoderm*. The primary endoderm originates in the sickle shaped, thickened germ wall at the caudal pole of the embryonic disc, from which the primitive streak also originates.

**3. Forward Growth of the Primitive Streak.** The position of the *primitive streak* and thus the position of the future body axis is determined by the position of the egg in the oviduct, which is influenced by gravity. The primitive streak is a thickening in the epiblast that arises in the *germ wall* at the caudal pole of the embryonic disc and grows cranially (**3a**). The primitive streak elongates cranially and after 20 hours of incubation, reaches the anterior third of the embryonic disc. The cells of the *ectoderm* are pushed in a medial direction at the surface and migrate through the *primitive streak* , where they leave the epithelium and form the definitive *mesoderm* and definitive *endoderm* (**3b**). The primary endoderm is displaced into the extraembryonic region of the embryonic disc.

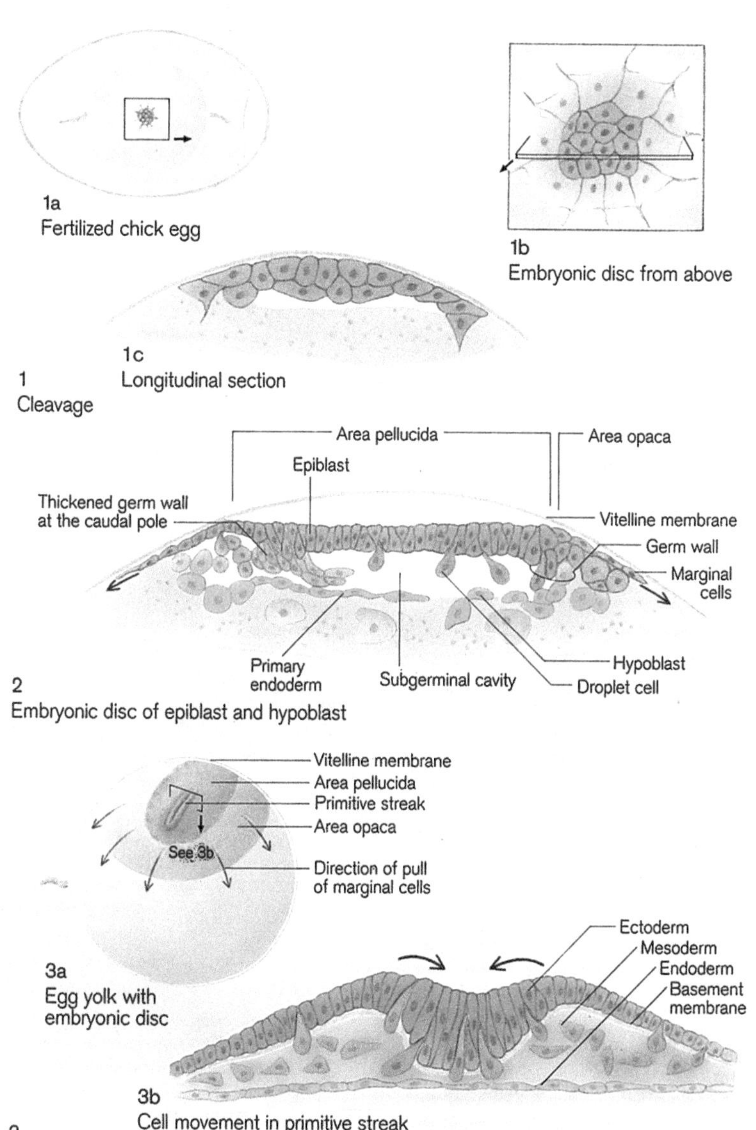
1a
Fertilized chick egg
1b
Embryonic disc from above
1c
Longitudinal section
1
Cleavage
Area pellucida
Area opaca
Epiblast
Thickened germ wall
at the caudal pole
Vitelline membrane
Germ wall
Marginal
cells
Primary
endoderm
Subgerminal cavity
Hypoblast
Droplet cell
2
Embryonic disc of epiblast and hypoblast
Vitelline membrane
Area pellucida
Primitive streak
Area opaca
See 3b
Direction of pull
of marginal cells
Ectoderm
Mesoderm
Endoderm
Basement
membrane
3a
Egg yolk with
embryonic disc
3b
Cell movement in primitive streak
3
Forward growth of primitive streak

A. Development of the embryonic disc in the chick embryo

## 3.8 Chick Emryo: Primitive Node

*Background*

The **primitive node** is a small thickening at the cranial end of the primitive streak. The primitive streak and primitive node may be considered an elongated blastopore through which mesodermal material migrates inward (→ 3.18). Later, the primitive node recedes caudally, inducing the organization of mesoderm into notochord, somites, and lateral plates. The retreating primitive node is an organization center that induces the reorganization of the primitive streak material into the axial organs of the embryo. If the primitive node is transplanted to another location in the embryonic disc, a second complete body axis, including notochord, neural tube, and somites, develops at this site. The primitive node, therefore, corresponds to the notochord-mesoderm complex in the amphibian embryo in its function as organizer of the body axis.

### B. The Primitive Node as an Organization Center

**1. Spread of Primitive Streak Mesoderm.** The prospective mesoderm lies initially in the ectoderm. It migrates medially to the *primitive streak* and is pulled inward through the primitive groove. In the primitive streak, the mesodermal cells detach from the epithelium and migrate between the ectoderm and endoderm, spreading laterally and cranially (arrows).

**2. Invagination of the Notochordal Process.** In the region of the *primitive node*, the primitive groove deepens to form the *primitive pit*. Cell material from the ectoderm enters the primitive pit and pushes forward cranially between the ectoderm and endoderm (arrow). The cells are organized immediately into the notochord, forming an extension of the primitive streak (notochordal process) that is visible through the ectoderm (**2a**). The notochordal primordium elongates caudally by continuous invagination of cell material through the primitive pit. In this process, the primitive node and primitive pit migrate caudally. In front of the primitive node, the paraxial (i.e., situated beside the midline) mesoderm becomes progressively organized from cranial to caudal into somites, the contours of which are visible on the surface of the embryonic disc (**3a**). The *ectoderm* thickens to form the *neural plate* above the notochord and the paraxial mesoderm.

**3. Establishment of the Head.** In front of the notochordal process, is a mesoderm-free region where the endodermal cells form a palisade structure (*endodermal palisade*, **2a**). The thickened endoderm and the neural plate lying above it rise from the surface of the embryonic disc as the head fold. During this process, the endoderm invaginates to form the foregut diverticulum, which opens into the yolk at the *anterior intestinal portal* (**3a**). With the establishment of the *head fold*, the neural plate becomes depressed and forms the neural groove. A cleft arises between the ectoderm and endoderm. Individual cells detach from the palisade structure of the foregut outpocketing and fill the space between ectoderm and endoderm as loose mesenchyme (*head mesoderm*) (**3a**, inset). Thus the endodermal palisade structure disintegrates.

The invagination of the head gut can be perceived as a special gastrulation process that is independent of the primitive streak and node. By this means, the head gut and head mesoderm arise.

**Prechordal Plate.** The structure in front of the notochord labeled *endodermal palisade* (**2a**), is known as the prechordal plate. This structure (independently of the primitive streak) gives rise to **head mesoderm** , which is later supplemented by "head mesenchyme" from the neural crest.

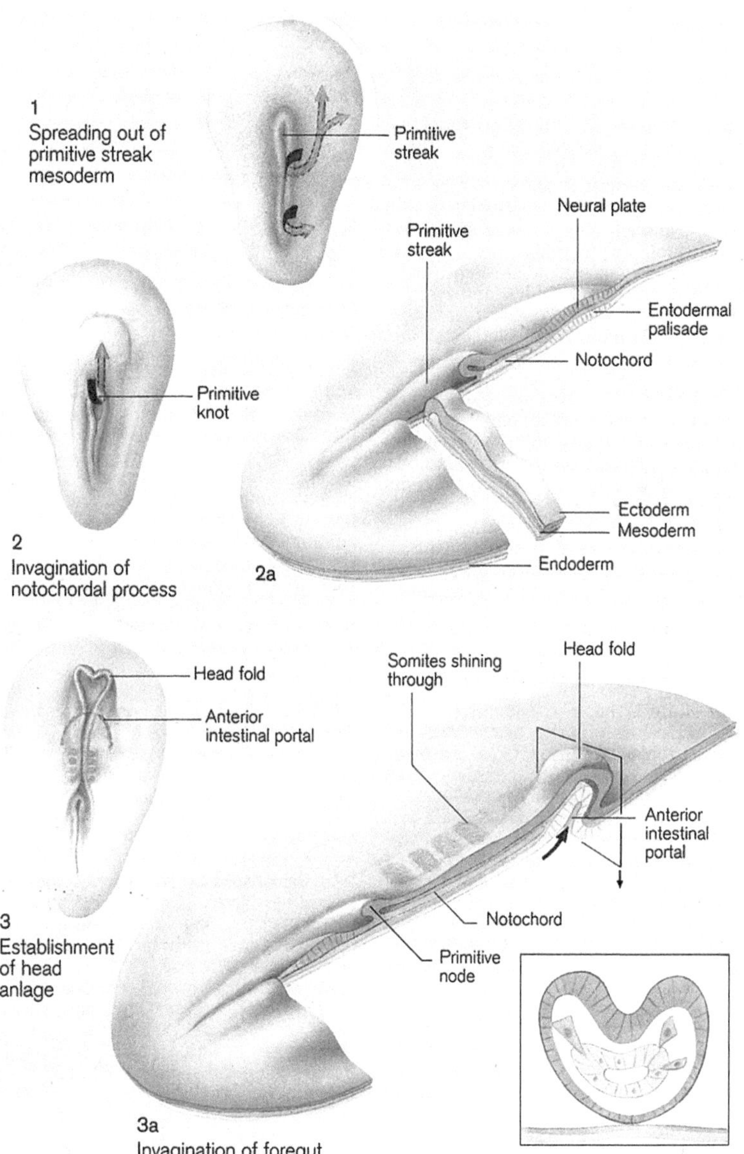


B. The primitive node as an organization center

## 3.9 Chick Embryo: Folding

*Background*

The formation of an **embryonic disc** is an adaptation of yolk-rich eggs, in which cleavage no longer can involve the entire egg. In the **folding process,** the embryo becomes raised from the yolk. On the ventral side, the endoderm closes into an intestinal tube and the yolk comes to lie in the newly formed, extraembryonically located yolk sac. In the **chick embryo**, the yolk sac is the nutritive and respiratory organ. In **mammals** with secondarily yolk-poor eggs, the nutritive and respiratory function is taken over by the placenta. Nevertheless, the mammalian embryo continues to develop as an embryonic disc and forms the embryonic body secondarily by a folding process. In mammals, the development of an embryonic disc and the folding process are necessary for the development of the extraembryonic organs. The formation of the placenta and of fetal membranes in mammals is homologous to the development of egg membranes in birds.

### C. Folding in the Chick Embryo

**1. 24-Hour Chick Embryo.** The folding process in chick embryos begins with the invagination of the foregut into the head fold (→ 3.8 B3a) and progresses from cranial to caudal. After 24 hours of incubation, the embryonic body is divided into three segments. In the anterior cranial segment, the *head* is lifted above the level of the embryonic disc. In the middle segment, the *primary organs* of the body axis—the neural tube, notochord, somites, and lateral plates—are progressively delimited from cranial to caudal. The blocks of somites are visible through the ectoderm. In the caudal segment, the *primitive streak* is still present. The material of the germ layers is still unsegmented. The arrows indicate three developmental processes occurring progressively in the embryonic disc from cranial to caudal. The primitive node (organization center) migrates caudally and induces the development of the primary organs. The caudal migration of the primitive node and the differentiation of the primitive organs is followed by a third wave, the folding of the embryonic body. At the anterior intestinal portal, the intestinal groove closes to form the intestinal tube. The fusion of the endodermal folds in the midline at the caudally migrating anterior intestinal portal can be compared to the closure of a zipper.

**a Head.** In front of the anterior intestinal portal, the embryonic body has detached completely from the extraembryonic portions of the germ layers. The *notochord* lies between the *neural tube* and the *foregut* .

**b Folding at the Intestinal Portal.** The embryo develops the mechanical force necessary for the closure of the digestive tube in morphogenetically active epithelial layers. The *visceral mesoderm* forms a palisade-like epithelium that rises and curves toward the midline, until the lips of the endoderm fuse with one another. The closure of the intestinal tube is followed, after a brief pause, by the closure of the ventral body wall, as the *lateral folds*, composed of ectoderm and a *parietal mesodermal layer*, curve inward. The cranial segment of the coelomic cavity forms the *pericardial cavity* (→ 6.2).

**c Primary Organs in Front of the Primitive Node.** Caudal to the anterior intestinal portal, is a body segment that still lies flat on the yolk. Here, the neural plate is raised into *neural folds* and the mesoderm is organized into *notochord, somites,* and *lateral plates*.

**d Unsegmented Germ Layers behind the Primitive Node.** The ectodermal epithelium of the *primitive streak* contains the prospective mesoderm for notochord and somites. The material for the neural plate lies laterally on both sides of the primitive streak. Later, after the primitive node has migrated caudally and the mesoderm has invaginated, the neural plate forms the neural groove in the midline of the embryo.

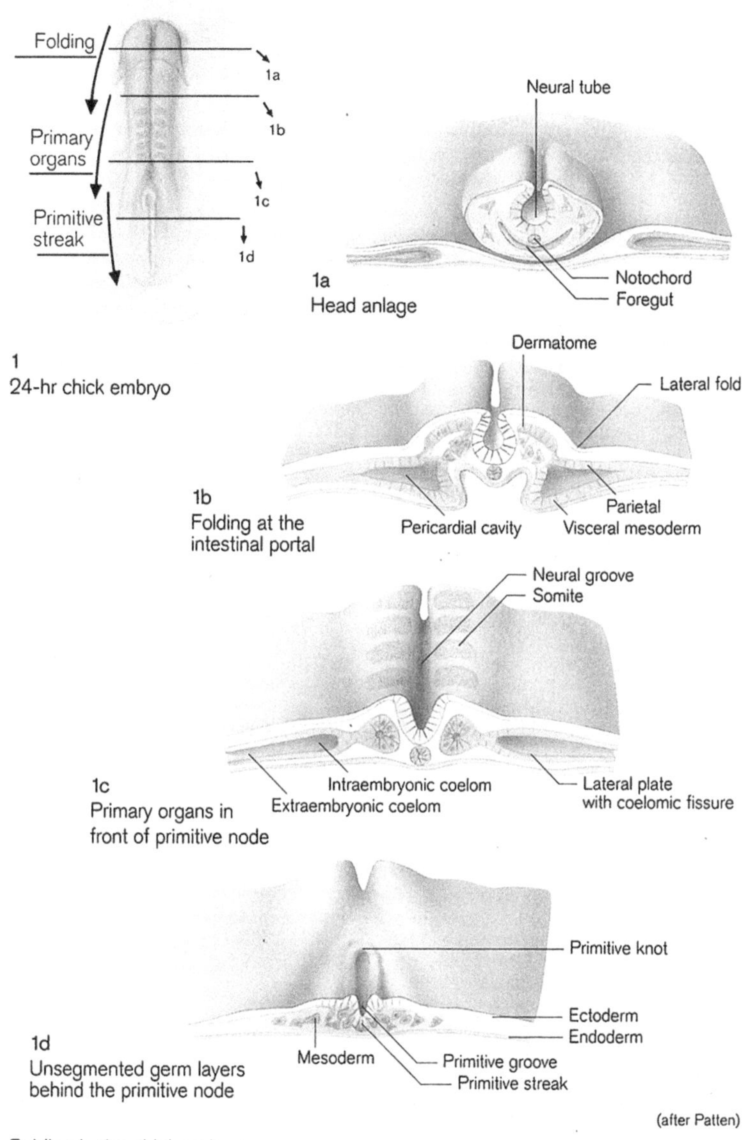
Folding
Primary organs
Primitive streak
1a
1b
1c
1d
1
24-hr chick embryo
Neural tube
Notochord
Foregut
1a
Head anlage
Dermatome
Lateral fold
Parietal
Visceral mesoderm
Pericardial cavity
1b
Folding at the intestinal portal
Neural groove
Somite
Intraembryonic coelom
Extraembryonic coelom
Lateral plate with coelomic fissure
1c
Primary organs in front of primitive node
Primitive knot
Ectoderm
Endoderm
Mesoderm
Primitive groove
Primitive streak
1d
Unsegmented germ layers behind the primitive node
(after Patten)

C. Folding in the chick embryo

# 3.10 Chick Embryo: Yolc Sac and Amniotic Cavity

## D. Conversion of the Primitive Node into the Tail Bud

**Tail Bud in the Chick Embryo.** In the 2½-day-old chick embryo, the primitive node (migrating caudally) reaches the end of the primitive streak (**D1**). The structure of the primitive node now diffuses into a broad area of undifferentiated tissue known as the blastema of the *tail bud* (**2b** and **c**). During further development, the tail bud gives rise to the notochord, somites, and neural tube in the lower half of the body. Neural tube and notochord form as complete structures directly from the tail bud blastema without the intermediate stages of neural groove formation (**2a**). In the tail bud, the development of the primary organs and the process of folding off via formation of lateral folds have caught up with (or even overtaken) the caudal migration of the primitive node. Beneath the tail bud, the digestive tube extends into the hind gut diverticulum, which opens into the yolk via the posterior intestinal portal.

A **tail bud is** already present in amphibian embryos (→ 3.18). In the chick embryo, the primitive pit does not break through into the gut. In contrast to the human embryo (→ 4.2), no axial canal arises and thus no neurenteric canal is formed.

## E. Yolk Sac and Amniotic Cavity

### 1. Growth over the Yolk Sac

The embryonic disc enlarges on the surface of the yolk sac between the vitelline membrane and the *yolk*. The margin of the embryonic disc consists of a thin ectodermal layer adhering to the vitelline membrane and an endodermal layer lying on the yolk. The *ectodermal marginal cells* move along the vitelline membrane by means of pseudopodia, pushing continuously over the large yolk-rich endodermal cells. The *mesodermal cells*, following at a distance, migrate inward between the ectoderm and *yolk endoderm* as a continuous layer. The mesodermal layer separates into a parietal layer, associated with the ectoderm, and a *visceral layer*, associated with the endoderm. The coelomic cavity (**E2**) arises between the two.

### 2. Fusion of Amniotic Folds

**Yolk Sac.** In the folding process, the definitive *intestinal tube* becomes constricted from the *yolk sac*, the two communicating only via the vitelline duct. The yolk comes to lie in the extraembryonic yolk sac, the wall of which consists of *yolk endoderm* and *extraembryonic visceral mesoderm*. Through the folding process, the small *intraembryonic coelom* separates from the large *extraembryonic coelom* (chorionic cavity).

**Amniotic Cavity.** During the folding of the embryonic body, the *amniotic folds* are formed laterally from the extraembryonic ectoderm and the *parietal layer of the mesoderm*. The embryo sinks slightly into the yolk and the amniotic folds fuse in the midline. The embryo thus becomes enclosed by the fluid-filled *amniotic cavity*. The fusion of the amniotic folds begins above the head and continues caudally with the folding of the embryonic body. In this zipper-like process, the amniotic folds ultimately fuse with the caudal amniotic fold above the tail bud of the embryo.

**Chorion.** After fusion of the amniotic folds and the complete enclosure of the yolk, there is no longer any connection between the embryo and the extraembryonic parietal mesoderm or ectoderm layers. The extraembryonic layers are known as the *chorion*, or in the case of birds, the *serosa*. Since the blood vessels lie in the visceral mesoderm, the chorion is primarily avascular. Through its connection with the allantois, it becomes the vascular-rich chorioallantois, which later dissolves the vitelline membrane and resorbs the white of the egg.

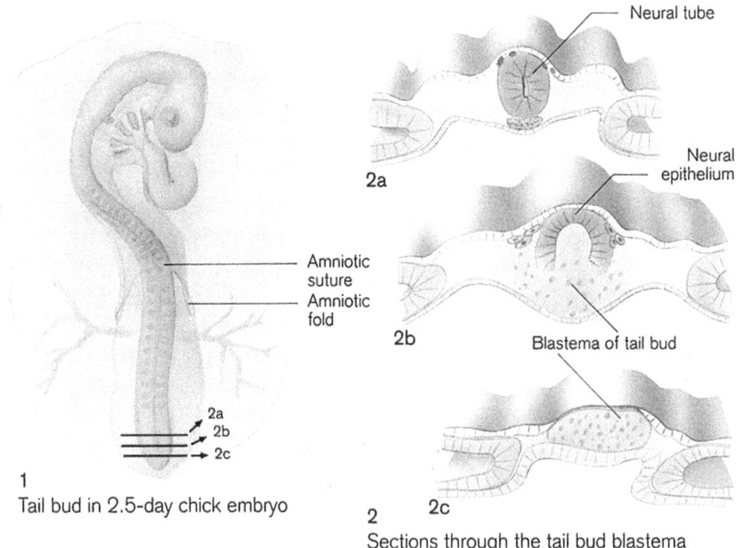


1
Tail bud in 2.5-day chick embryo

2
Sections through the tail bud blastema

D. Conversion of primitive knot into tail bud

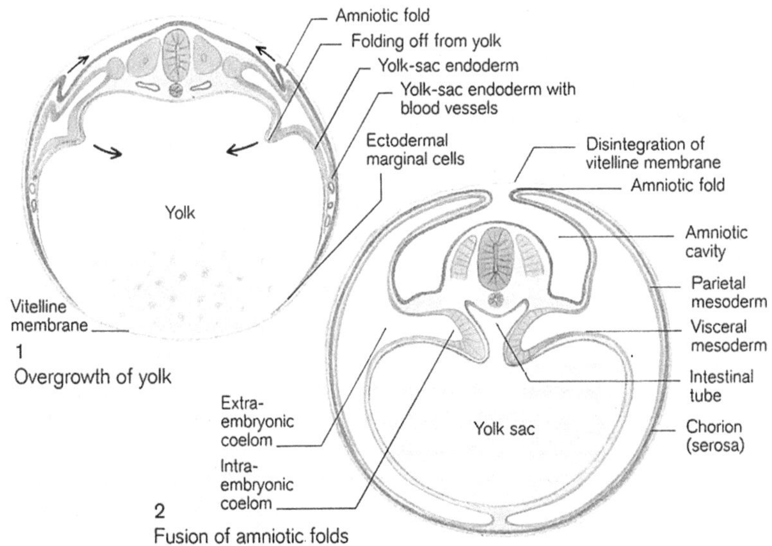


1
Overgrowth of yolk

2
Fusion of amniotic folds

E. Yolk sac and amniotic cavity

## 3.11 Chick Embryo: Fetal Membranes

*Background*

The **extraembryonic organs of the chick** have four **functions** in the egg: 1. **Nourishment** of the embryo. The embryo is nourished by the yolk, which is resorbed in the extraembryonic yolk sac and transported to the embryo via the vitelline vessels. 2. Establishment of an **aqueous environment,** in which morphogenetic movements can take place. This is accomplished by the amniotic fluid in the amniotic cavity where the embryo swims. 3. **Respiration**. The exchange of $O_2$ and $CO_2$ initially occurs in the capillary network of the yolk sac. As the yolk sac becomes smaller and the embryo larger, respiration is taken over by the chorioallantois, the forerunner of the placenta. 4. **Excretion** of metabolic end products. Before hatching, the chick cannot excrete substances that are usually eliminated with the urine. They are stored in the **allantois**, an extraembryonically located out-pocketing of the cloaca. The allantois consists of endoderm and highly vascularized visceral mesoderm. It fuses with the **chorion** and as the **chorioallantois**, takes over the respiratory function of the yolk sac from the 10th day of incubation until hatching on the 21st day. Since the chorion of the chick possesses no blood vessels, the embryo is connected with the chorioallantois only by the allantoic vessels.

### F. Position of the Embryo in the Egg

The chick embryo develops beneath the vitelline membrane and floats on the yolk (**F1**). The vitelline circulation is already formed on the 2nd day, when the embryonic disc covers just one-fourth of the yolk surface. Capillaries and blood islands arise in the mesodermal layer of the yolk sac. They are connected at the periphery with the *marginal sinus* and via vitelline arteries and veins with the beating heart, which arises below the anterior intestinal portal.

### G. Development of the Chorioallantois

**1. Formation of the Allantois.** On the 4th day, the allantois grows forward as an endodermal vesicle between the *cloacal membrane* and the vitelline duct, and enters the *extraembryonic coelom* (*chorionic cavity*) (**1a**). It evaginates from the part of the cloaca corresponding to the urinary bladder and is filled with urine from the embryonic mesonephros.

**2. Chorion and Chorionic Cavity.** After fusion of the *amniotic folds* and of the margins of the embryonic disc below the yolk (**G1**), the *extraembryonic coelom* is united above the *amniotic cavity* and below the *yolk sac* into an undivided *chorionic cavity* (**G3**). The external ectodermal layer, with its associated parietal mesoderm, becomes the *chorion* surrounding the embryo and the yolk sac. The chorion lies below the *vitelline membrane*, which disintegrates.

**3. Fusion of Chorion and Allantois.** The highly vascularized allantois finally fuses with the chorion, forming the **chorioallantois**, which replaces the diminishing yolk sac as the nutritive and respiratory organ. The vessels coursing in the visceral mesoderm of the allantois become the vascular stem of the chorioallantois and thus correspond to the umbilical vessels of mammals. The white of the egg is resorbed by the chorioallantois and is transported to the embryo as nutriment. As a respiratory organ, the chorioallantois lies closely apposed to the shell membrane and ultimately surrounds the entire embryo.

**Chorioallantoic Grafting.** The chick embryo is easily accessible for experimentation. By removal of a small amount of egg white (using suction), a second air chamber is formed over the embryo. A window can now be made in the calcareous shell and the shell membrane. The window is resealed with tape afterward. For chorioallantoic grafting, the egg is opened in this fashion at the beginning of the 3rd day of incubation. After the chorioallantois has formed on the 11th day, a test tissue can be transplanted onto the well-vascularized surface via the window and cultured up until the 20th day.

Calcareous shell
Shell membrane
Chorionic cavity
Vitelline membrane
Allantois
Marginal sinus
Egg white
Yolk
1
4 days old
Allantois
Amniotic cavity
Vitelline vessels
Yolk
2
5.5 days old

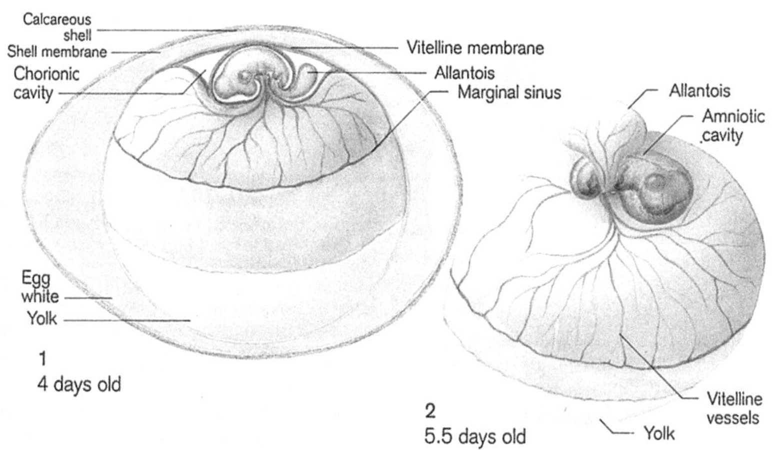

F. Position of chick embryo in egg

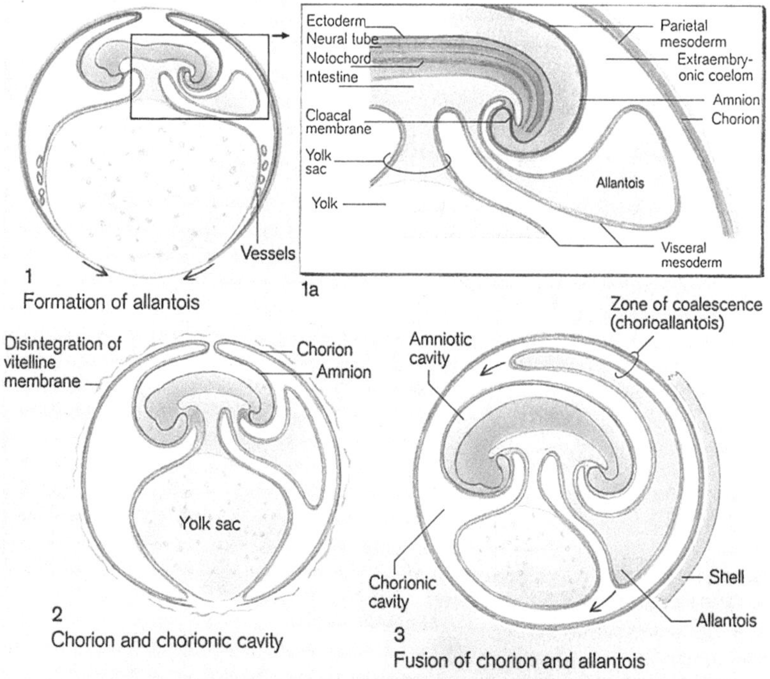

Vessels
1
Formation of allantois
Ectoderm
Neural tube
Notochord
Intestine
Cloacal membrane
Yolk sac
Yolk
Parietal mesoderm
Extraembry-onic coelom
Amnion
Chorion
Allantois
Visceral mesoderm
1a
Disintegration of vitelline membrane
Chorion
Amnion
Yolk sac
2
Chorion and chorionic cavity
Zone of coalescence (chorioallantois)
Amniotic cavity
Chorionic cavity
Shell
Allantois
3
Fusion of chorion and allantois

G. Development of chorioallantois

## 3.12 Quail-Chick Transplantation

*Background*

**Principle.** The technique of quail–chick transplantation (described by Nicole LeDouarin in 1969) is used to study the migratory movements of cells during embryonic development. The region of interest is transplanted from the quail embryo into the chick embryo. The transplanted tissue integrates without reaction while the chick undergoes further normal development. In paraffin sections, the quail and chick cells can be distinguished from each other by the Feulgen reaction. Whereas the nucleoli of quail cells are distinctly stained, the chick cell nuclei appear more homogeneous.

### A. Quail–Chick Transplantation

In a typical experiment to demonstrate the migration of neural crest cells (**A1**), a section of neural tube in a chick embryo at the somite stage is removed before emigration of neural crest cells and is replaced by a section of *neural tube* from a quail embryo of the same stage. The operation is carried out in a fenestrated egg through a small slit in the vitelline membrane, using needles of tungsten wire and small glass pipettes. The section of neural tube from the quail embryo undergoes normal development in the chick embryo. After 18 hours, the migration of *neural crest cells* can be observed in serial sections (**A2**). This method is also used to study migratory movements in the limb bud or in the origin of mesoderm. It is superior to the staining technique developed in amphibian embryos (→ 3.5) or the labelling of transplants with tritiated thymidine, since the marking cannot be lost by diffusion or by dilution during cell division.

### B. Experiments on the Derivation of the Peripheral Nervous System

#### 1. Autonomic Nervous System

The derivation of neurons of the autonomic ganglia can be determined by systematic transplantation of sections of neural tube from the quail embryo into the chick and histological study of the resulting quail–chick chimeras.

**Ciliary Ganglion.** The neurons of the ciliary ganglion arise from the neural crest of the mesencephalon.

**Parasympathetic System.** The neurons of the ganglia of the vagus, and in the parasympathetic ganglia along the gastrointestinal tract arise from the *neural crest* at the level of somites 1–7. This corresponds to the segments of origin of the vagus nerve. Below the umbilicus, parasympathetic neurons emerge from the neural crest caudal to the 28th somite (sacral portion of the parasympathetic system).

**Sympathetic System.** The autonomic neurons in the ganglia of the sympathetic nervous system originate from the neural crest below the 5th somitic segment. The chromaffin cells of the adrenal medulla are derived from somites 18 to 24 of the neural crest.

The experiments show that the functional organization of the autonomic nervous system is already determined at the time of migration of neural crest cells.

#### 2. Cephalic Ganglia

Transplantation of the *cephalic neural crest, otic vesicle,* or *epibranchial placodes* from the quail embryo into the chick makes it possible to determine the portion of neurons in the cephalic ganglia arising from the placodes (**2a**). The neurons and glial cells of the *spinal ganglia* arise exclusively from the *neural crest* (**2b**), whereas the *sensory ganglia* of the pharyngeal arch nerves are derived in part from the epibranchial placodes.

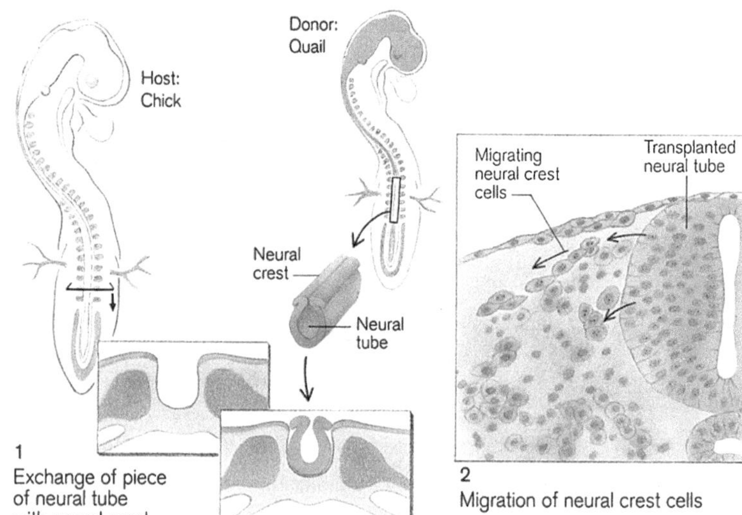


A. Quail-chick transplantation (after LeDouarin)

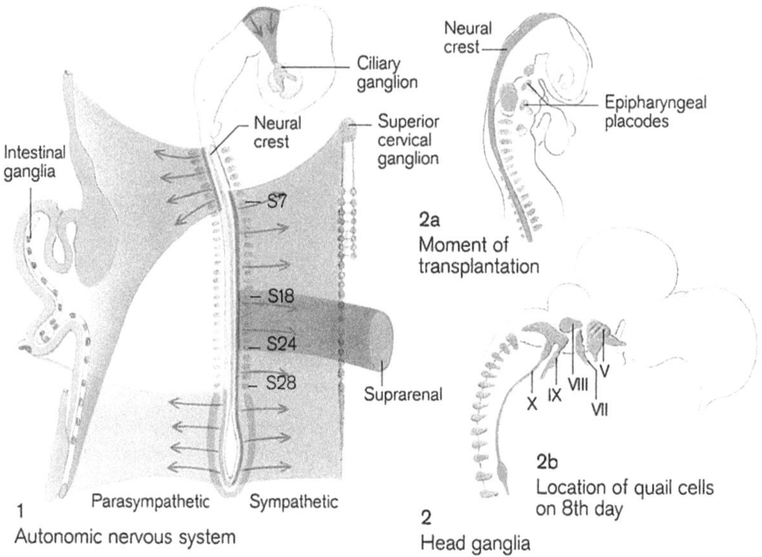


B. Experiments on the derivation of the peripheral nervous system

# Mammals

# 3.13 Early Development

*Background*

The **structure of the fetal membranes and placenta** indicate that mammals are derived from egg-laying ancestors. The embryo remains in the uterus (an expansion of the female genital duct) and is nourished via the placenta. Storage of yolk in the oocyte is therefore no longer necessary. The deposition of egg white and a calcareous shell during migration through the oviduct was replaced by the connection of the yolk sac vessels and ultimately of the chorioallantois to the maternal circulation.

## A. Early Development of Mammals

**1. Cleavage.** In the secondarily yolk-poor eggs of higher mammals, cleavage divisions produce equal-sized daughter cells (blastomeres). The blastomeres are pluripotent: Each cell can form all tissues, including germ cells. In sea urchins and amphibians, the differentiation of animal and vegetal poles is determined by maternal factors (mRNA in the cytoplasm of the oocyte). In mammals, this differentiation process is activated by regulatory factors produced by the embryonic cells themselves.

**2. Blastocyst.** After hatching from the zona pellucida, the blastocyst swims in the uterine lumen and is nourished by mucosal secretions. The *trophoblast cells* are therefore the first cells to differentiate and become distinct from the *inner cell mass*. They form an external epithelium with tight junctions, and actively transport fluid and nutrients into the blastocyst cavity.

**3. Bilaminar Embryonic Disc.** The embryonic disc originally developed in the wall of the blastocyst, a form of development that is preserved in species with superficial implantation, such as the hedgehog (Insectivora), many rodents, the pig, and the dog. The *trophoblast cells* above the inner cell mass degenerate. The inner cell mass, as a bilaminar embryonic disc, is intercalated into the epithelial layer of the trophoblast. The endodermal cells line the blastocyst cavity and form the extraembryonically situated yolk sac.

**4. Trilaminar Embryonic Disc.** The *mesoderm* arises in the embryonic disc via the *primitive streak*. It migrates laterally between the ectoderm and endoderm and, as extraembryonic mesoderm, penetrates between the trophoblast and the yolk sac. Blood vessels for the placenta can only arise in the mesoderm.

**5. Folding.** The mesodermal layer separates into a *parietal layer* facing the ectoderm and a *visceral layer* facing the endoderm; the body cavity arises between the two. The extraembryonic part of the cleft becomes the chorionic cavity. The embryonic body folds off from the yolk sac. The amniotic folds (arrows) are formed as in the chick embryo (→ 3.10) **(folding amnion)**.

**6. Embryonic Cavities.** Like the avian embryo, the mammalian embryo develops in an amniotic cavity and possesses an extraembryonic yolk sac that lies in the *chorionic cavity*. The chorion consists of an inner layer of extraembryonic mesoderm and an epithelial layer of extraembryonic ectoderm, derived from the trophoblast.

**7. Yolk Sac Placenta.** The placenta connects the fetal and maternal circulation so that nourishment, respiration, and excretion of metabolic products can take place. The simplest form of placenta is produced by the fusion of the vascularized yolk sac with the chorion (yolk sac placenta). Marsupials and lower mammals possess a yolk sac placenta.

**8. Allantois Placenta.** Fusion of the vascularized *allantois* with the chorion (allantois-placenta) is homologous to the formation of the chorioallantois in birds. In many mammals, formation of a yolk sac placenta is followed by formation of an allantois placenta (→ 3.14). In humans, only an allantois placenta develops. However, even in mammals with allantois placentas, the *yolk sac* is preserved as the site of blood formation and the site of origin of primordial germ cells.

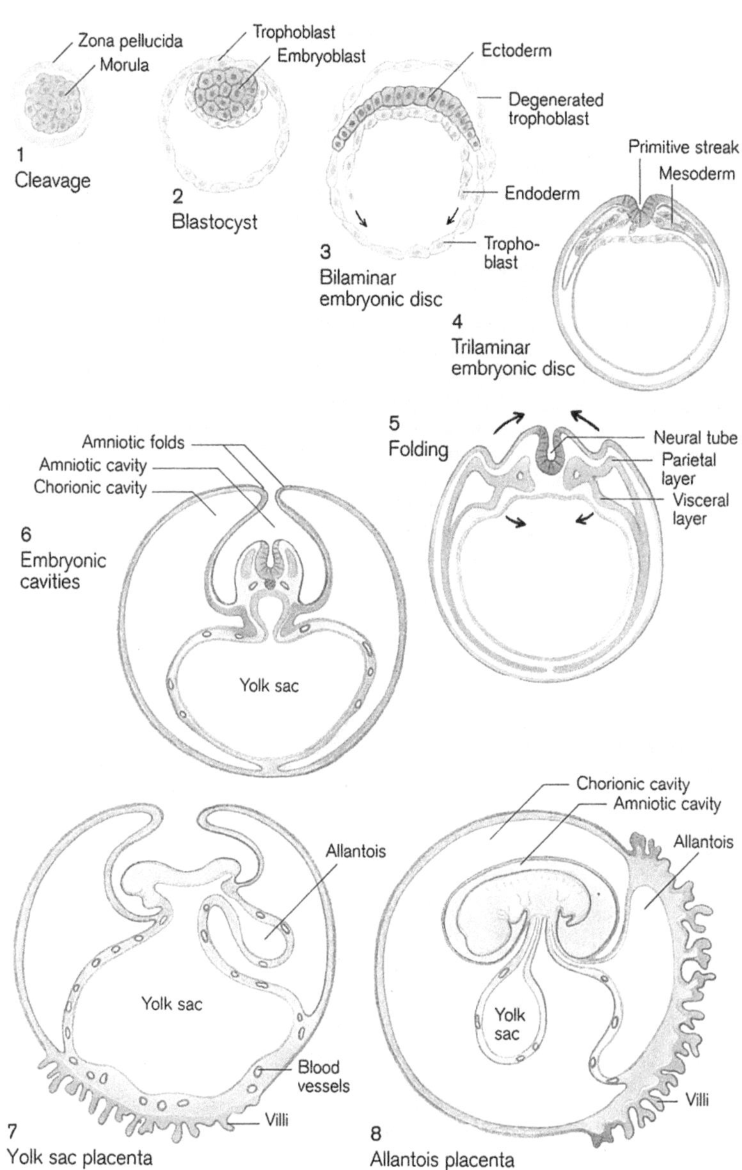
Zona pellucida
Morula
1
Cleavage
Trophoblast
Embryoblast
2
Blastocyst
Ectoderm
Degenerated trophoblast
Endoderm
Tropho-blast
3
Bilaminar embryonic disc
Primitive streak
Mesoderm
4
Trilaminar embryonic disc
5
Folding
Neural tube
Parietal layer
Visceral layer
Amniotic folds
Amniotic cavity
Chorionic cavity
6
Embryonic cavities
Yolk sac
Allantois
Yolk sac
Blood vessels
Villi
7
Yolk sac placenta
Chorionic cavity
Amniotic cavity
Allantois
Yolk sac
Villi
8
Allantois placenta

A. Early development of mammals

# 3.14 Mammals: Implantation

*Background*

**Implantation** is part of the **reproductive strategy** of a species. Cleavage and blastocyst development are very similar in all species. Implantation, in contrast, is highly species-specific. The **pig** and the **mouse** initially utilize the **resorption principle**, which is optimized in two quite different ways (→ 3.15). **Humans** form an allantois placenta directly, which functions according to the **diffusion principle.**

## B. Species-Specific Course of Implantation

**1. Superficial Implantation in the Pig.** In the pig, the original principle of intercalation of the *germinal disc* into the blastocyst wall is preserved. The blastocyst lies centrally in the uterine cavity and does not penetrate the mucous membrane (**1a**) (central superficial implantation). The extraembryonic mesoderm arises precociously and lines the chorionic cavity. As in the chick, the amniotic cavity forms by fusion of amniotic folds above the embryo (**folding amnion**). In the chorionic cavity, a well-developed *yolk sac* is first formed (**1b**). This is followed by the formation of the *allantois* (**1c**), which fuses with the chorion to form an *allantois placenta*. The chorionic vesicle of the pig grows enormously in length (over 1 m) before forming villi over its entire surface (*diffuse placenta*).

**2. Interstitial Implantation in the Human.** The human blastocyst implants in the connective tissue of the uterus (interstitial implantation) (**2a**). The trophoblast penetrates invasively into the mucosa. Afterwards, the embryonic disc arises simultaneously with the amniotic cavity (**2b**). A cleft appears between the inner cell mass and the trophoblast; at its base, the ectoderm of the bilayered embryonic disc forms. The cavity is secondarily lined by amnioblasts (**modified cavitation amnion**) (→ 2.8). Characteristic features are the enlargement of the chorionic cavity, which is accompanied by the transformation of the *primary* into the smaller *secondary* yolk sac (umbilical vesicle), and the early vascularization of the chorion. The vascularization of the chorion through the *body stalk* is preliminary to the development of an *allantois placenta* (**2c**). The body stalk is an allantoic stalk, into which a rudimentary allantoic diverticulum later grows. The vascularized trophoblast is, in effect, a *chorioallantois*, although it is conventionally defined as a chorion. In the narrow sense, the *chorion* consists of the trophoblast and the extraembryonic parietal mesoderm, which is still devoid of allantoic vessels.

**3. Inversion of Germ Layers in the Mouse.** Apart from interstitial implantation, the mouse exhibits specific adaptations that go beyond the specialization in humans. The blastocyst attaches itself at an endometrial gland of the decidua (**3a**). At the apical pole of the blastocyst, the trophoblast forms a cellular plug (*ectoplacenta, "ectoplacental cone"*) as precursor of the placenta. In the embryonic disc, a vertical cleft arises and widens into the *amniotic cavity* (**cavitation amnion**). The cleft that forms in the ectoplacenta is independent of the amniotic cavity and corresponds to an accessory blastocyst cavity. The embryonic disc protrudes into the primary *yolk sac*, which in turn extends into the trophoblast cavity and covers the trophoblast externally (*inversion of germ layers* ). The outer layer of the inverted yolk sac disintegrates together with the overlying trophoblast, so that the inner layer of the yolk sac contacts the uterine connective tissue. The dorsally concave curvature of the embryo that results from the inversion of the germ layers (**3b**) is reversed during the folding process (**3c**), when the embryo rotates around its body axis. Extraembryonic mesoderm invades the trophoblast of the ectoplacenta as stalk of vascular connective tissue without formation of an endodermal allantois. The **ectoplacenta** of the mouse is thus a precocious allantois placenta. Due to the inversion of the germ layers; the embryonic endoderm is in direct contact with uterine mucosa, from which it resorbs nutrients.

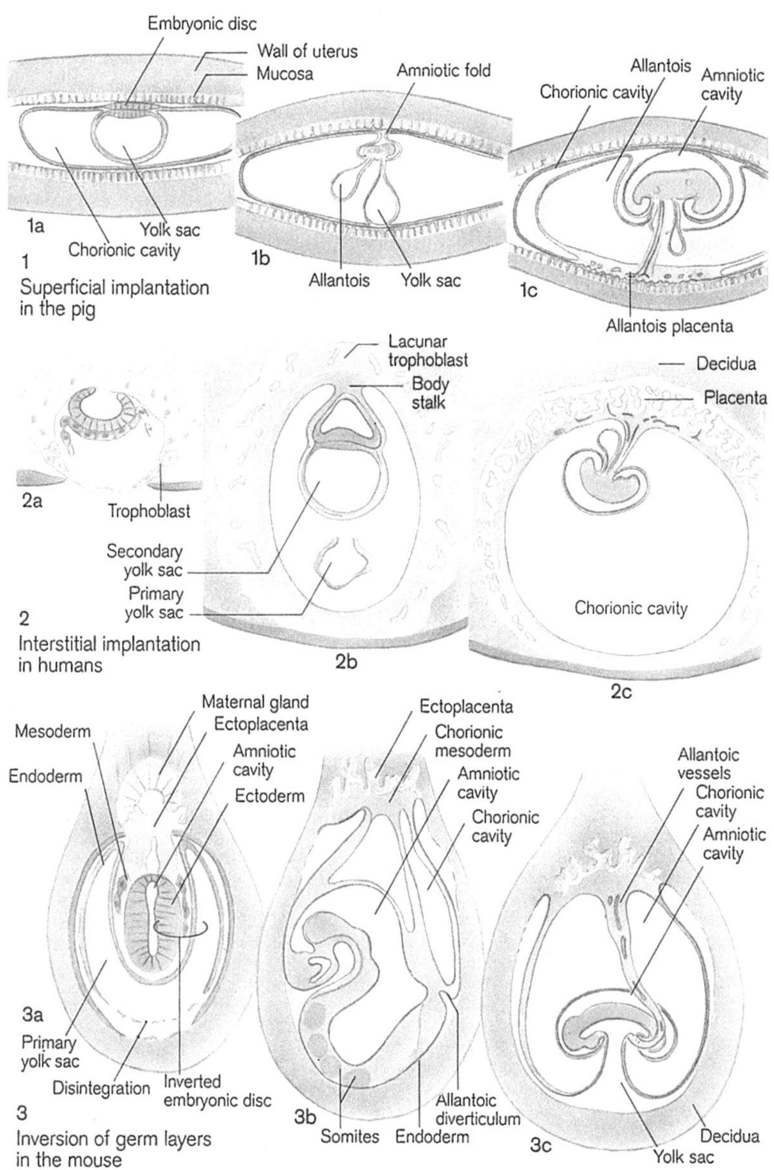
Embryonic disc
Wall of uterus
Mucosa
Amniotic fold
Allantois
Amniotic cavity
Chorionic cavity
1a
Yolk sac
Chorionic cavity
1
Superficial implantation in the pig
1b
Allantois
Yolk sac
1c
Allantois placenta
Lacunar trophoblast
Body stalk
Decidua
Placenta
2a
Trophoblast
Secondary yolk sac
Primary yolk sac
2
Interstitial implantation in humans
2b
Chorionic cavity
2c
Maternal gland
Ectoplacenta
Mesoderm
Amniotic cavity
Endoderm
Ectoderm
Ectoplacenta
Chorionic mesoderm
Amniotic cavity
Chorionic cavity
Allantoic vessels
Chorionic cavity
Amniotic cavity
3a
Primary yolk sac
Disintegration
Inverted embryonic disc
3
Inversion of germ layers in the mouse
3b
Somites
Endoderm
Allantoic diverticulum
3c
Decidua
Yolk sac

B. Species-specific course of implantation

# 3.15 Mammals: Placental Structure

## A. Contact between Chorionic Villi and Mucosa

### 1. The Principle of Resorption

The free-swimming blastocyst is nourished by **resorption of mucus,** which is secreted by the endometrial glands. After formation of a placenta, nutrition occurs by the diffusion of nutrients from the maternal to the fetal circulation. Diffusion takes place through the chorionic villi, which are in intimate contact with the uterine mucosa.

### 2. The Principle of Diffusion

Histological analysis of the mature placenta shows that the layers of maternal tissue lying between the maternal blood and the fetal villi have disappeared to different extents in different species. This observation can be interpreted as progressive **disintegration of diffusion barriers** on the maternal side in the course of evolution, while the fetal side remains intact. According to Grosser (1919), the following types of placentas may be distinguished:

**(a) Epitheliochorial Placenta.** All maternal layers are retained. The chorionic villi are closely apposed to the uterine epithelium. This type of placenta occurs, for example, in the pig. It is associated with superficial implantation of the blastocyst.

**(b) Endotheliochorial Placenta.** The trophoblast cells fuse into a syncytium and penetrate invasively into the decidua. The mucosal epithelium and the decidua disintegrate, but the endothelium of the maternal vessels is not degraded.

**(c) Hemochorial Placenta.** The endothelium of the maternal capillaries is additionally degraded by the syncytium. Maternal blood flows into the lacunae and bathes the chorionic villi directly.

## B. Labyrinthine Placenta and Villous Placenta in the Human

In a **labyrinthine placenta,** the maternal blood flows through the highly branched (labyrinthine) lacunae of the trophoblastic syncytium, which has grown invasively into the endometrium. A **villous placenta** is formed by the sprouting of branched chorionic villi. In humans, a *labyrinthine placenta* (**B1**) is initially formed. The invasive growth of the trophoblast stops, however, at the beginning of the third week, when the *stem villi* (**B2**) and the **cytotrophoblastic shell** develop (→ 2.40). *Villous trees* (**B3**) form between the trophoblast layer of the chorionic plate and the basal plate. The human placenta thus represents a combination between a labyrinthine placenta (formed by invasive growth) and a villous placenta (formed by sprouting).

## C. External Form of the Placenta

The placenta is the part of the chorion in which the chorionic villi differentiate and contact the maternal circulation. In the **pig** (**C1**), the villi are distributed over the entire chorion (*diffuse placenta*). In **humans** (**C2**), the placenta is disc shaped (*discoid placenta*). This structure arises by partial regression of villi, which initially cover the entire surface of the chorion. In the **rhesus monkey** (**C3**), the blastocyst is implanted centrally in the uterine lumen and penetrates the mucosa at two opposite poles. Thus, two placental discs are formed (*bidiscoid placenta* ). In the **mouse** (**C4**), the *discoid placenta* originates from trophoblast cells that separate precociously from the blastocyst (*ectoplacenta*). The remaining chorion regresses together with the maternal mucosal epithelium, causing the fetal membranes to be covered externally by the remnants of the primary yolk sac (→ 3.14).

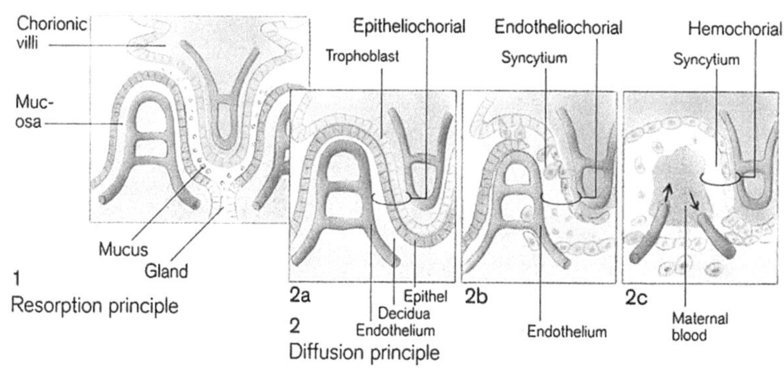


A. Contact between chorionic villi and mucosa

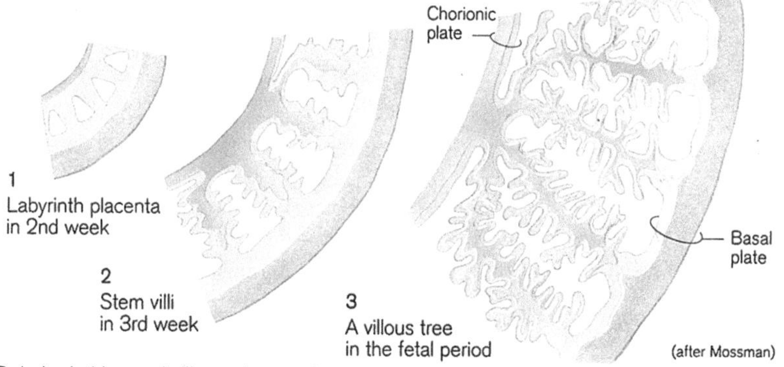


B. Labyrinthine and villous placenta in man

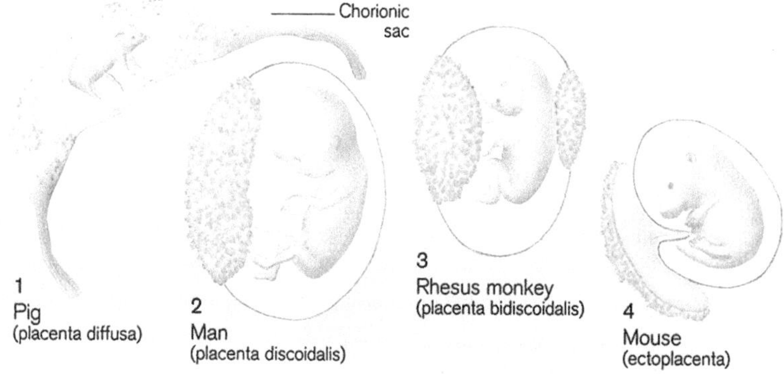


C. External forms of placenta

## 3.16 Transgenic Mice

*Background*

**Molecular Biology.** Isolated genes can be cloned and amplified in bacteria or amplified by means of a heat-stable bacterial DNA polymerase using the "polymerase chain reaction" (PCR). The function of an isolated **structural gene** can be tested in vitro. The DNA can be injected into tissue culture cells with a micromanipulator. The cells integrate one or more copies of the gene in their genome, duplicate it in the cell cycle, and express the gene product, which is under the control of promoter and operator sequences incorporated with the gene. The function of **regulatory genes** that control the determination of cells and tissues during embryonic development can only be tested in the whole organism. For this purpose, transgenic mice are used. An example is the demonstration of the function of the "sex-determining region" (Sry), which was isolated from the Y chromosomes of mouse and human cells.

### A. Production of Transgenic Mice

**1. Injection of DNA.** Fertilized oocytes are obtained from the uterine horn of a donor mouse by flushing. $10^{-10}$ mL (0.1 pL) of DNA solution (containing the gene of interest) are injected into the male or female pronucleus with a micromanipulator.

**2. Blastocyst transfer.** After passing through cleavage in vitro, the blastocysts are transferred to the uterus of a pseudopregnant mouse, where they complete development.

**3. Transgenic Mice.** About 10% to 30% of the newborn mice express the injected DNA in all body tissues, including the germ cells. Since the DNA was injected in only one of the pronuclei, the animals are heterozygotic for the transferred gene.

**4. Establishment of an Inbred Strain.** The transgenic animals are paired with normal mice. Half of the descendents are again heterozygotic for the injected gene. By backcrossing with the transgenic parent, a homozygotic mouse strain can be established for the transferred gene.

### B. Identification of the Sex-Determining Region (SRY)

**1. Cytogenetic Localization.** The sex chromosomes were discovered in 1959. In mammals, the Y chromosome induces the development of a testis and thus initiates male development (→8.5). The female phenotype is formed constitutively. In 1966, cytogenetic analysis of sex chromosomal aberrations (→8.10) in humans revealed that the male-determining region was confined to the short arm of the Y chromosome (Yp). Since the only known gene product of the Y chromosome was the weak *histocompatibility antigen HY*, this protein was long considered a candidate for the testis-determining factor. Analysis of XX male patients and of *sex reversed* mice (Sxr) led to the elucidation of the pairing region between the X and Y chromosomes, by which the testis-determining sequence could be transferred to the X chromosome. In 1986, this region was restricted in an XX male patient to 140 kb (kilobases). This DNA sequence contains a regulatory gene encoding a zinc-finger protein. Through the analysis of XX male patients lacking the *Zfy-region*, the region in question was reduced to 60 kb. Analysis of additional patients and omission of repetitive gene sequences reduced the **S**ex-determining **R**egion of the **Y**-chromosome to 35 kb (SRY, human sequence in capital letters).

**2. Transfection of Sry-sequence into a Mouse Strain.** By transfecting the 35 kb mouse sequence into an inbred strain, Koopman and co-workers (1991) succeeded in producing two transgenic XX males. The regulatory gene Sry (**2a**) that is injected into the zygote is activated in the Sertoli cells of the gonads in XX embryos (**2b**). It induces the development of a testis and thus a male phenotype (**2c**). The Sry gene possesses a highly conserved central HMG ("high mobility group") box, which binds to DNA without sequence specifity.

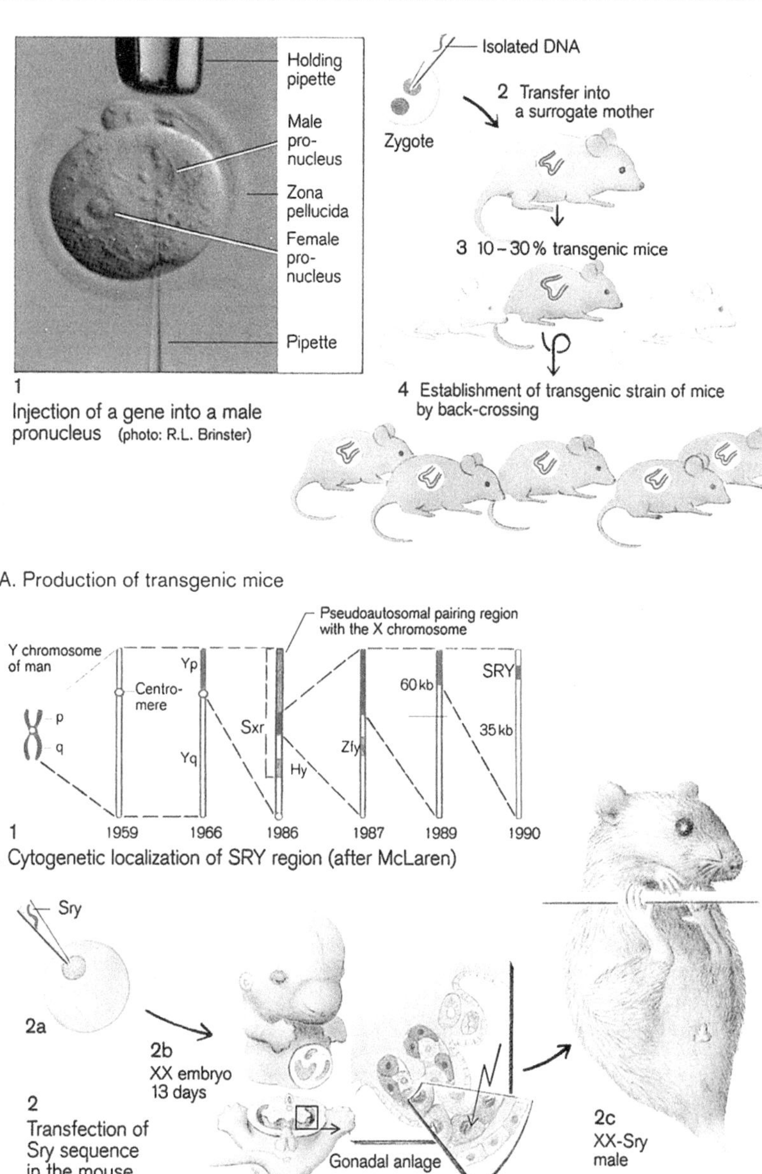


1
Injection of a gene into a male pronucleus (photo: R.L. Brinster)

A. Production of transgenic mice

1
Cytogenetic localization of SRY region (after McLaren)

2
Transfection of Sry sequence in the mouse

B. Identification of sex-determining region (Sry) on the Y chromosome

## Drosophila
# 3.17 Homeotic Genes

*Background*

In the fruit fly **(Drosophila melanogaster)** the genes determining segmentation of the embryo were analyzed genetically and characterized by molecular biology. The segmentation genes (**homeotic genes**) possess a common sequence, the homeobox domain. Segmentation genes are present in the genomes of all segmentally organized animals, including vertebrates. As regulatory genes in embryonic development, they induce the arrangement of the body into segments and determine which organs arise in the segments.

## A. Segmentation genes in Drosophila

**1. Syncytial Blastoderm and Expression of Segmentation Genes.** In the fertilized Drosophila zygote, "cleavage" occurs without the formation of cell boundaries. The cell nuclei migrate to the surface of the zygote, forming a syncytial blastoderm. At this stage, the body segments are determined by the segmentation genes. After *in-situ* hybridization with specific radioactive antisense DNA probes, the mRNA of the segmentation genes can be visualized by autoradiography in histological sections. Within an hour, a cascade of activation of four groups of segmentation genes takes place, giving rise to a complex "striped" pattern in the embryo. A representative gene is illustrated for each group (**1a**). The polarity of the embryo is determined by **maternal genes** that were already transcribed into mRNA before fertilization of the oocyte (maternal factors for embryonic development). The expression of the **"gap" genes** is induced by the diffusion gradients of the products of the maternal genes (**1b**). Mutations in the "gap" genes lead to gaps in the series of segments. The gene products of the "gap" genes in turn induce the **"pair-rule" genes**. These form a pattern of seven stripes that already reflects the prospective segmental arrangement of the larva.

The expression of two **"segment-polarity" genes** in the anterior and posterior portions of the segments determines the polarity of the segments. A pattern of 14 bands appears. After formation of cell boundaries (after 2.5h of development), the cascade of activation continues in essentially the same manner.

**2. Cellular Blastoderm and Expression of Antennapedia and Ultrabithorax.** The syncytial blastoderm is transformed into the cellular blastoderm. At the caudal pole, the *germ cells* (*pole cells*) differentiate first. Afterwards, the cell boundaries develop synchronously in the entire blastoderm, giving rise to an epithelial layer that surrounds the yolk. The segments of the larvae and the adult flies are now already determined and can be projected back to the stage of the cellular blastoderm.

The diffusion gradients of the gene products of **antennapedia (Antp)** and **ultrabithorax (Ubx)** (**1a**) determine the border between the thoracic and the abdominal segments. In the Antp mutation of the antennapedia gene, legs (instead of antennae) develop on the head. In the Ubx mutation of the ultrabithorax gene, an additional segment with wings arises in place of the third thoracic segment (**4a**, doubling of T2).

**3. Imaginal Discs in the Larva.** As the inner organs develop, the segments become visible on the surface of the larva. Each segment is functionally divided into an anterior and a posterior compartment. The *imaginal discs* are invaginations of the original blastoderm epithelium that contain the primordial material for the organs of the adult insect. They consist of stem cells that are determined to form wings, antennae, or gonads. Inside the imaginal disc, the pattern of the future organs is not yet determined.

**4. Adult Flies.** Metamorphosis into an adult insect is initiated during the last pupation by the pupation hormone ecdysone, which is produced by the endocrine prothorax gland. The imaginal discs evaginate and develop into the organs of the adult insect, while the body of the larva disintegrates, providing nutrition for the developing adult animal.

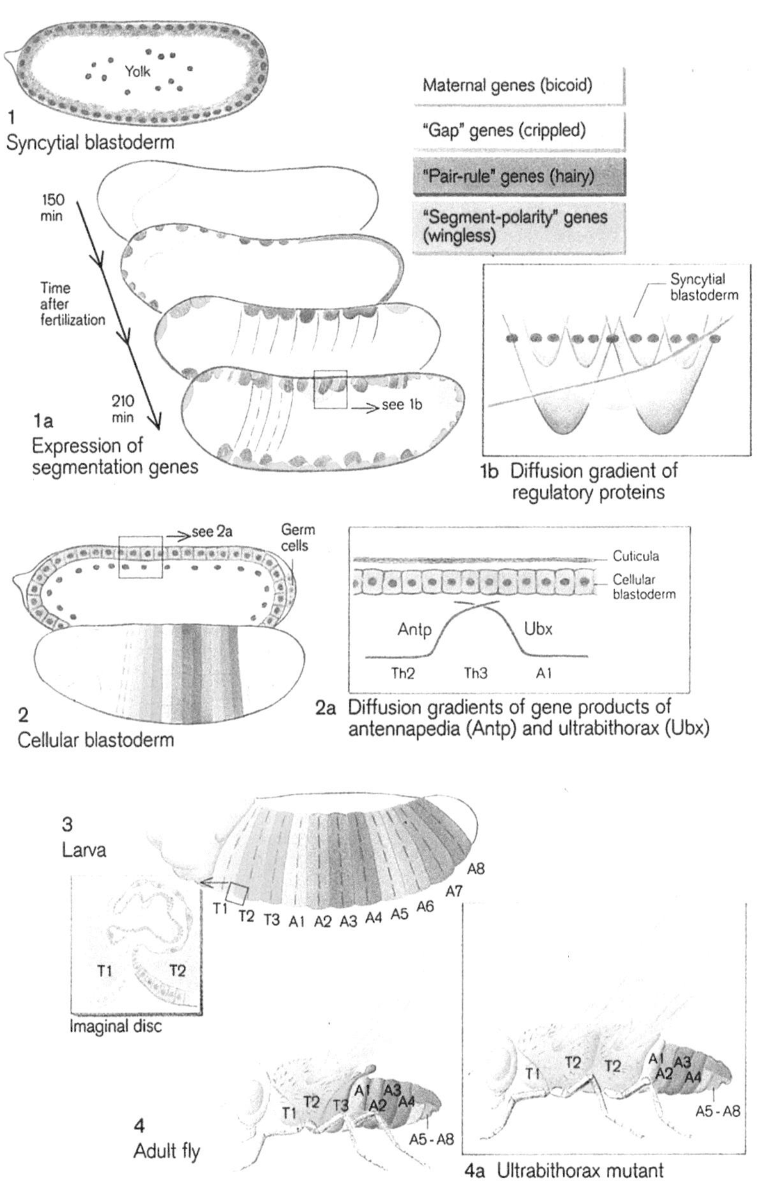

Yolk
1
Syncytial blastoderm
Maternal genes (bicoid)
"Gap" genes (crippled)
"Pair-rule" genes (hairy)
"Segment-polarity" genes (wingless)
150 min
Time after fertilization
210 min
see 1b
1a
Expression of segmentation genes
Syncytial blastoderm
1b Diffusion gradient of regulatory proteins
see 2a
Germ cells
Cuticula
Cellular blastoderm
Antp
Ubx
Th2
Th3
A1
2
Cellular blastoderm
2a Diffusion gradients of gene products of antennapedia (Antp) and ultrabithorax (Ubx)
3
Larva
T1 T2 T3 A1 A2 A3 A4 A5 A6 A7 A8
T1
T2
Imaginal disc
T1 T2 T2 A1 A2 A3 A4
A5 - A8
4
Adult fly
T1 T2 T3 A1 A2 A3 A4
A5 - A8
4a Ultrabithorax mutant

A. Segment genes of Drosophila

Basic Body Plan

## 3.18 Homology between Gastrula and Embryonic Disc

*Background*

The basic structure of the **vertebrate body**, consisting of a dorsally located neural tube, segmental muscular plates, and a ventrally situated digestive tube, is more distinctly expressed in the embryo than in the adult forms. In lower vertebrates with complete cleavage, the embryo arises by morphogenetic movements during **gastrulation** . The embryonic stage (e.g., tail bud stage in amphibia, **2a**) is transformed directly into the independently feeding, free-swimming juvenile form. The myotomes function as muscle plates and the notochord as an axial rod. At the end of the embryonic period, the embryos of reptiles, birds, and mammals bear a strong resemblance to each other and exhibit the same basic body plan as the embryos of lower vertebrates. The embryonic body develops from an **embryonic disc**. The morphogenetic movements in the embryonic disc fulfill the same function as gastrulation (i.e., development of body form). Comparison of gastrulation with the formation of germ layers in the embryonic disc illustrates the homologies in development and points out the basic body plan common to all vertebrates.

### A. Development of Body Form

**1. Gastrulation in Yolk-poor Eggs**

During gastrulation of lower vertebrates, a *blastopore* is formed. It corresponds to the mouth opening of coelenterates. The definitive mouth opening arises in the region of the *pharyngeal membrane* (**1a**). The mesoderm becomes detached from the roof of the archenteron (**1b**).

**2. Larval Stage in Amphibia**

In the tail bud stage of amphibia, the body form (corresponding to the basic structure of vertebrates) is already developed (**2a**). The body axis extends beyond the tail bud. Closure of the neural tube progresses caudally past the blastopore and into the *tail bud*. The blastopore opens into the neural tube and transiently connects the central canal of the spinal cord with the intestinal tube, forming the *neurenteric canal*. The definitive *anus* arises secondarily below the tail bud.

**Imaginary Widening into an Embryonic Disc.** As a “thought experiment,” one can take a transverse section through an amphibian embryo and cut open the ventral side (body wall and intestinal wall). The resulting body form is flat, resembling an embryonic disc. Such a form could arise, for example, by an increased amount of yolk in the intestinal tube.

**3. Development of Body Form via an Embryonic Disc**

**a Homology between the Blastopore and the Primitive Pit.** In longitudinal section through the germinal disc, the *primitive pit with the axial canal* resembles the blastopore, through which gastrulation takes place. As the primitive node migrates caudally (→ 3.8), the material of the notochord and the mesodermal material for the somites involute, migrating cranially and laterally. The primitive gut emerging from the axial canal opens widely into the yolk.

**b Human Embryo.** In species such as the human, which possess an axial canal, the developmental homology is more apparent than in the chick embryo, in which no structure comparable to the axial canal develops. In stage 9 of the human embryo (→ 2.13), the homology between the *pharyngeal membrane*, *cloacal membrane*, and *tail bud* and the corresponding structures in an amphibian embryo at the tail bud stage is clear. The notochord is intercalated into the roof of the archenteron, homologous to the notochord-mesoderm complex (→ 3.3 and 3.4).

**c The Body Form Arises by Folding.** In an embryo that begins its development by forming an embryonic disc, the basic body form is produced by a process of folding off from the yolk (→ 2.15 and 3.9). This developmental movement is the reverse of the imaginary expansion of the amphibian embryo cut open ventrally (represented in **2b**).

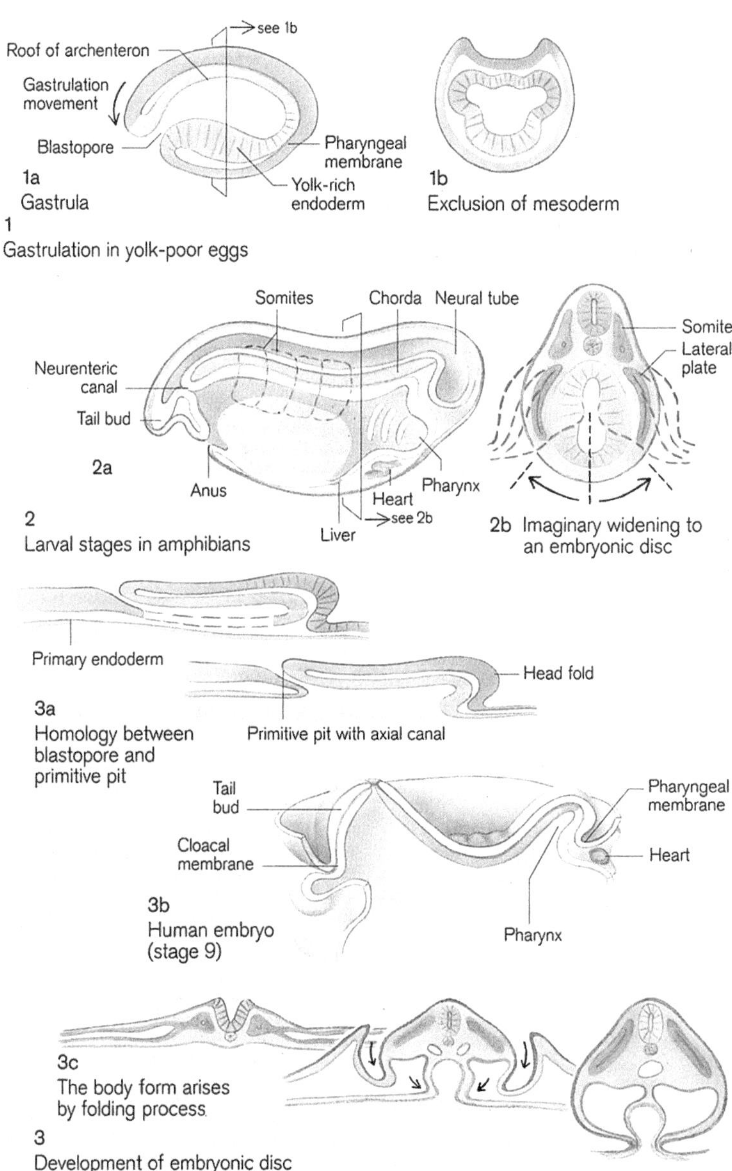
see 1b
Roof of archenteron
Gastrulation movement
Blastopore
Pharyngeal membrane
Yolk-rich endoderm
1a
Gastrula
1b
Exclusion of mesoderm
1
Gastrulation in yolk-poor eggs
Somites
Chorda
Neural tube
Somite
Lateral plate
Neurenteric canal
Tail bud
2a
Anus
Heart
Pharynx
see 2b
Liver
2
Larval stages in amphibians
2b Imaginary widening to an embryonic disc
Primary endoderm
Head fold
3a
Homology between blastopore and primitive pit
Primitive pit with axial canal
Tail bud
Cloacal membrane
Pharyngeal membrane
Heart
3b
Human embryo (stage 9)
Pharynx
3c
The body form arises by folding process
3
Development of embryonic disc

A. Development of body form

## 3.19 Basic Body Plan in Vertebrates

*Background*

The primitive form of the vertebrate body can be derived from the free-swimming larvae of filter feeders. The filter gut of the larva gives rise to the pharyngeal part of the vertebral body, which lengthens to form the gastrointestinal tract. The trunk moiety gives rise to the dorsally situated axial organs. Both parts of the body are segmented. The basic segment of the pharyngeal moiety is the pharyngeal arch. The trunk moiety is composed of somitic segments.

### A. Visceral Pharyngeal and Somatic Trunk Moieties of the Vertebral Body

The basic structure of vertebrates is found in the filtering gut of filter feeders (which serves in the absorption of food and in respiration) and in the trunk moiety formed from somites, which assists in locomotion.

**1. Prototype of an Ancestral Tunicate.** The original form of the pharyngeal gut can be recognized in the tunicate. The adult animal is firmly fixed to the sea bottom by a foot plate. Slits in the filtering gut filter out nutrients from the seawater entering through the mouth opening (arrow).

**2. Free-swimming Tunicate Larva.** Tunicates multiply by budding or by sexual reproduction, producing free-swimming larvae. In addition to the filtering gut, the larva possesses a trunk portion with muscle segments. The muscles are stabilized by a tough elastic axial rod. To coordinate movements, a neural tube is present. In the life cycle of the tunicate, the larva settles down as a sessile filter feeder at the sea bottom and loses its movement apparatus.

**3. Jawless Vertebrate.** The vertebrate body is composed of a visceral functional unit (filtering gut) and a somatic functional unit (axial organs). In chordates (Amphioxus) and in jawless vertebrates, the pharyngeal gut extends from the pharyngeal arch region into the gastrointestinal tract. This gives rise to the visceral functional unit, which also encloses the ventrally situated heart. It is innervated by the pharyngeal arch nerves. The trunk moiety gives rise to the axial organs, including the neural tube, the notochord, and the derivatives of the somites. This produces a somatic functional unit, which is innervated by spinal nerves and assists in locomotion.

**4. Functional Scheme of Branchial Vessels.** In fish, gills develop from the filtering gut. The blood from the heart flows through the pharyngeal arch arteries into a capillary network that lies in the finely branched gills. A current of water streams through the mouth of the fish, passing the gills and exiting through the gill slits. In fish, the pharyngeal arches thus develop into **branchial arches.**

### B. Base of the Skull and Visceral Skeleton

The cartilaginous arches of the primitive pharyngeal gut consist of two elements that are connected to each other by joints (**1a**). The first three cartilage arches unite into a definitive first pharyngeal arch (**1b**). The upper element of the first pharyngeal arch gives rise to the *maxilla* and the lower to the *mandible*. In fish, the maxillary element is attached to the central element of the base of the skull (*palatoquadrate*) by a joint and articulates with the mandible in the **primary jaw joint**. In terrestrial vertebrates, the maxillary element fuses with the base of the skull to form the definitive maxilla.

The vertebrate head is composed of the neurocranium and the visceral skeleton of the facial part of the skull. The neurocranium consists of an endochondral skull base and the *capsules* of the *central sense organs* (**1b**). In the course of evolution, the base of the skull appeared as an extension of the notochord and vertebral column, together with the cerebral vesicles, which are centers for the central sense organs.

Filtering pharyngeal gut

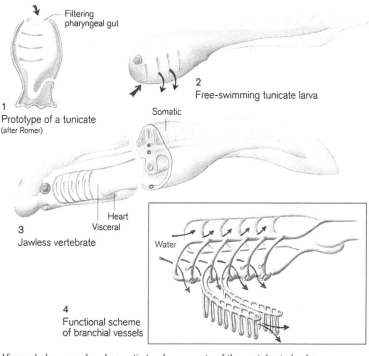

1
Prototype of a tunicate
(after Romer)

2
Free-swimming tunicate larva

Somatic

Heart
Visceral

3
Jawless vertebrate

Water

4
Functional scheme
of branchial vessels

A. Visceral pharyngeal and somatic trunk segments of the vertebrate body

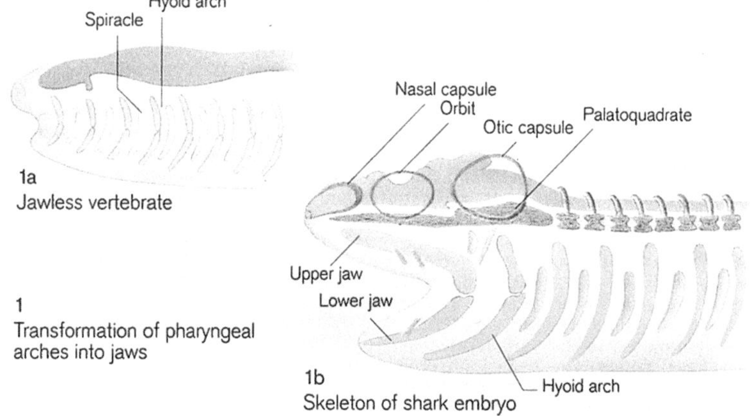


B. Base of skull and visceral skeleton

# 3.20 Pharyngeal Arches

*Background*

In the embryo, the **pharyngeal arches**, like the neural tube, somites, and notochord, are established as basic elements of the vertebrate body. Their original function as a filtering gut or as a gill apparatus can be inferred from their morphological expression and from phylogenesic analysis. In the embryo, the pharyngeal arches no longer possess these functions but represent the primordial material for the species-specific differentiation of the visceral skeleton and pharyngeal gut. They develop into the upper and lower jaw of the facial skeleton (→ 9.3), the middle ear (→ 5.10), and the hyoid bone and larynx (→ 7.3). The definitive pharynx and lungs finally arise from the pharyngeal gut.

## C. Pharyngeal Arches in the Embryo

### 1. Pharyngeal Arches in the Human Embryo

In a series of cross-sections through the human embryo, the *pharyngeal gut* and the pharyngeal arches are located between the *prosencephalon* and the spinal cord and come to lie directly above the *heart-liver bulge*. This location results from the expansion of the cerebral vesicles and the craniocaudal curvature of the embryo. Above the pharyngeal gut, the pontine flexure and cervical flexure develop (→ 2.28 stage 20). In the shark embryo large brain vesicles are not yet present. The pharyngeal gut and neural tube are thus straight (→ 3.19B).

### 2. Structure of the Pharyngeal Arches

**a Pharyngeal clefts and pouches.** In an isolated representation of the *ectoderm* and *endoderm* of the pharyngeal arch region, the relationship between ectodermal *pharyngeal clefts* and endodermal *pharyngeal pouches* is apparent. Deep in the pharyngeal clefts, the ectoderm is directly apposed to the endoderm of the pharyngeal pouch. The apposition of ectoderm and endoderm is a typical phenomenon in the formation of body openings; the pharyngeal membrane of the mouth and the cloacal membrane of the anus are other examples. The spaces between ectodermal pharyngeal clefts and endodermal pharyngeal pouches are filled by mesoderm in which the structures of the pharyngeal arches develop. The pharyngeal arch mesoderm originates from the neural crest of the head region.

**b Pharyngeal Arch Cartilage and Artery.** Each pharyngeal arch possesses a *cartilage* rod and a *pharyngeal arch artery.*

The original **cartilage rod** consists of a proximal and a distal element united by a joint (→ 3.19B). To open the upper and lower jaw units, or to open a whole row of branchial arches, the proximal and distal elements of the underlying pharyngeal arches are moved against each other by means of the primary articulation connecting the two elements. This is effected by the pharyngeal arch musculature, which arises from the mesenchyme of the pharyngeal arch. In the embryonic development of the vertebrate head, the proximal elements are already fused with the base of the future skull. The distal elements unite ventrally, forming the U-shaped skeletal elements of the mandible and the hyoid bone.

The **pharyngeal arch arteries** originate from the paired *ventral aorta* and open into the similarly paired *dorsal aorta*. The fourth pharyngeal arch artery gives rise to the definitive arch of the aorta (→ 6.7). The pharyngeal arch arteries are thus also known as aortic arches.

**c Pharyngeal Arch Nerves.** The pharyngeal arch nerves originate from the neural tube in the region of the rhomboid fossa (→ 4.12). *Ventral motor* roots enter the neural tube ventrally, and *dorsal sensory* roots are associated with a sensory ganglion and enter dorsally, as in the spinal nerves. As a derivative of the ectoderm, the *nerve* lies lateral to the *cartilaginous rod*. The *artery* (associated with the endoderm) lies medially.

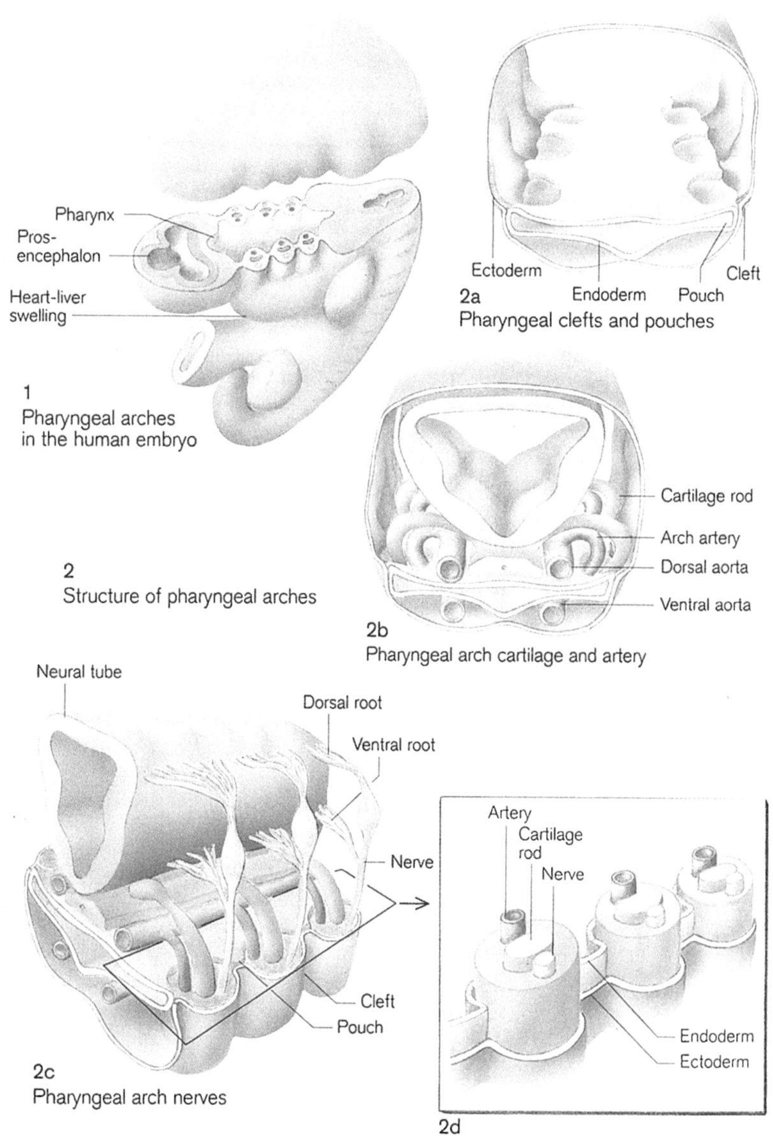
Pharynx
Pros-
encephalon
Heart-liver
swelling
1
Pharyngeal arches
in the human embryo
Ectoderm
Endoderm
Pouch
Cleft
2a
Pharyngeal clefts and pouches
2
Structure of pharyngeal arches
Cartilage rod
Arch artery
Dorsal aorta
Ventral aorta
2b
Pharyngeal arch cartilage and artery
Neural tube
Dorsal root
Ventral root
Nerve
Cleft
Pouch
2c
Pharyngeal arch nerves
Artery
Cartilage
rod
Nerve
Endoderm
Ectoderm
2d

C. Pharyngeal arches in the embryo

## 3.21 Somites

### A. Differentiation of Somites

**1. Origin of Somites in Paraxial Mesoderm.** The somites arise by segmentation—progressing from cranial to caudal—of the (paraxial) mesoderm (→3.9) located on both sides of the neural tube. In the loose mesenchymal mesoderm, the cells form discrete aggregates of columnar epithelium. The basal membranes lie externally and the apices of the cells are directed inward into the somitic cavity. Similar morphogenetic movements of cells occur in the mesoderm of the *lateral plate* , where the mesodermal cells become arranged into palisade-like epithelia in the parietal and visceral mesodermal layers (→3.24). The coelomic cavity arises between the two layers.

The **somites** are embryonic organs that are formed transiently in the embryo and disintegrate without differentiating further (primary organs). They function in the segmentation of the embryonic tissue and in the modelling of the embryonic body. They contain the cellular material for the vertebral column (**sclerotome**) and for all the striated musculature of the trunk and limbs (**myotome**), as well as the cellular material for the subcutaneous tissue (**dermatome**).

**2. Segmentation of Axial Organs.** The somites represent the basic element for the **metamerism** of the vertebrate body. The segmental organization of the vertebral column, of the *neural tube* with the spinal nerves, and of the body wall with the ribs arises from the somites. Although the metameric arrangement of the lateral plates that is still present in Amphioxus (→3.3) has disappeared in higher vertebrates, the somitic organization extends over the entire body wall. The path of neural crest cells and of the migrating nerve fibers of spinal nerves is determined by the segmental properties of the extracellular matrix (→3.25).

The primary role of the somites for the metameric organization of the vertebrate body is demonstrated by transplantation of a somite. This leads to the sprouting of an additional spinal nerve and to a corresponding change in the entire metameric pattern.

**3. Migration of Sclerotome Cells.** The disintegration of the somites begins with the emigration of *sclerotome cells*. The epithelial structure disintegrates in the medial, ventral corner, as individual cells migrate toward the notochord, where they eventually form the vertebral column.

**4. Differentiation of the Myotome.** Below the intact dorsolateral wall of the somite (the *dermatome),* the free margins of the somitic wall are united and form a new cellular plate, the *myotome*. The myotomic cells differentiate into myoblasts, which fuse with each other and form striated muscle fibers (→3.33). The muscle fibers run parallel to the neural tube. The segmental back musculature arises directly from the myotomes (→4.5). At the ventral wall of the *dermatomyotomes*, individual (nonfused) myoblasts begin to migrate ventrally as the sclerotome detaches. These are the stem cells of the striated musculature of the body wall and limb buds (→3.23). The mononuclear myoblasts cannot be distinguished histologically from the remaining mesodermal cells.

**5. Disintegration of the Dermatome.** The *dermatomes* at the dorsal wall of the somites are the longest-lasting somitic structures and determine the contour of the external body wall. Ultimately, these pseudostratified epithelial structures also disintegrate. The dermatome organization is preserved as an innervation region for the spinal nerves in the skin. Mesodermal cells form the subcutaneous tissue without leaving the area of the segment.

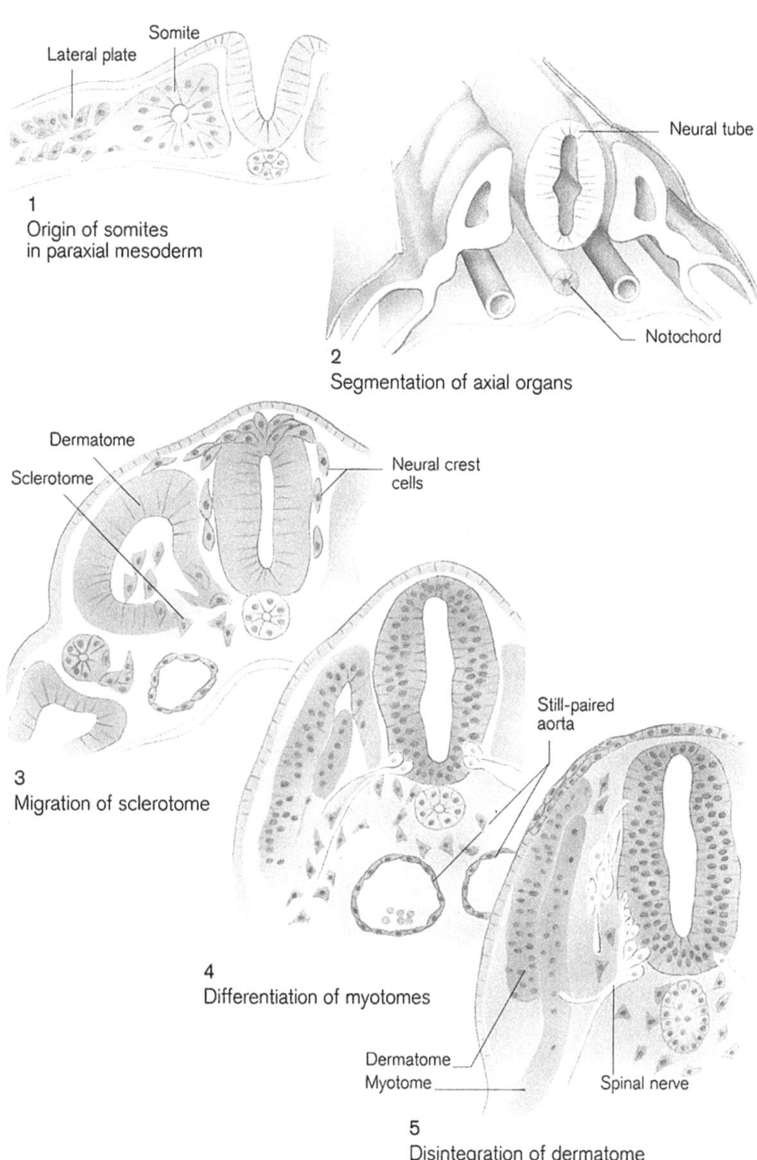


A. Differentiation of the somites

## 3.22 Resegmentation of Axial Organs

*Background*

The definitive **segmental organization** of the vertebrate body is based on the bony vertebrae. For functional reasons, the vertebrae arise by fusion of the cranial and caudal halves of two adjacent somites. By this fusion, the myotomes span over the intervertebral discs, enabling movement of the vertebral column. The segmental arrangement of the vertebral column is therefore not identical with the original somitic segmentation. The new arrangement of the body axis is called **resegmentation** (a term coined by Remak in 1855).

### B. Resegmentation of the Vertebral Column

**1. Subdivision of the Sclerotome.** The *somitic segments* are functionally divided, as in the segments of the Drosophila embryo (→ 3.17), into a *cranial* and a *caudal* subsegment. The craniocaudal polarity is already reflected in the differentiation of the *myotome*. The differentiation of striated muscle cells into the longitudinally organized myotomes begins in the cranial subsegment of the somite. The segmental arrangement of the *spinal ganglia* and of the bundles of *motor nerve fibers* leaving the spinal cord, is also determined by the polarity of the somitic mesoderm. The *cranial segment* promotes the migration of *neural crest cells* and permits the growth of the axons of motor neurons from the anterior column of the spinal cord. The mesodermal cells in the cranial segment of the somite synthesize a nerve-growth promoting factor which is deposited in the extracellular matrix. The *caudal subsegments* of somites, on the other hand, are impenetrable for neural crest cells and for the axons of motor neurons.

Because of the polarity of the somitic mesoderm, the neural crest cells emigrating from the neural tube and the axons of the motor neurons aggregate into *spinal ganglia* and into the roots of the spinal nerves at the level of the *cranial subsegments of the sclerotome*. The suborganization of the sclerotome is also visible microscopically. The cranial *sclerotomic subsegment* consists of loose tissue, in which tenascin can be demonstrated by immunohistochemistry. The caudal subsegment consists of thick, condensed mesenchyme.

**2. Resegmentation**. The myotome plates of the somites are oriented along the compact epithelial structure of the *dermatome* (**2a**). The intersegmental artery (which arises from the aorta) lies in the intersegmental space between the somites. Resegmentation begins with the reorientation of the muscle plates from the dermatome to the muscular processes of the *vertebrae* (**2b**). The *intervertebral discs*, which function as joints, are bridged over by the segmental muscle plates of the myotome. The dense *caudal sclerotomic* subsegment gives rise to the intervertebral disc, as well as the *vertebral arch*, the *transverse process*, and the *ribs* of the following vertebra.

The *cranial sclerotomic subsegment* gives rise to the caudal part of the vertebra. Muscle fibers attach to the transverse processes and vertebral arches of the vertebral column.

**3. Human Vertebral Column at Stage 16.** After the disintegration of the sclerotome, the sclerotome cells that have migrated ventrally to the notochord form a uniform tissue column around the notochord, causing the segmental arrangement of somites to disappear. The disc-shaped compressions of the *intervertebral discs* (→ 2.30) arise; in each disc, part of the notochord is preserved as a gelatinous nucleus (**B2**). The loose and cell-poor material situated between the discs is transformed into hyaline cartilage. In stage 16, the developing *vertebrae* (with their *transverse processes* and their still-open *vertebral arches*) and the *ribs* form a connected structure of hyaline cartilage. The exits for the spinal nerves remain open, lying at the level of the intervertebral discs. The organization into vertebrae and ribs (→ 2.36), which may be associated with functional stress, is concluded by endochondral ossification. The first *ossification center* appears in the 12th week of pregnancy (→ 2.35).

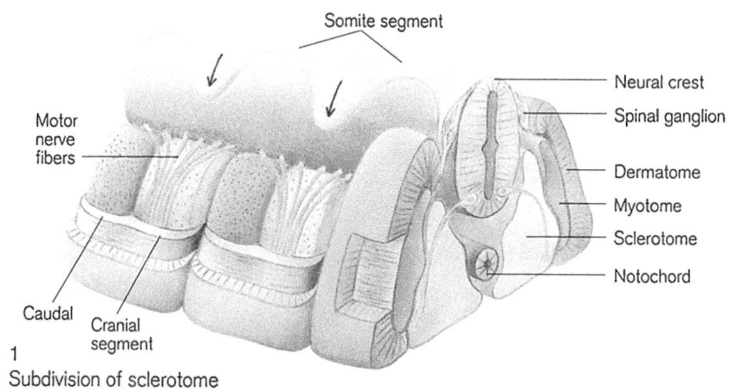


1
Subdivision of sclerotome

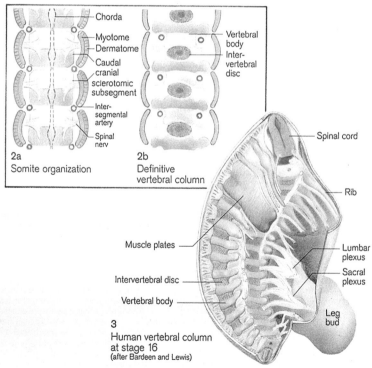

Chorda
Myotome
Dermatome
Caudal
cranial
sclerotomic
subsegment
Inter-
segmental
artery
Spinal
nerv

2a
Somite organization

Vertebral
body
Inter-
vertebral
disc

2b
Definitive
vertebral column

Spinal cord
Rib
Muscle plates
Lumbar
plexus
Sacral
plexus
Intervertebral disc
Vertebral body
Leg
bud

3
Human vertebral column
at stage 16
(after Bardeen and Lewis)

B. Resegmentation of axial organs

## 3.23 Pattern Formation in the Limb Bud

*Background*

Embryonic Cholinesterase. Embryonic cells communicate by means of the neurotransmitter acetylcholine during morphogenesis. In a phase-specific manner, they express muscarinic- acetylcholine receptors on the cell surface (Oettling et al. 1985) and synthesize the enzyme cholinesterase for the inactivation of the transmitter. Thus, morphogenetically active cell regions in the limb bud can be demonstrated histochemically by staining for cholinesterase (Drews, 1975). In microscopic sections, a brown precipitate is formed at the site of enzymatic activity.

### A. Embryonic Cholinesterase (ChE) in the Limb Bud

**1. Induction of the Limb Bud.** The mesoderm of the lateral body wall induces a ridge-shaped thickening known as the *apical-ectodermal ridge* in the ectoderm. This ridge in turn induces the outgrowth of the limb bud in the parietal mesoderm.

**2. Determination of Axes.** The *craniocaudal, dorsoventral,* and *proximodistal* axes are established early in limb bud development. The proximodistal axis is determined by the apical-ectodermal ridge and the craniocaudal polarity by the "posterior polarizing zone" (**B2**).

**3. Progress Zone.** The *apical-ectodermal ridge* induces the undifferentiated mesoderm located below the ectoderm to undergo further appositional growth. Thus, a distally advancing progress zone arises at the apex of the bud. From the progress zone, the central *skeletal elements* and the mantle of soft tissue emerge proximally. The *myoblasts* and the *nerve fibers* of spinal nerves (→ 4.5) originate in the corresponding somitic segments and invade the bud centrally.

**4. Differentiation.** After leaving the progress zone, the chondroblasts aggregate into the central *cartilage core*. Their cholinesterase activity remains for some time, but disappears as differentiation into hyaline cartilage takes place (→ 3.32). The cholinesterase activity in the muscle fibers represents the definitive enzyme that later is concentrated in the end plates, together with nicotinic receptors (→ 3.33).

**5. Development of Finger Rays.** As the hand and foot plates develop into the basic five-rayed pattern of all vertebrate limbs, zones of *physiological necrosis* arise in the apical-ectodermal ridge, continuing into the mesoderm of the interdigital spaces. During wing formation, the first and fifth ray recede.

### B. Experiments

**1. Self-Differentiation.** In a cell suspension of early limb buds, cell aggregates form and differentiate further into *hyaline cartilage*. At the periphery of the aggregate, fusion of myoblasts gives rise to multinucleated *muscle fibers* that encircle the cartilaginous central aggregate. The "sorting" of cartilage and muscle cells is accompanied by cholinesterase activity.

**2. Posterior Polarizing Zone.** A diffusible substance formed at the base of the limb bud is responsible for *craniocaudal polarity*. *Transplantation* of this zone into the anterior bud region of a *host embryo* leads to the doubling of the ulnar rays of the limb. A derivative of vitamin A (**retinoic acid**) is thought to be the polarizing diffusible substance.

**3. Expression of Hox Genes.** The regulator genes Hox 4.4–4.8 are expressed in a characteristic pattern in the limb buds of the mouse and chick (→ 3.27). The transfection of a mutated Hox 4.4 gene leads to a malformation corresponding to the transplantation of the posterior polarization zone.

**4. Hypothesis for Pattern Formation.** The apical ectodermal ridge determines whether the mesenchyme in the progress zone will form cartilage or soft tissue. The determination is retained as positional information during passage through the progress zone. The polarizer produces a diffusible factor (possibly retinoic acid), activating the cascade of Hox 4 genes, which determine the development of the ulna and radius and the finger rays.

Ecto-
derm
Apical-
ecto-
dermal
ridge
1
Induction of bud

Dorsal
Cranial
Proximal
Distal
Ventral
Caudal
ChE-activity
2
Determination of axes

Cartilage
blastema
3
Progress zone

Muscle
fiber
Cartilage
4
Differentiation of
muscle and cartilage

1
2
Physiological
necrosis
3
4
5
5
Demarcation of finger rays

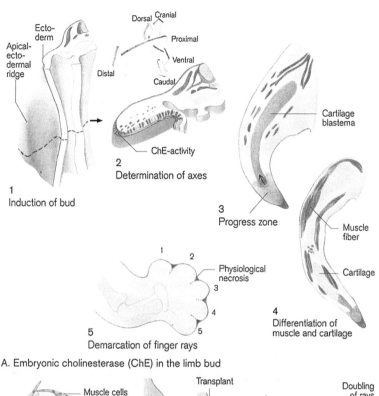

A. Embryonic cholinesterase (ChE) in the limb bud

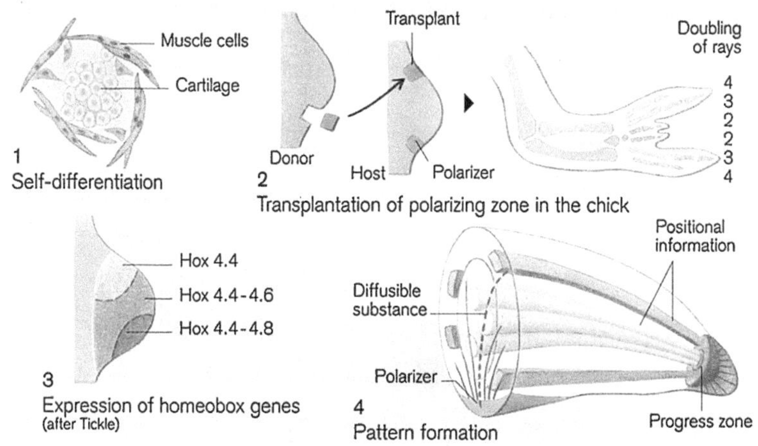


B. Experiments with limb bud

## 3.24 Differentiation of Germ Layers

*Background*

**Definition of Germ Layers.** In coelenterates, the body consists of two epithelial layers; an external ectodermal layer and an internal endodermal layer used for the absorption of food. This level of organization is attained in the embryonic development of vertebrates by gastrulation. Designation of the two layers as **ectoderm** and **endoderm** is derived from the homology between phylogeny and ontogeny (→ 3.1). At the next level of organization, an intermediate germ layer, the **mesoderm**, arises; skeletal elements and musculature are formed from this layer. In lower vertebrates, the germ layers originate by classical gastrulation. In vertebrates with yolk rich eggs, they arise via an embryonic disc and the formation of the primitive streak.

### A. Differentiation of Germ Layers

**1. Organization of Germ Layers in the Human Embryo.** The primary embryonic organs of the trunk, represented in the schematic cross section of the body (**A2**), are formed before folding in the *somitic region* of the stage 10 human embryo (**A1**). The *ectoderm* gives rise to the *neural tube* and to *surface ectoderm*. The mesodermal organs are the *notochord*, *somites*, and *lateral plates*. The latter have separated into a *visceral layer* that lies adjacent to the endoderm and a *parietal layer*, which lies close to the surface ectoderm. The body cavity lies between the *visceral* and *parietal mesodermal layers*. It opens laterally into the chorionic cavity and continues cranially into the pericardial cavity via the *coelomic canal* (arrow).

In the **somite region,** the germ layers and the primary organs arising from them are characterized not only by their position and their future function, but also by the mechanism of their formation in the primitive streak. Caudally (in the tail bud) and cranially (in the primordium of the head), the ectodermal, endodermal, and mesodermal components of the organs arise independently of the primitive streak. In the **tail bud**, notochord, neural tube, and somites arise directly from the tail bud blastema. The cell movements of gastrulation are replaced by the direct organization of the primary organs from a compact blastema. In the **head primordium,** the first mesodermal cells emerge from the endoderm of the foregut diverticulum (→ 3.8). The remaining **head mesoderm** is formed by migration of individual cells from the placodes and from the neural crest of the head.

**2. Differentiation of Germ Layers in the Somite Region.** In the schematic cross section, the structure of the **primary organs** is represented on the left side and the later **cellular differentiation** on the right side. The cells in the primary organs take part in morphogenetic movements. They do not differentiate; rather, they function in shaping the embryonic body. In this process, inductive interactions between the epithelial and mesenchymal tissue components determine cell fates within the morphological units (→ 3.38).

The diagram summarizes the derivation of tissues from the germ layers. The primary organs disintegrate and differentiate into tissues that perform functions related to the original role of the corresponding germ layer. Derivatives of the *ectoderm* protect the organism against external influences (surface ectoderm) and enable communication with the environment (sense organs and nervous system). Derivatives of the *mesoderm* form the inner supporting skeleton, the musculature, heart, and kidneys. The *endoderm* gives rise to the digestive tube and the digestive glands. The mesodermal palisades of visceral and parietal mesoderm produce the intestinal wall with its muscle layers and the body wall with the ribs. The myoblasts for the entire striated musculature originate from the myotomes of the somites. The inductive interactions between the germ layers are manifested in the structure of the *skin* and the *intestinal canal*, which are composed of an epithelial and a mesodermal component.

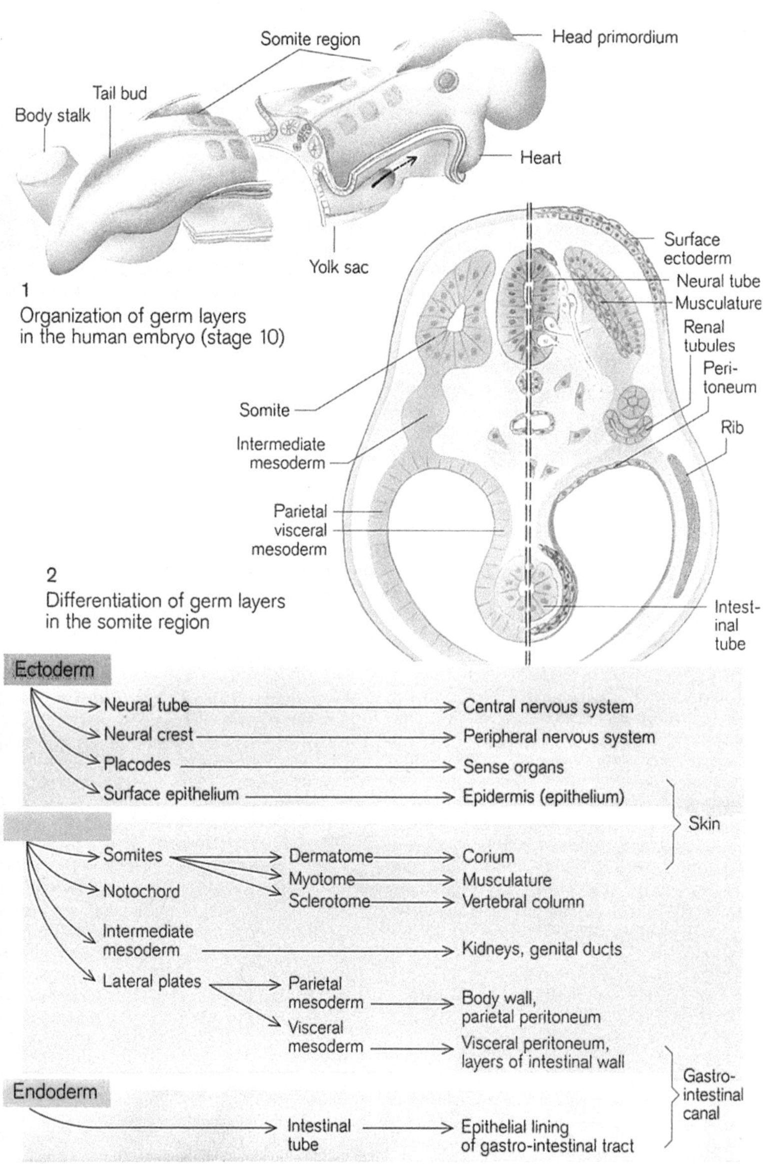
Somite region
Head primordium
Tail bud
Body stalk
Heart
Yolk sac
1
Organization of germ layers in the human embryo (stage 10)
Surface ectoderm
Neural tube
Musculature
Renal tubules
Peritoneum
Rib
Somite
Intermediate mesoderm
Parietal
visceral
mesoderm
2
Differentiation of germ layers in the somite region
Intestinal tube
Ectoderm
Neural tube → Central nervous system
Neural crest → Peripheral nervous system
Placodes → Sense organs
Surface epithelium → Epidermis (epithelium)
Skin
Somites → Dermatome → Corium
Myotome → Musculature
Sclerotome → Vertebral column
Notochord
Intermediate mesoderm → Kidneys, genital ducts
Lateral plates → Parietal mesoderm → Body wall, parietal peritoneum
Visceral mesoderm → Visceral peritoneum, layers of intestinal wall
Gastro-intestinal canal
Endoderm
Intestinal tube → Epithelial lining of gastro-intestinal tract

A. Differentiation of germ layers

## Regulation of Development

# 3.25 Mechanisms of Morphogenetic Movements

*Background*

Embryonic epithelial-cell layers can actively change their conformation. Within mesenchymal cell layers, individual cell populations travel great distances with amoeboid movements. Inductive interactions between mesenchymal and epithelial tissues are prerequisite for further differentiation.

## A. Epithelial Structures

In the **embryonic disc** of the blastocyst, cells aggregate (**A1**) and form a compact **epithelial structure (A2)**. In this process, the epithelium-specific "Cell Adhesion Molecule (CAM)" *E-cadherin* (→ 3.26) appears on the cell surface.

Cells that emigrate to form **mesoderm** (**A3**) do not express *E-cadherin*. It is expressed again during the epithelial rearrangement of mesodermal cells in the *somites* and in the *mesodermal palisades* (**A4**).

**Neural folding** (**A5**) is an example of the movement of embryonic epithelial structures. The cells are polarized in the epithelium. Basally, the cells are attached to a *basement membrane* secreted by the epithelial cells. The neural tube is formed by the contraction of *actin* and *myosin filaments* that extend between the *desmosomes* in the apical part of the cells. They cooperate with the *microtubules* and the intermediate *filaments* of the cytoskeleton, which give epithelial cells their shape. In neural epithelium, *N-cadherin* and *N-CAM* are the neuroepithial-specific variants of the epithelial-specific E-cadherin. The CAMs are concentrated in the desmosomes.

## B. Migration of Individual Cells

**1. Migration of Neural Crest Cells.** The neural crest cells that emerge from the neural tube lose their epithelial-specific adhesion molecule and express a new class of adhesive molecule with which they can recognize determinants in collagen and in the glycoproteins of the basal membrane. Pseudopodia appear basally and pull the cells through the basement membrane, while apically they still adhere strongly to the junctional complex of the epithelium. The neural crest cells use the basement membrane of the neural tube and of the surface ectoderm as guidance structures. The cells migrating along the neural tube become neurons and glial cells of the spinal ganglia, and form the autonomic nervous system. The cells migrating below the surface ectoderm become melanocytes and Merkel cells (→ 3.30). A specific glycoprotein of the basement membrane is **laminin**, which is a ligand for cell adhesion molecules of the **integrin** type (→ 3.26) on the neural crest cell surface.

**2. Organization of Mesenchyme.** The connective tissue cells (for example the *sclerotome cells)* emerge as individual cells from the mesodermal palisade-like epithelial layers and form a mesenchymal tissue. They secrete a small glycoprotein, **fibronectin,** which accumulates in the collagen of the intercellular matrix. Through *fibronectin receptors* of the integrin type (→ 3.26), adhesion sites form between the mesenchymal cells and the matrix. The intracellular region of the fibronectin receptors binds microfilaments and microtubules of the cytoskeleton. These molecules are responsible for the characteristic fibroblast shape of the connective tissue cells.

**3. Migration of Nerve Fibers.** The tip of a nerve fiber (*growth cone*) behaves like a pseudopodium, moving through tissues in amoeboid fashion by means of filopodia. The filopodia search the environment for contact points to which they can attach and pull the growth cone forward. Specific contacts are formed with the glycocalix of glial cells or of already developed nerve fibers. Between the growth cone and the nerve cell body, the axon is stabilized by means of microtubules, along which protein and metabolites are also transported.

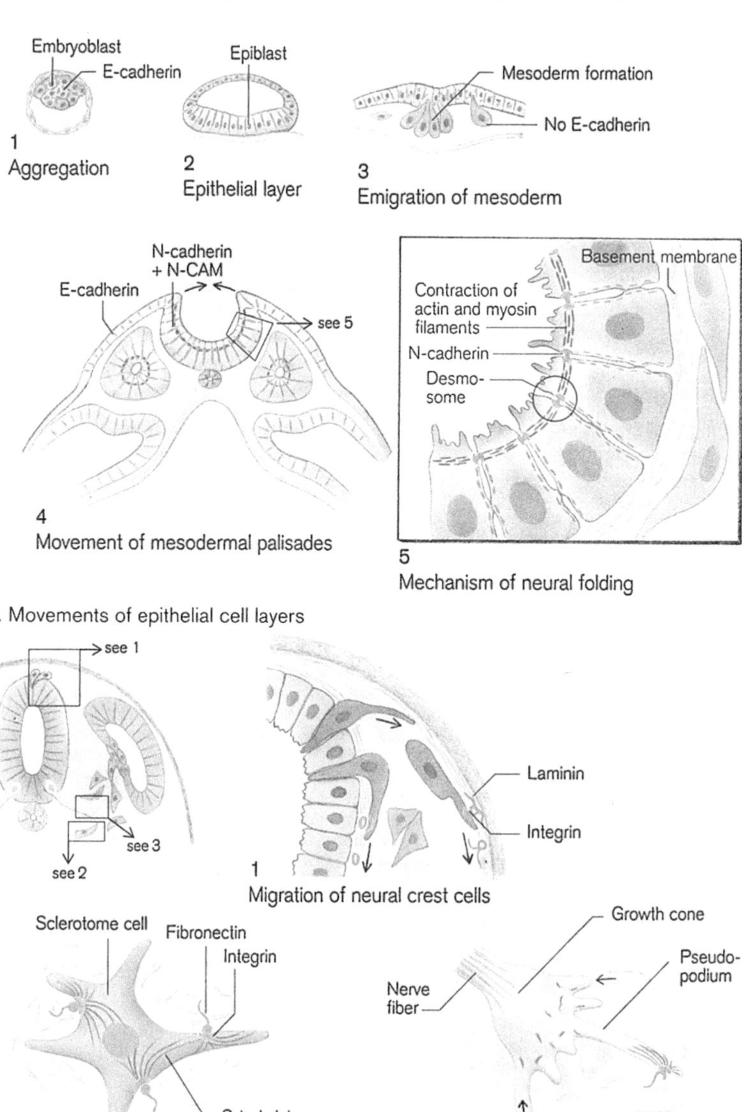


A. Movements of epithelial cell layers

B. Migration by individual cells

## 3.26 Cell Adhesion Molecules

*Background*

The **amoeboid movement of cells** can be observed directly in tissue culture. In culture, cells of different origin behave very similarly. They lose their differentiated properties, reenter the cell cycle, and migrate randomly with amoeboid movements along the floor of the culture dish. Because of the similarity with mesenchymal cells, dedifferentiated in vitro cells are often referred to as fibroblasts or fibrocytes.

### C. Amoeboid Movement

**1. Cytoplasmic Streaming.** A *migrating fibrocyte* pushes itself over the culture substrate with a broad front, pulling the cell nucleus and the remaining cytoplasm behind it. Contraction waves are formed in the cell membrane at the advancing front and spread over the cell body ("*ruffled membrane*"). In addition, thin cytoplasmic processes (*filopodia*) arise at the cell surface that "feel out" the environment of the cell. Depending on the adhesive properties encountered, the filopodia are either retracted or form focal contact points. The filopodia with contact points contract and pull the entire cell in their direction.

**2. Contact Points and Contraction.** The cortical cytoplasm of cells contains a network of *actin* and *myosin filaments,* which by local contraction and relaxation, produces contraction waves in the cell membrane and enables the extension of the filopodia. At the intracellular face of the contact points, actin filaments are inserted. These filaments, in concert with associated myosin lead to contraction of the filopodia.

**Contact Inhibition.** Through cell proliferation and migration, cultured cells eventually form a single layer of cells (monolayer) with many mutual cell contacts. These contact points cause the cells to cease their proliferation and migration, a phenomenon known as contact inhibition. T*ransformation* with an oncogene (→ 3.29) can prevent the arrest of cell division and cell movement and enable the cells to pile up and to form multilayered (stratified) nodules in an otherwise contact-inhibited cell culture.

### D. "Cell Adhesion Molecules" (CAM)

**1. Demonstration in a Cell Suspension.** Embryonic cells possess specific surface determinants, by means of which similar cells can adhere to each other (CAMs). If the individual cells from two different organs—for example, the liver and the kidney—are mixed in a cell suspension, the cell type with the stronger adhesive property—in our example, the liver cells—form an inner aggregate, and the cells of the second type (here the kidney cells) associate at the outside of the aggregate. The cell adhesion molecules thus lead to specific aggregation and to a separation of cell populations ("cell sorting").

**2. Molecular Forms.** CAMs are not organ-specific, but belong to three **supergene families** (→ 3.27). The various CAMs appear in different combinations and in specific phases of development.

The **selectins (2a)** possess a domain enabling calcium-independent binding, so that cells expressing selectins can undergo *homophilic adhesion* with cells of the same type. The binding sites, however, can also exhibit specificity toward other glycoproteins (heterophilic binding). The best-studied selectins are the CD-determinants on lymphocytes (→ 3.35).

The **cadherins (2b)** are responsible for tight contact between cells. This binding is calcium dependent. After cell aggregation, cadherin molecules are concentrated in the *desmosomes*. In the intracellular domain, cadherins associate with contractile actin filaments during movement of embryonic epithelia, or with intermediate filaments in static epithelia.

The **integrins (2c)** form contacts with collagen fibers in the basement membrane and with molecules of the extracellular matrix. **Laminin** (in the basement membrane) and **fibronectin** (in the extracellular matrix of the mesenchyme) are important ligands for integrins.

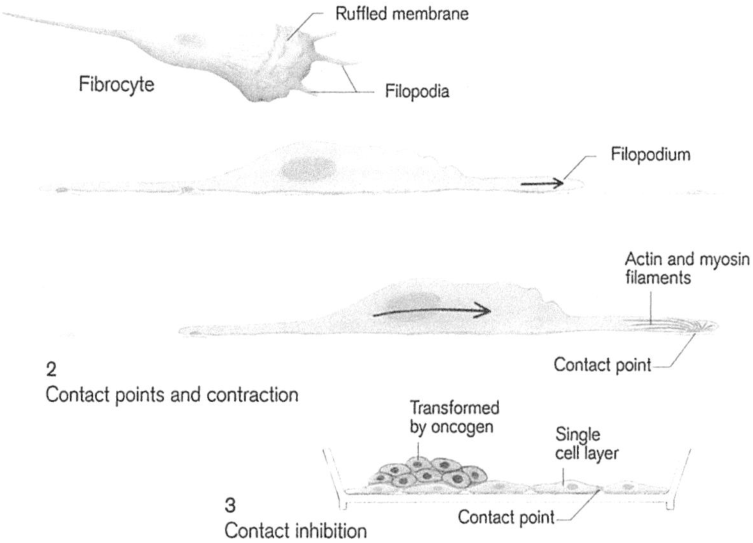

Ruffled membrane
Fibrocyte
Filopodia
Filopodium
Actin and myosin filaments
Contact point
2
Contact points and contraction
Transformed by oncogen
Single cell layer
Contact point
3
Contact inhibition

C. Amoeboid movement

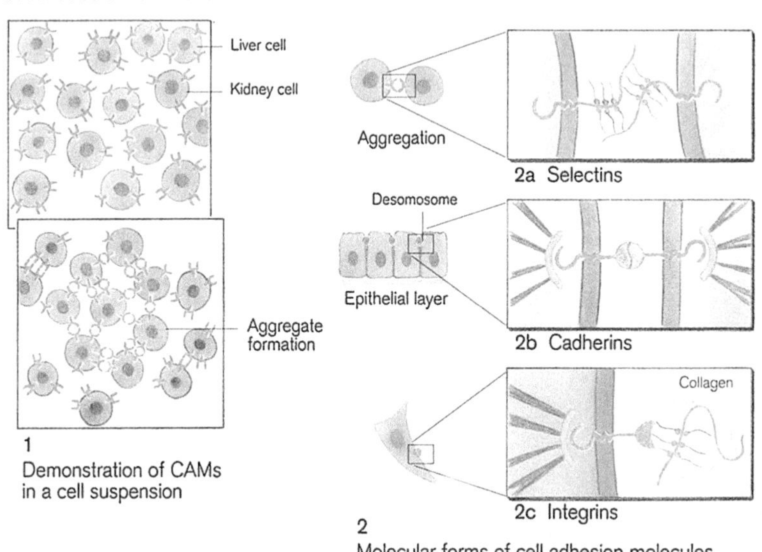

Liver cell
Kidney cell
Aggregate formation
1
Demonstration of CAMs in a cell suspension
Aggregation
2a Selectins
Desomosome
Epithelial layer
2b Cadherins
Collagen
2c Integrins
2
Molecular forms of cell adhesion molecules

D. Cell adhesion molecules (CAMs)

# 3.27 Organization of Genome and Cell Cycle

## A. Organization of the Genome

**1. Operon Principle of Bacteria and Gene Families of Eukaryotes.** Cells with nuclei (*eukaryotes*) have a genome organization more similar to that of simple *archeobacteria* than to aerobic *eubacteria*. The *ancestral gene* structure, common to all cells, consists of a binding site for RNA-polymerase (*promoter*), a *regulatory sequence*, and the *structural gene*.

In **eubacteria,** such as *E. coli*, the structural genes e.g. for enzymes are grouped into functional units called **operons (1a)**. The *transcription factor* can bind to the *regulatory sequence*; this association, in turn, is regulated by the binding of a central *metabolite* of the metabolic unit to the transcription factors. Thus, for example, lactose can regulate the functional state of the lac-operon. The transcription factor is encoded by a *regulatory gene*.

The genome of **eukaryotes** is about 100 times larger than that of eubacteria and contains the information for a large variety of differentiated states. In each cell, only a part of the genome is active. The basis for this organization is the development of **gene families** by **gene duplication.** Duplication of the *ancestral genes* of the cell gave rise to initially inactive gene copies, from which functionally significant variants could arise by mutation and selection. Thus for each cell type, a specific set of genes can be selectively activated. The seemingly chaotic and redundant increase in DNA is therefore the basis for the formation of multicellular organisms consisting of different differentiated cell types.

**2. Homeotic Genes.** The homeotic genes—so named because they determine "equal" segments—are *regulatory genes* that also arose by gene duplication. They possess a *consensus sequence* designated the **homeobox.** Homeotic genes code for *transcription factors* that bind to DNA. They lie in series on a chromosome, forming a gene cluster (Hox cluster). By sequentially switching on different homeobox genes, the set of structural genes characteristic for a certain cell type can be activated. The activity of transcription factors is dependent on the presence of specific *hormones* and *induction factors*. These are related to the metabolites and chemotactic factors that originally regulated the genes of ancestral cells. The originally exogenous stimuli are now derived from neighboring cells. The programmed, mutual dependence of cells on each other provides constant control of the spatial and temporal patterns in the development of a multicellular organism.

**3. Expression of the Hox-Cluster in the Mouse.** During segmentation of the axial organs of the mouse, Hox 1 (homologous to Ubx in Drosophila, → 3.17) is expressed. Although the fates of the individual cells in a segment are not yet determined, the fate of the entire segment is already irreversibly fixed, e.g., to form the thorax or abdomen. The limb bud is specified to become a leg or an arm even before the organ primordia are determined by progressive expression of the genes (e.g., Hox 4, → 3.23). In the differentiation of organs, further homeotic gene clusters are involved. An example are the **Pax genes** (with a "paired box"), which are activated during the induction of renal tubules and the development of the vertebral bodies.

## B. Regulation of the Cell Cycle

The cell cycle is an autonomous and highly conserved process in evolution. It is regulated by cyclic synthesis of the protein *cyclin*. At the G2/M-transition, the phosphorylation of cyclin by a *protein kinase* (phosphokinase) initiates the condensation of chromosomes and the disintegration of the nuclear membrane. During mitosis, cyclin is again degraded. In multicellular organisms, the cell cycle is subject to an endogenous suppression that inhibits the synthesis of cyclin in the G1 phase, inducing the cells to exit from the cell cycle (GO phase) and differentiate.

The cell cycle starts again automatically when cyclin levels exceed a threshold value in the G1 phase (*restriction point, R*). In embryonic cells, the endogenous arrest of the cell cycle is counteracted by exogenous growth factors.

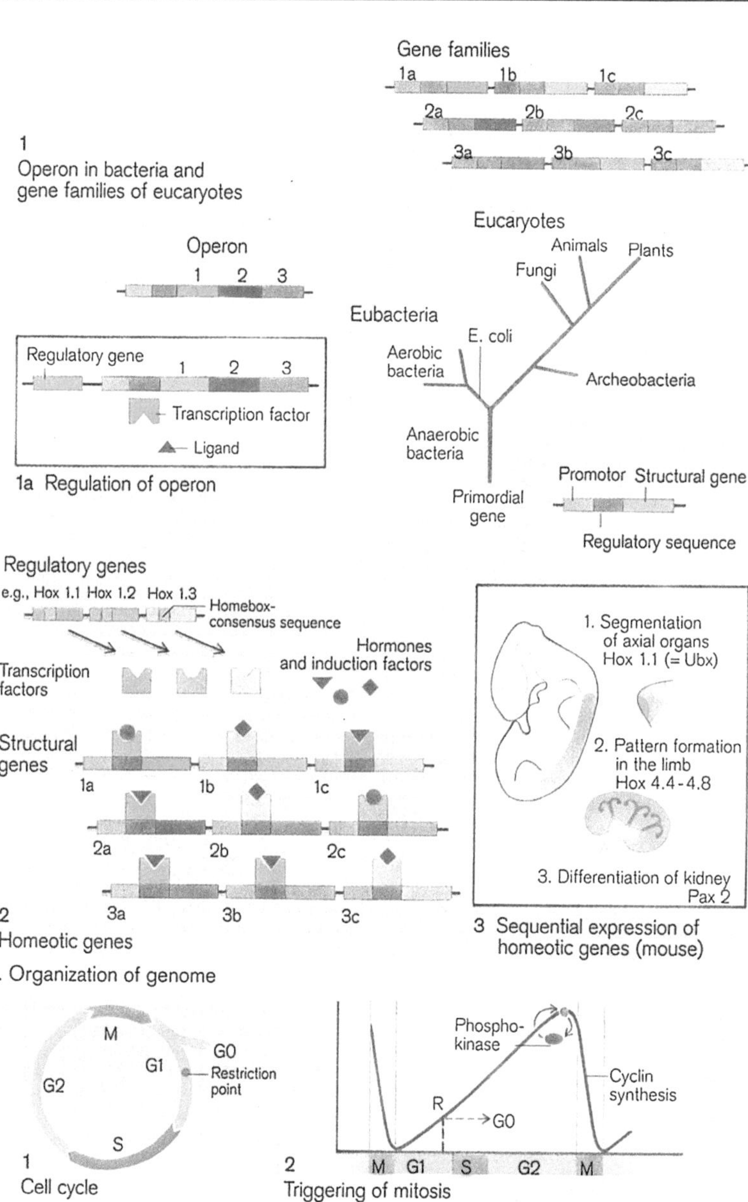


1a Regulation of operon

3 Sequential expression of homeotic genes (mouse)

A. Organization of genome

B. Regulation of the cell cycle

## 3.28 Hormonal Regulation

### A. Control of Growth and Differentiation

**1. Cell Lineage and Cell Interaction.** In embryonic development, cells go through phases of proliferation, giving rise to differently determined cells. Ultimately the determined cells exit from the cell cycle to begin *terminal differentiation.* In this process, the developmental potential of the initially pluripotent *embryonic stem cells* (ES) is successively restricted. In the terminally differentiated cells, only the structural genes characteristic of a specific cell type are active. A simple explanation for this developmental process would be the assumption of an inner clock in the cellular genome. After a fixed number of mitoses, a predetermined gene pattern would be activated in the daughter cells. Such an inner clock does not exist, however. The stepwise specification of the genome is controlled by cellular interactions between the daughter cells via growth factors and CAMs, a mechanism classically referred to as induction.

**2. Gene Regulation by Induction.** In general, both growth factors and CAMs (which may mediate induction through direct cell contact) bind at *tyrosine kinase linked receptors in the cell membrane.* They have three effects: **(1 ) Stimulation of proliferation.** They abolish the endogenous inhibition of the *cell cycle.* **(2) Irreversible specification of the genome** (*determination*). The potentially activatable genetic information in the embryonic cells is gradually and irreversibly limited to the set of genes characteristic for the differentiated cell. This occurs by the activation of *regulatory genes* (e.g., *Hox cluster*). The activation pattern is passed on to the daughter cells. Definitively inactivated regions of DNA (heterochromatin) may be methylated at the cytidine residues. **(3) Induction of CAMs and growth factors** for the next level of determination. In the special case of the syncytial blastoderm of **Drosophila** (→ 3.17), the transcription factors encoded by the regulatory genes build up diffusion gradients that directly switch on the regulatory genes of the next stage. After the formation of cell boundaries in Drosophila and in vertebrate embryos, successive steps in development are induced by the activation of genes for CAMs and for growth factors, which act via the cell membrane. For example, in the primitive node of the mouse, the gene *nodal*, which codes for an induction factor of the TGF-β type, is active. Nodal belongs to a large gene family that includes *activin* (→ 3.6), AMH (→ 8.5), BMP ("bone morphogenetic protein," an osteoblast-inducing factor), and other proteins.

In the **differentiated cell**, in contrast to the embryonic cell, the cell cycle is switched off. The functional state is regulated by hormones through reversible activation of specific structural genes. The remaining genome is irreversibly inactivated.

### B. Proliferation and Morphogenesis

**1. Blastemal Phase.** In an embryonic cellular blastema, proliferation, morphogenetic movement, and fate determination are closely linked. The responsiveness to specific CAMs or autocrine or paracrine growth factors is spatially and temporally limited (**phase specificity**).

**2. Control of Morphogenesis.** Morphogenetic movements are controlled by specific CAMs in the vicinity of the cells. Interactions between epithelium and mesenchyme lead to a regulated degradation and resynthesis of the basement membrane, which contains specific growth factors (→ 3.25). In addition, small metabolites such as ATP, amino acids, neuropeptides, neurotransmitters, and tissue hormones may be involved. The processes show some homology to chemotaxis in unicellular organisms.

**3. Differentiated Tissue.** In the adult organism, proliferation is mainly confined to **stem-cell populations** (e.g., hematopoietic stem cells, basal cells, germ cells). Proliferation is induced by secreted paracrine growth factors (e.g., from connective tissue) and is inhibited by feedback from differentiated cells, and by the development of definitive cell contacts.

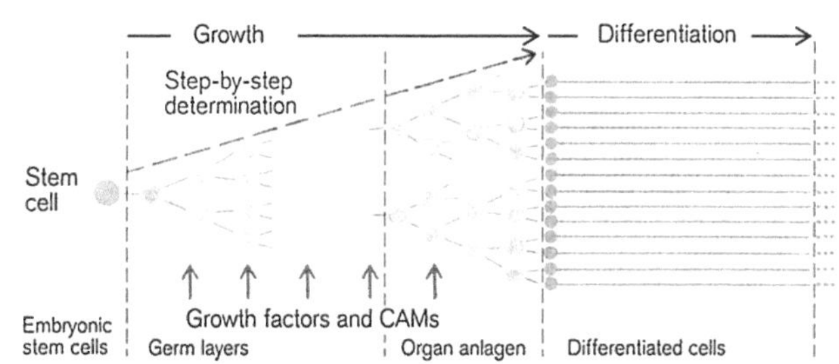


1 Cell lines and cell interaction

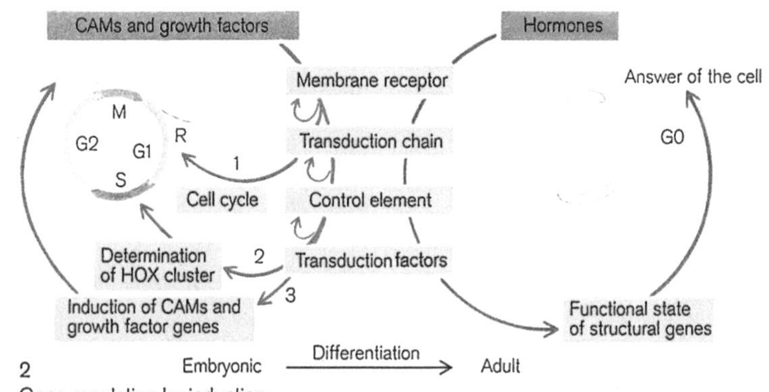


2
Gene regulation by induction

A. Growth regulation by induction

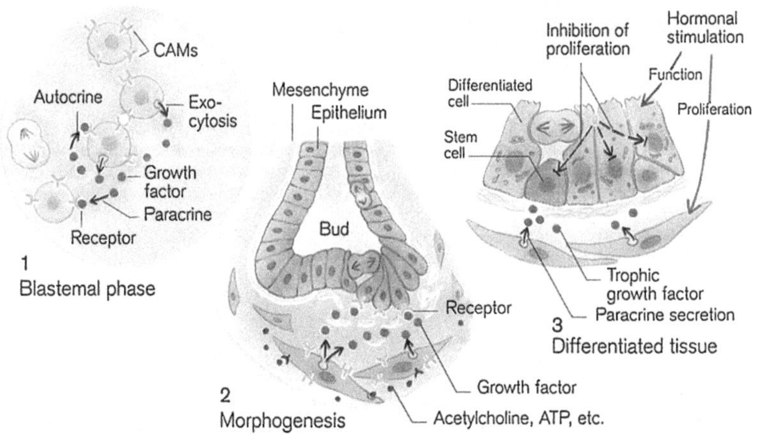


1
Blastemal phase

2
Morphogenesis

3
Differentiated tissue

B. Proliferation and morphogenesis

# 3.29 Transduction Chains

*Background*

Embryonic cells communicate by direct **cell contact**, by secreted autocrine or paracrine **growth factors**, and by local **transmitters**. In differentiated cells, this system is largely replaced by endocrine and nervous regulation of function.

## C. Transduction Cascades for Growth and Differentiation

**1. Membrane-permeable Hormones**
Hormones that can penetrate cell membranes bind to *cytoplasmic receptors* and are transported into the nucleus, where the hormone-receptor complex binds to transcription factors at the DNA. In this way, the hormones can activate specific genes. During embryonic development, hormones can induce morphogenesis and differentiation of entire organ systems. The steroid hormone *ecdysone* induces metamorphosis in insects. The metamorphosis hormone of amphibians is *thyroxine*. In higher vertebrates, thyroxine is necessary for the maturing of the brain. *Testosterone* induces the male sex organs. *Cortisone* is a cofactor for the differentiation of almost all organs. *Retinoic acid*, a newly discovered hormone related to Vitamin A, acts together with the Hox genes in determining the segmentation of the body axis and pattern formation in the limbs (→ 3.23).

**2. Tyrosine Kinase-linked Receptors**
Growth factors can be divided into various supergene families, e.g., TGF-βs. The structure of **growth factors** is related to the structure of **CAMs.** Hypothetically, a *growth factor* and its *receptor* can be derived by splitting off the distal extracellular domain from a CAM with homophilic binding (**2a**).

The stimulation of tyrosine kinase-linked receptors leads to *autophosphorylation* of tyrosine residues and to dimerization of receptors. Alteration of the tertiary structure of the receptor leads to altered binding properties. After a series of still unknown intermediate steps, *transcription factors* are induced and the cell cycle is activated. Phosphorylation of the *control elements* by kinases has the same effect as the binding of a ligand.

Receptors that couple with a GTPase activating protein (GAP) and with *phospholipase* C (PLC) induce the release of $InsP_3$ and $Ca^{2+}$. Stimulation by a growth factor can thus be coupled with changes in the cytoskeleton and with cell movements.

**3. G-Protein-linked Receptors.** The coupling of hormone receptors to a $G_o$ protein leads to the production of DAG (diacylglycerol) and $InsP_3$ (inositol trisphosphate) by the activation of PLC in the cell membrane. The $InsP_3$ induces *calcium release* from the endoplasmic reticulum, which in turn may trigger contraction of *actin* and *myosin* and thus *cell movement* or *exocytosis*. The DAG activates *protein kinase C* (PKC), initiating a series of complex phosphorylation reactions similar to those initiated by tyrosine kinases. In differentiated cells, hormone receptors can be coupled to G-proteins that stimulate ($G_s$) or inhibit ($G_i$) the enzyme cAMP-cyclase and thereby determine the functional state of the cell.

**Oncogenesis**. Oncogenes are mutated variants of specific members of the embyronic signal transduction chains. The corresponding cellular genes (c-oncogenes) can be incorporated by viruses into the viral genome (v-oncogenes). These viruses are thus able to imitate the embryonic signal transduction cascade and reinitiate cellular proliferation. Mutations in c-oncogenes induced by carcinogenic substances have the same effect.

**erbA:** **R**eceptor for thyroxine (**A**vian **er**ythro**b**lastosis virus).
**erbB:** EGF receptor.
**src:** Tyrosine kinase (Rous **Sarc**oma).
**ras:** GAP or G-protein (**Ra**t **S**arcoma virus).
**myc:** Transcription factor (Avian **My**elo**c**ytomatosis virus).
**Phorbol ester:** Carcinogen of skin, activates protein kinase C (PKC).

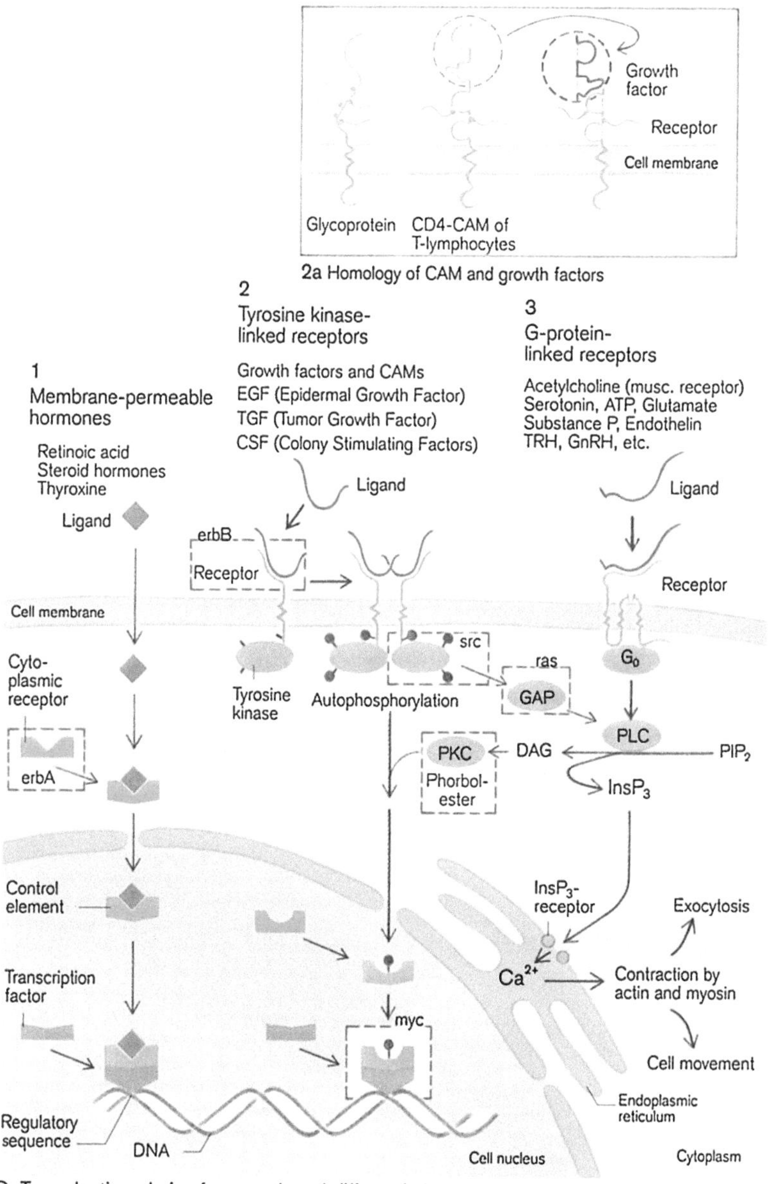


C. Transduction chains for growth and differentiation

## Differentiation of Tissues

## 3.30 Teeth, Skin and Hair

### A. Placoid Scales and Teeth

**1. Placoid scales in Lower Vertebrates.** Teeth are derived from the placoid scales of lower vertebrates. The placoid scales consist of an *enamel-like substance* that is formed basally by the epithelial cells of the epidermis. In armored reptiles and fish, the placoid scales are supplemented by membrane bones (exoskeleton), which are formed in the dermis by mesodermal cells. The exoskeleton is the basis for formation of **dentine** and **intramembranous ossification.**

**2. Tooth Development.** In mammals, two sets of teeth are formed during embryonic life by the **dental lamina** (**2a**). The dental lamina is a continuous, narrow depression of ectodermal epithelium in the oral cavity. Along the dental lamina, compact epithelial buds arise and are invaginated from below by condensed mesenchyme to form **dental bells** (**2b**). The condensed mesenchyme gives rise to the dentine-producing cells (*odontoblasts*) and the dental pulp. The inner layer of the dental bell contains the enamel-producing cells (*ameloblasts* ). The ectodermal cells in the interior of the bud loosen into a wide meshed *reticulum* of stellate cells.

**Enamel** is produced basally by the *ameloblasts*, and **dentine,** corresponding to bone, is produced apically by the *odontoblasts* (**2c**). Each odontoblast leaves behind a radially organized cell process in the dentine. The entire tooth primordium is surrounded by a *mesodermal sheath*, which guides the growth of odontoblasts and thus assists in the elongation of the tooth below the enamel cap (during teething). The bud of the *permanent tooth*, which also arises from the dental lamina during embryonic life, lies beside the deciduous tooth in a mesodermal dental sac.

### B. Skin and Hair

**1. Skin.** The *surface ectoderm* in the early embryonic period is covered by a single layer of flat cells, the *periderm*. Toward the end of the embryonic period, the surface ectoderm becomes stratified below the periderm. The epithelial cells multiply in the basal layer, differentiate during further cell divisions in the stratum spinosum, and synthesize *keratohyalin granules* in the stratum granulosum. These granules are released upon cell death, forming the cornified layer. Thus in the skin, the cycle of **proliferation, differentiation,** and **cell death** takes place continuously in specific compartments. The basal cell layer contains *melanocytes*, which have migrated in from the neural crest, and *Merkel cells*, which also come from the neural crest and function as simple target organs for sensory nerve fibers of the skin (→ 5.2). *Langhans cells,* which arise from the bone marrow, are related to macrophages.

**2. Development of Hair.** A hair is an invagination of the epidermis containing a conical cornification zone with a hair papilla at the base. The hair primordia are induced as solid **epidermal buds** (**2a**) by a mesenchymal condensation that gives rise to the **hair papilla** (**2b**). The cells in the basal layer of the hair follicle cornify and become displaced upward. This forms a hair shaft, which breaks through the neck of the compact hair bud. The neck of the bud gives rise to the **external epithelial root sheath** (**2c**). Two additional proliferation zones surround the central proliferation zone of the hair. In the *external zone,* the cells form a soft cellular horny layer (Henle's layer). In the *inner zone,* a layer of more cornified cells arises, which is pushed upward and breaks down at the surface as the hair exits (Huxley's layer). The two cell layers together are designated as the *inner root sheath*. They facilitate the outgrowth of the hair. At the end of the lifetime of a hair or during molting, the follicle falls out with the hair. A new follicle forms from the *epithelial bed*.

Ectoderm
Enamel substance
Bone substance

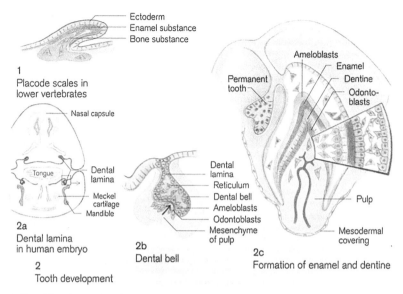

1
Placode scales in lower vertebrates

Nasal capsule
Tongue
Dental lamina
Meckel cartilage
Mandible

2a
Dental lamina in human embryo

Dental lamina
Reticulum
Dental bell
Ameloblasts
Odontoblasts
Mesenchyme of pulp

2b
Dental bell

Permanent tooth
Ameloblasts
Enamel
Dentine
Odonto-blasts
Pulp
Mesodermal covering

2c
Formation of enamel and dentine

2
Tooth development

A. Placoid scales and teeth

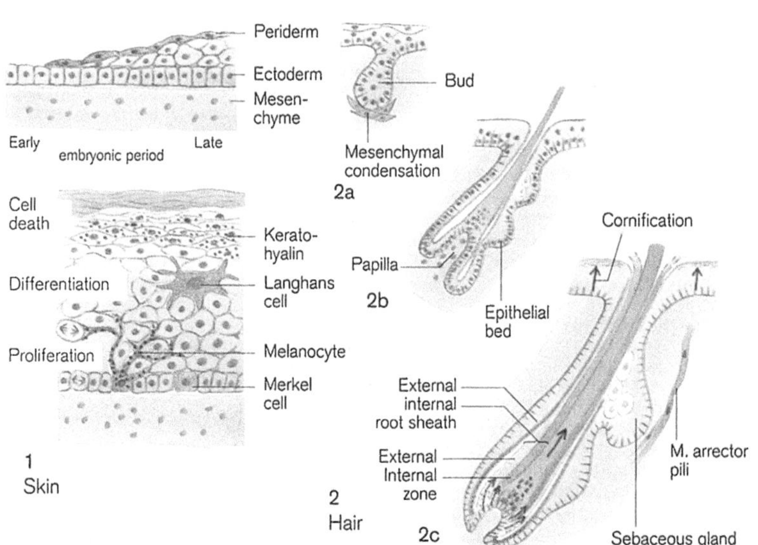


B. Skin and hair development

## 3.31 Ectodermal Glands

### A. Relationship between Ectodermal Glands

**1. Hair and Hypothetical Scale Pattern.** Teeth are derived from the scales of lower vertebrates. In mammals, the scales disappear as hair and glands arise. On surfaces possessing both scales and hair, such as the tail of the opossum, the hairs grow between the scales. They are originally formed as densely innervated tactile hairs. The arrangement of hair buds in the dorsal skin of the human fetus still shows the *original scale pattern*, although scales are no longer formed.

**2. Glands.** The ectodermal glands, like hairs, are induced as **buds (2a)** in the ectoderm by a mesenchymal condensation. Some glands are derived from **hair follicles (2b)**. The **holocrine sebaceous glands (2c)** on the nipple, below the preputium, and in the eyelids (Meibomian glands) are sebaceous glands in which the hair follicle has receded. The **mammary glands (2e)** are derived from the **odoriferous glands (2d)**, as indicated by their *apocrine secretion* and the presence of *myoepithelial cells*. The tubular, unbranched eccrine **sweat glands (2f)** are a recent development that first appeared in primates (Romer/Parsons). This development is accompanied by reduction of the hair coat and increase in subcutaneous fat, which now functions in temperature regulation.

### B. Development and Cyclic Growth of the Mammary Gland

**1. Prenatal Growth.** Like the teeth, the mammary glands arise along a continuous epithelial ridge. The **mammary ridge (1a)** is an elevated ectodermal thickening that extends (in the human embryo at stage 18) from the axillae to the inguinal region. This ridge gives rise to the **buds (1b)** of the mammary glands and later regresses. The epithelial buds slowly grow into the underlying mesenchyme and form 15–20 **lactiferous ducts (1c)** with compact end buds at their apices. At the opening of the ducts, the surface epithelium is depressed into a pit that is evaginated shortly before birth (**eversion of nipple, 1d**).

**2. Androgen Dependence in the Mouse.** In the mouse, in contrast to humans, the mammary gland is already sexually dimorphic in the embryonic period. Mesenchymal cells in the condensed mesenchyme of the developing mammary gland express *androgen receptors* in their nuclei. In male embryos, testosterone causes the mesenchymal cells in the neck region of the bud to contract, so that the bud constricts and disappears.

**3. Pregnancy and Lactation.** After puberty, female steroid hormones (estrogens) induce the development of subcutaneous fat in the female breast. In successive **cycles**, estrogen induces a growth spurt in the duct system (proliferative phase), while progesterone induces an abortive differentiation of the terminal buds (secretory phase). **Duct growth** occurs by proliferation and branching of the compact *end buds*. The pattern of ramification is determined by the connective tissue.

During the first two-thirds of **pregnancy**, estrogen and growth hormone induce an **extensive duct growth**. In the last third of pregnancy under the influence of progesterone and prolactin, the *end buds* differentiate into *alveoli* (**differentiation**). Milk secretion (**lactation** ) is initiated by hormonal stimulation (oxytocin) and nervous stimulation (suckling). After weaning, the entire secretory tissue recedes (**involution**) and only the duct system is preserved. It contains extensive segments of undifferentiated embryonic cells, from which **new end buds** emerge during continuing cycles and in further pregnancies. The existence of embryonic cells with proliferative potential within the duct system of the mammary gland explains why these organs are so susceptible to **malignant growth**.

Hair anlage
1
Hair and hypothetical scale pattern (after Arey)
2a
Epithelial bud
2f
Eccrine sweat gland
Rudimentary hair follicle
2e
Mammary gland
2b
Hair anlage
2c
Holocrine sebaceous gland
2d
Odoriferous gland
Apocrine secretion
Myoepithelial cell
2
Glands

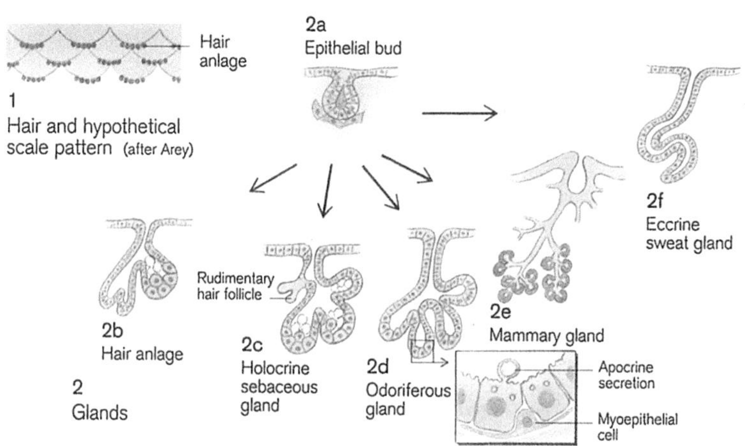

A. Relationship between ectodermal glands

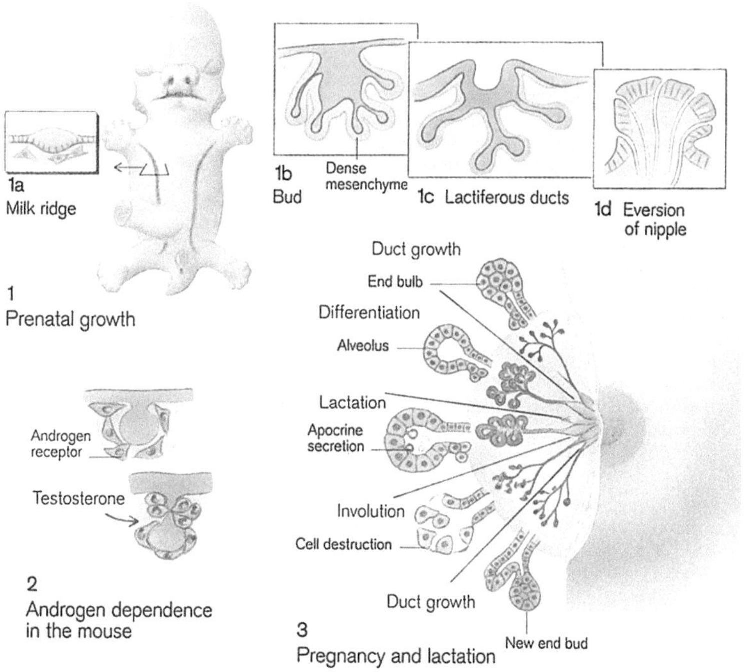

1a
Milk ridge
1b
Bud
Dense mesenchyme
1c Lactiferous ducts
1d Eversion of nipple
1
Prenatal growth
Duct growth
End bulb
Differentiation
Alveolus
Lactation
Apocrine secretion
Involution
Cell destruction
Duct growth
New end bud
Androgen receptor
Testosterone
2
Androgen dependence in the mouse
3
Pregnancy and lactation

B. Development and cyclic growth of mammary gland

## 3.32 Supporting Tissue

### A. Differentiation of Supporting Tissue

**1. Mesenchyme.** The connective tissues and supporting tissues of the body develop from mesoderm. Mesodermal cells form a loose, cellular network known as mesenchyme between the epithelial organs.

**2. Fibroblasts in Connective Tissue.** Within connective tissue, mesenchymal cells differentiate into fibroblasts. They synthesize *protocollagen and glycosaminoglycan*, which are secreted into the extracellular space by exocytosis. The subunits of protocollagen aggregate into *collagen fibrils* that are enveloped by glycosaminoglycans.

**3. Tendon.** Collagen fibers dominate in tendons; their organization determines the position and shape of the fibroblasts.

**4. Cartilage.** Cartilage arises by the aggregation of mesenchymal cells into a cartilage blastema, in which chondroblasts synthesize *collagen* and a hyaline ground substance. The ground substance gradually covers the network of collagen fibers and ultimately encloses the cells, now known as *chondrocytes*.

**5. Bone.** During *intramembranous ossification*, bone arises directly within a mesenchymal cell layer. The cells form a ground substance similar to hyaline cartilage, in which collagen fibers are enclosed. This material contains crystallization centers where calcium salts can be deposited, leading to bone formation. *Osteoblasts* thus become enclosed as *osteocytes* and are ultimately connected with each other only via long cell processes in the canaliculi of bones.

**Types of Collagen.** The collagen genes represent a *gene family* (→ 3.27) that evolved by gene reduplication and now contains many collagen variants. Each tissue expresses a specific type of collagen. Connective tissue, tendon, and bone produce type I; cartilage, type II; and embryonic mesenchyme, type III. Type III collagen occurs in the adult organism in the reticulin fibers of reticular connective tissue, which are unusally delicate and can be impregnated with silver salts.

### B. Endochondral Ossification.

The skeletal elements of the **endoskeleton**, i.e., the vertebral column, the skull base, shoulder, and pelvic girdles, as well as the limbs, are preceded by **cartilage models** that form bones by endochondral ossification. The viscerocranium, the covering bones of the skull, and the superficial elements of the shoulder girdle are derived from the **exoskeleton** of vertebrates (→ 3.30) and ossify dermally (intramembranously).

**1. Cartilage Model.** Endochondral ossification begins with a swelling of the chondrocytes in the interior of the cartilage model.

**2. Bony Collar and Ossification Centers.** As the developing bone is stabilized by the deposition of a periosteal *bony collar*, a *vascular bud* penetrates into the cartilage model. Macrophages and *osteoblasts* accompany the bud. The intact chondrocytes are stimulated to divide and become arranged into columns, in which the cells hypertrophy (**B3**). At the border to the vascular connective tissue, the *lacunae* containing the chondrocytes open. Bone is formed by osteoblasts on the already internally calcified trabeculae of hyaline cartilage between the opened lacunae. Precise synchronization of bone deposition by *osteoblasts* and bone resorption by *osteoclasts* permits the bone to retain its definitive morphology during progressive fetal and postnatal growth.

**3. Epiphysial Disc.** In developing long tubular bones, *ossification centers* arise at the ends (epiphyses) and in the shaft (diaphysis). Cartilage tissue is embedded between the two, forming a growth zone (*epiphysial disc*). Stimulation by growth hormone induces the chondrocytes to enter a *proliferative* phase, followed by a terminal *differentiation* phase, and a programmed *cell death* while bone is successively deposited on the trabeculae. At puberty, the acceleration of differentiation by sexual steroids leads to a growth spurt and to exhaustion and ossification of the disc.

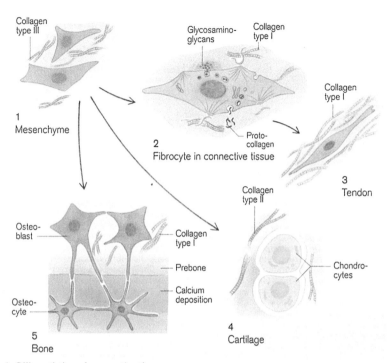

Collagen type III
1 Mesenchyme
Glycosamino-glycans
Collagen type I
Proto-collagen
2 Fibrocyte in connective tissue
Collagen type I
3 Tendon
Collagen type II
Chondro-cytes
4 Cartilage
Osteo-blast
Collagen type I
Prebone
Calcium deposition
Osteo-cyte
5 Bone

A. Differentiation of connective tissue

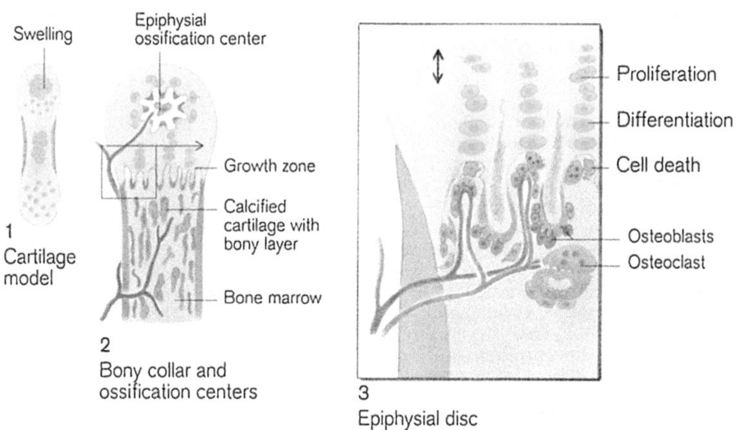


B. Endochondral ossification

## 3.33 Skeletal Muscle

### A. Development of Skeletal Muscle

**1. Determination in the Myotome.** Skeletal muscle arises from the somites. The myoblasts for the autochthonous back musculature fuse in the *myotomes* into segmentally organized muscle fibers, which after innervation, are converted into the definitive back muscles. The myoblasts for the ventral body wall and the limbs migrate as individual cells from the transitional zone between the *myotome* and *dermatome*. The masticatory and facial musculature originate from the corresponding segments of the pharyngeal arches (→ 9.0, "head problem"). In front of the pharyngeal arch region lie still rudimentary somitic segments that give rise to the myoblasts for the extrinsic eye muscles (**pro-otic myotomes** ).

Of the **regulatory genes** (**1a**) responsible for the determination of the myoblasts, the *MyoD gene* was the first to be discovered. Since transfection with MyoD can cause other cells to be transformed into myoblasts in tissue culture, MyoD was considered a master gene that switched on all the genes necessary for the development of skeletal muscle. Analysis of transgenic mice defective for MyoD revealed, however, that MyoD is only one member of an entire family of regulatory genes. The regulatory gene Myf-5 is involved in the specification of myoblasts in the myotomes, and the regulatory gene MyoD is involved in the terminal differentiation of muscle tubes. Myf-5 may act to switch on MyoD, which in turn switches off Myf-5. The ligands interacting with these transcription factors are currently unknown (Hughes, 1992).

**2. Migration of Myoblasts.** The migration of myoblasts into the limb buds is apparently directed by a segment-specific combination of CAMs. Hypothetically, this combination is imparted as position information to parietal mesodermal cells moving through the progression zone (→ 3.23) and subsequently serves to guide the growth of segmental nerve fibers (→ 3.25).

In the myotome and during migration, the myoblasts, like other embryonic cells that undergo morphogenetic movements, express **muscarinic acetylcholine receptors** (**2a**). Stimulation of these receptors leads, via InsP3, to mobilization of intracellular calcium (→ 3.29), which possibly regulates the contraction of the actin-myosin filaments during amoeboid movement.

**3. Terminal Differentiation.** In the muscle primordium, the myoblasts stop proliferating and begin to fuse with one another. The multinucleated cells differentiate into muscle fibers. The *muscarinic acetylcholine receptor* disappears and a *nicotinic receptor* is expressed (**3a**). Between the muscle fibers, some resting myoblasts remain as *satellite cells*, which can be activated to regenerate the muscle after damage.

When a muscle fiber is innervated by a nerve fiber originating from the *same* segment, it forms an endplate (**3b**) in which *nicotinic receptors* are concentrated. The endoplasmic reticulum of the myoblast becomes the sarcoplasmic reticulum of the muscle fiber. The cell membrane invaginates to form the T-tubular system. The *triad* is occupied by the ryanodine receptor, a member of the gene family of $InsP_3$ receptors of the endoplasmic reticulum. This receptor responds to an *action potential* propagated from the end plate by inducing calcium release.

During the differentiation of myoblasts, all major cellular components, from receptors to actin-myosin filaments, are replaced by specific (differentiated) variants from the corresponding gene families. The correct contact between nerve fibers and muscle fibers, generated by a "trial and error" approach, is secured by continued synthesis of CAMs (which function as trophic factors). Denervation leads to the loss of endplates and to the distribution of nicotinic receptors over the entire muscle cell membrane. Similarly, destruction of the muscle fiber causes degeneration of the nerve fiber.

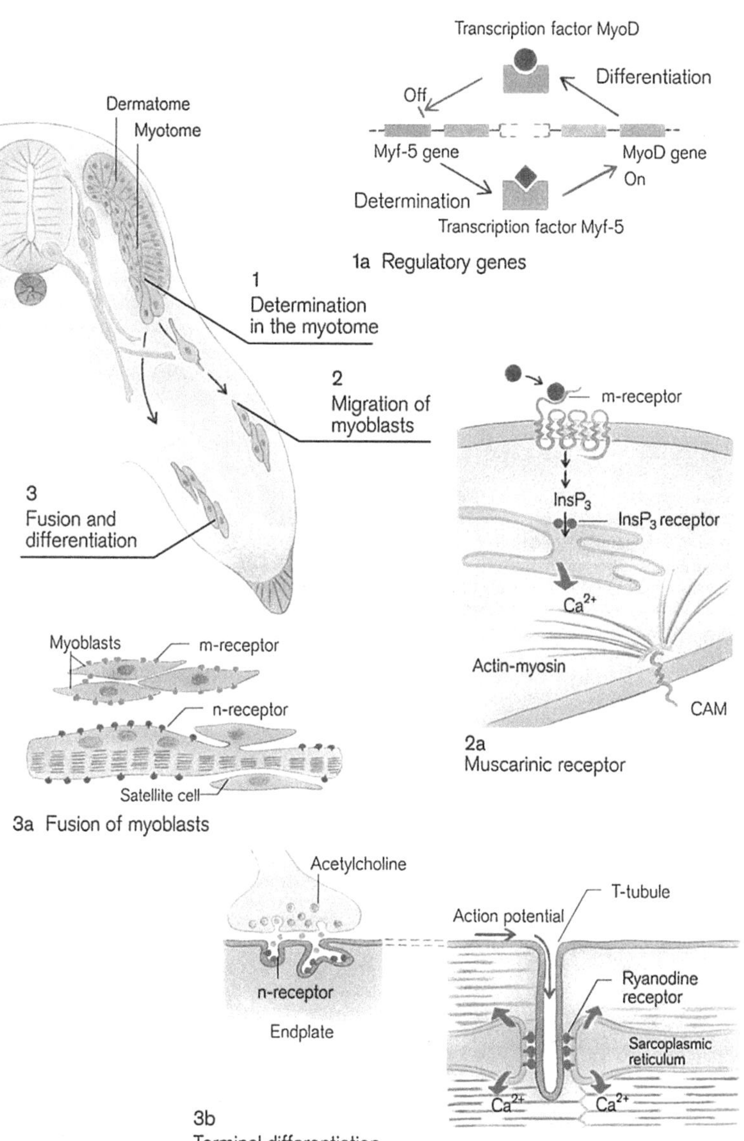


A. Development of skeletal musculature

## 3.34 Hemopoiesis and Lymphopoiesis

### A. Blood Islands and Hemopoiesis

**1. Blood Islands in the Yolk Sac.** Blood islands are induced in the *visceral mesoderm* by the *endoderm*. They contain the *stem cells* of hemopoiesis and produce daughter cells that differentiate in cell nests into *erythrocytes*. The blood islands are surrounded by *endothelial cells*. The endothelial tubes for the *dorsal aorta* and the heart are induced in the visceral mesoderm by the endoderm of the intestinal groove and the pharynx. The tubes are connected with the blood islands in the yolk sac by capillary sprouts. As the cardiac tube begins to pulsate, capillary networks are converted into vascular channels. Experiments with quail–chick transplantations (→ 3.12) and labelling with specific antibodies revealed that endothelial cells arise only in the visceral mesoderm and spread from there into the parietal mesoderm (Pardanaud and Dieterlen-Lievre, 1993). The amniotic and chorionic mesoderm, which originate from parietal mesoderm, are correspondingly deficient in blood vessels (→ 3.14). In the human, the function of the primary yolk sac could thus be the induction of vessels in the chorionic mesoderm (→ 2.10).

**2. Phases of Hemopoiesis.** Erythrocytes are terminally differentiated cells that ultimately synthesize only hemoglobin and subsequently inactivate their entire genome. During embryonic development, distinct hemoglobin molecules are successively expressed. Each of them has an oxygen-binding capacity adapted to the circulatory conditions prevailing in the embryo and fetus. In the **embryonic phase**, erythrocytes differentiate in the blood islands of the yolk sac. The embryonic erythrocytes are large, contain embryonic hemoglobin with ζ- and ε-chains, and retain their inactivated cell nucleus. (In amphibians and birds, the adult animals also possess nucleated erythrocytes.) After regression of the yolk sac, hemopoiesis is taken over by the liver and spleen (**hepatolienal phase**). The erythrocytes contain fetal hemoglobin (HbF with α- and γ-chains). During fetal life, erythropoiesis is shifted to the **bone marrow**. There, adult hemoglobin (HbA with α- and β-chains) is formed.

### B. Lymphatic System

**1. Bone Marrow.** The stem cells for *erythropoiesis* , *myelopoiesis* (granulocytes, general defense functions), and *lymphopoiesis* are found in the bone marrow. In humans, **lymphopoiesis** begins in the 11th week of pregnancy and **myelopoiesis** in the 12th.

**2. Thymus.** The thymus (→ 7.3) is colonized around the llth week of pregnancy by *dendritic cells* and *lymphocytes* from the liver and bone marrow, which migrate into the thymus primordium via the bloodstream.

The lymphocytes settle in the intercellular spaces between the epithelial cells and differentiate into T-lymphocytes, which are again taken up into the bloodstream.

**3. Tonsils.** Dendritic cells and B-lymphocytes settle in the reticulated, endodermal epithelium of the tonsils, where they produce IgA against bacterial and viral antigens. Clonal proliferation of B-lymphocytes occurs in the lymphatic nodules within the mesenchyme of the tonsils.

**4. White Pulp of Spleen.** Macrophages settle in the wall of the *encapsulated capillaries*, where they present hematogenic antigens for the T-lymphocytes that settle in the surrounding nodules of the malpighian body.

**5. Lymph Nodes.** Lymphatic vessels arise at the end of the embryonic period, when intercellular spaces are lined with lymphatic endothelium. They first appear at the junction of the jugular vein and then spread throughout the entire body. *Lymph nodes* are formed by the accumulation of dendritic cells at the branchings of the lymphatic vascular system, where T- and B-lymphocytes settle. The hilum of ingrowing blood vessels and the connective tissue capsule of the lymph nodes develop secondarily.

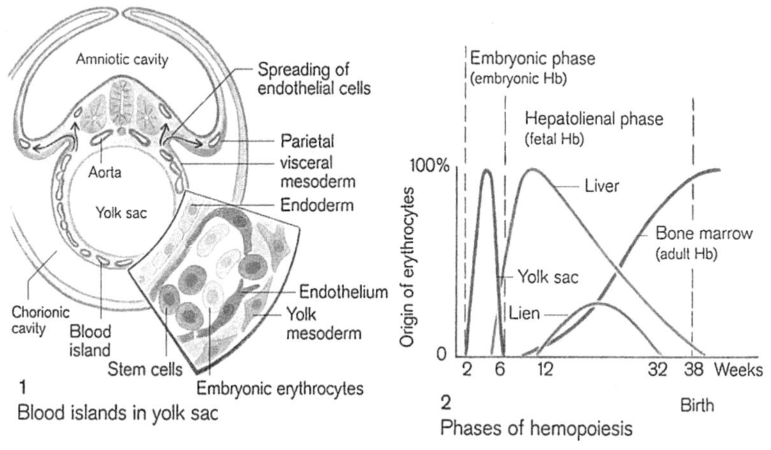


1
Blood islands in yolk sac

2
Phases of hemopoiesis

A. Hemopoiesis

Thymus

Epithelial cells
T-lymphocyte
Dendritic cell

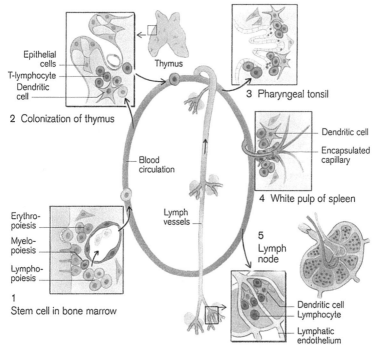

2 Colonization of thymus

3 Pharyngeal tonsil

Dendritic cell
Encapsulated capillary

4 White pulp of spleen

Blood circulation

Lymph vessels

Erythro-poiesis
Myelo-poiesis
Lympho-poiesis

1
Stem cell in bone marrow

5
Lymph node

Dendritic cell
Lymphocyte
Lymphatic endothelium

B. Lymphatic system

## 3.35 Immunoglobulins

### C. Determination and Differentiation of Lymphocytes

**Immunoglobulin Superfamily**

The immunoglobulin superfamily is derived from a cell membrane glycoprotein. The membrane-bound members are related to the cell adhesion molecules (CAMs) of the **selectin** type (→ 3.26). Together with the growth factors of the lymphatic system, the **cytokines**, they are the best-studied examples of molecules that induce determination and differentiation.

The fully matured **immunoglobulin M (IgM)** molecule is located in the cell membrane of B-lymphocytes and functions as a receptor for antigens. The **T-cell receptor (TCR)** is the corresponding receptor in the membrane of T-lymphocytes. The **histocompatibility complex** (MHC, "major histocompatibility complex") codes for the antigens involved in immunological self-recognition. **MHC I** is expressed in all cells, **MHC II** only in the antigen-presenting macrophages, dendritic cells, and lymphocytes. The **ancestral gene** probably encoded a protein with a subunit (domain) of the **$\beta_2$-microglobulin ($\beta_2$M)** type. In the course of evolution, replication of subunits within the gene and repeated duplication of the entire gene took place, giving rise to a superfamily of immunoglobulin genes. **CD4 and CD8** are molecules that characterize a stem-cell line. CD4 is expressed on T-helper cells and CD8 on cytotoxic T-cells. All hematopoietic stem cells are characterized by CD-determinants (cluster of differentiation). The **poly-Ig receptor** is a membrane protein used in the placenta for transcellular transport of maternal antibodies into the fetus. The **carcinoembryonic antigen (CEA)** occurs in cancer cells of the gastrointestinal tract and in embryonic endoderm. As a tumor marker, it is used in the diagnosis of tumors. Its function is unknown.

**Determination and Differentiation**

**Determination in Bone Marrow.** Like the stem cells of lymphopoiesis, the *dendritic cells* in the lymphatic nodules and the macrophages come from the bone marrow. There, direct contact between these cells may specify the determinants for later "homing in" in the lymphatic organs.

**Differentiation in the Thymus.** The precursors of T-cells migrate into the thymus. During this "**homing in**," CD7 functions as a CAM. After **somatic recombination** in the variable region of the T-cell receptor gene, each lymphocyte expresses an individual T-cell receptor. Differentiation is followed by selection. In this process, the cell surface determinants characteristic of an individual are represented in the thymus by the MHC complex on the epithelial cells (MHC I) and the dendritic cells (MHC II). All T-lymphocytes that possess T-cell receptors recognizing endogenous determinants are eliminated by *autolysis*. The immature T-cells in the thymus still carry both T-cell specific determinants CD4 and CD8. Binding to MHC I induces differentiation of CD8-positive cytotoxic T-cells, while binding to MHC II induces CD4-positive T-helper cells. The differentiation of B-lymphocytes takes place analogously in bone marrow (equivalent to the **bursa of birds**).

**Terminal Differentiation.** Lymphocytes migrate into the T-cell and B-cell regions of lymphatic organs. Terminal differentiation is induced by antigen contact (**Inset**). The processed antigen is presented in a groove on the surface of the MHC protein. The lymphocyte receptor binds to the antigen, and the CD4- or CD8-molecule to MHC II or MHC I. The CD determinants and the T-cell receptor are linked to a *tyrosine kinase* of the src-oncogene family. Activation initiates the secretion of growth factors (*interleukines)*, which elicit clonal proliferation.

The **B-cells** ultimately differentiate into plasma cells that secrete IgG or IgA. For activation of B-cells, *cooperation* with *T-helper* cells is necessary. B-cells present the antigen with MHC II to T-helper cells, which induce clonal expansion of the B-cell by secretion of *interleucins*. "Memory cells," retained after a primary reaction, correspond to the determined stem cell "reserve" also found in other tissues.

For activation of B-cells, *cooperation* with *T-helper* cells is necessary. B-cells present the antigen with MHC II to T-helper cells, which induce clonal expansion of the B-cell by secretion of *interleucins*.

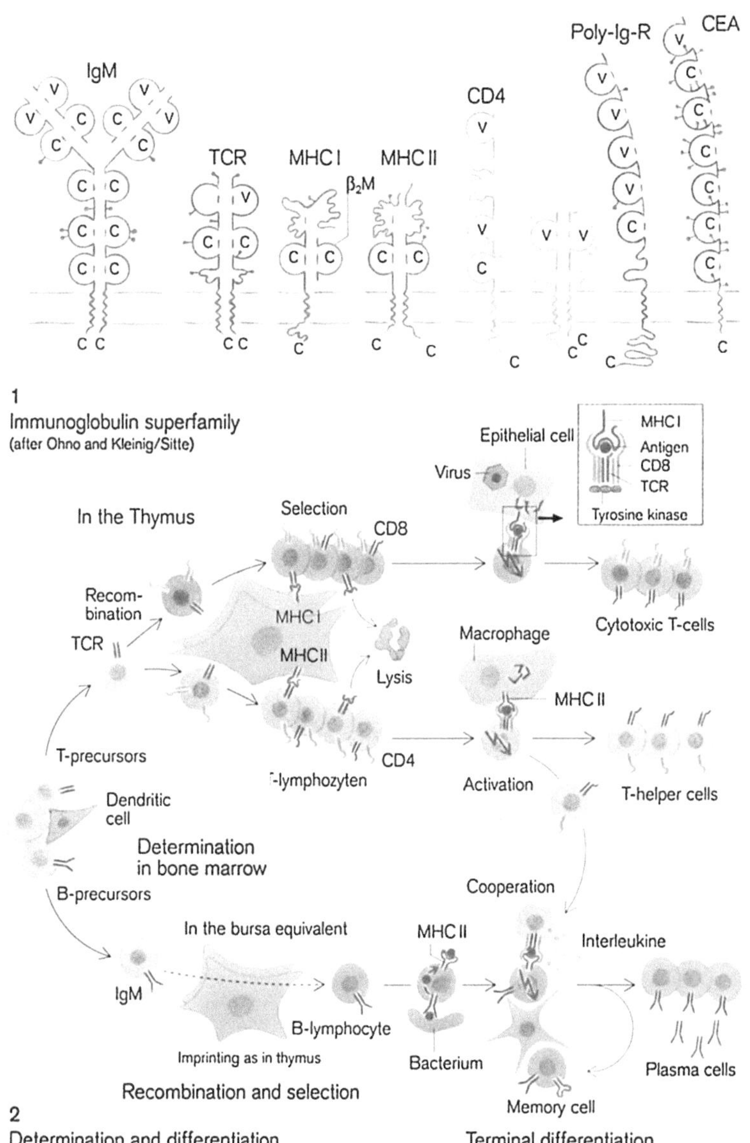


C. Determination and differentiation of lymphocytes

# Chapter 4: Nervous System

## Introduction

**Aim of the Chapter.** The goal of this chapter is to clarify the complex anatomy of the brain by analyzing its embryological development. Early in embryogenesis, the neural tube gives rise to the brain vesicles, which are the basis for the definitive organization. The anatomy of the brain can thus be reconstructed from its embryonic development.

**Structure and Function.** Anatomy is most easily understood when anatomical structures are studied in terms of their functions. Embryonic structures are not yet differentiated and have no function; however, their (prospective) functions can be deduced by comparison with the corresponding structures in phylogeny.

**Phylontotractus.** The phylontotractus is utilized to relate the functions observed in the phylogenetic series to homologous structures in the embryo (→ 4.1). The Phylontotractus is an abstraction, a system of thought in which parallels between phylogeny and ontogeny are emphasized. For example, the basic anatomical and functional organization of the spinal cord can be understood by relating it to the function of the segmental unit of spinal nerve, vertebral body, and muscle plate in the swimming movements of aquatic vertebrates. The basic unit of somite and spinal nerve is found in the human during embryonic life. It represents the starting material for the differentiation of a locomotor system appropriate for life on land.

**Basic Organization of the Neural Tube.** All parts of the central nervous system arise from the neural tube. The basic histological structure is the neuroepithelium. In the *spinal cord* (→ 4.3), the neuroblasts lie as a mantle layer (gray matter) above the matrix zone around the central canal. The axons of the nerve cells extend outward in the marginal zone (white matter) beneath the original basement membrane of the neuroepithelium. In the *brainstem* (→ 4.10), the central nuclei, like the gray matter of the spinal cord, develop in the mantle layer of the neuroepithelium. In the *cerebral cortex* (→ 4.17), the neuroblasts migrate through the mantle layer into the marginal layer beneath the basement membrane of the neuroepithelium. This process gives rise to the cortical plate, which undergoes further development to form the cerebral cortex. In the cerebellum ( → 4.14), the cells migrating into the "cortical plate" retain their mitotic capability and form an external matrix zone at the outer surface, where postmitotic neuroblasts arise.

**Basal and Alar Plate**. In the spinal cord, the organization of the neural tube into a motor basal plate and a sensory alar plate, and into somatic and autonomic functional components, is readily discernible (→ 4.10). The attempt to apply this organizational scheme to the brainstem meets with a number of difficulties. The assembly of neurons into the nuclei of origin of the cranial nerves is more pronounced than the organization into functionally defined columns. The transitions between somatic and autonomic, and between sensitive and sensory functions are blurred. In general, such categorizations are not appropriate for the brainstem. The renaissance of the neuromeres, on the other hand, indicates that the assumption of a fundamental homology between spinal cord and brain is justified.

**Neuromeres.** It has been known for over a hundred years that the developing brain is organized into neuromeres (→ 4.7). In relation to the theory of brain vesicles, however, the significance of the neuromeres has been unclear (→ 9.0, head problem). The expression of segmentation genes in the neuromeres, in homologous fashion to the homeotic genes of Drosophila, indicates that neuromeres represent metameric segments that correspond to the somites. In the body, the segmental pattern appears primarily during the organization of somites in the paraxial mesoderm. Outgrowth of the spinal nerves is induced by the caudal sclerotome segment (→ 3.22). In the head, on the other hand, the segmental pattern develops primarily in the neural tube. The cranial nerves obtain their positional information already in the cranial neuromere of the pharyngeal arch segment (→ 4.7). The difference in the determination of metamerism between trunk and head may be due only to a different temporal or spatial pattern of expression of homeotic genes (→ 3.17).

**Brain Vesicles.** The appearance of brain vesicles in evolution coincides with the centralization of sensory organs and the development of the head. The lancelet fish (→ 3.3) has neither head nor brain and possesses dispersed sensory cells, for example, light-sensitive cells distributed in the spinal cord (→ 5.1). The expansion of the neural tube into cerebral vesicles can be interpreted as a functional enlargement of the neural tube for the central representation of the sensory organs of the head (→ 4.1 and 4.9). With this concept, the course of the central sensory pathways in the brainstem can be meaningfully described.

**Hierarchy with Cerebrum.** During evolution, the primitive system of the spinal cord and medulla oblongata is subordinated to the control of the higher centers of the basal ganglia, which in turn become controlled by the cerebral cortex. The cerebral cortex, in turn, consists of three hierarchical levels, the paleo-, archi-, and neocortex. The preexisting systems are integrated at a lower level with newer, more complex structures. The hierarchical organization is apparent in the extension of the sensory pathways of the brainstem into the cerebrum, as well as in the organization of motor innervation at the level of spinal cord and medulla oblongata, at the level of the brainstem (extrapyramidal system), and finally at the level of the cerebral cortex (→ 4.25).

**Hemispheric Rotation.** Hemispheric rotation (→ 4.15) is not a true rotational movement, but comes about by the insertion of a large, wedge-shaped segment of neocortex (frontal brain) in front of the primordial hippocampus, which originally lies on the apex of the telencephalon(→ 4.20). The size of the inserted neocortical segment can be recognized by the extension of the corpus callosum. In the mouse, the hippocampus still lies in the apical region. In humans, it is shifted into the temporal lobe. During hemispheric rotation, the tip of the temporal lobe containing the amygdaloid nucleus does not actually move, but is fixed to the root of the olfactory bulb. The original position of the hippocampus can be recognized from the course of the fornix, the hippocampal fiber tract. The nerve fibers of the fornix are already connected with their target regions in the hippocampus before hemispheric rotation begins. As the hippocampus becomes displaced, the fiber tract elongates but retains its original position in the medial wall of the ventricle (→ 4.21).

**Pineal Gland (Epiphysis).** The function of the pineal gland ( → 4.23) as generator of an endogenous rhythm (which was originally linked to the length of the day and night) is evidenced by glands that still contain light-sensitive cells. The development of a light-opaque scalp led to the formation of a "sensory tract" from the eye to the pineal gland, using the preexisting pathways of the sympathetic nervous system.

**Conserved Ventricles and Progressive Cerebral Tracts.** In the ventricular system of the definitive brain, the organization of the embryonic brain vesicles is preserved (→ 4.8). The fiber tracts of the cerebrum, on the other hand, are progressive structures that do not conform to the structural organization of the brainstem, as determined by the cerebral vesicles and by the hemispheric rotation (→ 4.22). They connect their regions of origin with their target sites by the shortest possible connection. Examples are the projection of the central sensory pathways into the cerebral cortex, the corpus callosum as a commissure between the two cerebral hemispheres, and the corticobulbar and corticospinal tracts that pass through the internal capsule and the cerebral crura.

## 4.1 Overview: Phylontotractus

### A. Archaic Organization of the Nervous System

The central nervous system consists of three parts that develop sequentially in the course of vertebrate phylogeny. They are represented in the fictitious "*phylontotractus* " (**A1** and **A2**): The **spinal cord** functions in the regulation of body movements; the **hindbrain** regulates food intake, digestion, and respiration; the **true brain** processes olfactory, visual, and auditory stimuli from the central sense organs.

The **spinal cord** coordinates the original sinuous serpentine movements of the trunk via a simple movement program based on local reflex arcs. The trunk is made up of segmentally arranged muscle plates that are attached to the vertebrae and are innervated by spinal nerves.

The branchial nerves originate in the **hindbrain** and pass to the pharyngeal arches. The pharynx can be traced back to a primitive branchial gut (→ 3.19), which is transformed into a gill apparatus in aquatic vertebrates. In the transition to life on land, the pharyngeal arches were transformed and became adapted to food intake on land. The pharynx is closely associated with the posterior part of the rhombencephalon.

The true brain originates from **three cerebral vesicles,** to which the central sense organs are linked. Olfaction and vision are localized in the first vesicle. It consists of the rhinencephalon with the olfactory bulb—the thickened root of which gives rise to the *telencephalon-* and the visual brain, the future *diencephalon*, from which the eyeballs evaginate.

The middle brain vesicle (*mesencephalon* ) contains the centers in which input from the eyes and ears are transformed into impulses directing eye and head movements. Thus the ancestral portions of the *visual tract* terminate in the *superior colliculus* of the *corpora quadrigemina* and the *auditory tract* relays in the *inferior colliculus*.

The auditory and vestibular organs arise from the otic vesicle, which is associated with the third primary brain vesicle (*rhombencephalon*). The anterior part of the rhombencephalon serves in the processing of auditory and equilibrium information, whereas the posterior portion is associated with the pharyngeal arch nerves. The two parts overlap.

### B. Embryonic Organization of the Central Nervous System

In the **embryonic period** (stage 17), the developing central nervous system occupies more than half of the total embryo. The organization is analogous to that of the "phylontotractus." The brain vesicles are established in corresponding fashion, although they are not yet functionally differentiated. At this time, they consist of neuroepithelium in which morphogenetic movements still occur; differentiation begins later. In contrast, the nervous system of an organism at this level of organization in phylogeny already consists of differentiated neurons that are optimally adapted to the environment of the species.

The trunk of the embryo (**B1**) is organized metamerically into myotomes, vertebral bodies, and spinal nerves. The branchial nerves pass to the pharyngeal arches lying beneath them.

In the **fetal period** (**B2**), the brain takes on its definitive shape, in which the primordial organization remains recognizable. The three portions of the brainstem are covered by the *telencephalon*, which grows from the original prosencephalon at the *interventricular foramen*. The prosencephalic vesicle becomes the third ventricle in the *diencephalon,* which is continuous with the *mesencephalon* (containing the pons and the corpora quadrigemina). The cerebellum, functionally connected to the auditory and vestibular organs, develops above the *rhombencephalon*.

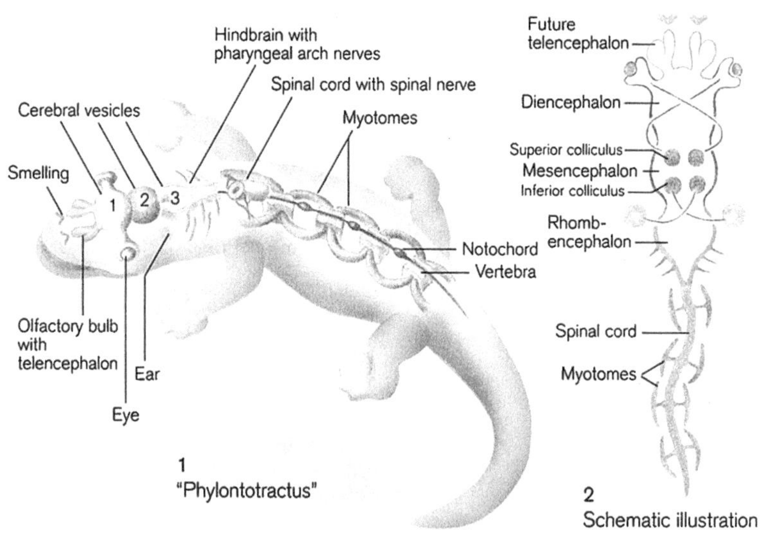


1
"Phylontotractus"

2
Schematic illustration

A. Archaic organization of nervous system

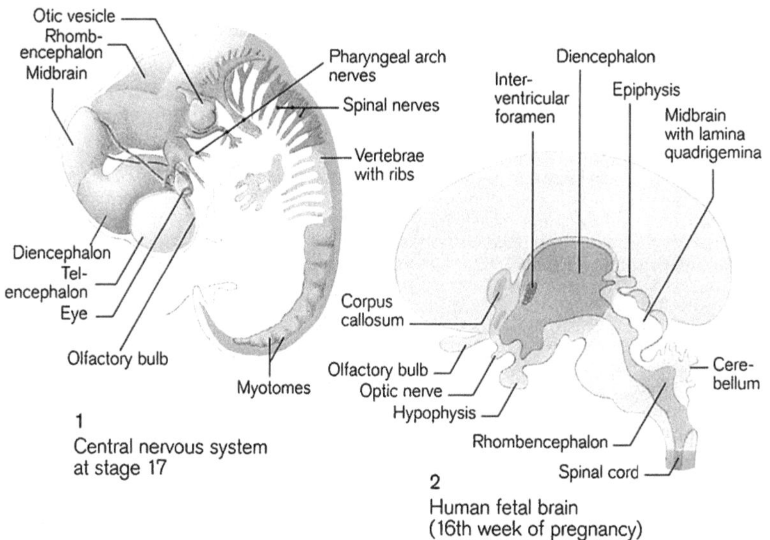


1
Central nervous system at stage 17

2
Human fetal brain (16th week of pregnancy)

B. Embryonic organization of the central nervous system

# Neural Tube and Spinal Cord

## 4.2 Neural Tube

*Background*

The neural tube arises from the neural plate. The **neural plate** is induced in the ectoderm by the notochord-mesoderm complex (→ 3.4) the correlate of which in birds and mammals is the head process and the mesoderm involuting through the primitive node. The ectodermal cells form a thick pseudostratified epithelium (**neuroepithelium**), which rises to form a **neural groove** and then closes by fusion of the **neural folds,** forming the **neural tube.** During fusion, the neural crest cells migrate outward from the neural folds.

### A. Neural Folding in Stage 10

In the human embryo, the neural plate is induced in the ectoderm (anterior to the primitive node) in the 3rd week, at stages 7 and 8 (→ 2.10). Neural folds arise at the beginning of the 4th week in stage 10, at the time when somite formation occurs, initiating the delineation of the embryonic body. Closure of the neural tube begins cranially and like the formation of somites, follows the migration of the primitive node in the caudal direction. Above the expanding head region, the neural plate is so broad that closure of the neural tube is delayed relative to the trunk. Therefore, the neural tube closes first in the waist region of the embryo at the level of the fourth somite. From there, the closure of the neural tube advances cranially and caudally. The rostral opening of the tube is designated the *anterior neuropore*; the caudal opening, the *posterior neuropore* (**B1**).

**a Formation of Neural Groove.** The neural groove develops anterior to the primitive node and directly above the notochordial process. The inductive relationship between the notochord-mesoderm complex and the neural plate is indicated by the close apposition between the neuroepithelium and the notochordal process.

**b Neural Groove with Neural Crest.** Contraction of intracellular actin-myosin filaments, located between the apical desmosomes of neuroepithelial cells (→ 3.25), causes the neural folds to move toward each other. The V-shaped neural groove becomes tub shaped.

The neural folds contain the neural crest material. During the fusion of the neural folds, the neural crest cells migrate outward from the neuroepithelium. These cells are the progenitors for the pigment cells of the body, the spinal ganglia, the cells of the autonomic nervous system, and the Schwann cells of peripheral nerves.

**c Closed Neural Tube.** The *neural crest cells* migrate from the neural tube along two pathways. On the *lateral path,* they use the underside of the surface epithelium as a guiding structure; these neural crest cells become the melanoblasts of the skin. The *medial path* is located between the neural tube and the somites. It is taken by the cells of the peripheral autonomic nervous system and by the Schwann cells of the spinal nerves. The neural crest cells for the spinal ganglia settle down in their final position on the medial path directly beside the neural tube.

### B. Displacement of Anterior and Posterior Neuropores

As the embryo folds off from the umbilical vesicle, it gains a pronounced ventral curvature. The driving force for the curving of the embryo is the rapid growth of the brain. The *anterior neuropore* comes to lie above the cerebral vesicles (**B1**). The optic vesicles begin to evaginate (*optic sulci*) even before the prosencephalon has closed. The *posterior neuropore* is displaced caudally above the tail bud, which is directed upward due to the embryonic curvature.

The primitive node is transformed into the **tail bud,** which gives rise directly to the notochord, the somites, and the neural groove (**B2**). After closure of the posterior neuropore, the remainder of the neural tube arises as a complete structure from the blastema of the tail bud (→ 3.10).

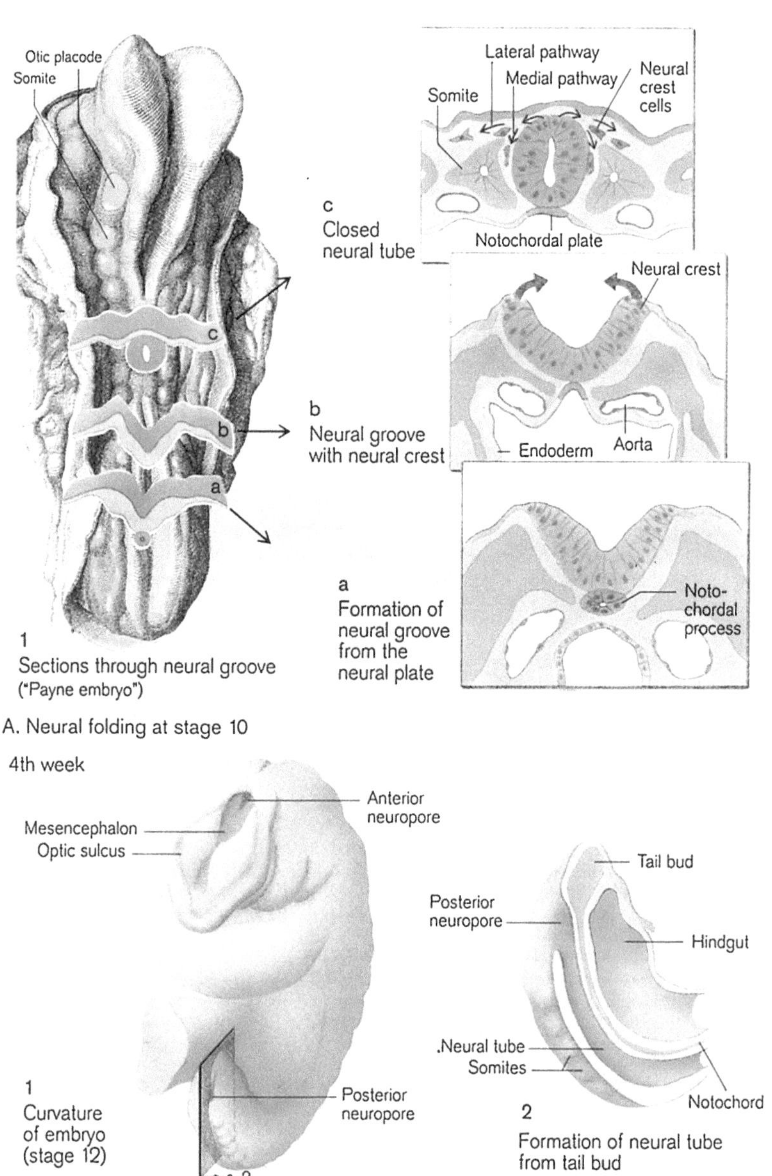


c
Closed neural tube

b
Neural groove with neural crest

a
Formation of neural groove from the neural plate

1
Sections through neural groove ("Payne embryo")

A. Neural folding at stage 10

4th week

1
Curvature of embryo (stage 12)

2
Formation of neural tube from tail bud

B. Movement of anterior and posterior neuropores

# 4.3 Spinal Cord

## A. Proliferation of the Neuroepithelium

**1. Position of the Basement Membrane.** After closure of the neural tube, the *basement membrane* of the neuroepithelium lies on the exterior of the neural tube (**1a**) and the cell apices are directed inward toward the central canal (**1b**). The *external limiting membrane* is the basement membrane of the neuroepithelium. The *internal limiting membrane*, which is visible by light microscopy, is an internal boundary formed by the junctional complexes of the neuroepithelial cells at the border of the central canal.

**2. Cell Division.** In the *neural tube*, differentiation of the *neuroepithelial cells* is preceded by a phase of proliferation. As in other pseudostratified epithelia, the neuroepithelial cells become rounded before mitosis, detach from the *basement membrane*, and migrate upward to the cell apices. Metaphase cells are therefore found near the *central canal*. A single neuroepithelial cell gives rise to two neuroepithelial daughter cells that again extend processes between the basal and apical regions of the epithelium (**2a**).

## B. Differentiation of Nerve Cells and Glial Cells

**1. Cellular Differentiation**

The differentiation of neuroblasts and glial cells takes place within the neuroepithelium. As the wall of the neural tube increases in thickness, it loses its epithelial character.

**a Neurons**. Neurons arise by an unequal division **(critical mitosis)** of neuroepithelial cells. The critical mitosis gives rise to an additional neuroepithelial cell, which is capable of division and a *neuroblast* that is no longer capable of division, but undergoes further differentiation to form a neuron. The neuroblast becomes rounded into a cell with a large, light nucleus and a distinct nucleolus. It separates from the internal limiting membrane, whereas the neuroepithelial daughter cell becomes stretched out again, extending processes that span the whole epithelium. The mitotic spindles of the critical mitoses are oriented radially around the internal limiting membrane.

**b Glial Cells.** Glial cells also originate from neuroepithelial cells. *Astroglia* are stellate, branched supporting cells. *Oligodendroglia* are supporting cells with thick processes that become closely apposed to neurons and later form myelin sheaths in the central nervous system. The regular epithelial structure of the neuroepithelium disintegrates as neuroblasts and glial cells form. Some neuroepithelial cells extend outward as *pillar cells* (radial fibers) between the internal and external limiting membranes. The radial fibers serve as migration supports for neuroblasts and glioblasts. Their nucleus lies at the central canal. The long cell processes of the original neuroepithelial cells that span between the external and internal limiting membrane ultimately disintegrate. A layer of cuboidal cells remains, in which the cell apices are oriented toward the central canal (*ependymal cells*).

**c Spinal Ganglia.** The spinal ganglia arise from neural crest cells. The spinal ganglion cells project one axon back to the neural tube (central process) and one axon to the periphery along the spinal nerves (peripheral process). The roots of the two axons gradually migrate toward one another and fuse into a single stem, forming a *pseudounipolar ganglion cell*.

**2. Gray and White Matter of the Spinal Cord**

The cell nuclei of proliferating neuroepithelial cells are shifted toward the central canal. They form the **matrix zone,** from which neuroblasts and glial cells originate. When the matrix zone is exhausted, only the **ependyma** persists. The neuroblasts form an intermediate layer of cell nuclei in the wall of the neural tube that surrounds the matrix zone like a mantle (**B1**) and is therefore known as the **mantle layer**. It becomes the **gray matter** of the spinal cord (**B2**). Below the external limiting membrane, a nucleus-free marginal zone arises in which the ascending and descending axons of the neuroblasts spread out. This delicate marginal zone is called the **marginal layer** (**B1**). It becomes the **white matter** of the spinal cord.

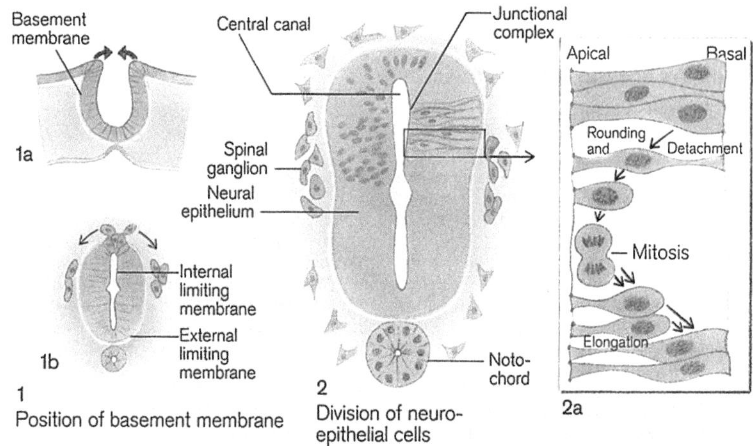

Basement membrane
1a
Central canal
Junctional complex
Spinal ganglion
Neural epithelium
Apical
Basal
Rounding and
Detachment
Mitosis
Elongation
Internal limiting membrane
External limiting membrane
1b
Noto-chord
1
Position of basement membrane
2
Division of neuro-epithelial cells
2a

A. Proliferation of neuroepithelium

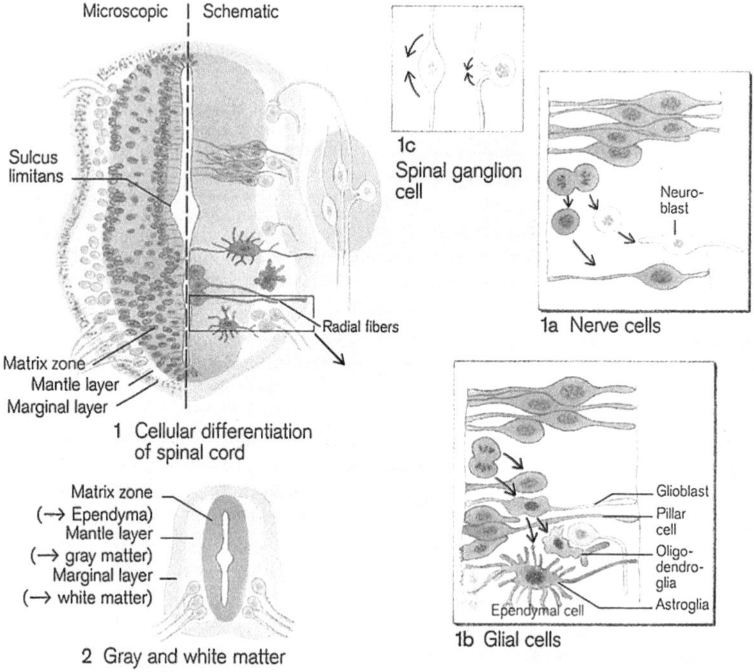

Microscopic
Schematic
Sulcus limitans
Radial fibers
Matrix zone
Mantle layer
Marginal layer
1 Cellular differentiation of spinal cord
1c
Spinal ganglion cell
Neuro-blast
1a Nerve cells
Matrix zone (→ Ependyma)
Mantle layer (→ gray matter)
Marginal layer (→ white matter)
2 Gray and white matter
Glioblast
Pillar cell
Oligo-dendro-glia
Ependymal cell
Astroglia
1b Glial cells

B. Differentiation of nerve cells and glial cells

## 4.4 Spinal Nerves

### A. Spinal Cord and Spinal Nerves

**1. Outgrowth of Pioneer Fibers**

The axons of neurons of the *motor anterior horn* emerge from the neural tube when the first striated muscle fibers form in the myotomes by cell fusion. The tips of the growing axony form *growth cones* from which pseudopodia constantly extend, seeking a path along the sclerotome cells. Axon growth ceases when the pseudopodia contact a muscle fiber with which the neuron can form a synapse (→3.25). Further axons follow; since their growth cones move along the already advanced *pioneer fibers*, they have a greater chance of reaching the target organ. Incorrectly targeted axons or axons that fail to find appropriate targets (i.e., noninnervated muscle fibers) perish. The peripheral processes of the sensory spinal ganglion cells in the *spinal ganglia* join the motor nerve tracts, whereas their central processes form synapses with sensory neurons in the alar plate. The axons of the ventral branch of the spinal nerve follow the *myoblasts*, which migrate into the ventral body wall and the *limb buds*. Synapses develop only when the myoblasts have reached their destination and fuse to form muscle fibers (→3.33).

**2. Development of Segmental Spinal Nerves**

**a Basal and Alar Plates.** As the neurons differentiate, the mantle layer (→4.3) increases in thickness and determines the shape of the neural tube. The ventral protrusion of the mantle layer is designated as the *basal plate*, the dorsal as the *alar plate*. Basal and alar plates protrude into the central canal so that the *limiting sulcus* arises between the two. In the basal plate lie cells of the *motor anterior horn* (**A1**), the axons of which exit from the spinal cord via the ventral roots. The alar plate contains *sensory neurons* (**A1**), which receive the terminals of the afferent axons of the spinal ganglion cells.

**b Peripheral Nerve Pathways.** Successful pioneer fibers determine the paths for the axons of the spinal nerves by guiding subsequent axons along the shortest route to the target cells that develop from the somites. Each somite thus induces the formation of a spinal nerve (→4.5). *Spinal* nerves are connected to the spinal cord by a *dorsal sensory* and a *ventral motor root*; their axons segregate into a mixed *dorsal branch* and a mixed *ventral branch* for the *dorsal* and *ventral musculature* and the corresponding cutaneous regions.

**c Myelin Formation.** *Schwann cells*, the supporting cells for the axons of the spinal nerves, arise from the neural crest. They migrate along the axons of developing spinal ganglia into the periphery, where they become supporting cells for the peripheral nerve fibers. Initially, the Schwann cells surround the axons and incorporate them in deep invaginations of the cell membrane (as in "nonmyelinated" fibers); later, they wrap the invaginated cell membranes around the axons ("myelinated" fibers).

### B. Development of the Cauda Equina

In the embryonic period, the central nervous system grows faster than the other organ systems and therefore occupies about one third of the embryo. In the fetal period, on the other hand, the vertebral column and the rest of the fetal body grows faster than the neural tube (→8.2). The lower end of the spinal cord is thereby shifted cranially relative to the vertebral column, while the spinal ganglia remain fixed in the intervertebral foramina of their primordial segments. The roots of the spinal nerves are extended considerably. At birth, the end of the spinal cord lies at the level of the 3rd lumbar vertebra (L3), whereas in the adult it ends at the level of L2. Below L2, the spinal cord continues into the *filum terminale*, which contains no nerve cells. The roots of the spinal nerves descending in the dural sac of the spinal canal are called the cauda equina (site of *lumbar puncture*).

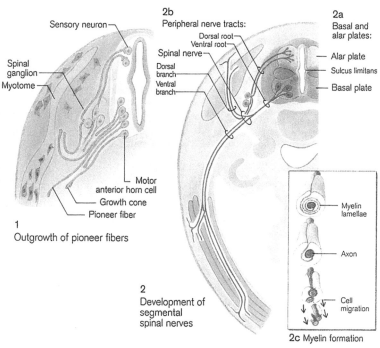

Sensory neuron
Spinal ganglion
Myotome
Motor anterior horn cell
Growth cone
Pioneer fiber

1
Outgrowth of pioneer fibers

2b
Peripheral nerve tracts:
Dorsal root
Ventral root
Spinal nerve
Dorsal branch
Ventral branch

2a
Basal and alar plates:
Alar plate
Sulcus limitans
Basal plate

Myelin lamellae
Axon
Cell migration

2c Myelin formation

2
Development of segmental spinal nerves

A. Spinal cord and spinal nerves

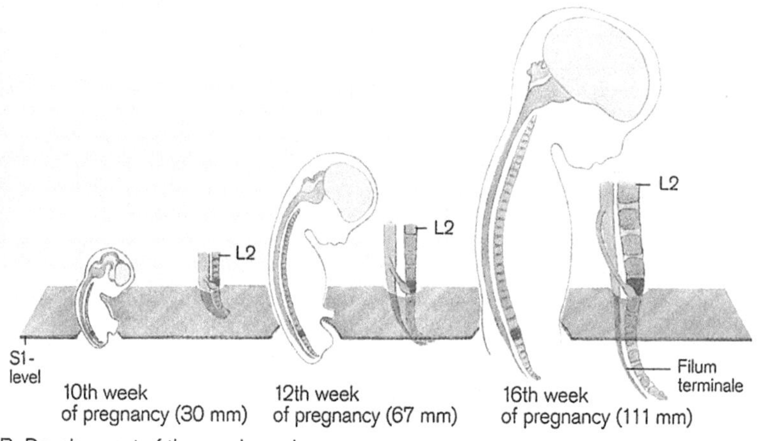


B. Development of the cauda equina

# 4.5 Dermatomes

## A. Spinal Nerves and Dermatomes

**1. Spinal nerves.** The reconstruction shows the course of the spinal nerves at stage 20. The spinal nerves extend perpendicularly from the spinal cord and do not yet show their (later obliquely) descending course. The thin dorsal rami branch off immediately behind the swelling of the spinal ganglion. The much thicker ventral rami maintain their segmental arrangement between the ribs, where they later form the intercostal nerves. Where no ribs are present, they form **nerve plexuses** and give rise to peripheral nerves that are not identical with the spinal nerves. In the cervical region, the *cervical* and *brachial plexuses* are formed and in the lumbar region, the *lumbar* and *sacral plexuses* are formed.

**2. Dermatomes.** The motor fibers of a spinal nerve innervate the musculature derived from a single somite; sensory fibers innervate the corresponding cutaneous region. The subcutaneous tissue that overlies the somites arises from the dermatomes (→ 3.22). The subcutaneous tissue of the ventral body wall and the limbs arises from the parietal mesoderm of the lateral plate, into which the myoblasts have migrated from the somites (→ 3.33). In extensions of the concept of the dermatome as part of the somite, the area of innervation of each pertinent spinal nerve is referred to as a **dermatome.** In the embryo dermatomes can be represented as horizontal stripes on the body surface

## B. Peripheral Nerves and Dermatomes

### 1. Segmental Arrangement of Spinal Nerves and Somites

The first motor axons that grow out from the neural tube innervate the muscle cells that arose from the corresponding myotome, forming the dorsal ramus of the spinal nerve. The axons that grow ventrally follow the myoblasts that migrated from the myotome into the ventral body wall and into the limb buds. In the periphery, the myoblasts from adjacent somites unite into individual muscle primordia that are innervated by axons from the segments of origin. Nerve fibers with muscle contacts become displaced together with the muscle, while new axons continue to extend into the periphery along the existing tracts. Thus the target area of the axons is apparently determined by the myoblasts arising from the same segment, but the path of axon growth is not. The axons orient themselves along the pathways of the pioneer fibers and at the same time seek the shortest route. In this way, nerve plexuses are formed.

### 2. Segments and Peripheral Nerves

The areas of innervation of peripheral nerves are not identical to the dermatomes.

**Roots of Spinal Nerve.** The spinal nerve is a mixed nerve consisting of a dorsal, sensory and a ventral, motor root.

**Dorsal Rami.** The dorsal back musculature, which is innervated by the dorsal branches of the spinal nerves, arises from the myotomes and retains its segmental arrangement.

**Ventral Rami and Plexus Formation.** The axons of the ventral branches form nerve plexuses that give rise to peripheral nerves. Each peripheral nerve contains contributions from different spinal nerves.

**Peripheral Nerves.** The peripheral nerves innervate muscles and cutaneous regions derived from more than one somitic segment.

**Dermatomes.** The regions innervated by the spinal nerves, which can be reconstructed by tracing back the nerve fibers, are referred to as dermatomes.

**Neuromeres and Motor Columns in the Spinal Cord.** In the somatomotor basal plate of the neural tube, the motor anterior horn cells form a segmental pattern of *neuromeres* that correspond to the somites. In the definitive spinal cord, the motor neurons assemble into nuclei of origin (*motor columns*), which represent definitive functional units (muscles and muscle groups).

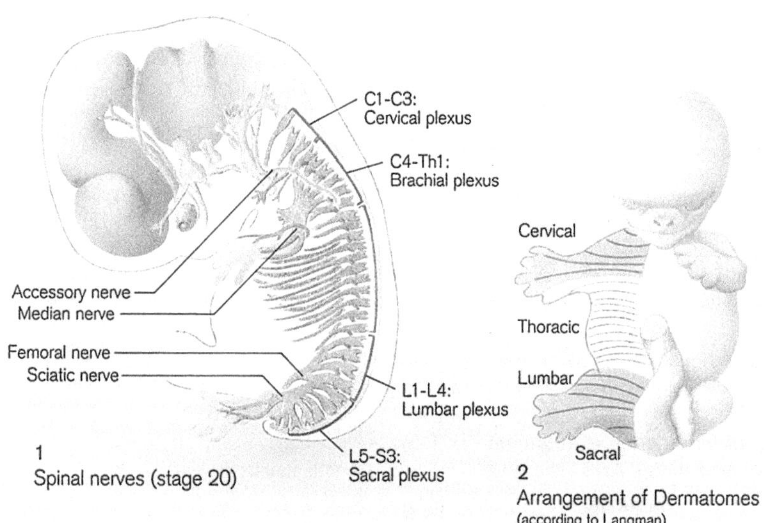


1
Spinal nerves (stage 20)

2
Arrangement of Dermatomes
(according to Langman)

A. Spinal nerves and dermatomes

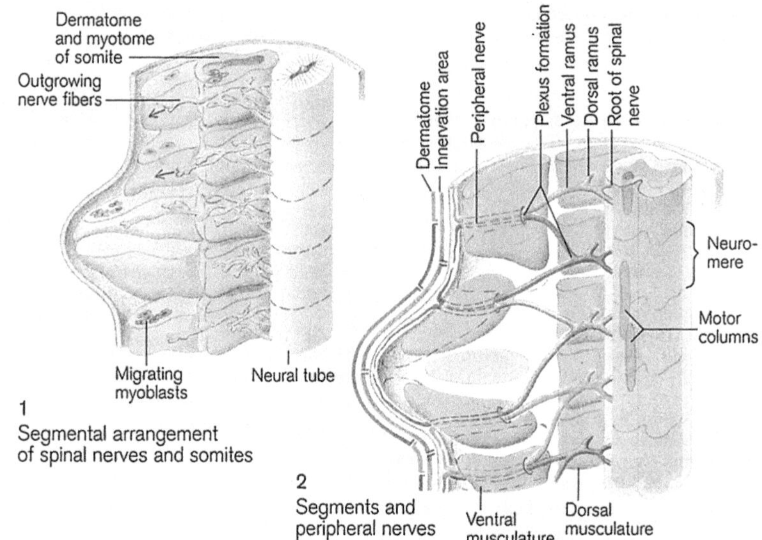


1
Segmental arrangement
of spinal nerves and somites

2
Segments and
peripheral nerves

B. Peripheral nerves and dermatomes

# 4.6 Autonomic Nervous System

## A. Segmental Development of the Autonomic Nervous System

### 1. Migration of Neural Crest Cells

The cells of the autonomic nervous system originate from the neural crest. They migrate ventrally between the somites and neural tube and form the primordia of the *spinal ganglia*. Some of the cells proceed further ventrally and form ganglia on both sides of the vertebrae (*sympathetic trunk*), as well as in the root of the mesentery (*preaortic ganglia*). Laterally, a stream of cells branches off for the adrenal medulla. The main migratory path leads further through the mesentery and up into the intestinal wall (*intramural ganglia*).

### 2. Differentiation of Autonomic Ganglia

**a Local Reflex Arcs.** The functional unit of the autonomic nervous system is localized in the periphery: In the wall of the intestinal tract, the neural crest cells form an autonomic, intramural nervous system consisting of ganglia (*submucous plexus* and *myenteric plexus*) and local reflex arcs that sustain the basic pattern of peristaltic movements.

**b Regional Control.** Regional autonomic ganglia arise along the migratory path of the neural crest cells. From these centers, nerve fibers travel to the heart, intestinal tract, or to the genital organs, as well as to the skin via the gray rami communicantes of the spinal nerves.

**c Central Control.** The central representation of the autonomic nervous system in the *lateral horn* of the spinal cord inhibits or stimulates the peripheral autonomic ganglia via efferent (*visceromotor*) nerve fibers. The fibers exit from the spinal cord with the motor root of the spinal nerve, leave the spinal nerve as myelinated white *rami communicantes*, and pass to the ganglia of the sympathetic trunk or to the *preaortic ganglia*. The *viscerosensory* fibers travel in the opposite direction to the viscerosensory centers in the ventral part of the alar plate. The corresponding sensory nerve cells lie in the spinal ganglia as pseudounipolar ganglion cells.

## B. Functional Organization

### 1. Sympathetic and Parasympathetic Nervous Systems in the Embryonic Period

Local environmental influences induce the neural crest cells in the intestinal wall to differentiate into muscarinic-cholinergic neurons, whereas the neural crest cells in the sclerotomic material at the dorsal body wall become adrenergic neurons. Thus the neurons become functionally arranged into cholinergic *parasympathetic ganglia*, associated with the intestinal tract, and into adrenergic *sympathetic ganglia* (sympathetic trunk), associated with the dorsal body wall and the large arteries.

The cholinergic neurons of the intestinal tract in the area innervated by the vagus arise from the neural crest of the rhombencephalon (→ 4.10). Correspondingly, the visceromotor column of the neural tube (A2c) and of the rhomboid fossa is functionally organized into a *sympathetic portion* (shown in pink) that extends from the first thoracic to the third lumbar segment and into a *parasympathetic portion* (shown in green) that is localized in the lateral horn of the rhomboid fossa and in the second to fourth sacral segment of the spinal cord. All target organs are innervated by both systems.

**a Linkage of Autonomic Ganglia in the Head.** The parasympathetic fibers for the lacrimal and salivary glands exit from the rhombencephalon with the glossopharyngeal or facial nerve. They reach the lacrimal gland and the nasal mucosa (associated with the maxillary nerve) via the *greater petrosal nerve* and the *pterygopalatine ganglion*, the parotid gland via the *lesser petrosal nerve* and the *otic ganglion* (associated with the mandibular nerve), and the submandibular gland via the *chorda tympani* and the *submandibular ganglion* (associated with the lingual nerve) (→ 4.12).

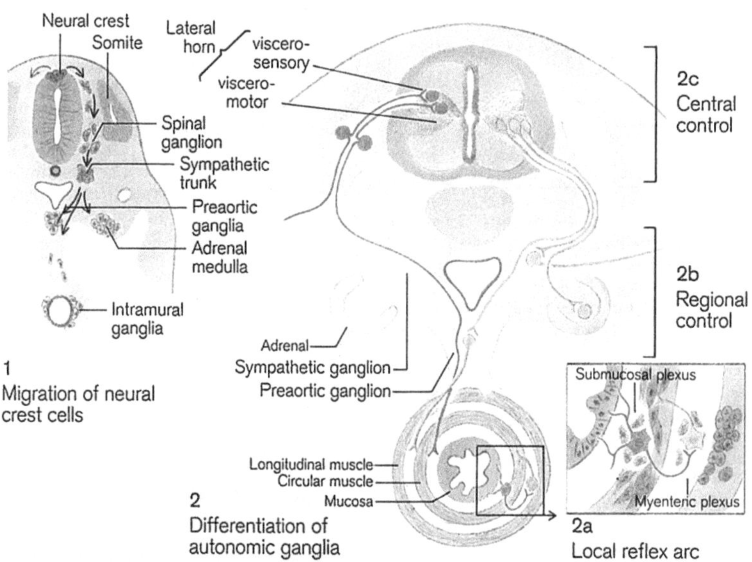


1
Migration of neural crest cells

2
Differentiation of autonomic ganglia

2a
Local reflex arc

A. Segmental development of autonomic nervous system

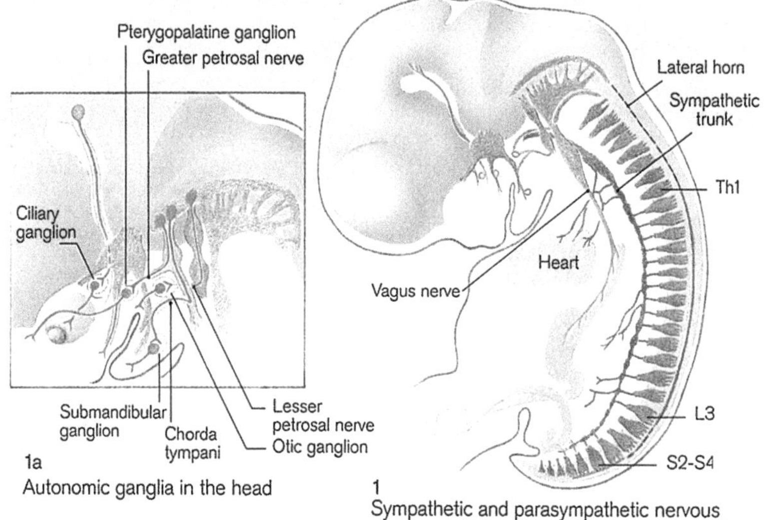


1a
Autonomic ganglia in the head

1
Sympathetic and parasympathetic nervous systems in the embryonic period (stage 17)

B. Functional organization

# Brain Vesicles

# 4.7 Neuromeres and Placodes

*Background*

Before the cerebral vesicles develop, the neural tube of the head has a metameric organization corresponding to the organization of the trunk into somitic segments. These segments in the neural tube are known as **neuromeres.** They reflect the primary segmentation of the head, while the development of the cerebral vesicles is already related to the functional morphogenesis.

The first head mesoderm arises from the prechordal plate (→ 3.8). It is supplemented by mesenchyme from the **neural crest**, which forms the mesodermal component of the pharyngeal arches (→ 5.2), including the pharyngeal arch cartilages.

Additional mesenchyme arises from the **placodes**, thickenings in the ectoderm that are located lateral to the neural tube. In their developmental potential, the placodes correspond to the neuroepithelium of the neural crest (→ 5.2). The placodes are associated with the pharyngeal arches. A *dorsolateral series of placodes* lies above the sensory ganglia of the pharyngeal arch nerves and contributes cell material to the ganglia. An *epipharyngeal series* lies in the ectoderm of the pharyngeal arches themselves. In contrast to the sensory placodes, the pharyngeal arch placodes disappear as the cells emigrate.

## A. Neuromeres and Placodes in Stage 11

**1. Head with Placodes.** In stage 11, closure of the neural tube has reached the region of the mesencephalon. In the reconstruction of the head folds of the "Blechschmidt embryo" 3.1 mm (**A1**, → 2.20), the surface ectoderm is removed, exposing the *dorsolateral* and *epipharyngeal placodes*, as well as the thickened *neural crest material* for the maxillary process and the first and second pharyngeal arches. The **section** passes dorsally through the *mesencephalon* and ventrally through the prosencephalon with the *optic sulci.* It illustrates the migration of cells from the *neural crest* and the *dorsolateral placodes.*

**2. Neuromeres.** The boundaries of the *neuromeres* can be recognized as notches in the lumen of the neural tube. Two neuromeres (*D1* and *D2*) lie in the region of the future diencephalon. Neuromeres *M1* and *M2* lie in the region of the mesencephalon and neuromeres *Rh1* to *Rh7* reside in the future rhombencephalon. Aggregations of *neural crest cells* that have already emigrated are indicated above the neuromeres.

The *olfactory placode* lies in the ectoderm above the future telencephalon. In the midline, the interface between surface ectoderm and neural ectoderm grows upward as the *lamina terminalis*, contributing to the closure of the *anterior neuropore*.

## B. Segmental Organization of the Pharyngeal Arch Nerves

**1. Neuromeres and Head Ganglia in Humans.** At stage 12, the nerves of the pharyngeal arches grow out. The projection onto the neuromeres shows that a pharyngeal arch nerve originates from every second neuromere: from Rh2, the trigeminal (**V**), from Rh4 the facial (**VII**), and from Rh6 the glossopharyngeal (**IX**). The root of the vagus (**X**) arises in the region of the occipital somites and extends past Rh7.

**2. Outgrowth of Motor Neurons in the Rhombencephalon of the Chick Embryo.** By selective staining of the motor nerve cells and their growing axons with a monoclonal antibody (represented in yellow), the relationship to the neuromeres can be recognized. The motor nerve fibers of pharyngeal arch nerves V, VII, IX, and X heed the segmental boundaries of the rhombencephalic neuromeres. Each motor nerve emerges from the cranial neuromere associated with the respective pharyngeal arch (Lumsden and Keynes 1989). The outgrowth of the nerve fibers is regulated by local factors inherent to the neuromeres. This is reminiscent of the expression of the pair rule genes in the segmentation of Drosophila (→ 3.17), as well as of the outgrowth of spinal nerves (→ 3.22).

Optic sulcus
Mesencephalon
Neural crest material
Dorsolateral placode
Epipharyngeal placode
Lamina terminalis
Maxillary process

Neural crest
Mesenchyme
Dorsolateral placode
Optic sulcus

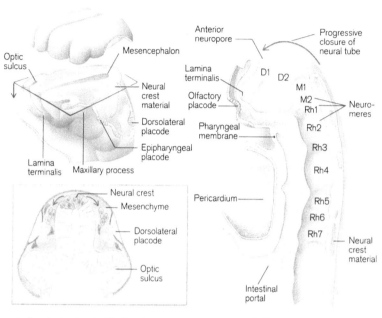

1 Developing head with placodes

Anterior neuropore
Progressive closure of neural tube
Lamina terminalis
Olfactory placode
Pharyngeal membrane
D1
D2
M1
M2
Rh1
Neuro-meres
Rh2
Rh3
Rh4
Pericardium
Rh5
Rh6
Rh7
Neural crest material
Intestinal portal

2 Neuromeres

A. Neuromeres and placodes at stage 11

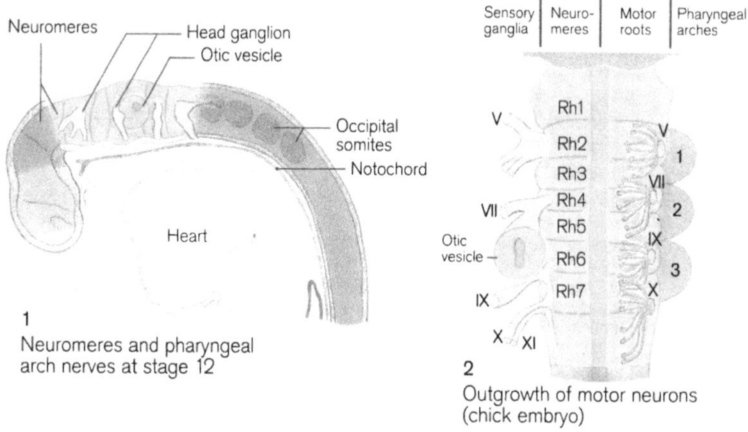


1
Neuromeres and pharyngeal arch nerves at stage 12

2
Outgrowth of motor neurons (chick embryo)

B. Segmental organization of pharyngeal arch nerves

## 4.8 Brain Vesicles

*Background*

The development of the brain vesicles is superimposed on the organization of the neural tube into neuromeres. Initially, three **primary brain vesicles** are formed (**A1**). With the outgrowth of the telencephalic vesicles from the prosencephalon, the brain obtains its definitive organization. The **ventricular system** (**A3**) arises from the brain vesicles.

### A. Brain Vesicles

**1. The Three Primary Brain Vesicles**

They are the centers for the central sense organs: olfaction (smell), vision (sight), and audition (hearing). From the first vesicle, the *prosencephalon* (forebrain), the optic vesicles evaginate laterally and induce the lens placodes in the surface ectoderm. In the ectoderm of the frontal process (→9.1), the prosencephalon induces the olfactory placodes. The second vesicle corresponds to the future *mesencephalon* (midbrain). The third primary brain vesicle is the *rhombencephalon* (hindbrain). The otic vesicles are associated with the rhombencephalon and develop from the ectoderm by invaginations of the otic placodes.

**2. Cephalic and Cervical Flexures**

At stage 12 (**A2a**), the *cephalic flexure* forms above the midbrain; it represents the highest point in the measurement of the greatest length. Only in stages 14 and 15 (**A2b**), the *cervical flexure* lies higher than the cephalic flexure (→ 2.4).

**3. Definitive Parts of the Brainstem**

**Subdivision of the Prosencephalon.** The anterior part of the prosencephalon is the rhinencephalon, which gives rise to the *olfactory bulb* and the *telencephalon*. Through the growth of the telencephalic vesicles, the primordial prosencephalon (as the diencephalon) is enclosed between the telencephalic vesicles. The telencephalic vesicles form the lateral ventricles, while the unpaired forebrain vesicle becomes the III. ventricle in the diencephalon. The *lamina terminalis*, which is the anterior boundary of the prosencephalon, is included with the telencephalon.

**Telencephalon.** The telencephalic hemispheres leave the diencephalon at the *interventricular foramen* and ultimately grow over the entire brainstem.

**Diencephalon.** The diencephalon is primarily a visual brain, from which the optic vesicles evaginate. The *thalamus* in the wall of the diencephalon serves in the processing of visual information.

**Mesencephalon.** The *quadrigeminal plate* (corpora quadrigemina) forms in the mesencephalon. It is functionally divided into the superior colliculi, which process visual information, and the inferior colliculi, which process auditory and vestibular information into postural and visual movements. The mesencephalic vesicle becomes constricted to form the *cerebral aqueduct*.

**Subdivision of the Rhombencephalon.** The posterior portion of the rhombencephalon can be perceived as an elongated spinal cord that gives rise to the pharyngeal arch nerves. It is called the *myelencephalon*. The last segment of the true brain is the *metencephalon*, the anterior part of the rhombencephalon.

**Metencephalon.** The metencephalon contains the central representation of the auditory and vestibular organs. The cerebellar swelling arises in the superior lips of the rhomboid fossa. Functions of the cerebellum include fine-tuning of posture in collaboration with the vestibular organ and coordination of skilled movements.

**Myelencephalon.** The myelencephalon (as the brain of the pharynx) contains the nuclei for the nerves of the pharyngeal arches 1–5.

**4. Development of the Pontine Flexure**

The neural tube bends in the ventral direction, giving rise to the pontine flexure and the rhomboid structure, with its laterally protruding corners. During this process, the roof of the fourth ventricle becomes stretched into a thin lamina.

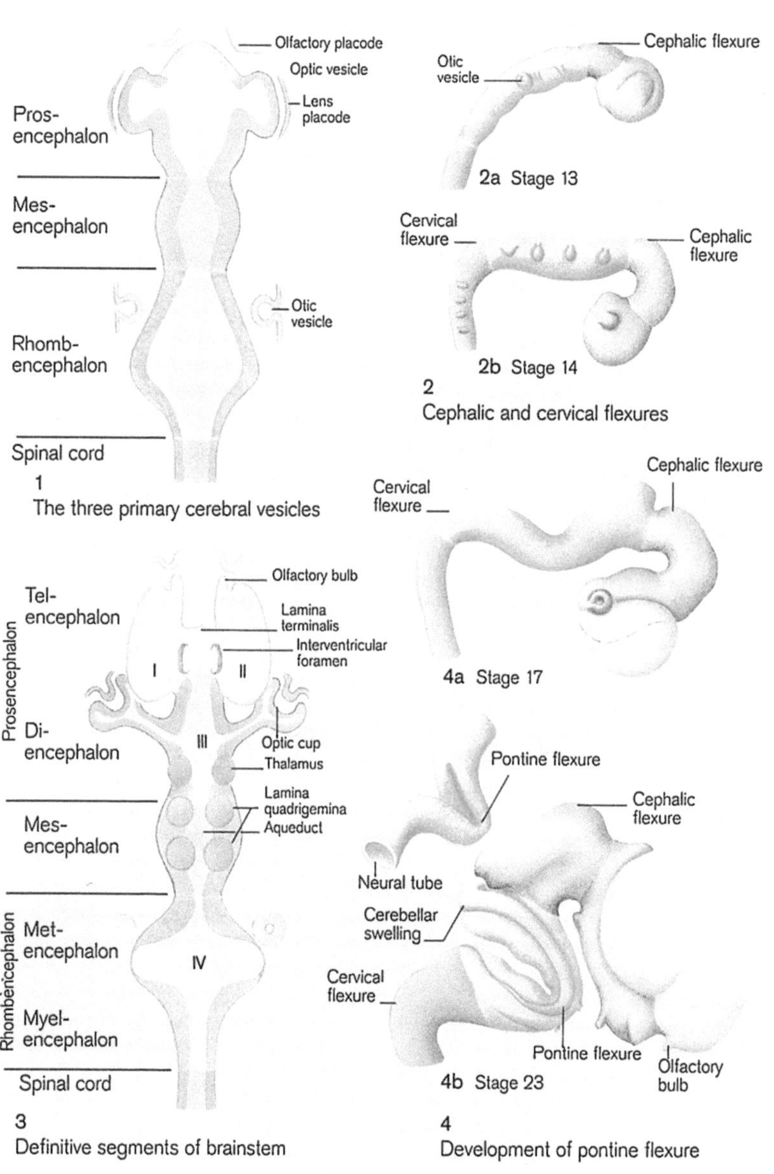


1
The three primary cerebral vesicles

2
Cephalic and cervical flexures

3
Definitive segments of brainstem

4
Development of pontine flexure

A. Cerebral vesicles

# 4.9 Central Sensory Pathways

## A. Course of the Central Sensory Pathways in the Brainstem

**1. Olfactory Tract.** The epithelial cells of the *olfactory placode* differentiate into sensory cells and supporting cells (→ 5.5). The *sensory cells* send a nerve process centrally and synapse with neurons in the *olfactory bulb*. The olfactory placode is shifted deep into the primary choana and finally comes to lie on and above the uppermost nasal concha. The olfactory bulb is the first central representation of the olfactory tract. From there, one crus of the olfactory tract passes to the medial, another crus to the lateral olfactory center in the wall of the telencephalic vesicle.

**2. Visual Pathway.** The optic vesicles grow out from the forebrain and induce the ectoderm to form the *lens placode*, which develops into the ocular lens (→ 5.6). The optic vesicle invaginates to form the optic cup. The neuroepithelium of the inner layer of the optic cup gives rise to the *sensory cells* of the retina (rods and cones), as well as to the *bipolar neurons* that link them to the *ganglion cells* of the retina. The axons of the ganglion cells converge in the stalk of the optic cup as the *optic nerve*. The nerve fibers from the nasal half of the optic cup cross over the midline in the *optic chiasma*, whereas the fibers from the temporal half do not decussate; thus the right visual field is projected to the left half of the brain and the left to the right half of the brain. Most of the fibers end in the *thalamus* (within the wall of the diencephalon), which is primarily a visual center. Some of the visual fibers extend to the *superior colliculus* in the roof of the mesencephalon. Processing of visual information in the superior colliculus serves to coordinate eye movements. Nerves innervating the ocular muscles therefore arise from the motor basal plate of the mesencephalon (→ 4.11).

**3. Auditory Pathway.** The sensory cells of the auditory and vestibular organs develop in the epithelium of the *otic vesicle*, which is formed by the invagination of the ectodermal otic placode lateral to the rhombencephalon (→ 5.9). The *sensory cells* in the inner ear possess cilia that can register movements of the endolymph. The information is conducted centrally via bipolar ganglion cells of the *spiral ganglion* (CN VIII). The first central representation of the auditory and vestibular pathway is the *vestibulocochlear nucleus* in the alar plate of the rhombencephalon. From there, auditory fibers pass to the inferior colliculus, where the auditory and vestibular information is processed for the regulation of movement. Some of the fibers extend into the thalamus.

## B. Projection into the Cerebral Cortex

The cerebral hemispheres overgrow the brainstem. The central sensory tracts extend as *optic* and *auditory* radiation from the thalamus into the corresponding projection fields of the cerebral cortex. The nerve fibers take the shortest route and thus cross the border between the diencephalon and telencephalon. The thalamus becomes the relay station of the cerebral cortex where all afferent tracts except the olfactory tract are synapsed. Since the telencephalon arises from the rhinencephalon, the olfactory pathway is already primarily represented in the telencephalon.

**1. Olfactory Tract.** The olfactory tract ends with a medial and lateral crus in the phylogenetically oldest parts of the telencephalon (paleocortex). The olfactory tract proceeds uncrossed.

**2. Visual Pathway.** The nerve fibers for conscious visual perception synapse in the *lateral geniculate body*, a nucleus of the thalamus. From the lateral geniculate body, the fibers of the *visual pathway* pass over the medullary layer of the occipital lobe and terminate in the *visual cortex*.

**3, Auditory Pathway.** Like the fibers of the visual pathway, the auditory and vestibular fibers for conscious perception pass to the thalamus and after synapsing in the *medial geniculate body*, continue on to the auditory area in the temporal lobe. In the visual pathway the mesencephalic projection (superior colliculus) is a parallel fiber tract; in the auditory pathway it serves as relay station (inferior colliculus).

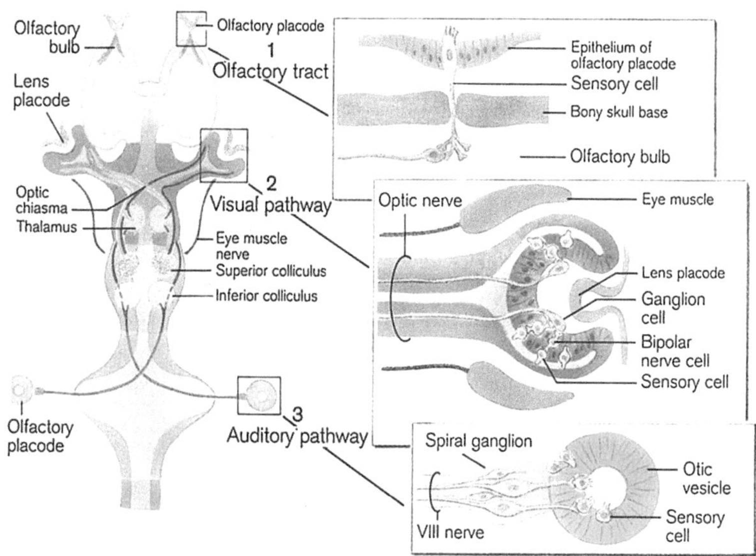


A. Course and circuitry of the central sensory pathways in the brainstem

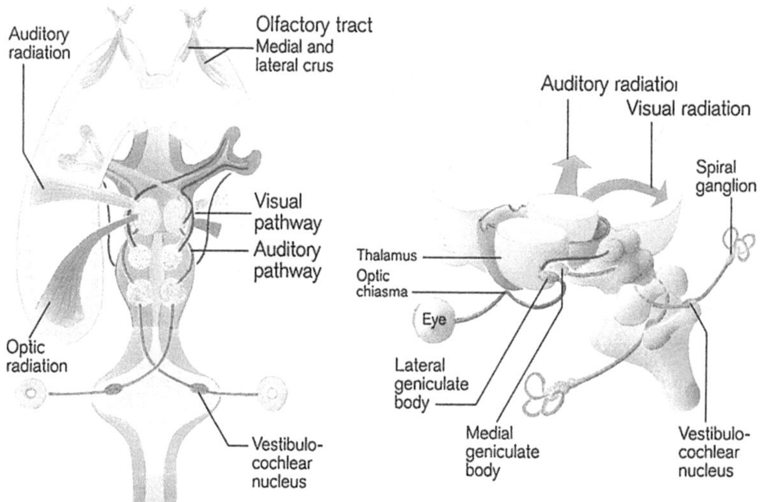


B. Projection of central sensory pathways into the cerebral cortex

# Brainstem

# 4.10 Basal and Alar Plates

## A. Basal and Alar Plates in the Brainstem

### 1. Organization of Basal and Alar Plates in the Spinal Cord and Rhombencephalon

The neural tube has the same fundamental organization in the spinal cord and in the brainstem. Motor centers lie in the basal plate, sensory centers in the alar plate.

**a Spinal Cord.** The **basal plate** of the spinal cord contains two types of motor nuclei (→ 4.4A and 4.6A). The nuclei for the somatic musculature lie in the motor anterior horn (*somatomotor column*) and those for autonomic functions reside in the lateral horn (*visceromotor column*) (**A1**). The **alar plate** contains the *somatosensory* and *viscerosensory* nuclei of the spinal nerves. The visceromotor and viscerosensory columns in the lateral horn, which are located on both sides of the *sulcus limitans* (→ 4.6), form a functional unit in the central representation of the autonomic nervous system.

**b Rhombencephalon.** The functional organization into a basal motor plate and a sensory alar plate continues in the brainstem. In the rhomboid fossa, the neural tube is opened like a book so that the basal and alar plates (separated by the *sulcus limitans)* appear as flat, longitudinal bulges at the floor of the **fourth ventricle**. The basal plate contains the motor nuclei and the alar plate contains the sensory nuclei of the pharyngeal nerves. As in the spinal cord, the autonomic nuclei are located at the sulcus limitans.

Neuroblasts from the matrix zone at the edge of the alar plate (**rhomboic lips**) migrate ventrally and form the *basal nuclei* of the brainstem. The basal nuclei of the brainstem include the *reticular formation* (containing centers for respiration and deglutition), nuclei associated with the extrapyramidal system (*red nucleus* and *substantia nigra*), and nuclei associated with the cerebellum (nucleus olivarius, pontine nuclei). The *vestibulocochlear nerve* arises at the lateral corner of the rhomboic fossa. The cerebellum emerges from the upper rhombic lips (→ 4.13). The roof plate of the neural tube is stretched to become the thin roof of the IV. ventricle.

### 2. General and Special Centers of Pharyngeal Nerves in the Brainstem

The basal and alar plates of the rhomboid fossa, like the spinal cord, contain somatic and visceral columns. Additional columns, specific to the pharyngeal nerves, are inserted between somatic and visceral columns. These additional *branchiomotor* and *branchiosensory* columns, which are only present in the rhombencephalon, are referred to as *special visceral efferent* and *special visceral afferent*. This contrasts them from the *somatomotor* and *somatosensory* columns that are also present in the spinal cord and are therefore referred to as *general somatic efferent* and *general somatic afferent*.

**Basal Plate.** In the inferomedial region of the basal plate, is a nuclear region that represents a continuation of the somatomotor column of the spinal cord and which innervates muscles derived from the occipital somites (tongue musculature, hypoglossal nerve XII). Laterally above this column, lies a motor column innervating the (branchial) musculature derived from the pharyngeal arches. It is designated the special branchiomotor column and occurs only in the brainstem. It contains motor nuclei for the skeletal pharyngeal musculature (IX), facial musculature (VII), and masticatory musculature (V3). Attached to the branchiomotor column at the sulcus limitans is the general visceromotor column, which is also present in the spinal cord. It contains the visceral efferent nuclei of the vagus (X) and the nuclei for the parasympathetic cranial ganglia (VII, IX).

**Alar Plate**. In the alar plate, the special branchiosensory nuclei involved in the perception of taste (e.g., chorda tympani from VII), are present only in the brainstem, and are situated between the general visceral afferent area of the parasympathetic nervous system and the general somatic afferent nuclear region of the trigeminal nerve (V).

Rhomb-
encephalon
Trigeminal nerve
Somato-
sensory
column
Hypoglossal nerve
see
1b
Somato-
motor
column
Spinal cord
see
1a

1b
Rhombencephalon

1a
Spinal cord

Rhombic lip
Alar plate
Viscerosensory
Visceromotor
Basal plate
Sulcus limitans
Basal
nuclear region
Central canal
Migration of cells
from the rhombic lip

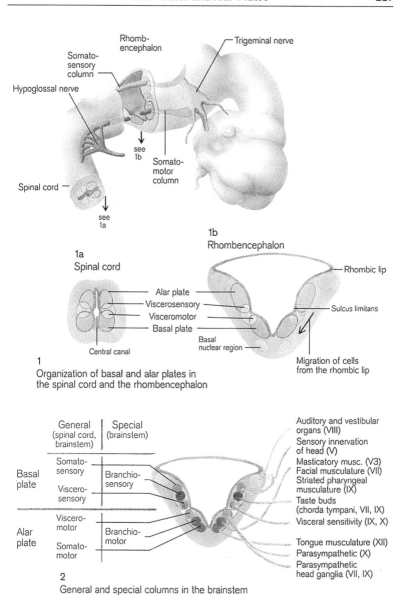

1
Organization of basal and alar plates in the spinal cord and the rhombencephalon

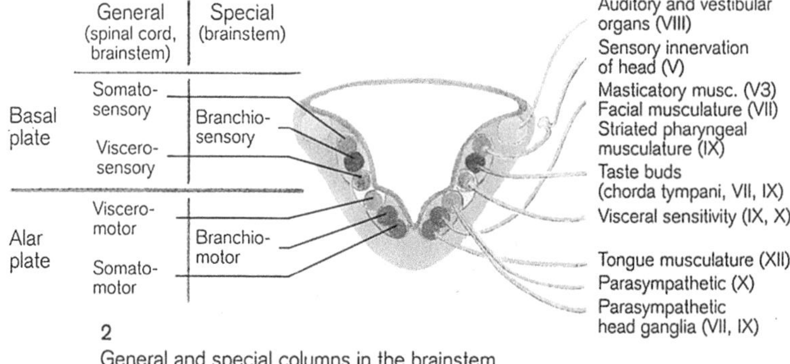


2
General and special columns in the brainstem

A. Basal and alar plates in the brainstem

# 4.11 Brain Stem

## A. Modifications of Basal and Alar Plates in the Brainstem

The illustration emphasizes the organization of the basal and alar plates into somatic, branchial, and visceral columns. For comparison, sections of the major subdivisions of the brain at 14 weeks of pregnancy (**A1**) are aligned along a straight axis.

**a Myelencephalon.** The myelencephalon (medulla oblongata = extended spinal cord) contains the nuclei of origin of the pharyngeal arch nerves and includes the posterior part of the rhomboid fossa. During the early development of the hind brain, however, the nuclei of the pharyngeal nerves are shifted far into the metencephalon. In the motor basal plate, the nucleus of the *hypoglossal nerve* lies in the somatomotor column and the nucleus of the *accessory nerve* resides in the branchiomotor column, ascending from C1-C4. The visceromotor column at the sulcus limitans is formed by the visceromotor nuclei of the *vagus nerve* and *glossopharyngeal nerve*. Both cranial nerves contain in addition branchiomotor and branchiosensory portions. The descending nucleus of the *trigeminal nerve* lies in the somatosensory column of the alar plate. It extends beyond the metencephalon into the mesencephalon.

**b Metencephalon.** The metencephalon is the cranial part of the rhombencephalon. It primarily contains the central representation of the auditory and vestibular organs (*vestibulocochlear nucleus*). The cerebellum develops in the spatial and functional vicinity of the latter, in the upper rhomboic lips. Its original function is the processing of information from the vestibular organ for postural correction.

The branchiomotor column contains the nucleus of the *facial nerve* and the motor root of the *trigeminal nerve*, which supplies the masticatory muscles. The *chorda tympani* contains parasympathetic visceroefferent fibers and branchiosensory taste fibers. The somatomotor column gives origin to the *abducens nerve*, which innervates an ocular muscle and therefore belongs functionally to the mesencephalon.

**c Mesencephalon.** The midbrain serves in the control of eye movements and of visual movements involving the head and body. The nuclei for *ocular muscle nerves* (III and IV) reside in the somatomotor column. The *Edinger-Westphal nucleus*, from which pupillary reaction and accommodation are regulated, lies in the visceromotor column.

The *lamina quadrigemina* arises in the alar plate. The upper laminated nuclear region of the superior colliculus contains a topical representation of the field of vision. In the inferior colliculus, impulses from the auditory and vestibular organs are processed in a similar manner. At the base of the cerebral crus, the *red nucleus* and the *substantia nigra*—parts of the extrapyramidal system—arise from neuroblasts that migrate downward from the matrix zone of the alar plate (– 4.10).

**d Diencephalon and Telencephalon.** In the diencephalon, the primitive organization into basal and alar plates is modified. The *hypothalamic nuclei*, which control endocrine functions via the hypophysis, arise in the basal plate. The *thalamus* arises in the alar plate. The *basal ganglia* arise at the floor of the telencephalon. Functionally, the thalamus can be perceived as a higher sensory center and the basal ganglia as a higher motor center; thus these structures correspond to the basal and alar plates of the neural tube in the prosencephalon of a primitive vertebrate that does not have higher order cortical centers.

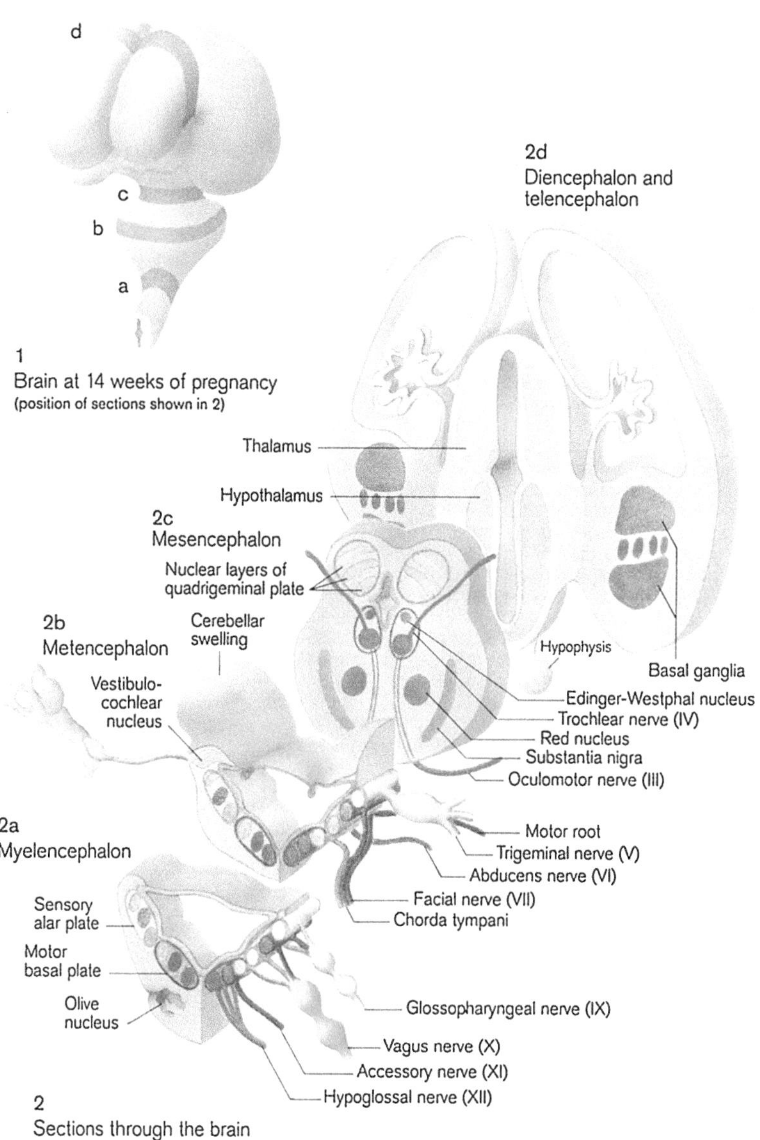
d
c
b
a
1
Brain at 14 weeks of pregnancy
(position of sections shown in 2)
2d
Diencephalon and telencephalon
Thalamus
Hypothalamus
2c
Mesencephalon
Nuclear layers of quadrigeminal plate
2b
Metencephalon
Cerebellar swelling
Vestibulo-cochlear nucleus
Hypophysis
Basal ganglia
Edinger-Westphal nucleus
Trochlear nerve (IV)
Red nucleus
Substantia nigra
Oculomotor nerve (III)
2a
Myelencephalon
Motor root
Trigeminal nerve (V)
Abducens nerve (VI)
Facial nerve (VII)
Chorda tympani
Sensory alar plate
Motor basal plate
Olive nucleus
Glossopharyngeal nerve (IX)
Vagus nerve (X)
Accessory nerve (XI)
Hypoglossal nerve (XII)
2
Sections through the brain

A. Modifications of basal and alar plates in the brainstem

# 4.12 Cranial Nerves

## A. Cranial Nerves and Pharyngeal Arches

The twelve cranial nerves are designated with roman numerals in the order in which they arise from the base of the brain. At the primary brain vesicle stage **in the 5th week** (**A1**), the association of the cranial nerves with the central sense organs, with the midbrain, and with the pharyngeal arches is clearly visible. **At the end of the embryonic period** (A2), the nerves have reached their definitive locations. The cranial nerves are organized functionally into three groups:

(1) Nerves for the **central sense organs**: smell, (I) *olfactory bulb*; vision, (II) *optic nerve*; hearing, (VIII) *vestibulocochlear nerve*.

(2) **Nerves for the Ocular Muscles:** (III) *oculomotor nerve*; (IV) *trochlear nerve*; (VI) *abducens nerve*, and

(3) **Pharyngeal Arch Nerves:** The *trigeminal nerve* (V) is the nerve of the first pharyngeal arch, from which the maxillary process and the mandible emerge (**A1**). The third branch of the trigeminal nerve contains motor fibers for the muscles of mastication. The *facial nerve (VII)* is the nerve of the second pharyngeal arch and innervates the muscles of facial expression. The *chorda tympani* conducts parasympathetic fibers to the *submandibular ganglion* and *taste fibers* from the anterior two-thirds of the tongue.

The *glossopharyngeal nerve (IX)* is the nerve of the third pharyngeal arch and contains taste fibers, as well as sensory and motor fibers for the pharynx and the root of the tongue.

The *vagus nerve (X)* is the nerve of the fourth pharyngeal arch and conducts parasympathetic fibers to the gastrointestinal tract (viscera). Its companion, the *accessory nerve (XI)*, innervates the sternocleidomastoid and trapezius muscles, which move the head (e.g., toward food). The *XII cranial nerve (hypoglossal nerve)* arises from the fusion of occipital spinal nerves and provides motor innervation to the tongue.

## B. Nuclei of Origin in the Brainstem

### 1. Motor Nuclei

**Ocular Muscle Nerves.** The nuclei of the nerves supplying the ocular muscles emerge from the **somatomotor column** of the mesencephalon. Parasympathetic fibers for the pupillary reaction pass with the oculomotor nerve to the *ciliary ganglion*. They originate in the **visceromotor column** in the *Edinger-Westphal nucleus*. Due to the growth of neighboring fiber bundles, the origin of the *trochlear nerve* is shifted to the dorsal side of the brainstem. The nucleus of the *abducens nerve* is displaced caudally into the metencephalon so that its exit comes to lie below the pons (hence the long course of the abducens nerve in the base of the brain).

**Pharyngeal Arch Nerves.** The branchiomotor column for the musculature of the pharyngeal arches is composed of the motor nucleus of the *mandibular nerve* (V3, masticatory muscles) and the nucleus of the *facial nerve* (facial musculature). The *facial nerve* passes around the nucleus of the *abducens nerve* and thereby forms its inner genu. The branchiomotor nuclei of the *glossopharyngeal, vagus,* and *accessory* nerves (supplying the skeletal pharyngeal musculature) are united with the **visceromotor nuclear regions** of these nerves (supplying the smooth pharyngeal musculature) to form the **nucleus ambiguus**, in front of which lie the visceromotor nuclei of the *facial nerve* and the *glossopharyngeal nerve* (**salivatory nucleus**). The fibers for the *hypoglossal nerve* originate in the lower **somatomotor column.**

### 2. Sensory Nuclei

The long **sensory nucleus of the trigeminal nerve**, which extends from the mesencephalon to the myelencephalon, lies in the **somatosensory column** of the alar plate (→ 4.10 A1). The nuclei of the **branchiosensory column** (taste fibers) for the chorda tympani—the pseudounipolar ganglion cells lie in the *geniculate ganglion of the facial nerve*—, for the *glossopharyngeal nerve*, and for the *vagus nerve* are united with the parasympathetic, viscerosensory nuclei of the *glossopharyngeal nerve* and *vagus nerve* to form the **nucleus solitarius**.

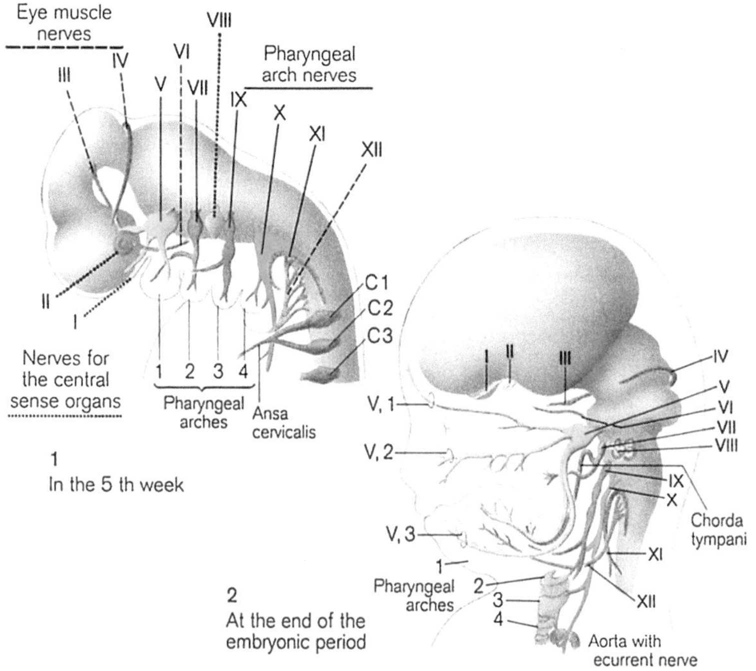

Eye muscle nerves
III
IV
V
VI
VII
VIII
IX
X
XI
XII
Pharyngeal arch nerves
II
I
Nerves for the central sense organs
1 2 3 4
Pharyngeal arches
Ansa cervicalis
C1
C2
C3

1
In the 5 th week

I II III
IV
V, 1
V, 2
V, 3
V
VI
VII
VIII
IX
X
Chorda tympani
XI
XII
1
2
3
4
Pharyngeal arches
Aorta with ecurrent nerve

2
At the end of the embryonic period

A. Cranial nerves and pharyngeal arches

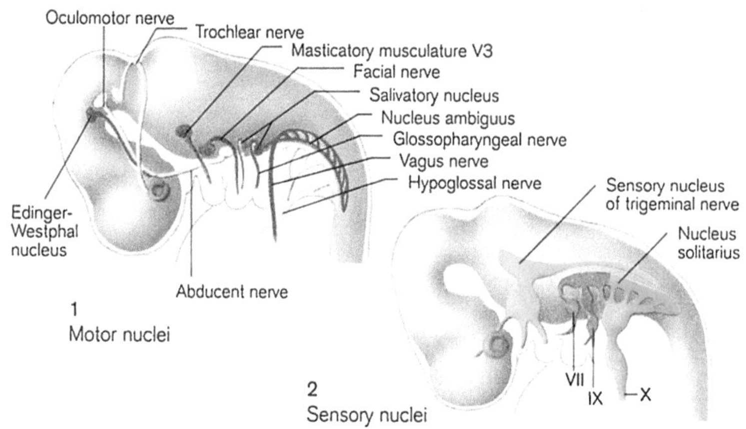


1
Motor nuclei

2
Sensory nuclei

B. Nuclei of origin in the brainstem

## Cerebellum

## 4.13 Gross Development

### A. Development and Functional Organization of the Cerebellum

**1. Anlage of Cerebellum in Stage 23**

The cerebellum arises at the end of the embryonic period from the upper *rhombic lips*. As the rhombencephalon bends to form the pontine flexure (**1a**), the lips become oriented transversely and form a swelling that projects into the ventricle and extends across the roof of the rhomboid fossa (**1b**). The border between the extraventricular and intraventricular parts is formed by the edge of the thinly stretched roof of the fourth ventricle. The basal and alar plates of the myelencephalon can be recognized at the floor of the fourth ventricle (**1b**).

**2. Anlage of Cerebellum at 16 Weeks of Pregnancy**

In the fetal period, the cerebellar swelling bulges outward. The hemispheres of the *neocerebellum* protrude on both sides, while the central segment lags behind in growth and forms a wormlike structure (*vermis*) in the longitudinal axis. Transverse grooves in the cerebellum separate the phylogenetically old parts (*nodulus* and *flocculus*) from the younger cerebellar hemispheres.

In frontal section (**2a**), the *fourth ventricle* and the *olive* can be seen below the anlage of the cerebellum. The cerebellar cortex develops at the surface of the cerebellar hemispheres. The *dentate nucleus* originates in the center of the hemispheres on both sides.

The *choroid plexus* of the fourth ventricle arises from a transverse invagination in the roof of the rhomboid fossa. At the lateral corners of the fourth ventricle the plexus bulges externally (**2a**). Villi of the plexus extend cranially and caudally from the choroid fissure, parallel to the longitudinal axis of the rhomboid fossa (without separate invagination). The *median* and *lateral apertures* arise toward the end of the fetal period by local dissolution of the ventricular roof (**2b**). In the lateral aperture, the roof of the ventricle disintegrates below the bulge of the plexus (**2a**) so that the villi of the plexus protrude from the opening into the subarachnoid space.

**3. Functional organization**

**Paleocerebellum.** The cerebellum is a motor center that automatically adjusts the position of the body in response to impulses from the vestibular organ ( *vestibulocerebellum*). In addition to afferents from the vestibular organ, it receives afferents from muscle and tendon spindles (*spinocerebellum*). These phylogenetically old segments lie at the lower (nodulus and flocculus) and upper root of the cerebellar swelling and are called the *paleocerebellum*. Failure of this region leads to ataxia.

**Neocerebellum.** Parallel to the development of the cerebrum, the cerebellum enlarges by extroversion and widening of the cerebellar swelling and forms the *neocerebellum*. The neocerebellum receives a parallel input of motor impulses from the cerebral cortex and the extrapyramidal system and preferentially regulates the fine motor movements of the hands and fingers. Failure of this region leads to intention tremor and rigidity.

**Classification according to Afferents.** The afferents from the vestibular organ arrive at the *vestibulocerebellum* via the *inferior cerebellar peduncle*. The afferents from the spinal cord and the olive enter through the *superior and inferior cerebellar peduncle* and end in the *spinocerebellum*. The vestibulo- and spinocerebellum together correspond to the *paleocerebellum*. The afferents from the cerebral cortex and the extrapyramidal system synapse in the pontine nuclei, enter through the *middle cerebellar peduncle*, and terminate in the *pontocerebellum*, which corresponds to the *neocerebellum*. The **efferents** of the neocerebellum originate from the *dentate nucleus* and leave the cerebellum via the superior and inferior cerebellar peduncles.

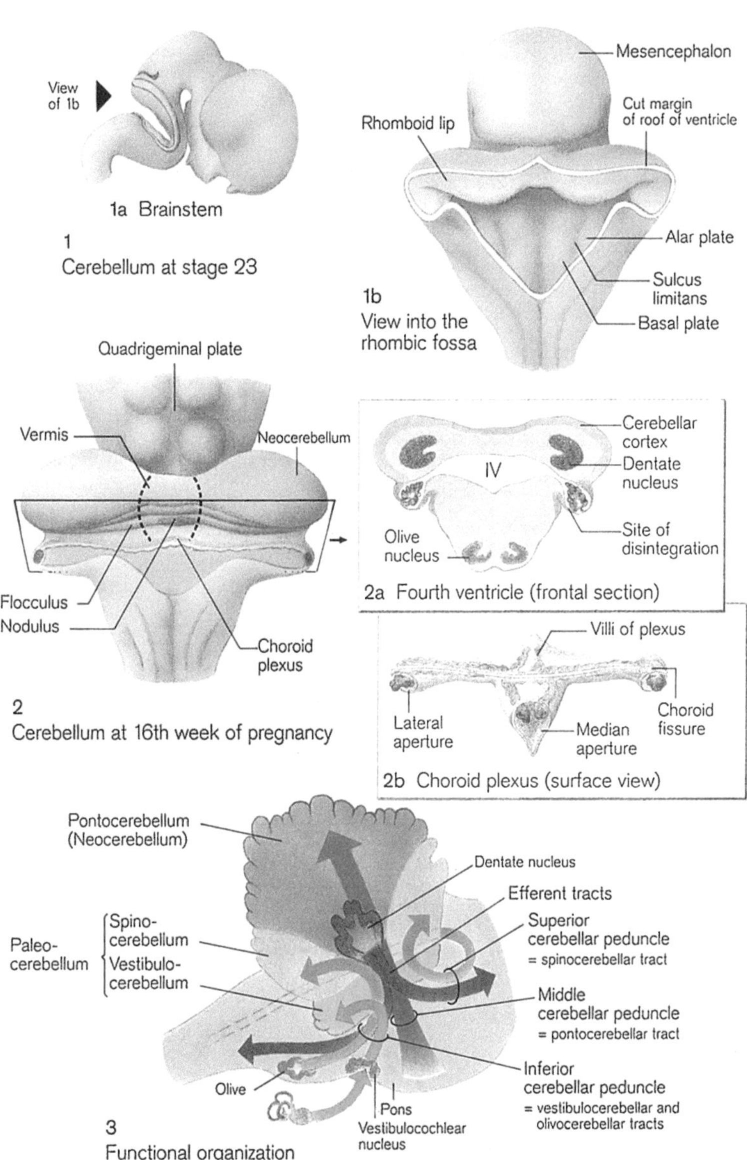
View of 1b
1a Brainstem
1
Cerebellum at stage 23
Mesencephalon
Rhomboid lip
Cut margin of roof of ventricle
Alar plate
Sulcus limitans
Basal plate
1b
View into the rhombic fossa
Quadrigeminal plate
Vermis
Neocerebellum
Flocculus
Nodulus
Choroid plexus
2
Cerebellum at 16th week of pregnancy
Cerebellar cortex
Dentate nucleus
IV
Site of disintegration
Olive nucleus
2a Fourth ventricle (frontal section)
Villi of plexus
Lateral aperture
Median aperture
Choroid fissure
2b Choroid plexus (surface view)
Pontocerebellum (Neocerebellum)
Dentate nucleus
Efferent tracts
Paleo-cerebellum
Spino-cerebellum
Vestibulo-cerebellum
Superior cerebellar peduncle = spinocerebellar tract
Middle cerebellar peduncle = pontocerebellar tract
Inferior cerebellar peduncle = vestibulocerebellar and olivocerebellar tracts
Olive
Pons
Vestibulocochlear nucleus
3
Functional organization

A. Development and organization of cerebellum

# 4.14 Cerebellar Cortex

## B. Histological Development of the Cerebellar Cortex

The basal nuclei and the cerebellar cortex differentiate from the *neuroepithelium* of the upper rhombic lip (**B1**). The basement membrane of the neuroepithelium lies at the surface of the brain; the cell apices are directed toward the lumen of the fourth ventricle. Analogous to the differentiation of the neural tube into the spinal cord (→4.3), a zone of proliferation (*inner matrix zone*) is formed at the ventricular lumen where the neuroblasts arise by critical mitoses. In the *mantle zone*, corresponding to the gray matter of the spinal cord, the neuroblasts differentiate into the *basal (central) cerebellar nuclei*. In the externally situated marginal zone, the cerebellar cortex is formed from neuroepithelial cells ascending from the inner matrix zone. In contrast to the cerebral cortex, which is formed by neuroblasts no longer capable of dividing, the cerebellum develops an *external matrix zone* in which the neurons and glial cells of the cerebellar cortex arise (**B2**). Only the large *Purkinje cells* characteristic of the cerebellum ascend directly from the inner matrix zone.

**1. Basal Cerebellar Nuclei.** From the matrix zone of the neuroepithelium located at the ventricle, the neuroblasts for the basal nuclei of the cerebellum are the first to migrate out and settle down in the *mantle layer* of the neuroepithelium. They form the bilaterally located *dentate nucleus* (**B3**) of the cerebellar hemispheres (neocerebellum), as well as the *fastigial*, *globose*, and *emboliform nuclei* of the paleocerebellum.

**2. External Matrix Zone and Purkinje Cells.** In a second migratory wave, the Purkinje cells and still mitotically active neuroepithelial cells leave the internal matrix zone near the ventricle and travel externally along the supporting cells of the neuroepithelium, which become transformed into *pillar cells* (radial fibers). The *Purkinje cells* remain connected with the neurons in the basal nuclei by their axons. Other cells, still capable of division, form the *external matrix zone* (**B2**) at the surface of the cerebellar anlage.

The initial growth of the cerebellar swelling is directed into the fourth ventricle (**A1**). The direction of growth is now reversed and the bulge of the cerebellum extends externally (*eversion of cerebellum*).

**3. Molecular and Granular Layer.** The neuroblasts for the cerebellar cortex form two cellular layers at the surface, an outer granular layer (*stratum moleculare*, "molecule" = grain, here cell nuclei) and an inner granular layer (*stratum granulosum*, granule, grain, here also equivalent to cell nuclei). Between the two layers lie the large Purkinje cells characteristic of the cerebellum. The dendritic tree of the Purkinje cells receives afferents from climbing fibers and mossy fibers. The *climbing fibers* belong to neurons of the olive nucleus, the surface of which possesses a topical representation of the total body. The climbing fibers lead to a localized excitation of the Purkinje cells. The *mossy fibers* are the terminal ramifications of all other fibers entering the cerebellum. They extend over a larger region of the cerebellar cortex.

The afferents of the cerebellum arriving via the climbing and mossy fibers are processed at the small dendritic tree of the Purkinje cells into impulses that are conducted to the basal nuclei of the cerebellum (*dentate nucleus*) via the long main axon of the *Purkinje cells*. The basal cerebellar nuclei are topically organized and influence fundamental muscle tone by a continuous innervation. Activity of the Purkinje cells in the cerebellar cortex inhibits the activity of neurons in the basal nuclei and thus adjusts the action of agonists and antagonists to movements initiated by the cerebral cortex and the extrapyramidal system. The cerebellar impulses are generated "on line" and are effected in parallel to general motor impulses by influencing the tonus of specific muscles. In contrast to the cerebrum, the cerebellum does not function in memory.

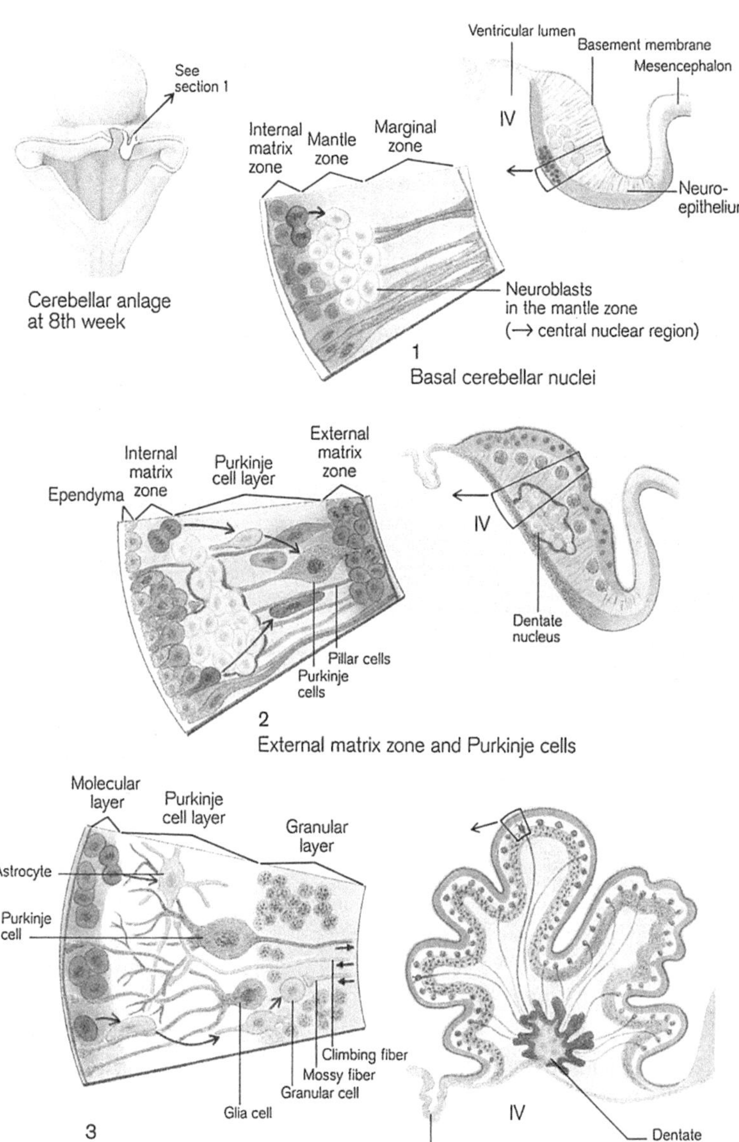
See section 1
Cerebellar anlage at 8th week
Internal matrix zone
Mantle zone
Marginal zone
Ventricular lumen
Basement membrane
Mesencephalon
IV
Neuro-epithelium
Neuroblasts in the mantle zone (→ central nuclear region)
1
Basal cerebellar nuclei
Ependyma
Internal matrix zone
Purkinje cell layer
External matrix zone
IV
Dentate nucleus
Pillar cells
Purkinje cells
2
External matrix zone and Purkinje cells
Molecular layer
Purkinje cell layer
Granular layer
Astrocyte
Purkinje cell
Climbing fiber
Mossy fiber
Granular cell
Glia cell
IV
Dentate nucleus
Choriod plexus
3
Molecular and granular layer

B. Histological development of cerebellar cortex

# Cerebrum

## 4.15 Overview: Rotation of Hemispheres

### A. Outgrowth of the Hemispheres

**1. Rotation of Hemispheres**

**a Outgrowth of the Telencephalic Vesicles.** The cerebrum or telencephalon develops from the *telencephalic vesicles*, which evaginate from the forebrain vesicle at the root of the *olfactory bulb* (**1a**). The cerebral vesicles grow out like the horns of a ram, in an arch directed backward and spirally outward (arrow in **1a** and **3c**). This developmental movement is known as *rotation of the hemispheres*. The midpoint of the movement is the thalamus with the basal ganglia and the surrounding *insular cortex* (**3c**). Through the rotation, the ventricle is drawn up into the temporal lobes. The hemispheric rotation is not a true rotary movement but is caused by the disproportional growth of the *neocortex* (**1b**).

**b Medial View of Telencephalic Vesicle.** The *paleocortex* and the *archicortex* lie in the inner wall of the telencephalic vesicle. The paleocortex and the amygdaloid nucleus enclose the *interventricular foramen* from below and the archicortex with the *hippocampus structure* from above. The *neocortex* is inserted between the paleocortex and the archicortex. The expansive growth of the neocortex (→4.20B) shifts the archicortex (hippocampus) into the temporal lobe. The apex of the temporal lobe—marked by the position of the amygdaloid nucleus—does not move but forms a fixed point in the "rotation of hemispheres." During the outgrowth of the cerebral vesicle, the paleo- and archicortex change their position only slightly and therefore come to lie on the inner- and underside of the cerebrum in the region of the cerebral crura (**A2**).

**2. The Rhinencephalon as Origin of the Cerebrum**

In the course of evolution, the cerebral vesicle developed at the base of the olfactory bulb and was originally a part of the rhinencephalon (paleocortex) that enlarged by the expansion of the vesicle, giving rise first to the archicortex and afterwards to the neocortex (**1b**). In humans the *olfactory bulb* does not become delimited as an independent structure on the underside of the telencephalic vesicle until the end of the embryonic period.

After the cerebral hemispheres grow out, the rhinencephalon forms a continuous complex at the base of the brain. It consists of the *medial* and *lateral olfactory convolutions* connected to the olfactory bulb. The lateral olfactory cortical field continues as an arch into the insular cortex and is connected with the cortical region of the *uncus*, below which lies the *amygdaloid nucleus*. The *hippocampus* (archicortex), which was displaced into the temporal lobe during the rotation of hemispheres, is attached posteriorly.

**3. The Cerebrum Overgrows the Brainstem**

In the fetal period, the cerebrum grows much more rapidly than the rest of the brain and covers the brainstem like a mantle (pallium). The originally external wall of the telencephalic vesicle (above the basal ganglia) is overgrown by the neocortical portions of the cortex and becomes displaced deep into the brain as the insula (**3c**). From the 32nd week of pregnancy onward, the surface of the brain enlarges still further by the development of gyri and sulci (**3d**).

The **paleo- and archicortex** (**A2**) originate directly from the rhinencephalon and are covered by the neocortex. These regions contain functional centers for escape, aggression, rest, and sex, thus regulating the basic functions of the individual and the species. The higher centers for *hearing* and *vision* lie in the **neocortex,** as do the *motor and sensory association fields*. The latter are connected with the precentral and postcentral gyri, which in turn are separated from one another by the *central sulcus*. Emotional awareness is localized in the paleo- and archicortex, whereas epicritical consciousness is localized in the neocortex.

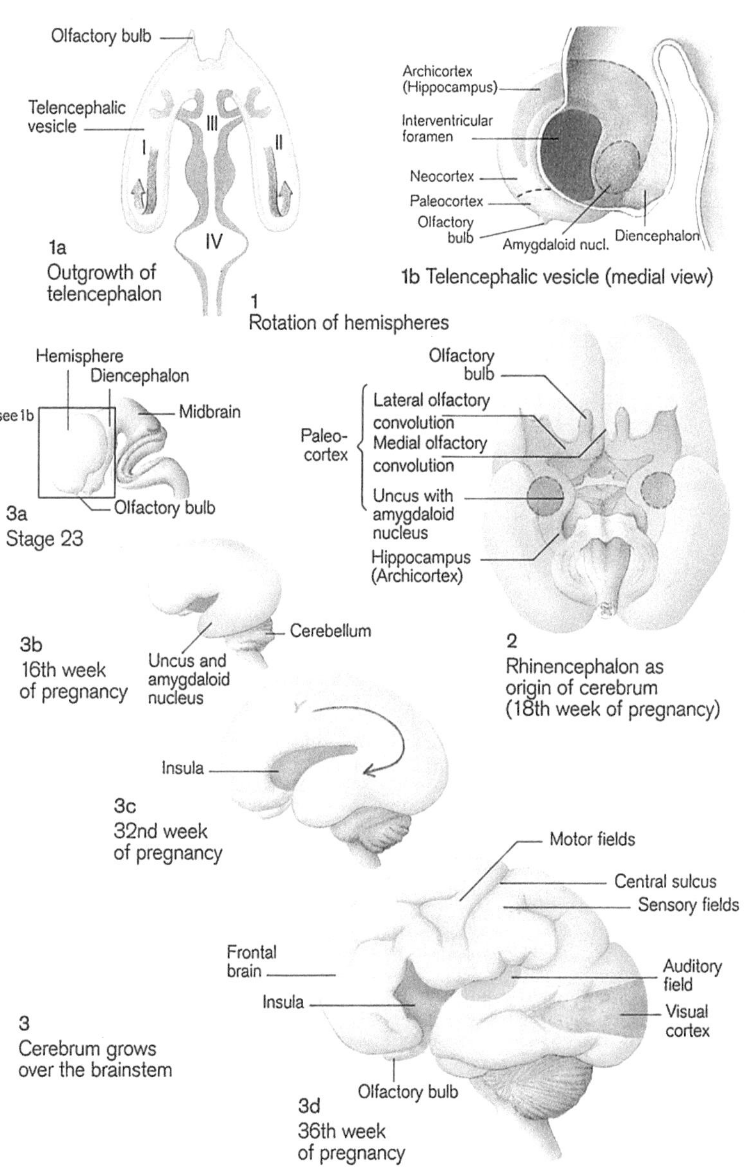
Olfactory bulb
Telencephalic vesicle
III
I
II
IV
1a
Outgrowth of telencephalon
Archicortex (Hippocampus)
Interventricular foramen
Neocortex
Paleocortex
Olfactory bulb
Amygdaloid nucl.
Diencephalon
1b Telencephalic vesicle (medial view)
1
Rotation of hemispheres
Hemisphere
Diencephalon
see 1b
Midbrain
Olfactory bulb
3a
Stage 23
Olfactory bulb
Paleo-cortex
Lateral olfactory convolution
Medial olfactory convolution
Uncus with amygdaloid nucleus
Hippocampus (Archicortex)
Cerebellum
3b
16th week of pregnancy
Uncus and amygdaloid nucleus
2
Rhinencephalon as origin of cerebrum (18th week of pregnancy)
Insula
3c
32nd week of pregnancy
Motor fields
Central sulcus
Sensory fields
Frontal brain
Auditory field
Insula
Visual cortex
3
Cerebrum grows over the brainstem
Olfactory bulb
3d
36th week of pregnancy

A. Outgrowth of hemispheres

# 4.16 Overview: Nuclei and Tracts

## A. Nuclei and Tracts in the Cerebrum

### 1. Ganglionic Hillock and Cortical Plate

**Ganglionic Hillock.** The telencephalic vesicles, like the rest of the neural tube, consist of neuroepithelium. At the floor of the cerebral vesicles, the neuroblasts, as in the rest of the brainstem and in the spinal cord (→ 4.3), form a mantle layer, that attaches directly to the matrix zone. In this layer, the central nuclei of the cerebrum develop (*basal ganglia*). The cell aggregations for the basal ganglia bulge into the ventricle as a *ganglionic hillock*. The basal ganglia form below and lateral to the *interventricular foramen* (**A1**) and extend posteriorly at the floor of the ventricle. There, they lie lateral to the *thalamus* (**A2**), which arises in the alar plate of the diencephalon.

**Cortical Plate.** At the end of the embryonic period, the neuroblasts for the cerebral cortex migrate out of the inner matrix zone located at the ventricular lumen and enter the marginal zone of the ventricular wall, where they form the *cortical plate* (→ 4.17). The neuroblasts in the cortical plate are no longer able to divide. The cortical plate grows by the immigration of neuroblasts from the matrix zone. The medial wall of the cerebral vesicles remains thin and is invaginated into the lateral ventricle as *choroid plexus*.

### 2. Central Nuclei and Internal Capsule

**Nuclei.** The protrusions of the thalamus and basal ganglia narrow the interventricular foramen from behind and displace it forward so that in the 16th week of pregnancy—in frontal sections of the brain—the foramen is not found in the same plane as the thalamus (compare sections 1 and 2). The *lateral division of the ganglionic hillock* (**A1**) is formed by the motor nuclei of the cerebrum, the *caudate nucleus*, and the *putamen*. Together with the *globus pallidus* ("pale nucleus"), which arises from the basal plate of the diencephalon, they form the motor nuclei of the extrapyramidal system. The *medial division* of the ganglionic hillock (**A1**) contains the matrix zone of the *paleocortex* and of the *amygdaloid body*. The neuroblasts migrate deeply and lose contact with the ventricle (arrow in A1). The *amygdaloid nucleus* remains at the apex of the temporal lobe as a fixed point during rotation of hemispheres (→ 4.15). It belongs to the rhinencephalon and with its lamellated, stratified arrangement, is a structure that can be classified as intermediate between a primitive cortical area and a central nucleus.

**Internal Capsule.** The fiber tracts passing from the thalamus to the cerebral cortex and from the cortex to the brainstem and the spinal cord (e.g., the *pyramidal tract*) penetrate the basal ganglia. These tracts form the *internal capsule*, separating the *putamen* and the *globus pallidus* from the *caudate nucleus* (→ 4.19). In the region of the penetrating fiber tracts, the medial wall of the cerebral hemisphere fuses with the wall of the diencephalon. The *claustrum* is delimited from the putamen by the external capsule.

### 3. Corpus Callosum and "Limbus"

**Corpus Callosum.** The fiber tracts connecting the cerebral hemispheres (commissures) first pass through the lamina terminalis (→ 4.22). The largest of the commissures is the *corpus callosum*, which extends posteriorly via a fusion zone in the medial walls of the cerebral hemispheres.

**Limbic Structures.** After the *rotation of the hemispheres* (arrow), the most primitive cortical portions in direct vicinity of the ventricle come to lie around the center of the *thalamus*, *lentiform nucleus*, and *insula* like a border (limbus). In a frontal section, the structures lying in the wall of the ventricle—the *caudate nucleus*, the line of attachment of the *choroid plexus*, and the *hippocampus*—appear in the inferior horn of the ventricle in the temporal lobes in reverse order (→ 4.21).

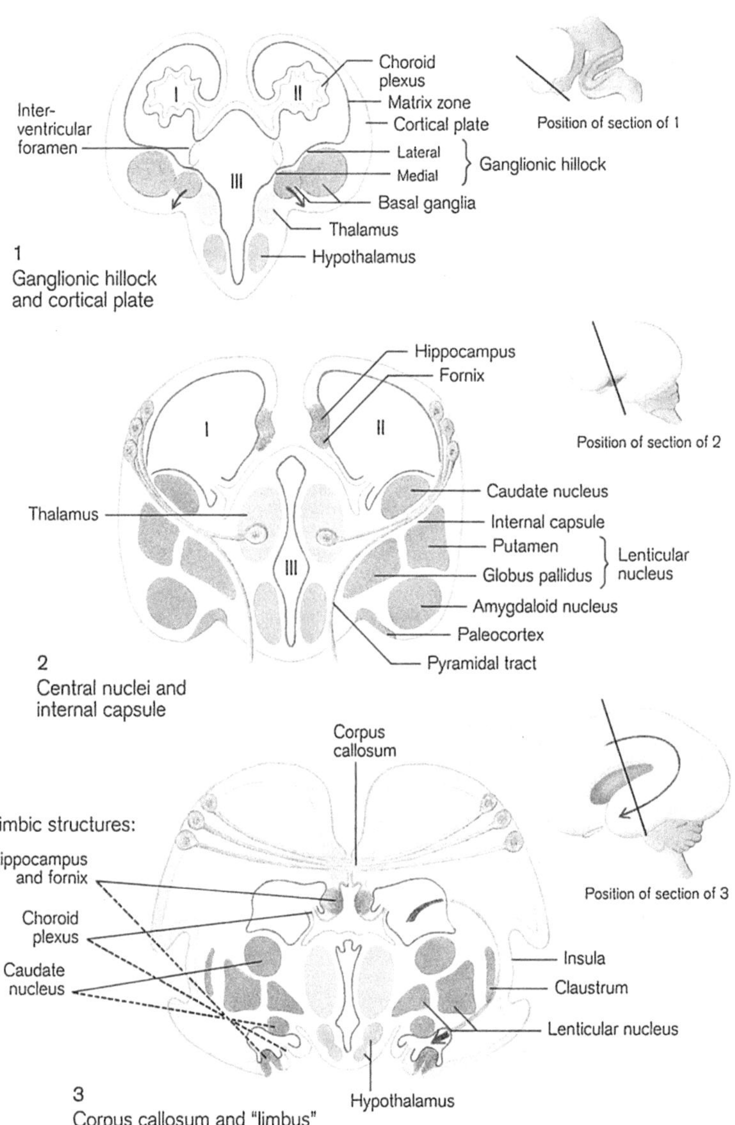
Choroid
plexus
Matrix zone
Cortical plate
Inter-
ventricular
foramen
I
II
III
Lateral
Medial
Ganglionic hillock
Basal ganglia
Thalamus
Hypothalamus
Position of section of 1
1
Ganglionic hillock
and cortical plate
Hippocampus
Fornix
Position of section of 2
Caudate nucleus
Thalamus
Internal capsule
Putamen
Globus pallidus
Lenticular
nucleus
Amygdaloid nucleus
Paleocortex
Pyramidal tract
2
Central nuclei and
internal capsule
Corpus
callosum
Limbic structures:
Hippocampus
and fornix
Choroid
plexus
Caudate
nucleus
Position of section of 3
Insula
Claustrum
Lenticular nucleus
Hypothalamus
3
Corpus callosum and "limbus"

A. Nuclei and tracts in the cerebrum

## 4.17 Cerebral Cortex

### A. Development of Cerebral Cortex from Neuroepithelium

**1. Mantle Layer and Cortical Plate.** The cerebral cortex develops in the roof of the telencephalic vesicle and ultimately covers the entire brainstem including the *basal ganglia*, which arise from the basal portion of the telencephalic vesicle (→ 4.15). By translocation of neurons to the enlarging surface of the brain, the number of possible synaptic connections in association fields is enormously increased. The basic organization of neurons in the mantle layer of the neural tube ( → 4.3) is retained in the basal ganglia, but is modified by the development of the *cortical plate*. The cortical plate differentiates into the cerebral cortex, the fiber tracts of which now pass into the intermediate zone between the matrix zone and the cortical plate (*white matter*).

**a Neuroepithelium and Matrix Zone.** The wall of the cerebral vesicle consists of pseudostratified neuroepithelium, with the basement membrane lying externally and the cell apices directed toward the ventricle. During cell division, the neuroepithelial cells round off and migrate apically. Mitoses therefore lie on the side of the neuroepithelium facing the ventricular lumen. The proliferating neuroepithelial cells form a proliferative zone (*matrix zone*) from which *neuroblasts* and *glial cells* arise. Some postmitotic neuroblasts initially lie in the intermediate zone (**1b**), whereas the marginal zone contains no cell nuclei. The pia mater is formed from the loose vascular connective tissue surrounding the cerebral vesicles.

**b Development of the Cortical Plate.** At the end of the embryonic period, the recently added postmitotic neuroblasts accumulate between the *intermediate* and *marginal* zones, where they form a thick layer of cells called the *cortical plate*. This plate first arises in the region of the insula (**A1**) and spreads from there to the vertex of the hemisphere. In the 12th and 13th week of pregnancy, the first nerve fibers ascend from the *thalamus* (thalamocortical fibers) into the cortical plate and develop contacts with the most differentiated (mature) neuroblasts.

**c Origin of Cortical Stratification by "Inside-out layering."** Between the 13th and 15th week of pregnancy, the first *pyramidal cells* differentiate at the underside of the cortical plate. Emigration of additional neuroblasts and growth of the fiber layers gives rise to the six-layered cerebral cortex from the cortical plate. The neuroblasts of recently added layers migrate from the matrix zone through the already existing layers of differentiated neurons and become deposited on the external side of the cortical plate ("inside-out layering"). The layers of the cerebral cortex are therefore internally further differentiated than externally. In the 28th week of pregnancy, the six layers can already be recognized in the neocortex.

During their passage from the matrix zone into the external layers of the cortical plate, the postmitotic neuroblasts use the *pillar cells* or *radial fibers* stretched between the fiber mass of the developing medullary layer as guiding structures. From the 15th week of pregnancy onward, a renewed burst of proliferation occurs. The center of proliferation now lies in the subventricular zone, which has arisen by expansion of the matrix zone. When the matrix zone is exhausted, new nerve cells can no longer arise. A single layer of *ependymal cells* remains behind and lines the ventricle.

The surface of the brain is covered by loose, vascularized connective tissue derived from the mesenchyme of the neural crest. The myelin sheaths of nerve fibers in the white matter are formed by the cell processes of *oligodendroglia*. Myelin sheath formation begins in the 16th week of pregnancy and does not terminate until the first year of postnatal life.

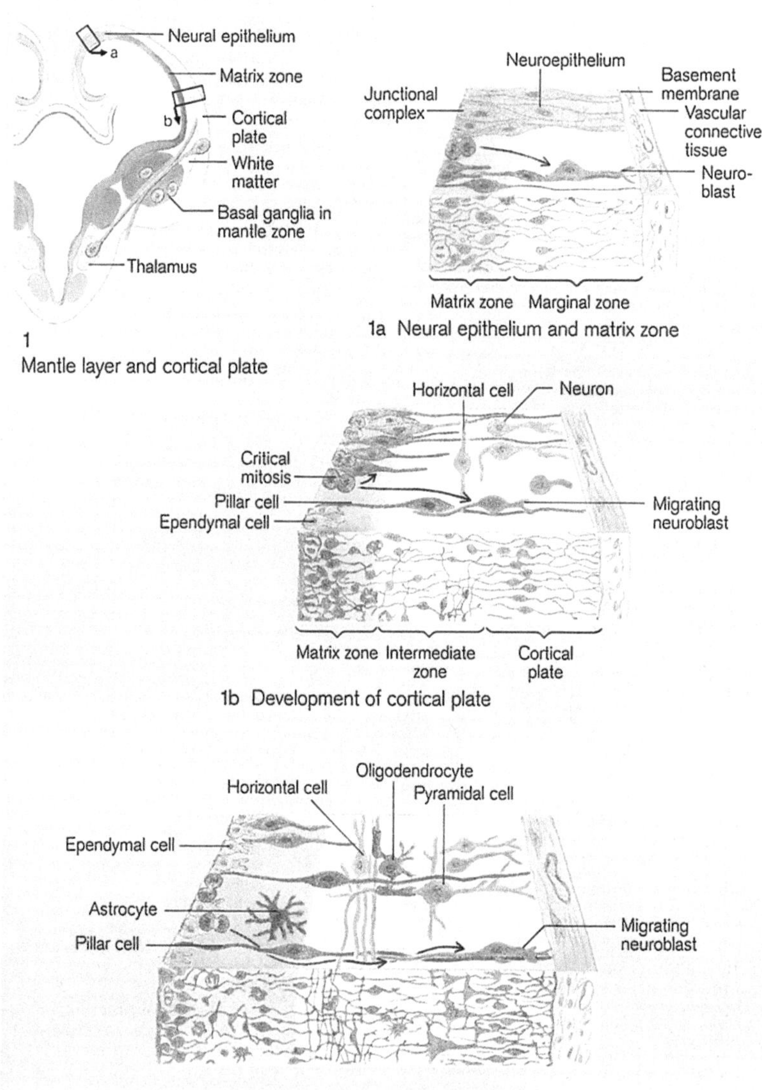


1
Mantle layer and cortical plate

1a Neural epithelium and matrix zone

1b Development of cortical plate

1c Stratification of cortex by "inside-out-layering"

A. Development of cerebral cortex from neural epithelium

# 4.18 Paleo-, Archi- and Neocortex

*Background*

In vertebrate **phylogeny**, the size of the telencephalon increases significantly, whereas the brainstem, including the basal ganglia, undergoes relatively little change.

The **paleocortex** is the primordial rhinencephalon at the root of the olfactory bulb. The **archicortex** arches posteriorly around the interventricular foramen and includes the hippocampus region and the cingulate gyrus located above the corpus callosum. The paleo- and archicortex are responsible for instinctive behavior patterns required for eating, reproduction, aggression, and defense. The **neocortex** contains cortical regions with an analytical and associative (conscious) representation of sensory perceptions and of the sensory and motor areas of the body.

## A. Phylogeny of the Cerebrum

In **reptiles**, the telencephalon consists of a swelling at the root of the large olfactory bulb (**A1**). In **lower mammals**, it already covers the midbrain (**A2**). In **higher mammals**, the surface is further increased by the formation of gyri and sulci (**A3**), which in the case of the olfactory-centered dog even extend into the olfactory bulb. The *central sulcus* in the dog lies in the anterior third of the hemisphere. In the human, it is shifted to the apex of the brain by the enlargement of the frontal brain.

The **transverse sections** show that the cerebral hemispheres are enlarged by the development of the *neocortex* in the crown of the telencephalic vesicle. The neocortex displaces the *paleocortex* (**A1**), which is initially situated in the roof of the telencephalic vesicle, in the medial direction (double arrow in **A2**), and finally the underside of the brain (**A3**). The *archicortex* (**A1**), located in the medial wall of the telencephalic vesicle, is shifted into the temporal lobe by the hemispheric rotation (→ 4.15).

## B. Paleo-, Archi-, and Neocortex at the End of the Embryonic Period

**1. Organization of the Matrix Zone** (according to Kahle). In **ontogeny**, the segments of the cerebrum corresponding to the paleo- and archicortex develop before the phylogenetically younger neocortex. The regions of the cerebrum (represented on the right side) can be projected back to the *matrix zone* of the ventricular wall (represented on the left).

The ventricular wall directly below the interventricular foramen, at the transition between the diencephalon and telencephalon, contains the matrix zone for the paleocortex. The cortical zone of the **paleocortex** is pushed away from the ventricular lumen by the basal ganglia and is shifted to the ventral side of the frontal brain.

The matrix zone of the paleocortex is followed laterally by the matrix zone of the **corpus striatum** (nucleus caudatum and putamen). The lateral ganglionic hillock arises by the accumulation of neurons for the basal ganglia in the mantle layer of the neuroepithelium. The lateral wall of the ventricle contains the matrix zone for the **insula.** The cortical plate of the insula is already developed. It detaches from its matrix zone and migrates caudally (arrow in **B1**) so that it comes to lie above the corpus striatum. The stratification of the insular cortex (*mesocortex*) forms a transition between archi- and neocortex.

The matrix zone of the **archicortex** forms the *hippocampus* in the medial wall of the telencephalic vesicle above the interventricular foramen. The cortex of the hippocampus is invaginated into the ventricle, so that the hippocampal sulcus arises on the medial wall of the cerebral vesicle (→ 4.21).

The early **neocortex** lies in the roof of the cerebral vesicle. It enlarges in the fetal period and in humans, ultimately covers the entire brainstem.

**2. Enlargement of the Telencephalic Vesicle.** The expansion of the telencephalic vesicle resembles the inflation of a balloon: The wall segments at the neck (*paleo-* and *archicortex*) remain as fixed points while the balloon is stretched at the crown (*neocortex*).

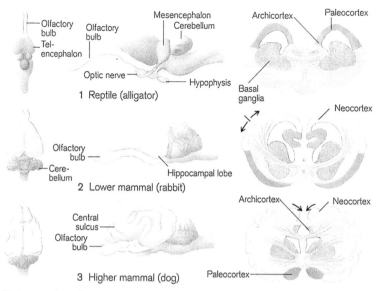

Olfactory bulb
Tel-encephalon
Olfactory bulb
Mesencephalon
Cerebellum
Optic nerve
Hypophysis
1 Reptile (alligator)
Archicortex
Paleocortex
Basal ganglia
Neocortex
Olfactory bulb
Cere-bellum
Hippocampal lobe
2 Lower mammal (rabbit)
Archicortex
Neocortex
Central sulcus
Olfactory bulb
3 Higher mammal (dog)
Paleocortex

A. Phylogeny of cerebrum

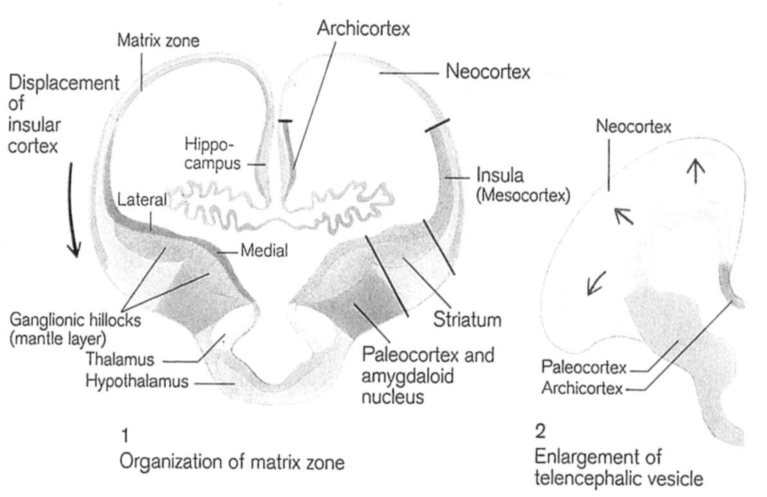


B. Paleo-, archi-, and neocortex at the end of the embryonic period

# 4.19 Pyramidal Tract

## A. Course of the Pyramidal Tract

The *pyramidal tract* links the cerebral cortex with the motor anterior horn cells of the spinal cord. The emerging axons of the pyramidal cells in the motor cortex take the shortest route through the brainstem. They penetrate the nuclear region of the *basal ganglia*, leave the cerebrum via the *crus of the cerebrum*, and pass through the pons to the spinal cord. In the fiber mantle of the neural tube within the medulla oblongata, they form two pyramid-shaped protrusions (*pyramids*) that give the tract its name. Ninety-five percent of the fibers cross over (*pyramidal decussation*) in the floor of the pyramid.

The white matter in the region where the pyramidal tract passes through the basal ganglia is called the *internal capsule*. In addition to the fibers of the pyramidal tract, all ascending and descending fiber systems of the telencephalon pass through the internal capsule. The fibers descending from the cerebrum to the cerebellum cross over in the pons before they enter the middle cerebellar peduncle.

## B. Nuclear Regions of the Extrapyramidal System

The thalamus and basal ganglia form a functional unit superordinate to the spinal cord, generating unconcious complex behavior and movement patterns. With the development of the cerebral cortex, the sensory center of the thalamus becomes an input station. The motor nuclei of the basal ganglia become the extrapyramidal system and are subordinate to the motor system of the cerebral cortex, which is characterized by the pyramidal tract.

### 1. Derivation

The caudate nucleus and the putamen arise from the *lateral ganglionic hillock* in the wall of the telencephalic vesicle (**1a**). The originally continuous nuclear region of the *caudate nucleus* and *putamen* is perforated by the nerve fibers of the internal capsule (**1b**). The penetrating bundle of myelinated fibers give the nuclear complex a striated appearance, so that the caudate nucleus and the putamen are grouped together as the striate body (*corpus striatum*) (B**2**). Behind the interventricular foramen, the medial wall of the telencephalon is fused with the wall of the diencephalon (here shown separated). The motor nuclei of the *globus pallidus* are separated from the thalamus by fiber tracts of the internal capsule. Like the thalamus, the globus pallidus is derived from the wall of the diencephalon.

### 2. Anatomical and Functional Arrangement

**Anatomy.** The *caudate nucleus*, *putamen*, and *globus pallidus* are grouped together as the basal ganglia. The *tail of the caudate nucleus* (shown in **A**) participates in the hemispheric rotation and therefore ends in the temporal lobe at the *amygdaloid body*. The putamen and globus pallidus fit like a lens in the arch of the caudate nucleus and are therefore together designated the *lentiform nucleus*.

**Function.** The extrapyramidal system regulates the fundamental tonus of the musculature. It is responsible for involuntary movements such as automatic movements associated with movements intended in the pyramidal system, as well as for learned and coordinated movement sequences stored subconsciously. Apart from the basal ganglia, the extrapyramidal system also includes the *substantia nigra* and the *red nucleus* in the midbrain, which arise from the rhombic lip (→ 4.9).

**Parkinson's disease**, a senile disease of the extrapyramidal system, begins with the degeneration of neurons in the substantia nigra. From the substantia nigra, dopaminergic fibers pass to the striatum, which in turn has a modulating and inhibiting influence on the pallidum. The pallidum is connected with the thalamus via the fiber bundle of the *ansa lenticularis* (**1b**). By this path, the efferents of the extrapyramidal system are conducted to the frontal brain via the thalamus, thus modulating the movements induced via the pyramidal tract.

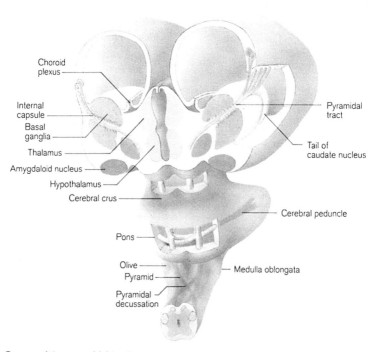

Choroid plexus
Internal capsule
Basal ganglia
Thalamus
Amygdaloid nucleus
Hypothalamus
Cerebral crus
Pyramidal tract
Tail of caudate nucleus
Cerebral peduncle
Pons
Olive
Pyramid
Pyramidal decussation
Medulla oblongata

A. Course of the pyramidal tract

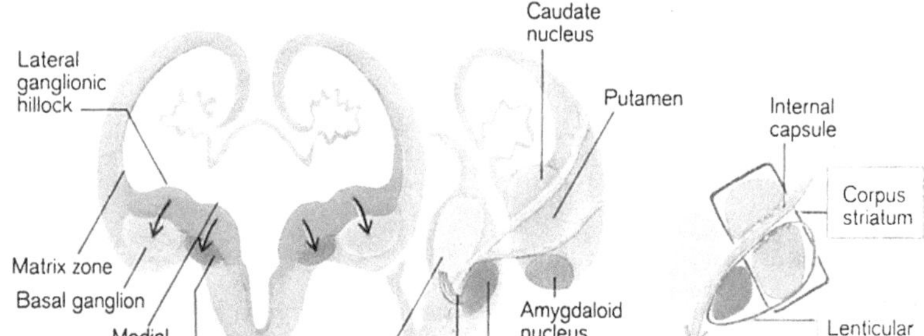


1a At the level of the foramen

1b Behind the foramen

1 Derivation

2 Anatomical and functional organization

B. Nuclear regions of the extrapyramidal tract

# 4.20 Limbic System

## A. Development of the Lateral Ventricles

### 1. The Zone of Fusion with the Diencephalon

The lateral ventricles (representing the first two ventricles) arise from the telencephalic vesicles (→ 4.8). The ventricular inlet, the *interventricular foramen*, is constricted by the thalamus into a comma-shaped fissure. The *thalamus* in the wall of the diencephalon and the *basal ganglia* at the floor of the telencephalon fuse with one another and extend posteriorly. As they protrude into the ventricle from below, they spread the ventricles apart posteriorly (**A3**). Below, the *cerebral crura* grow out and extend to the pons. The *root of the choroid plexus* passes from the *interventricular foramen* in the medial wall of the *lateral ventricle*, between the *thalamus* and the *basal ganglia*, to the *inferior horn* of the ventricle (**A2**) in the *temporal lobe*. The root of the plexus follows the rotation of the hemispheres.

### 2. Ventricular System in the 14th Week of Pregnancy

The disproportional growth of the ventricular wall in the roof of the ventricle during the development of the neocortex gives rise to three outpocketings of the lateral ventricle that extend into the newly formed portion of the cerebrum. The *anterior horn* of the lateral ventricle extends into the frontal brain. Posteriorly, the ventricle widens into the *posterior horn*, which extends into the occipital lobe. The *inferior horn* is pushed forward into the temporal lobe.

### 3. Expansion of Anterior and Posterior Horns

In the adult, the original medial wall of the lateral ventricle is marked by the attachment line of the *choroid plexus* behind the interventricular foramen. The central parts of the lateral ventricels and the posterior and inferior horns are pushed laterally by the expansion of thalamus and basal ganglia. The roof of the ventricle is formed by fibers of the *corpus callosum* that connect the hemispheres. The anterior horns are only separated by the septum pellucidum and contain no plexus.

## B. Overgrowth of the Limbic System by the Neocortex

The limbic system encompasses the brain areas that lie like a margin (limbus) in the medial wall of the lateral ventricle. Following the hemispheric rotation, they form a ring around the center of the brain, i.e., around the *thalamus*, the basal ganglia, and the insula. The limbic structures are phylogenetically old brain areas derived from the paleo- and archicortex, and the limbic system is distinguished from the rest of the cerebrum.

In the 16th week of pregnancy, the limbic structures still surround the entrance into the ventricle (interventricular foramen) and the *thalamus* (**B1**) as a closed ring. The structures of the paleocortex that are derived from the rhinencephalon lie anteriorly: the olfactory bulb, the medial crus of the olfactory tract, which passes to the *septal nuclei* in the medial wall of the frontal brain, and the lateral crus, which passes to the *amygdaloid nucleus* at the apex of the temporal lobe. Posteriorly, the ring is closed by the hippocampus, the cortical region of the archicortex.

The *growth of the cerebrum* (double arrow in **B1**) is apparent in the enlargement of the *corpus callosum*, which connects the neocortical parts of the two hemispheres with each other (**B2**). The new brain portion is inserted like a segment between the *septal nuclei* and the *hippocampal area* and thus between the paleo- and archicortex. The enlargement of the new brain segment displaces the hippocampal cortex into the temporal lobe (hemispheric rotation). The hippocampal tract, known as the *fornix* (vault), remains as a fiber bundle in the medial wall of the lateral ventricle and connects the hippocampus with the mamillary body in the hypothalamus. The crus of the fornix, branching off in front of the interventricular foramen, passes to the septal nuclei. The expansion of the frontal brain leads to the development of the *septum pellucidum*, the thinly stretched wall of the lateral ventricle between the corpus callosum and fornix (**B3**).

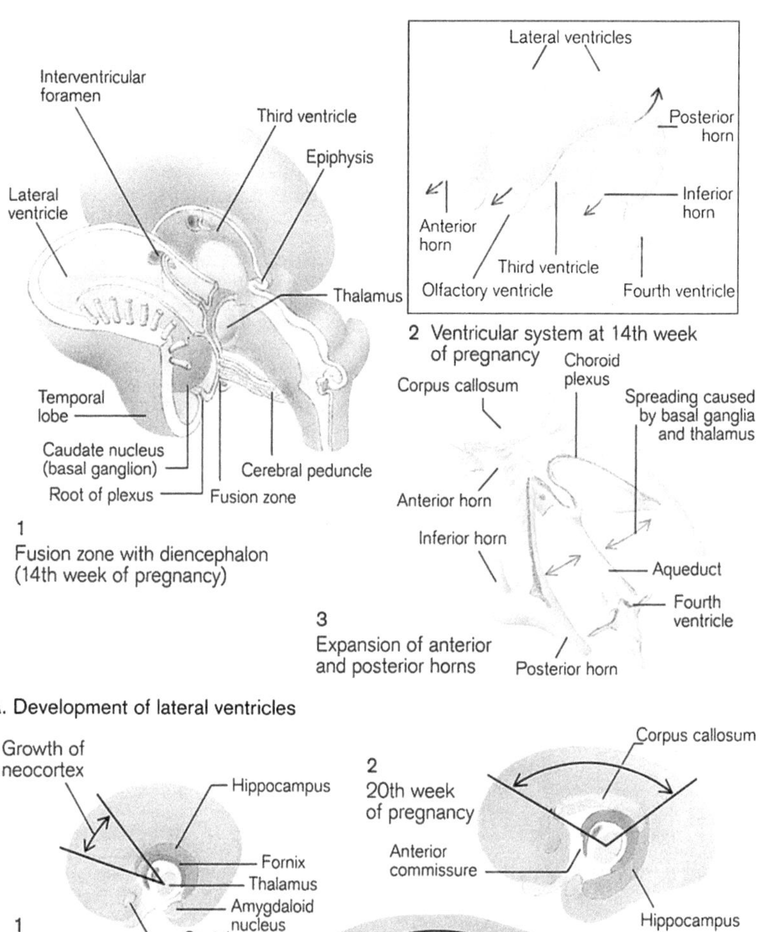
Interventricular
foramen
Third ventricle
Epiphysis
Lateral
ventricle
Thalamus
Temporal
lobe
Caudate nucleus
(basal ganglion)
Root of plexus
Fusion zone
Cerebral peduncle
1
Fusion zone with diencephalon
(14th week of pregnancy)
Lateral ventricles
Posterior
horn
Inferior
horn
Anterior
horn
Third ventricle
Olfactory ventricle
Fourth ventricle
2 Ventricular system at 14th week
of pregnancy
Corpus callosum
Choroid
plexus
Spreading caused
by basal ganglia
and thalamus
Anterior horn
Inferior horn
Aqueduct
Fourth
ventricle
Posterior horn
3
Expansion of anterior
and posterior horns
Growth of
neocortex
Hippocampus
Fornix
Thalamus
Amygdaloid
nucleus
Septal
nuclei
1
16th week
of pregnancy
Corpus callosum
2
20th week
of pregnancy
Anterior
commissure
Hippocampus
Septum
pellucidum
Septal
nuclei
3
30th week
of pregnancy

A. Development of lateral ventricles

B. Enclosure of limbic system by neocortex

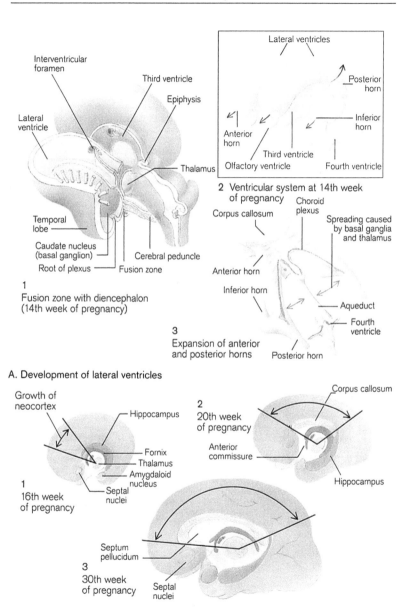

# 4.21 Choroid Plexus and Hippocampus

## A. Development of the Choroid Plexus

### 1. Invagination of the Plexus

The choroid plexus is an invagination from the venous plexus of the brain surface into the ventricles. In the choroid plexus, cerebrospinal fluid is formed. The invagination of the plexus into the telencephalic vesicle begins in the 5th week (stage 17) above the still-wide *interventricular foramen*. The bulge of *hippocampus* lies above the plexus.

### 2. Position in the Ventricular Wall

The choroid plexus and hippocampus take part in the hemispheric rotation. In this process, the position of the plexus relative to the hippocampus is reversed in the inferior horn of the lateral ventricle. The plexus comes to lie above the hippocampus (**B1**).

### 3. Origin of the Tela, Tenia, and Lamina Affixa

The plexus of the lateral ventricle merges into the choroid plexus of the third ventricle in the interventricular foramen. In a section posterior to the interventricular foramen (12th week of pregnancy), the thin roof of the diencephalon bulges like a dome between the hemispheres and is invaginated by many small venous tufts (**3a**) that later give rise to an efferent vein for each lateral ventricle and to the paired choroid plexus of the third ventricle. Behind the interventricular foramen, the plexus of the thin medial wall of the lateral ventricle becomes apposed to the thalamus and merges with it. The portion of the medial ventricular wall that has grown together with the thalamus is called the *lamina affixa*, the vascular connective tissue passing into the plexus, the *tela* (= connective tissue layer) *choroidea*, and the torn edge that arises by removal of the plexus (during preparation of the brain), the *tenia choroidea*.

**Inset (3a).** The space above the roof of the third ventricle is filled with loose connective tissue and large veins. Vascular connective tissue invaginates medially into the thin dome-shaped roof of the third ventricle (choroid plexus of the 3rd ventricle) and laterally into choroid plexus of the lateral ventricle. The venous plexus in the ventricles is covered by a single layer of *ependymal cells* that blends laterally with the matrix zone of the *caudate nucleus*. Between the root of the plexus and the caudate nucleus, the ependymal layer forms the medial wall of the lateral ventricle on the thalamus (*lamina affixa*); superiorly, it goes over into the hippocampal cortex, forming a *cortical plate* and a *matrix zone*. At the inferior border of the hippocampal cortex, nerve fibers of the *fornix* course longitudinally in the ventricular wall.

**Vascular Supply of the Plexus.** The choroid plexus is connected to the veins of the transverse fissure (→ 4.22) at the interventricular foramen. Above the thalamus, the connection to the venous plexus at the brain surface is interrupted. The plexus follows the lateral ventricle into the temporal lobe. In the temporal lobe, the medial wall of the ventricle is detached from the thalamus so that pial vessels can again medially enter into the *choroid fissure*.

## B. Development of the Hippocampus

The hippocampus contains the cortical area of the archicortex (→ 4.18). In the embryo, the hippocampus is a continuous structure in the medial wall of the ventricle, extending from the interventricular foramen into the temporal lobe (**B1**). With the development of the neocortex and corpus callosum, the hippocampus becomes displaced entirely into the temporal lobe. Only the *fornix* (**2a**) remains below the corpus callosum as the fiber tract of the hippocampus (→ 4.20). The mature hippocampus is a convoluted, seahorse-shaped structure that lies at the floor of the ventricle (**2b**). As the hippocampus invaginates, the *hippocampal sulcus* arises on the external side of the brain. The hippocampal sulcus runs parallel to the *choroid fissure*. A segment of the cortical plate involutes together with the hippocampal invagination and forms the cortical zone of the inwardly directed *dentate gyrus* (**2b**).

Hippocampus
Choroid plexus
Epiphysis
Diencephalon
Inter-ventricular foramen
Ganglionic hillock

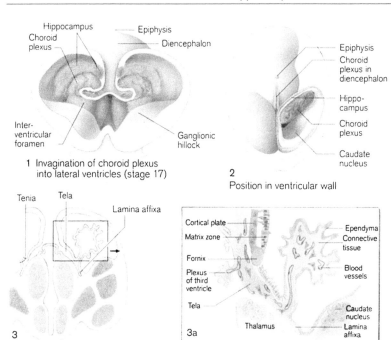

1 Invagination of choroid plexus into lateral ventricles (stage 17)

Epiphysis
Choroid plexus in diencephalon
Hippo-campus
Choroid plexus
Caudate nucleus

2
Position in ventricular wall

Tenia
Tela
Lamina affixa

3
Origin of tela, tenia, and lamina affixa (12th week of pregnancy)

Cortical plate
Matrix zone
Fornix
Plexus of third ventricle
Tela
Thalamus
Ependyma
Connective tissue
Blood vessels
Caudate nucleus
Lamina affixa

3a

A. Development of choroid plexus

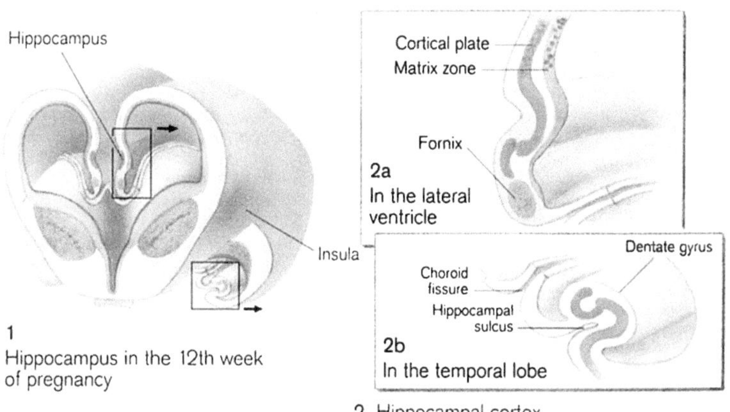


1
Hippocampus in the 12th week of pregnancy

2a
In the lateral ventricle

2b
In the temporal lobe

2 Hippocampal cortex

B. Development of hippocampus

# 4.22 Commissures

## A. Commissures of the Telencephalon

### 1. Origin of the Commissures in the Lamina Terminalis

Commissures are fiber tracts that unite the two hemispheres with each other. They arise in the *lamina terminalis*, the inherent connection between the two halves of the brain. The upper portion of the lamina terminalis is thereby transformed into the *commissural plate*.

**Anterior Commissure.** The anterior commissure is the commissure of the paleocortex. It connects the centers of the rhinencephalon with one another and retains its original position in the lamina terminalis.

**Fornix and its Commissure.** The *fornix* is a fiber tract of the archicortex that links the hippocampal cortex with the *mamillary body*. It travels anteriorly below the hippocampus in the medial wall of the hemisphere and enters the *lamina terminalis* in front of the *interventricular foramen*. From there, the fornix continues its path in the wall of the diencephalon up into the mammillary body of the hypothalamus. Some of the fibers cross to the opposite side. The fusion of the columns of the fornix in the lamina terminalis is called the *commissure of the fornix* or the *hippocampal commissure*. The rotation of the hemispheres and the outgrowth of the corpus callosum cause the fornix to extend into the temporal lobe. The commissure of the fornix becomes displaced posteriorly below the corpus callosum.

**Corpus Callosum.** The fibers of the *corpus callosum* link the neocortex of the left and right hemisphere. The corpus callosum is the largest structure in the commissural plate (**1b**). Its fibers first descend steeply in the medial wall of the frontal brain (**1a**) and subsequently take a more horizontal course (**1b**).

### 2. Growth of the Corpus Callosum

Anteriorly, the corpus callosum extends by arching between the enlarging lobes of the frontal brain; posteriorly, it extends into the fusion zone between the hemispheres (→ 4.16).

**Septum Pellucidum.** The part of the commissural plate located in the genu of the corpus callosum is stretched into a transparent lamella, the septum pellucidum. Before the expansion of the corpus callosum, the *septum* (**A2**) lies between the *corpus callosum* and the *anterior commissure*; afterwards, it lies in the medial wall of the cerebral ventricles (**2a**). A fluid-filled cavity (*cavity of the septum pellucidum*) arises secondarily in the septum. The *septal nuclei* lie below the septum pellucidum and in front of the lamina terminalis. They belong to the paleocortex.

**Transverse Fissure.** Behind the septum pellucidum, the corpus callosum expands posteriorly into a fusion zone of the hemispheric walls above the roof of the third ventricle. The *septum pellucidum* ends at the posteriorly arched columns of the fornix. Between the corpus callosum and the roof of the third ventricle lies a space filled with pial connective tissue (*transverse fissure* in **2a**, arrow in **A2**), which opens posteriorly above the epiphysis and quadrigeminal plate. There, below the splenium of the corpus callosum, is the origin of the great cerebral vein, which collects blood from the thalamostriate vein and from the choroid plexus of both sides and carries it to the confluence of the sinuses. Anteriorly, the space filled with pial connective tissue ends at the fused columns of the fornix. The columns, which enter the lamina terminalis from the original medial wall of the hemispheres, form the roof of the interventricular foramen.

The corpus callosum penetrates the archicortex and divides it into two regions. The *fornix*, the tract of the archicortex, lies below the corpus callosum. Above the corpus callosum, lies the original hippocampal fissure, and over it the *cingulate gyrus* (also derived from the archicortex). The *posterior commissure* arises together with the *habenular commissure*, independently of the commissural plate (→ 4.23).

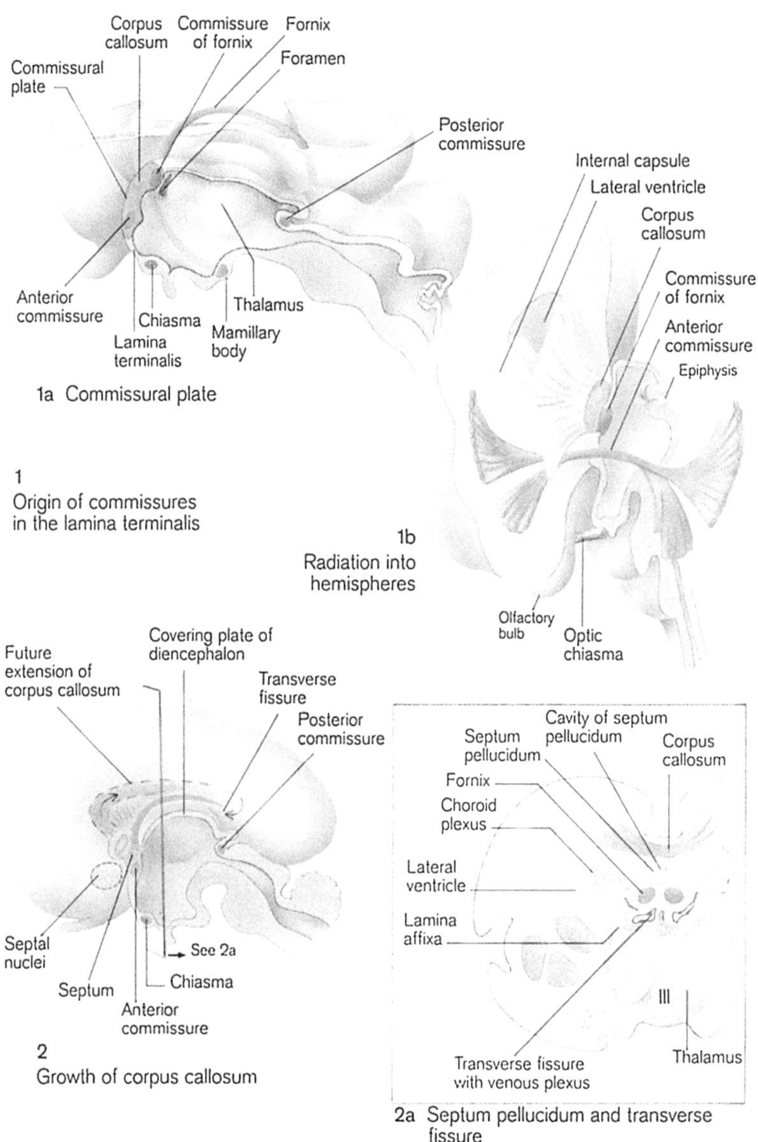


A. Commissures of telencephalon

## 4.23 Pineal Gland

*Background*

The **pineal gland** (epiphysis) and **pituitary gland** (hypophysis) are neuroendocrine organs. They contain neuroendocrine cells that are related to sensory cells and nerve cells. The neuroendocrine cells do not release their "neurotransmitters" at synapses, however, but secrete them into the blood as hormones.

### A. From the Light-Sensitive Cells to the Pinealocytes

The pineal gland (epiphysis) was originally an unpaired light-sensitive sense organ in the roof of the diencephalon. The unpaired epiphysial "eye" served in sensing the length of the day/night (light/dark) cycle and thus in regulating the circadian rhythm and the reproductive cycle. This explains why light-sensitive cells are found in the epiphysial vesicle of many lower vertebrates.

In the **Tuatara** (**A1**) (Sphenodon, ancestral vertebrate from New Zealand), an additional unpaired, primitive eye with an optic cup and lens arises from the epiphysial vesicle. It lies in the skull roof between the parietal bones and is known as a *parietal eye*. From the light-sensitive cells, nerve fibers pass to the diencephalon (*pineal nerve*) (**A2**). The lens originates from the connective tissue. The primitive optic cup is filled with large ganglion cells. The pineal eye is a specialized organ that is derived from the epiphysis and clearly demonstrates the light-sensing function.

In the course of evolution, the *light-sensitive cells* in the epiphysial diverticulum developed into neuroendocrine *pinealocytes* (**2a**), which secrete the neurohormone melatonin (an indole derivative) into the blood. Transition forms between the light-sensitive cells with synapses and the pinealocytes, showing progressive involution of the apical receptor processes and synapses, can be found in different species (**2b**).

### B. Development of the Pineal Gland in Humans

In the embryonic period, the epiphysis forms a neuroepithelial *diverticulum* in the roof of the diencephalon. In the fetal period, cells leave the matrix zone and differentiate into *pinealocytes* and *glial cells* (**1a**). Differentiated *pinealocytes* possess cell processes from which they release the melatonin directly into the ventricle or into the capillaries that sprout in from the pial plexus. Above and below the epiphysial diverticulum, the commissures of the diencephalon—the *habenular commissure* and the *posterior commissure*—arise in the marginal zone of the neuroepithelium. The commissures are not functionally connected with the pineal gland.

In higher vertebrates and mammals, the vault of the cranium is closed over the epiphysis and the light receptors are no longer formed, so that the pineal gland consists only of melatonin-synthesizing neuroendocrine cells. The gland retains its function in correlating for circadian rhythm and the reproductive cycle with the day-night cycle. The pineal gland is secondarily connected with the *definitive eyes* (the lateral eyes) (**B1**). The optic afferents are conducted over sympathetic fibers to the *superior cervical ganglion* of the sympathetic nervous system, parallel to the light stimulus for the pupillary reaction. From there, the optic information arrives at the pineal gland via sympathetic pathways along the small arteries and parallel to the great cerebral vein. This sympathetic innervation of the pineal gland is projected on the embryonic brain in **B1**.

**Melatonin** in lower vertebrates causes a retraction of melanin granules in the melanocytes; it is the antagonist of melanocyte-stimulating hormone (MSH) produced by the intermediate lobe of the hypophysis and inhibits gonadal functions via the hypophysis. Secretion of melatonin is increased by darkness. Overall, the pineal gland is a control center by means of which the activity or the depression of an organism is correlated with light. (The "time lag" after long distance flights can be influenced by strong illumination via this pathway.)

Parietal eye
Skull
Epiphysis
Midbrain
Rhinencephalon
Cerebellum
Olfactory bulb
Optic nerve
Hypophysis

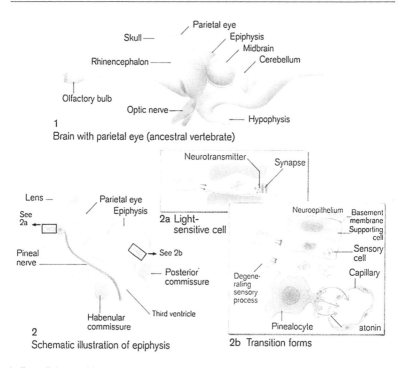

1
Brain with parietal eye (ancestral vertebrate)

Neurotransmitter
Synapse

2a Light-sensitive cell

Lens
Parietal eye
Epiphysis
See 2a
See 2b
Pineal nerve
Posterior commissure
Habenular commissure
Third ventricle

2
Schematic illustration of epiphysis

Neuroepithelium
Basement membrane
Supporting cell
Sensory cell
Capillary
Degene-rating sensory process
Pinealocyte
atonin

2b Transition forms

A. From light-sensitive cells to pinealocytes

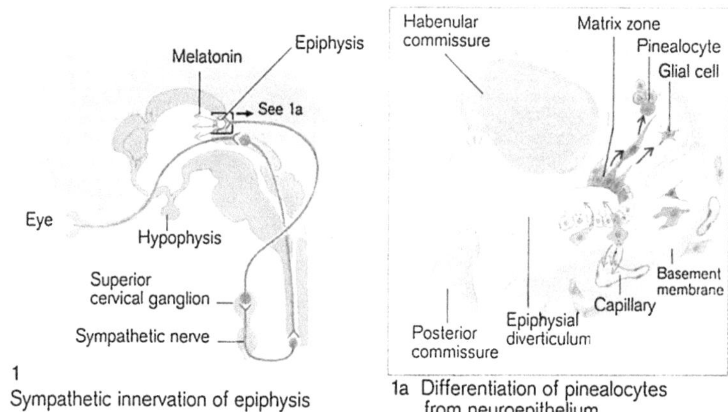


1
Sympathetic innervation of epiphysis

1a Differentiation of pinealocytes from neuroepithelium

B. Development of human pineal gland

## 4.24 Pituitary Gland

*Background*

The anterior lobe of the pituitary gland (**adenohypophysis**) arises from the hypophysial pouch (Rathke's pouch) in the roof of the stomodeum. The posterior lobe of the pituitary (**neurohypophysis**) is an evagination of the diencephalon.

### A. Development of the Pituitary Gland

**1. Placode Stage.** In stage 13, the ectodermal roof of the stomodeum becomes closely apposed to the floor of the *diencephalon* in front of the *pharyngeal membrane* and thickens. The primordium of the anterior lobe of the pituitary (hypophysis) is therefore not a derivative of the primitive gastrointestinal tract, but rather a placode of the head.

**2. Hypophyseal Pouch and Infundibulum.** The *hypophyseal pouch* develops from the placode-like thickening in stage 17. The neurohypophysis evaginates from the floor of the diencephalon and becomes apposed to the side of the hypophyseal pouch. This gives rise to an outpocketing of the third ventricle, the *infundibulum* (**2a**).

**3. Abscission from the Pharyngeal Roof.** In stage 22, the hypophysis becomes separated from the roof of the pharynx by the cartilaginous base of the skull. The hypophysis comes to lie in the recess of the sella turcica in the *sphenoid bone* and remains connected to the brain via the hypophyseal stalk.

**Pharyngeal Hypophysis.** At the end of the embryonic period, the remains of the original connection between the hypophysis and the roof of the oral cavity are still visible in the cartilaginous base of the cranium. The remains of the hypophyseal pouch can give rise to a pharyngeal hypophysis or to a tumor known as a **craniopharyngioma.** Both lie within the cranium and cause symptoms similar to those caused by a tumor of the anterior lobe of the hypophysis. The symptoms generally appear before the 15th year of life.

**4. Anterior, Middle, and Posterior Lobes of the Hypophysis.** The *anterior lobe of the hypophysis* and the *pars tuberalis* surrounding the hypophyseal stalk arise from the anterior wall of the hypophyseal pouch. The epithelium of the hypophyseal pouch sprouts out into the meningeal connective tissue. The buds and epitheleal cords are vascularized and differentiate into endocrine cells that produce peptide hormones. The secretion of hormones (ACTH, LH, FSH, TH, STH, and prolactin) is regulated by the hypothalamus. Neurons in the hypothalamus produce *releasing factors*, which are axonally transported to the hypophyseal stalk. Here, they are taken up by venous capillaries (portal circulation of the hypophysis) and are transported to the anterior lobe of the hypophysis.

The posterior wall of the hypophyseal pouch develops into the *middle lobe* of the hypophysis, in which melanocyte-stimulating hormone (MSH) is synthesized. The hypophyseal stalk and the *posterior lobe of the hypophysis* arise from the diencephalic portion of the anlage. The matrix zone of the outpocketing of the third ventricle gives rise only to *glial cells* (pituicytes) and not to neurons. The hormones of the posterior lobe (oxytocin and vasopressin) are synthesized in neurons of the hypothalamus, axonally transported to the posterior lobe, and secreted directly into capillaries penetrating into the pituitary gland from the pial vascular plexus.

**Molecular Biology.** In the TSH, STH, and prolactin-secreting cells of the adenohypophysis, a regulatory gene (pit-1) was discovered on the basis of its structural similarity to the homeotic genes of Drosophila (→ 3.17). This gene regulates determination and morphogenesis of the pituitary gland in the embryo.

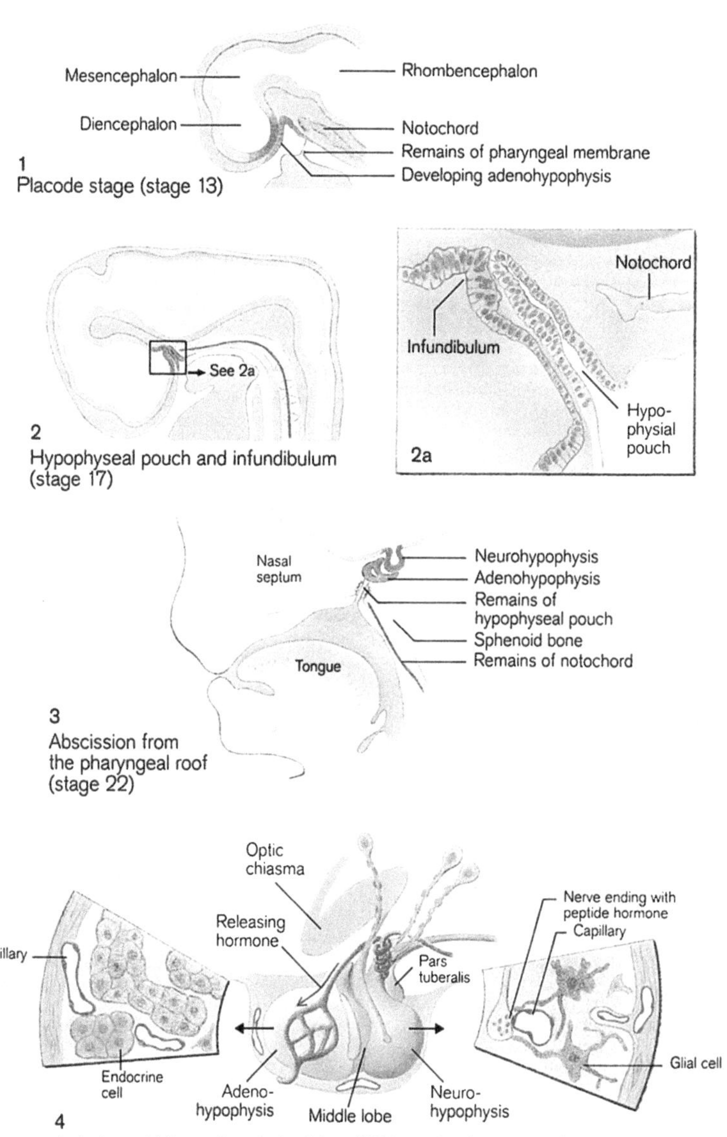
Mesencephalon
Diencephalon
Rhombencephalon
Notochord
Remains of pharyngeal membrane
Developing adenohypophysis
1
Placode stage (stage 13)
See 2a
2
Hypophyseal pouch and infundibulum (stage 17)
Notochord
Infundibulum
Hypo-physial pouch
2a
Nasal septum
Tongue
Neurohypophysis
Adenohypophysis
Remains of hypophyseal pouch
Sphenoid bone
Remains of notochord
3
Abscission from the pharyngeal roof (stage 22)
Optic chiasma
Releasing hormone
Pars tuberalis
Capillary
Endocrine cell
Adeno-hypophysis
Middle lobe
Neuro-hypophysis
Nerve ending with peptide hormone
Capillary
Glial cell
4
Anterior, middle, and posterior lobes (16th week of pregnancy)

A. Development of pituitary gland

# Summary

# 4.25 Synopsis of the Brain

## A. Hierarchical Organization of Central Regulation

### 1. Regulation of Motor Response

The central regulation of movement is organized into three hierarchical levels. At the lowest level are reflex arcs in the spinal cord, at the intermediate level are centers in the brainstem (extrapyramidal system), and at the highest level is the cerebral cortex with the pyramidal tract.

**Reflex arcs in the Spinal Cord.** The afferent fibers for the reflex arc enter through the posterior root of the spinal cord. The efferent fibers are the axons of the motor anterior horn cells. Injury of these cells leads to *flaccid paralysis*. Central inputs regulate motor response by inhibitory impulses. Interruption of the central inputs therefore leads to increased spontaneous activity of the motor anterior horn cells (*spastic paralysis*).

**Reflex arcs in the Rhombencephalon.** The pharyngeal arch nerves arising in the rhombencephalon play an important role in regulating involuntary motor activity required for respiration and swallowing. The respiratory center and the deglutition center are localized in the nuclear regions of the *reticular formation*.

**Precentral Gyrus and Pyramidal Tract.** The conscious motor response is regulated from the motor *precentral gyrus*. Axons of the pyramidal cells form the pyramidal tract, which passes directly to the motor anterior horn cells in the spinal cord and in the rhombencephalon. The corresponding *afferent tracts* (deep sensitivity, epicritical sensitivity) synapse in the *thalamus* before proceeding forward to the *postcentral gyrus*.

**Extrapyramidal System.** In the thalamus, a general, emotional awareness of the individual's physiological state is already present. The *basal ganglia*, together with the motor nuclei in the brainstem (red nucleus and substantia nigra), represent the motor system associated with the thalamus, in which subcortical, complex, coordinated movements arise. After the development of the superordinate cerebral cortex, the thalamus becomes the central input station for all afferents to the cortex. The thalamus and basal ganglia become the extrapyramidal system, supplementing the voluntary movements elicited in the motor cortex by automatic coinnervation.

**Cerebellum.** The cerebellum originally processes impulses from the vestibular organ. It supplements the impulses from the motor cortex and the extrapyramidal system by "on line" fine-tuning of agonists and antagonists.

### 2. Central Sensory Tracts

The cerebrum arises from the rhinencephalic vesicles. The *olfactory tract* therefore ends directly in the basal nuclear regions of the telencephalon (septal nuclei, amygdaloid nucleus). The **optic tract** and the **auditory tract** synapse in the thalamus (lateral and medial geniculate body, respectively). From there, the optic tract passes to the visual cortex and the auditory radiation to the auditory gyri in the temporal lobe. Parallel to the optic tract, fibers pass to the *superior colliculus* in the midbrain, where ocular movement and spatial position are controlled by means of reflexes. The center for the auditory and vestibular tracts lies in the metencephalon. The auditory pathway possesses a relay station in the inferior colliculus and is connected directly to the cerebellum.

The branchiosensory *taste fibers* pass to the *nucleus solitarius* in the metencephalon.

### 3. Limbic System

The central autonomic and emotional functions are localized in the phylogenetically old parts of the telencephalon and diencephalon. Since the *paleocortex*, the *archicortex*, and the *hypothalamus* are organized into a marginal zone (limbus) around the thalamus and the interventricular foramen, they are anatomically and functionally grouped together as the "limbic system." The limbic system is an archaic "emotional brain," in contrast to the epicritical *neocortex*.

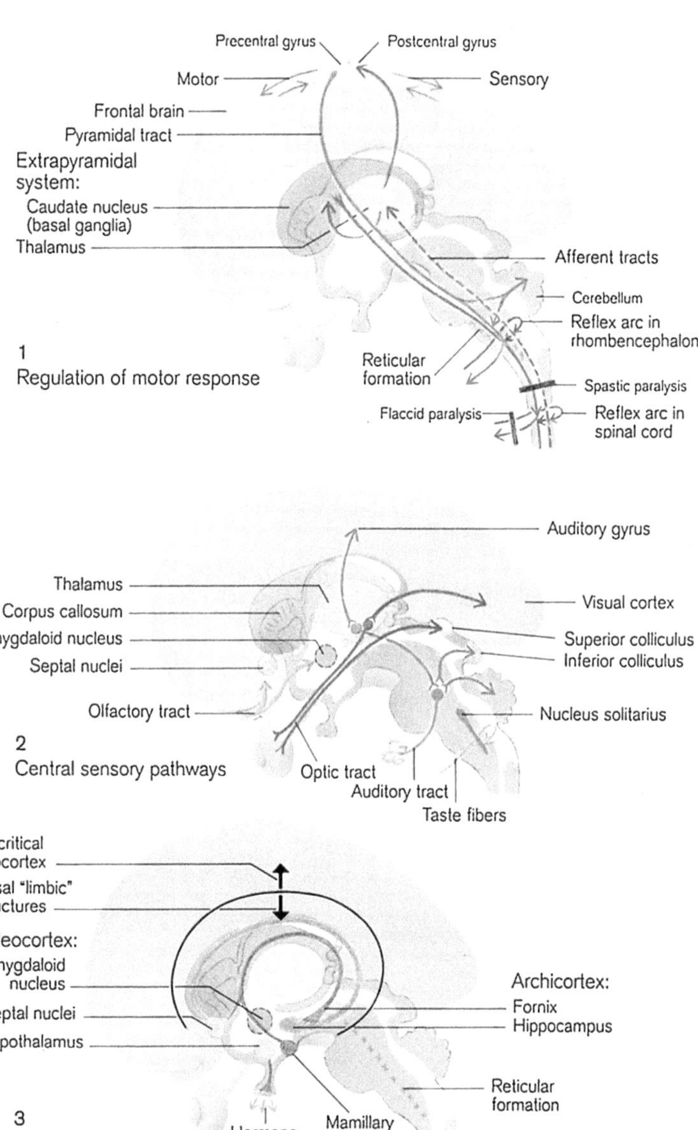
Precentral gyrus
Postcentral gyrus
Motor
Sensory
Frontal brain
Pyramidal tract
Extrapyramidal system:
Caudate nucleus (basal ganglia)
Thalamus
Afferent tracts
Cerebellum
Reflex arc in rhombencephalon
1
Regulation of motor response
Reticular formation
Spastic paralysis
Flaccid paralysis
Reflex arc in spinal cord
Auditory gyrus
Thalamus
Corpus callosum
Amygdaloid nucleus
Septal nuclei
Olfactory tract
Visual cortex
Superior colliculus
Inferior colliculus
Nucleus solitarius
2
Central sensory pathways
Optic tract
Auditory tract
Taste fibers
Epicritical neocortex
Basal "limbic" structures
Paleocortex:
Amygdaloid nucleus
Septal nuclei
Hypothalamus
Archicortex:
Fornix
Hippocampus
Reticular formation
3
Limbic system
Hormone release from the pituitary gland
Mamillary body

A. Brain synopsis

# Chapter 5: Sense Organs

## Introduction

**5.1 Evolution.** The occurrence of dispersed sensory cells in simple, multicellular organisms suggests that the sense organs originated by the assemblage of sensory cells into sensory fields. The analogous development of a lenticular eye in unrelated animal classes points to the selection pressure exerted by the physical properties of light. Primary light-sensitive cells found in the neural tube of lancetfish may be forerunners to the light-sensitive cells in the pineal gland, which supplement the definitive eyes of vertebrates *(lateral eyes)* (→ 4.23). The development of *secondary sensory cells*, i.e., the segregation of sensory cells and conducting nerve cells, is a specialization found only in vertebrates. It allows stimuli to be processed by means of complex circuitry in the sense organs themselves.

**5.2 Placodes.** Placodes may be viewed as primitive sensory fields in the embryonic ectoderm. The placodes of the head give rise to the central sense organs. The *dorsolateral placodes* are the primordia for sense organs of the lateral line type, which are reduced to the auditory and vestibular organs in terrestrial vertebrates. The *epipharyngeal placodes* are primordia for the taste buds, which were also shifted inward and greatly reduced during the transition to life on land. In addition to sensory cells, the placodes give rise to associated peripheral nerve cells. For example, they form the vestibulocochlear ganglion and the double ganglionic series of the cranial nerves. The neural crest can be viewed as a placode for the sensory cells of the skin and the afferent nerve fibers, as well as for the receptors and nerve plexuses of the digestive tract.

**5.3 Transduction chains**. The sensory cells for olfaction, vision, and hearing bear transformed kinocilia and thus may have descended from ciliated cells of the ectoderm. Taste cells, on the other hand, do not possess cilia. Only in the hair cells of the auditory and vestibular organs does ciliary movement still serve in the reception of stimuli; all other sensory cells possess membrane receptors analogous to hormone receptors. The receptor proteins, which possess seven transmembrane domains, are members of a family that also includes the muscarinic acetylcholine receptor, α-adrenergic receptors, and $GABA_B$-receptors. These are all coupled to a *G-protein*. The olfactory receptor forms a variety of epitopes at the cell surface for the different odorous substances, a phenomenon reminiscent of the receptor diversity found in the immune system.

G-proteins in the sensory cells regulate the functional state of the cell by means of adenylate cyclase and cAMP or cGMP levels. This corresponds to the hormonal control of differentiated cells. The G-protein coupled receptors that appear in specific phases of embryonic development influence phospholipase C activity, thereby affecting the regulation of the cell cycle, cell determination, and morphogenesis (→ 3.29).

**5.4 Lateral Lines.** In aquatic vertebrates, the lateral line organs of the head (facial system) and of the trunk (lateral nerve associated with the vagus), as well as the vestibular organ, arise from dorsolateral placodes. Epipharyngeal placodes give rise to the taste buds, which can occur in both the ectoderm of the pharyngeal cleft and the pharynx (endoderm of the pharyngeal pouches). Taste buds are associated with the inferior ganglion series of the facial, glossopharyngeal, and vagus nerves. The sensory cells in the taste buds are not derived directly from the placodes; rather, they are induced by the axons of afferent neurons derived from the epipharyngeal placodes. The innervation of the taste buds is continous with the sensory innervation of the pharynx by the glossopharyngeal and vagus nerves and the general sensory innervation of the digestive tract by neural crest-derived parts of the autonomic nervous system.

**5.5 Olfaction**. During the induction of the olfactory placode, the wall of the prosencephalon and the future olfactory epithelium are closely apposed. This inductive contact is essential for the functional connection between the olfactory epithelium and the olfactory brain and enables regenerative outgrowth of olfactory fibers into the olfactory bulb even in the adult.

Initially, the neuroepithelium of the *olfactory bulb* is completely integrated into the wall of the prosencephalon. In the embryonic period, the bulb forms a downward outpocketing that later (in the fetal period) forms the horizontally lying olfactory bulb. The shift of the olfactory bulb into the horizontal position is caused by the growth of the frontal brain and the corpus callosum. The olfactory fibers are the only afferents of the cerebrum that do not synapse in the thalamus.

The complex circuitry that connects the primary olfactory sensory cells with the mitral cells in the *glomeruli of the bulb* corresponds to the circuitry of secondary sensory cells in the retina and in the spiral ganglion of the auditory and vestibular organs.

**5.6 and 5.7 Eye.** The derivation of the eye and its accessory organs from the optic cup, the surface ectoderm, and the head mesoderm is a classic concept, dating back to the reconstructions of Mann (1928). Here it is supplemented only by a discussion of recent molecular data indicating the role of fibroblast growth factor (FGF) as a secondary embryonic inductor in lens development.

**5.8 Derivation of Internal, Middle, and External Ear.** The overview of ear development from the otic vesicle, the pharyngeal cleft, and pouch follows the description by Patten, in which the labyrinth and the auditory ossicle chain are already symbolically included in the histological section of an embryonic stage.

**5.9 Inner Ear.** The transformation of the otic vesicle into the labyrinth with semicircular ducts and cochlea is described with reference to the wax plate reconstructions of Streeter (1906). A number of cellular details are pointed out in each section shown. The endolymphatic space, like the subarachnoid space, is formed in the loose mesenchyme, which separates the neuroepithelium of the otic vesicle from the cartilage capsule and the subsequently ossified petrous bone. The cupula in the vestibular organ and the tectorial membrane in the cochlea arise by extracellular, surface differentiation of supporting cells in the sensory epithelium. The three-dimensional drawing of the ampulla after Werner (1960) shows that the sections usually made through the ampulla are flat sections that cannot reveal the movement of the cupula in relation to the cuticular plate.

**5.10 Chain of Auditory Ossicles.** The shifting of the primary jaw articulation into the chain of auditory ossicles is illustrative of the entirety of vertebrate evolution. Fusion of the anterior cartilaginous rods of the filtering gut of the lancetfish gives rise to the primary upper and lower jaws, which remain attached to the following cartilages and can open in a scissor-like fashion. With the development of the skull base and the transition to life on land, the upper element becomes free and can develop into an auditory ossicle (columella), which in the former spiracle connects the primitive cochlea (lagena) and the tympanic membrane. With the development of a secondary jaw articulation in mammals, two additional bony elements become free, and the primary jaw joint is relieved of its function. Together with the stapes, which represent the transformed columella, the two bones become arranged into the chain of auditory ossicles.

The development of the pinna from the auricular hillocks, on the other hand, is an embryological development specific to humans and therefore is treated in terms of pure descriptive human embryology.

# Sensory Cells and Placodes

## 5.1 Evolution

### A. On the Evolution of Sensory Cells

**1. Sensory Nerve Cells.** In simple animals like the *polyp (Hydra),* the surface epithelium contains cells specialized for the reception of external chemical or physical stimuli (**1a**). They send out an axon that penetrates the basement membrane of the epithelium and takes part in the formation of a diffuse nerve plexus. A sensory cell with its own axon is called a *sensory nerve cell*, since it possesses properties of both sensory and nerve cells (**1b**).

**2. Assemblage of Sensory Cells into Sensory Fields.** In more highly developed animals, the sensory cells in the surface epithelium are assembled into sensory fields and invaginated into primitive sensory organs. The *visual pit of the snail* in this way enables directional vision with limited spatial resolution (**2a**).

*Amphioxus* (lancetfish, Branchiostoma lanceolatum, → 3.3) possesses a segmentally organized trunk but has neither a brain nor central sense organs (Acrania). Primary sensory cells for chemical and physical stimuli reside in the skin. The neural tube contains *light-sensitive sensory cells* that are associated with light-impermeable *pigment cells* and are arranged in such a way that they can sense the direction of light (**2b**).

**3. The Structure of Sense Organs.** The *lenticular eye of the octopus (cuttlefish)* (**3a**) arises from a sensory field in the surface epithelium that is depressed into an optic vesicle. The *lenticular eye of vertebrates* (**3b**) arises from a sensory field in the neuroepithelium of the already invaginated neural tube. The outgrowth of the optic vesicle and the invagination into an optic cup cause the light-sensitive cells of the vertebrate eye to be oriented inward. If the neuroepithelium could be stretched out from the neural tube and optic cup and integrated into the surface epithelium, it would form a sensory field with the light-sensitive cells directed outward. Different primordia with different genetic information can give rise to lenticular eyes with almost identical functional structures, suggesting that the physical properties of light exert a selective pressure. In evolutionary theory, these various lenticular eyes are examples of *analogous development.*

In the vertebrate eye, reception of stimuli and transmission of impulses are functions of different cells. Sensory cells without axons are known as *secondary sensory cells*; in evolution, these cells first appear in the central sense organs of vertebrates. Primary sensory cells (= sensory nerve cells) are retained only in the olfactory epithelium of vertebrates.

### B. Stimulus Conduction in Primary and Secondary Sensory Cells

**1. Primary Sensory Cells.** A physical or chemical *stimulus* is recognized by a *membrane receptor* and transmitted via an intracellular *transduction chain*. $Na^{+}$channels open and cause the *membrane potential* of the sensory cells to decrease (depolarization). In primary sensory cells, the change in membrane potential is transformed at the root of the axon into propagated *action potentials* with a frequency proportional to the depolarization. The terminal of the axon contains synapses. Action potentials arriving at the terminal cause a reduction in the presynaptic membrane potential, which via $Ca^{++}$ influx triggers exocytosis of the respective *neurotransmitters*.

**2. Secondary Sensory Cells.** A secondary sensory cell possesses no axon of its own. Stimulation of the membrane receptors leads to depolarization and release of *neurotransmitter*, producing a postsynaptic potential in the conducting central or peripheral *nerve cell.* This is converted into propagated action potentials.

Transmission of signals through synapses allows a complex circuitry to be established between secondary sensory cells and propagating nerve cells by additional pre- and postsynaptic contacts and thus enables local impulse processing, which is not possible in the case of primary sensory cells.

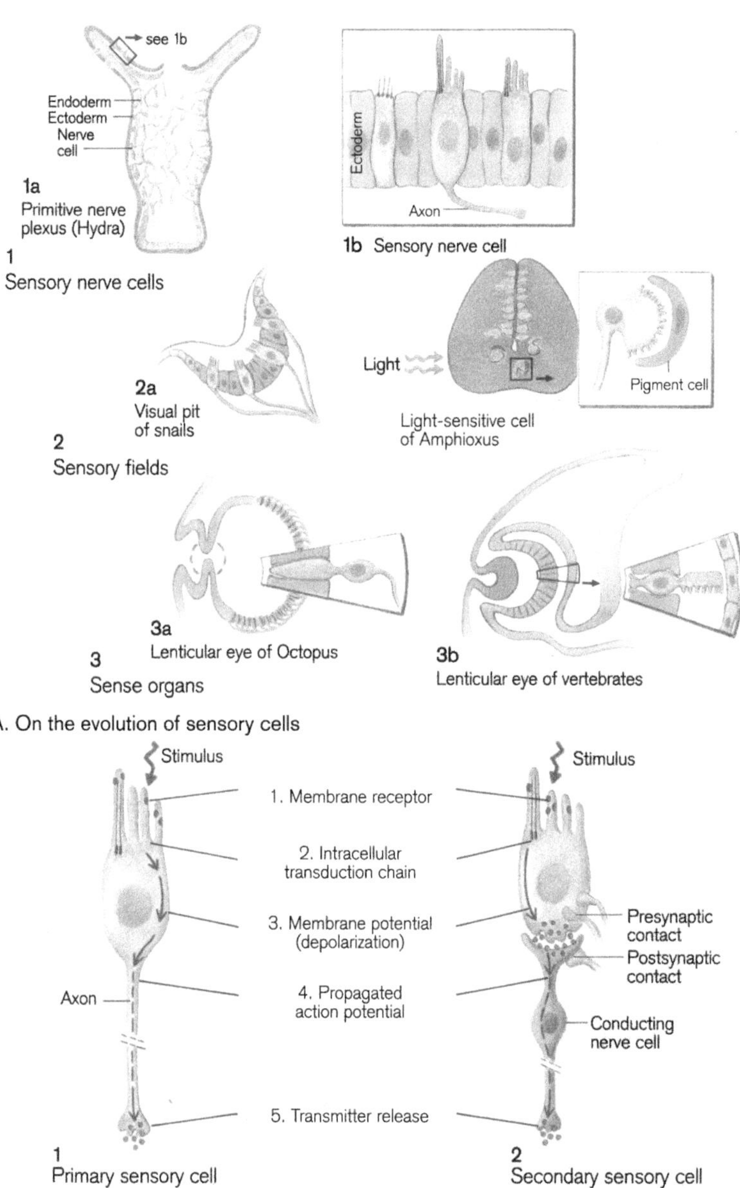


A. On the evolution of sensory cells



B. Stimulus conduction in primary and secondary sensory cells

## 5.2 Placodes

*Background*

**Placodes** are ectodermal thickenings that differentiate into sensory epithelium and sensory ganglia. They give rise to sensory cells and to peripheral nerve cells. Placodes originally represent embryonic sensory fields. The neural plate may be considered a large placode that separates from the ectoderm and becomes transformed into the central nervous system. It contains the efferent motor neurons and in the neural crest (at its margins), the afferent sensory neurons. The neural crest cells migrate outward and form the sensory ganglia and the peripheral nervous system.

### A. Classification of Placodes

**1. Sensory Placodes**

Sensory placodes are the origin for the central sense organs. They are induced in the ectoderm by contact with a specific region of the neural tube that later functions in the central representation of sensory input. As development continues, the placodes become separated from the neural tube. However, the nerve fibers emerging from the placode material find their way to the brain segment that initially induced the placodes.

**Olfactory Placode.** The olfactory placode is induced by the prosencephalon, invaginates into an olfactory pit, and is ultimately integrated as olfactory epithelium into the nasal mucosa. The olfactory placode gives rise to a sensory epithelium with primary sensory cells.

**Optic Vesicle and Lens Placode.** The light-sensitive cells do not reside in the epithelium of the placode, but in the neuroepithelium of the *optic vesicle*. The placode induced by the optic vesicle develops into the lens.

**Otic Placode.** The otic placode is induced by the neuroepithelium of the rhombencephalon and invaginates to form the otic vesicle, which gives rise to the inner ear.

**2. Dorsolateral and Epipharyngeal Placodes.** At the level of the rhombencephalon, two series of placodes associated with the pharyngeal arches—a superior *dorsolateral* and an inferior *epipharyngeal* series—arise. The *otic placode* is one of the dorsolateral placodes, although it is not connected to the pharyngeal arches.

### B. Differentiation of the Placodes

**Migration of Mesoderm.** Apart from sensory cells and neuroblasts, all placodes (**B1** and **2**) give rise to *mesenchymal cells* that leave the placodes and form **head mesoderm**.

**1. Otic Vesicle**. Secondary sensory cells differentiate in the epithelium of the otic vesicle. The associated nerve cells in the *vestibulocochlear ganglion* migrate out from the epithelium, linking the sensory cells in the otic vesicle to centers in the rhombencephalon. The remaining **dorsolateral placodes (B2)** contribute neuroblasts to the superior ganglia of the pharyngeal arch nerves.

**2. Epipharyngeal Placodes.** *Taste buds* are derived from the epipharyngeal placodes. These placodes also contribute neuroblasts to the *inferior ganglia* of the cranial nerves supplying the taste buds (→ 3.12). The taste cells of land-living vertebrates do not arise from the ectoderm, but are induced by nerve endings in the endodermal pharynx.

**3. Neural Crest.** The ganglion cells of the *spinal ganglia* originate in the neural crest. Their axons terminate e.g., on the tactile sensory cells (*Merkel cells*) in the skin. It is uncertain whether Merkel cells, like pigment cells, come from the neural crest or whether they originate in the ectoderm. The axons of afferent neurons in the spinal ganglia also form free nerve endings with receptors for specific transmitters (such as the pain mediator Substance P). Finally, they innervate end organs such as muscle spindles and *tactile corpuscles*.

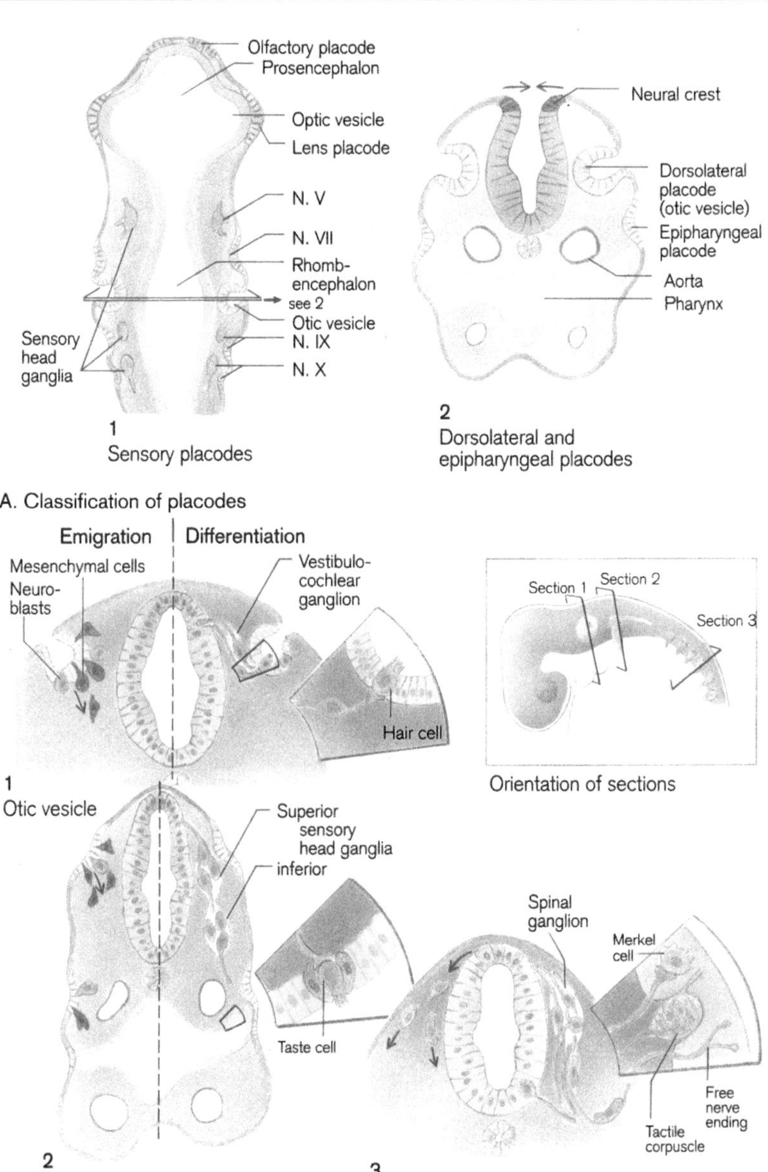


A. Classification of placodes

B. Migration of head mesoderm and differentiation of placodes

## 5.3 Transduction Chain

*Background*

**Sensory cells** can be derived from ciliated cells in the external epithelial layer. In the course of evolution, they formed sensory fields in the ectoderm, and appear as placodes in vertebrate embryos. The transduction cascade can be perceived as a hormone receptor-like mechanism in electrically excitable cells.

### A. Transduction Cascade of the Central Sensory Cells

**Olfactory sensory cells (A1)** arise in the *olfactory placode*; **light-sensing cells (A2)** in the neuroepithelium occupying the inner layer of the *optic cup;* and **hair cells (A3)** of the auditory and vestibular organs in the *otic vesicle*. **Taste cells (A4)** are induced in the endoderm of the pharynx by the gustatory nerves.

**Common Features in the Transduction Chain.** In *olfactory sensory cells* and *light-sensing cells,* the stimulus-sensitive apical segment is derived from a kinocilium that has lost its individual motility. *Hair cells* possess one kinocilium and many stereocilia; *taste cells* possess only stereocilia. In olfactory, visual, and gustatory sensory cells, extracellular stimuli are converted into intracellular signals via a *membrane receptor* coupled to a *G-protein* (guanine-nucleotide-binding protein). The G-protein consists of an α and a β/γ-subunit. The transduction cascade is similar to that of G-protein-coupled hormone receptors. The *hair cells* are excited (depolarized) by passive ciliary movement. Like nerve cells and muscle cells, all sensory cells are electrically excitable: they respond to a stimulus by depolarizing and releasing neurotransmitter at the base of the cell.

At their apical poles, **olfactory sensory cells (A1)** have cilia that project into the mucous layer above the epithelium. The cilia possess receptors for odorous substances. These receptors are bound to a G-protein (inset), which is coupled to the adenylate cyclase (AC). Stimulation of the receptor causes the α-subunit of the G-protein to bind GTP in place of GDP and thus to become activated. The α-subunit is released from the β/γ-complex and activates adenylate cyclase, inducing a rise in cellular cAMP levels and consequently depolarization of the cell. Propagated action potentials are released at the root of the axon of the olfactory sensory cell.

The origin of **light-sensing cells (A2)** from ciliated cells can be deduced from the presence of ciliar structures (a basal body and microtubules) in the neck segment. The cell membrane above the cilium invaginates serially, forming a stack of membrane invaginations that eventually lose contact with the plasma membrane and form an intracellular membrane stack. The invaginated membranes contain *rhodopsin* (visual purple). Rhodopsin consists of retinal, a visual pigment derived from vitamin A that functions as a ligand, and of opsin, the receptor molecule that is coupled to a G-protein (*transducin*). In darkness, the ligand (retinal) occupies the receptor (opsin) in the 11-*cis*-form. Exposure to light causes the 11-cis-retinal to switch into its isomer, all-*trans-retinal*, and to be released from the receptor. The α-subunit of the transducin activates cGMP-phosphodiesterase (PDE), which lowers cellular cGMP levels and thereby opens the sodium channels in the membrane. The light-sensing cell reacts by hyperpolarizing. In the *refractory phase* retinal leaves the receptor and is recycled via the pigment epithelium.

The cilia of the **hair cells (A3)** in the auditory and vestibular organs are activated by the movement of endolymph. Displacement of the stereocilia relative to the kinocilium induces the depolarization of hair cells. Hair cells with mechanoelectrical coupling are related to the sensory cells in the lateral line organs of fish, which detect currents and pressure waves in the surrounding water.

The sensory cells in the **taste buds (A4)** possess microvilli with membrane-bound receptors for *flavored substances*. As in olfactory cells, stimuli are conducted via a G-protein coupled to adenylate cyclase.

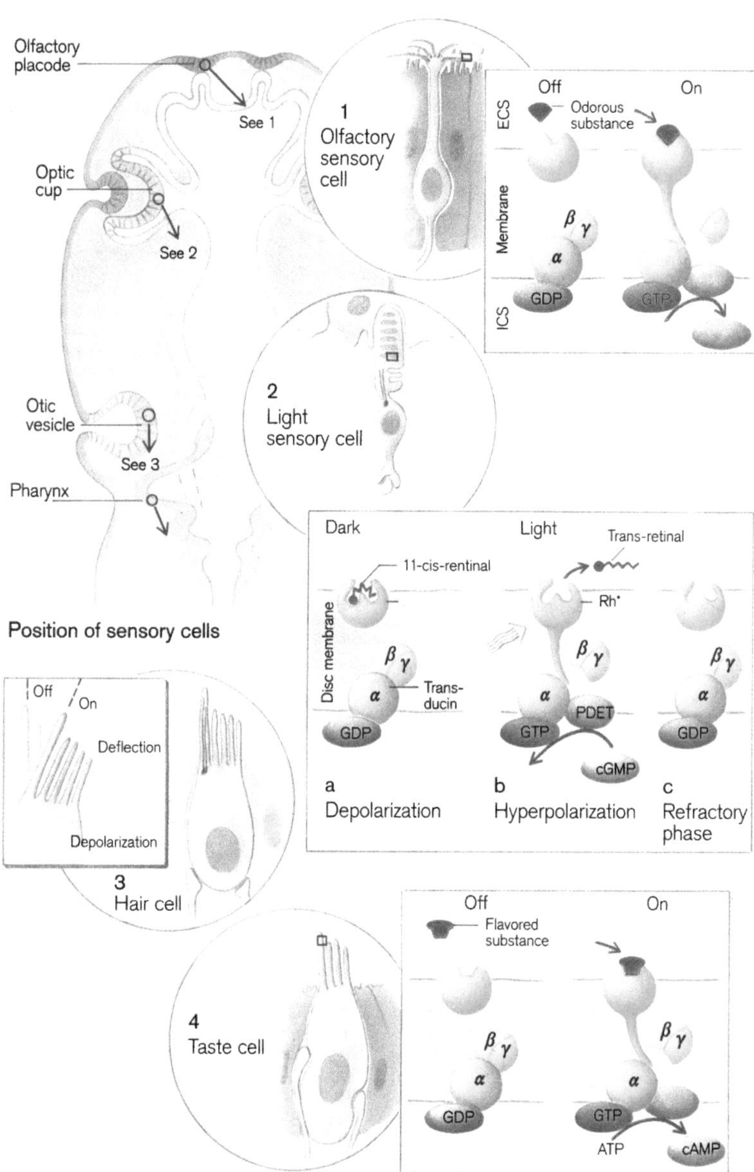


A. Transduction chain of central sensory cells

# Sense ot Taste

## 5.4 Lateral Line Organs and Taste Buds

*Background*

In their ectoderm, fish possess extensive **sensory fields** by which currents and "flavored substances" in the water can be perceived. These sensory fields disappeared in the transition to life on land. Of the dorsolateral placodes (for detection of currents), only the semicircular duct system persists, while of the epipharyngeal placodes (for taste), only the taste buds of the 2nd, 3rd, and 4th cranial nerves remain. These are now internalized into the endoderm.

### A. Placodes and Sensory Fields

In aquatic vertebrates, the **dorsolateral placodes** (**A1**) give rise to the sensory fields of lateral line organs. The respective sensory cells and the sensory ganglion cells migrate from the placodes during the embryonic period and form the **lateral line organs** of the head and the trunk (**A2**). In *fish*, the lateral line organs consist of a canal system sunken into the skin, into which the sensory cilia of the sensory cells project. In the *amphibian larvae* (**2a**), the *cilia* of the *sensory cells* of the lateral line are embedded in a *cupula*, which projects from the body surface. The lateral lines enable pressure waves in the water to be perceived.

The vestibular organ is a special form of lateral line organ, in which the canal system is closed off from the surface so that changes in the position of the body can be perceived through movement of the endolymph.

The *lateral line organs of the head* (**A2**) originate from the dorsolateral placodes located in front of the otic vesicle. The associated sensory ganglia and nerves derive from the *facial nerve*. The *lateral lines of the trunk* arise from placodes situated behind the otic vesicle. They are supplied by the *lateral nerve*, which is considered a branch of the vagus. The lateral line organs disappeared completely during the transition to life on land, whereas the semicircular ducts (equilibrium) were supplemented by the development of the cochlea (hearing).

**Taste buds** are sensory fields containing sensory cells for chemical stimuli and are sunken into the surface epithelium (**2b**). In aquatic vertebrates, they are arranged in the ectoderm and in the endoderm of the oral cavity and of the pharyngeal clefts. In some fish, such as the catfish, they are distributed over the entire surface of the body.

The **epipharyngeal placodes** (**A1**) contribute ganglion cells to the *epipharyngeal ganglia* (**A2**) of the cranial nerves VII (geniculate ganglion); IX and X that innervate the taste buds. The sensory cells for the taste buds do not migrate from the epipharyngeal placodes, but are induced by the terminal branches of the gustatory nerves. The significance of the epipharyngeal placodes in the development of the sense of taste is illustrated by the fact that species with many taste buds possess highly developed epipharyngeal placodes during embryonic life.

### B. Taste Buds in Humans

The development of taste buds is induced in the tongue and in the entire pharyngeal space by the terminal branchings of the facial, glossopharyngeal, and vagus nerves. Taste buds consist of *secondary sensory cells*, *supporting cells*, and *basal cells*. The sensory cells are continuously renewed (**B2**). The development of the taste buds peaks between the 5th and 7th fetal month; toward the end of the fetal period and after birth, most taste buds atrophy. This regression during fetal development recapitulates the regression in the course of phylogeny. The taste buds are concentrated at the base of the tongue, in the pits of the *vallate papillae* (circumvallate papillae) (**B3**). In the *development of the papillae* (**B1**), taste buds initially also arise on the surface (**1a**), but these taste buds atrophy, and only those in the pits of the vallate papillae are preserved (**1c**). The taste buds at the base of the tongue are sensitive to bitter tastes; those at the margin, to acidic and salty tastes; and those at the tip of the tongue, to sweet tastes.

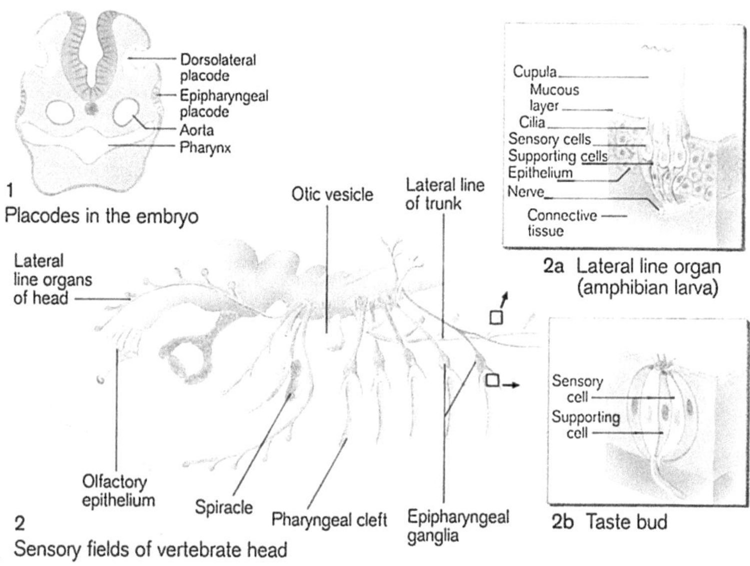
Dorsolateral placode
Epipharyngeal placode
Aorta
Pharynx
1
Placodes in the embryo
Otic vesicle
Lateral line of trunk
Cupula
Mucous layer
Cilia
Sensory cells
Supporting cells
Epithelium
Nerve
Connective tissue
2a Lateral line organ (amphibian larva)
Lateral line organs of head
Sensory cell
Supporting cell
Olfactory epithelium
Spiracle
Pharyngeal cleft
Epipharyngeal ganglia
2b Taste bud
2
Sensory fields of vertebrate head

A. Placodes and sensory fields

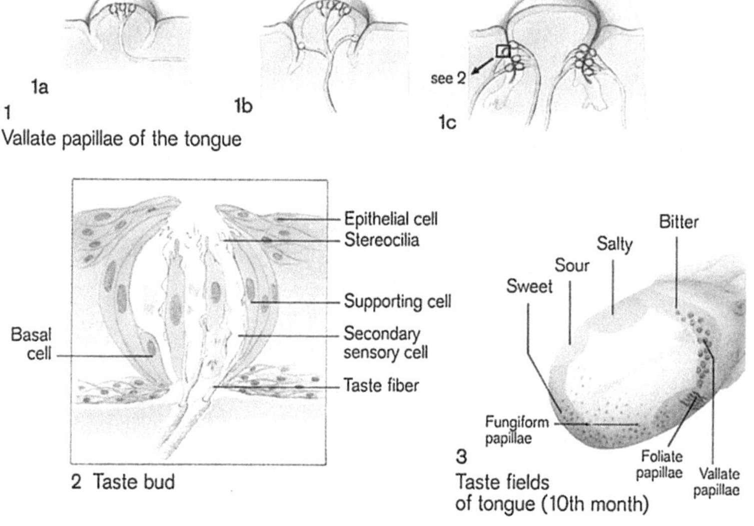
1a
1
1b
see 2
1c
Vallate papillae of the tongue
Epithelial cell
Stereocilia
Supporting cell
Basal cell
Secondary sensory cell
Taste fiber
2 Taste bud
Bitter
Salty
Sour
Sweet
Fungiform papillae
Foliate papillae
Vallate papillae
3
Taste fields of tongue (10th month)

B. Development of taste buds in the human

Sense of Smell

# 5.5 Olfactory Organ

## A. Development of the Sense of Smell

**1. Induction of the Olfactory Placode.** The olfactory placode is induced in stage 9, when the surface ectoderm makes direct contact with the prosencephalic vesicle. The thickened ectoderm of the olfactory placode gives rise to the olfactory epithelium.

**2. Invagination of the Olfactory Pit.** Migration of *head mesenchyme* causes the epithelium to detach from the wall of the prosencephalon (**2a**). Proliferation of the mesenchyme leads to the formation of the *lateral* and *medial nasal swellings*, between which the olfactory epithelium sinks in and forms the olfactory pit. The *nasal septum* forms between the apposed medial nasal swellings.

The epithelium of the olfactory pit forms a *medial* and a *lateral*, upward-directed *outpocketing* (**2a**). The roof of the dorsolateral outpocketing of the olfactory pit gives rise to the definitive olfactory epithelium, while the medial outpocketing forms the **vomeronasal organ** (Jacobson's organ). This organ contains olfactory cells for pheromones involved in reproduction and brood care. In humans, the vomeronasal organ recedes during fetal life (→ 2.31, 1b). A small blind-ending process may persist in the lower segment of the nasal septum.

**3. Nasal Cavity.** The olfactory pit enlarges posteriorly, and in stage 19 it breaks through into the oral cavity (*primary choanae*) (→ 9.1). Fusion of the *palatal processes* extends the nasal cavity posteriorly (*secondary choanae*). The olfactory epithelium comes to lie in the roof of the nasal cavity.

**4. Olfactory Bulb and Olfactory Fibers.** In stage 16, the axons of the primary sensory cells of the *olfactory epithelium* grow outward and contact the nerve cells in the anterior wall of the *prosencephalon* (**4a**), which becomes the telencephalon. At this stage, the olfactory bulb has not yet developed. In stage 22, a *bulb* begins to differentiate from the telencephalon (**4b**). It initially grows in the inferior direction, but turns back medially in stage 23 (→ 4.8, A4). During the fetal period, it is shifted into the sagittal plane and comes to lie on the *ethmoidal plate* (**4c**). The ventricular lumen in the olfactory bulb is obliterated.

The *ethmoidal plate* of the ethmoid bone is a part of the cartilaginous nasal capsule (**A3**) that surrounds the invaginated olfactory epithelium. Olfactory fibers connect the olfactory bulb and the olfactory epithelium before the nasal capsule develops. Cartilage forms only between the olfactory fiber, so that the nerve canals remain open after endochondral ossification of the ethmoid has taken place.

The olfactory epithelium, which consists of supporting cells and *sensory cells* (**4c**), forms the olfactory area in the respiratory epithelium of the nose, above the superior nasal concha. The olfactory cells are primary sensory cells (→ 5.1). Their axons are not myelinated. In the olfactory bulb, their ramified ends form a meshwork of synaptic contacts (*glomerulus*) with the dendritic processes of *mitral cells*. Dendritic glomeruli are specific to primary olfactory sensory cells and enable stimulus processing analogous to that in central sense organs with secondary sensory cells (→ 5. 1B).

The **life span of olfactory sensory cells** is about 3 weeks. Sensory cells regenerate from stem cells in the olfactory epithelium. The new axons grow along the preformed nerve pathways through the ethmoidal plate to the bulb. The olfactory area is larger in the fetal period than after birth and continues to regress throughout life. The olfactory sense is poorly developed in man. The regression of the olfactory area during ontogeny reflects the phylogenetic regression of the sense of smell.

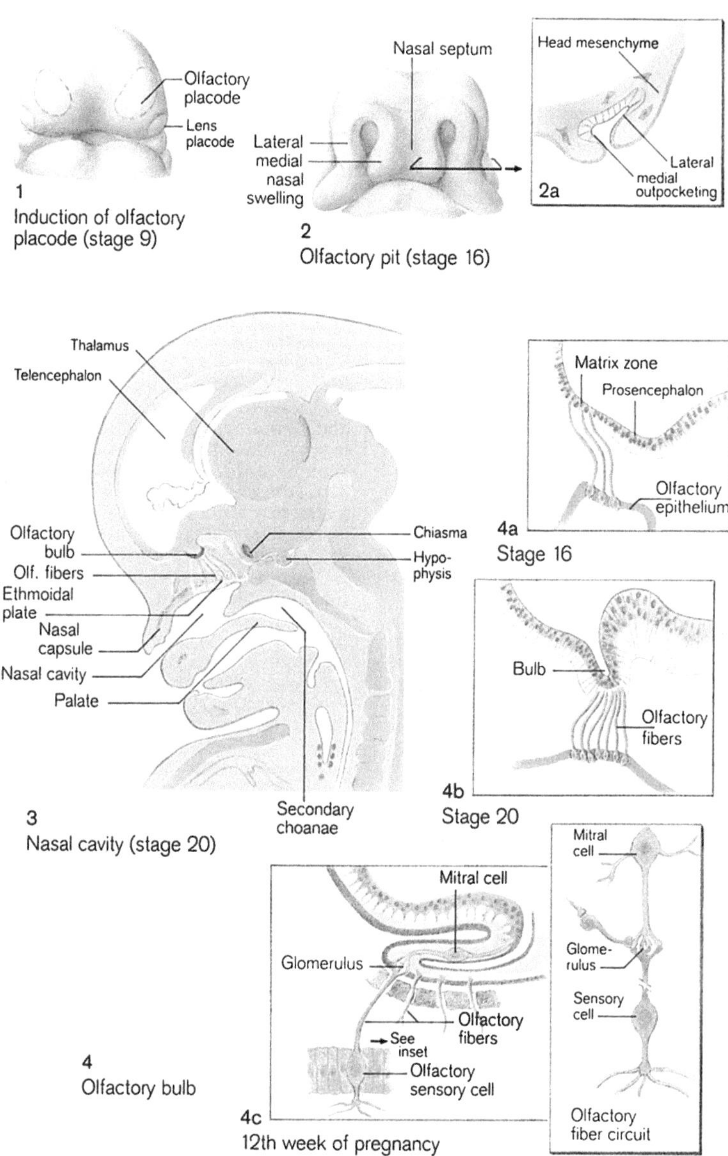

Olfactory placode
Lens placode
1
Induction of olfactory placode (stage 9)
Nasal septum
Lateral
medial
nasal
swelling
2
Olfactory pit (stage 16)
Head mesenchyme
Lateral
medial
outpocketing
2a
Thalamus
Telencephalon
Olfactory bulb
Olf. fibers
Ethmoidal plate
Nasal capsule
Nasal cavity
Palate
Chiasma
Hypophysis
Secondary choanae
3
Nasal cavity (stage 20)
Matrix zone
Prosencephalon
Olfactory epithelium
4a
Stage 16
Bulb
Olfactory fibers
4b
Stage 20
Mitral cell
Glomerulus
Olfactory fibers
See inset
Olfactory sensory cell
4c
12th week of pregnancy
Mitral cell
Glomerulus
Sensory cell
Olfactory fiber circuit
4
Olfactory bulb

A. Development of sense of smell

# Sense of Vision

# 5.6 Optic Cup

## A. Development of the Optic Cup

**1. Optic Sulcus.** The rudiments of the eye evaginate from the wall of the forebrain (*prosencephalon*). Evagination begins before the neural tube has closed; in stage 11, the optic sulcus is visible through the open anterior neuropore. On account of the strong curvature of the embryo, the optic sulci are directed downward (→ 2.17 A3 and 4.7 A1).

The cells of the cephalic neural crest migrate out before the neural tube has closed and form *head mesoderm*. The emigration is not restricted to the fold between neuroectoderm and surface ectoderm, but extends over the entire primordium of the optic vesicle.

**2. Optic Vesicle and Lens Placode.** After the closure of the neural tube in stage 12, the optic vesicle induces the lens placode in the surface ectoderm by direct contact (→ 3.6).

**3. Optic Cup.** In stage 14, the *optic vesicle* invaginates to form the *optic cup* and the *lens placode* invaginates to form the *lens vesicle*. A stalk connects the optic cup to the diencephalon, which arises from the prosencephalic vesicle (→ 4.8).

## B. Optic Cup and Optic Cup Fissure.

**1. Retina.** The *inner layer* of the optic cup gives rise to the actual *retina*, while the *outer layer* forms the *pigment epithelium* of the retina. The two layers are separated by a space, the *optic ventricle*, which continues into the third ventricle via the stalk of the optic cup. In the inner layer of the optic cup, the neuroepithelial cells differentiate into *sensory cells* (rods and cones), *bipolar nerve cells*, and *ganglion cells*, which send their axons centrally to the thalamus and into the quadrigeminal plate. The sensory cells are directed externally into the optic ventricle, whereas the nerve fibers, travelling on the internal surface of the retina, converge at the stalk of the optic cup.

**2. Optic Nerve and Optic Cup Fissure.** The *nerve fibers* that pass to the diencephalon from the retina ultimately fill the *optic stalk* and transform it into the optic nerve. The optic ventricle is obliterated (**2a** and **b**).

The interior of the optic cup and the lens vesicle are supplied with blood from the surface of the developing brain. The *hyaloid artery*, a branch of the ophthalmic artery, enters the optic cup at its medial and inferior side through a fissure in the optic cup. This *optic cup fissure* (choroid fissure) later closes around the vessels, so that the hyaloid artery courses in the optic nerve. After obliteration of the branches that pass through the vitreous body into the lens, the hyaloid artery becomes the *central artery of the retina*.

**Malformation:** In rare cases, the embryonic optic cup fissure fails to close, leading to an **anomaly (coloboma)** of the optic cup. A mild form is a cleft in the iris (**coloboma iridis**) directed medially and inferiorly.

**3. Lens.** The *lens vesicle* separates from the ectoderm. Cells in the posterior layer of the lens vesicle elongate and become organized into parallel lens fibers. This forms the *lens hillock*. The lens fibers produce lens crystallins, specific proteins that are deposited intracellularly and determine the refractive properties of the lens.

**Inset:** Lens cells divide in the anterior layer of the lens vesicle. At the equator, they migrate posteriorly, elongate, and begin to differentiate. *Proliferation, migration,* and *differentiation* are regulated by gradients of fibroblast growth factor (FGF).

The lens fibers in the lens hillock form the *lens nucleus*, which is covered anteriorly by cuboidal lens epithelium derived from the anterior layer of the lens vesicle. New lens fibers are formed mitotically in the equatorial zone and are added to the lens nucleus up to the 20th year of life.

Pros-
encephalon
Head
mesoderm
1 Optic sulcus
Lens
placode
2 Optic vesicle
Invagination
of
lens placode
3 Optic cup

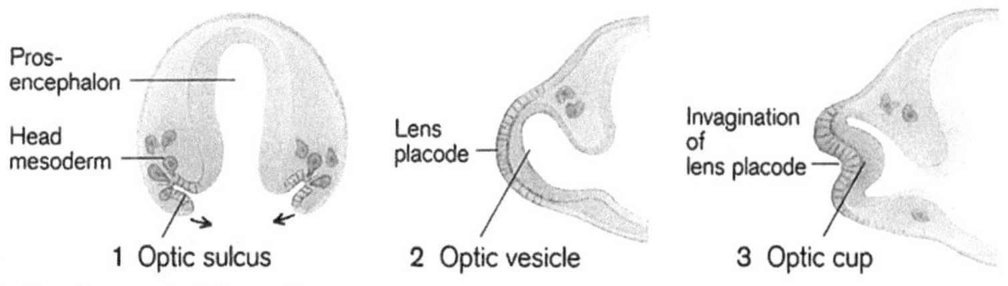

A. Development of the optic cup

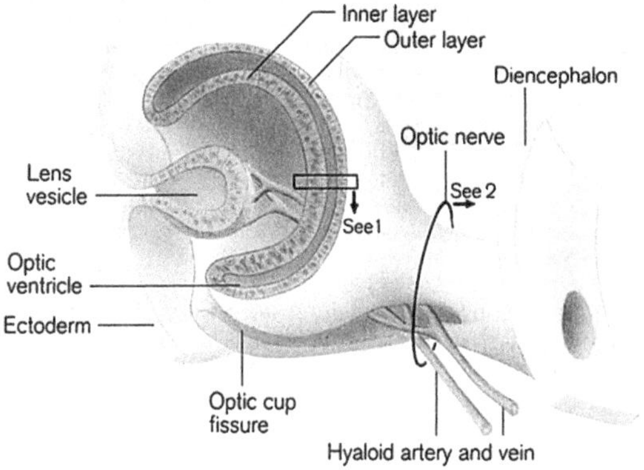

Inner layer
Outer layer
Diencephalon
Optic nerve
Lens
vesicle
See 2
See 1
Optic
ventricle
Ectoderm
Optic cup
fissure
Hyaloid artery and vein

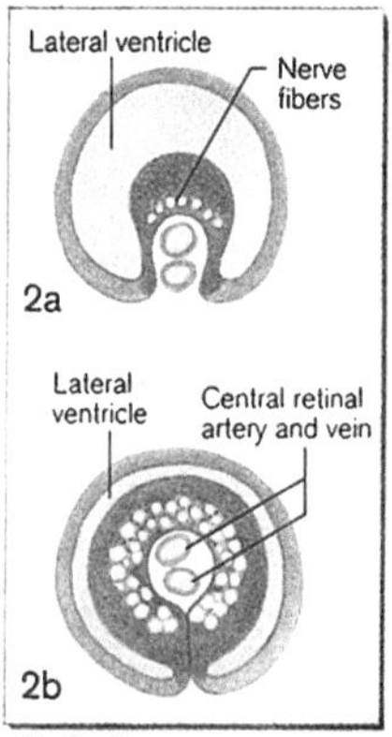

Lateral ventricle
Nerve
fibers
2a
Lateral
ventricle
Central retinal
artery and vein
2b

2 Optic nerve

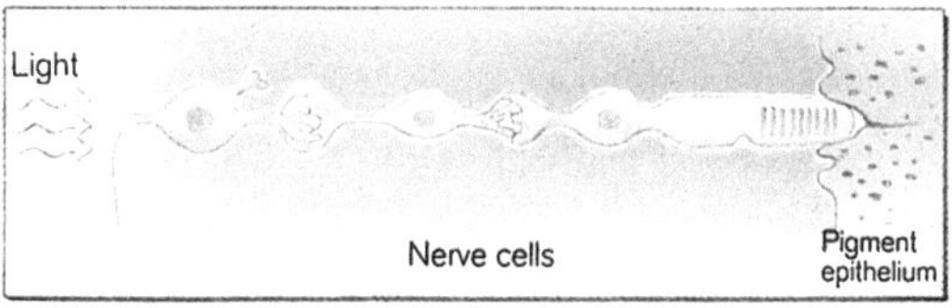

Light
Nerve cells
Pigment
epithelium

1 Retina

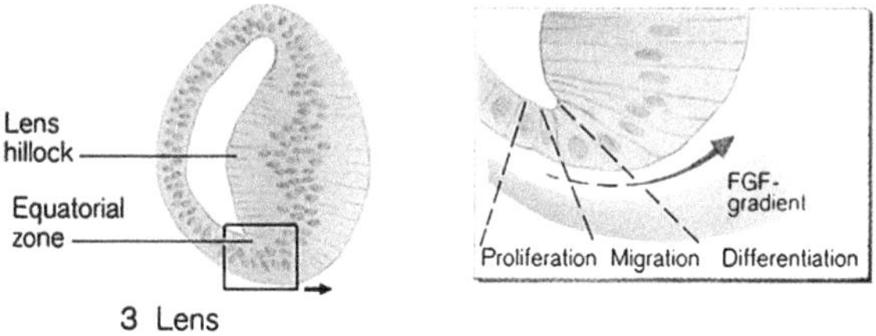

Lens
hillock
Equatorial
zone
FGF-
gradient
Proliferation
Migration
Differentiation

3 Lens

B. Optic cup and optic fissure

## 5.7 Accessory Organs of the Eye

### C. Sclera, Cornea, and Iris

**Choroid and Sclera.** At the end of the embryonic period, the optic cup and the lens are still supplied solely by the *hyaloid artery* (**C1**). Then, the terminal branch passing through the vitreous body to the lens is obliterated, and the stem of the vessel becomes the *central retinal artery*. The blood supply is taken over by a richly vascularized layer surrounding the pigment epithelium of the optic cup. This layer, known as the *choroid* (**C2**), corresponds to the pia mater of the brain. In addition to blood vessels, it contains many pigment cells.

Closely surrounding the choroid is a rigid, collagen-rich tissue, the *sclera*, which corresponds to the *dura mater* of the brain and is continuous with the dural covering of the optic nerve. The extrinsic ocular muscles are derived from the "preotic myotomes." They insert into the sclera and take origin in the dura of the optic nerve at the optic foramen (**C2**).

**Cornea.** Anteriorly, the sclera is continuous with the stroma of the *cornea*. In the loose connective tissue between the cornea and the lens, a space—the *anterior chamber*—arises (**C2**). It is lined by a flat epithelium of mesenchymal origin (*mesothelium*). Externally to internally, the cornea consists of three layers: an epithelial layer derived from *surface ectoderm*, a layer of dense connective tissue called the *substantia propria* (which is continuous with the sclera), and the *mesothelium*, which lines the anterior chamber. The transparency of the cornea is due to its turgescence, which is maintained by ATP-dependent ionic pumps.

The richly vascularized, loose connective tissue between the anterior chamber and the lens is a continuation of the choroid and is known as the *iridopupillary (pupillary) membrane*. After the eye has differentiated, it normally disappears and leaves the pupil free of obstruction.

**Malformation: Persistence of the Pupillary Membrane** is a frequent anomaly. A network of connective tissue fibers lies in the pupil in front of the lens.

**Iris and Ciliary Body.** The *iris* and the *ciliary body* develop from the margins of the optic cup (**C2**). The *pigment epithelium* of the retina continues into the iris, and the inner layer of the optic cup persists as a single layer of cells containing no neurons (**2a**). The internal ocular muscles—i.e. the *sphincter* and *dilator pupillae* and the *ciliary muscles*—are derived from the neural ectoderm of the optic cup and lie in the mesenchyme, which surrounds the iris.

The loose mesenchyme between the lens and *ciliary body* gives rise to the *suspensory ligaments* of the lens (**2a**), which function in regulating the lens curvature in response to contraction or relaxation of the ciliary muscles (accomodation). The mesenchyme and the gelatinous ground substance then disappear, so that a posterior chamber arises around the lens. After the obliteration of the *hyaloid artery* (**C2**), the mesenchyme in the optic cup is transformed into the clear gelatinous ground substance, forming the *vitreous body* of the eye.

The folds of the ciliary processes secrete *aqueous humor*, which passes from the posterior chamber through the pupil to the anterior chamber, where it is discharged into the canal of Schlemm, a circular lymphatic vessel in the angle of the anterior chamber.

**Eyelids and Lacrimal Apparatus.** The *eyelids* are folds of ectoderm and associated mesoderm that slide over the eye from above and below (**C1**). At the end of the embryonic period, the eyelids are still open (→ 2.32). In the fetal period, however, the eyelids close and become fused (**C2**, → 2.37), opening again only shortly before birth. The underside of the eyelid is lined by a delicate ectodermal epithelium with loose, richly vascularized connective tissue that continues onto the sclera of the eyeball as the *conjunctiva*.

The **lacrimal gland** and the nasolacrimal duct are ectodermal structures. The nasolacrimal duct arises as a compact, epithelial duct between the frontal process and the maxillary process. Its lumen forms only shortly before birth (→ 9.1).

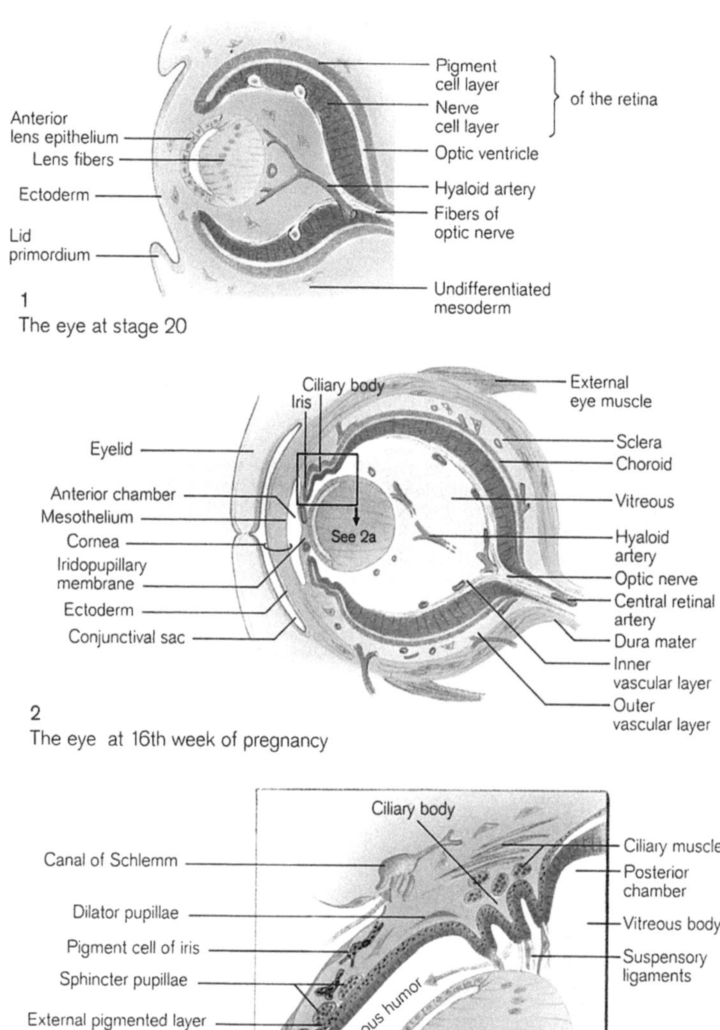


1
The eye at stage 20



2
The eye at 16th week of pregnancy



2a Iris and ciliary body

C. Accessory organs of the eye

# Auditory and Vestibular Organs

## 5.8 Derivation of the Ear

### A. Development from Otic Vesicle and Pharyngeal Arches

**1. Otic Vesicle and Pharynx in Stage 13**

The inner ear develops from the *otic vesicle*, the middle ear from the *first pharyngeal pouch*, and the external auditory meatus from the *first pharyngeal cleft* (**A1**). In stage 13 (4.6 mm), the otic vesicle and the pharynx with the pharyngeal clefts are established independently of each other (→ 2.22).

**2. Transformation into the Inner Ear and Middle Ear**

**Inner Ear.** In stage 11, the otic placode (**2a**) is induced in the ectoderm of the wall of the rhombencephalon; in stage 12, it invaginates to form the *otic pit* (**2b**). Neuroblasts for the *vestibulocochlear ganglion* (**2c**) migrate out from the otic vesicle. Superiorly, the *endolymphatic duct* (**2d**) grows out. Its upper end possesses an ampullary dilatation, which after closure of the otic vesicle, comes to lie underneath the dura at the bony petrous bone and serves as a pressure-equalizing vessel for the endolymph. Further development of the otic vesicle produces the semicircular ducts and the cochlea of the inner ear (**2e**).

**Middle Ear and Auditory Ossicles.** The middle ear arises from the first pharyngeal pouch (**2c**); the connection to the pharynx persists as the *auditory tube*. The *tympanic membrane* originates from the endoderm of the first pharyngeal pouch and the ectoderm of the first pharyngeal cleft. First, however, the contact zone (**2c**) between the endoderm and ectoderm disappears and mesoderm migrates in between the epithelial layers (**2d**). In the extension of the first and second pharyngeal pouches, loose mesoderm condenses into the primordia of the auditory ossicles. The *hammer* (malleus) and the *anvil* (incus) are derived from the cartilage of the first pharyngeal arch, the *stirrup* (stapes) from that of the second.

The ampullary dilatation at the end of the first pharyngeal pouch (*auditory tube*) (**2e**) extends out into the loose mesenchyme in the interior of the cartilaginous otic capsule (arrow), forming the *tympanic cavity*. The endoderm of the pharyngeal pouch then covers the auditory ossicles and becomes closely apposed to the inner side of the future *tympanic membrane* (dotted lines). In the same fashion, the chambers in the mastoid process are "pneumatized" and lined with endoderm as the paranasal sinuses widen after birth.

The *inner ear*, containing the labyrinth, becomes enclosed by the cartilaginous otic capsule. Between the inner ear and the middle ear, a canal in the future petrous bone contains the *facial nerve*. Since the facial nerve comes from the second pharyngeal arch, already in stage 13 (**A1**) it takes its course between the otic vesicle and the first pharyngeal pouch.

**External Auditory Meatus.** The external auditory meatus develops from the first *pharyngeal cleft* (**2c**). After dissolution of the original contact zone between the endoderm and ectoderm (**2d**), the external auditory meatus grows inward as a compact ectodermal epithelial cone (*meatal plug* ) (**2e**) that becomes canalized secondarily in the 7th month. The *tympanic membrane* is covered on the inner side by the endoderm of the tympanic cavity and on the outer side by the ectoderm of the external auditory meatus. The two layers enclose a layer of mesoderm in which the handle of the malleus is embedded.

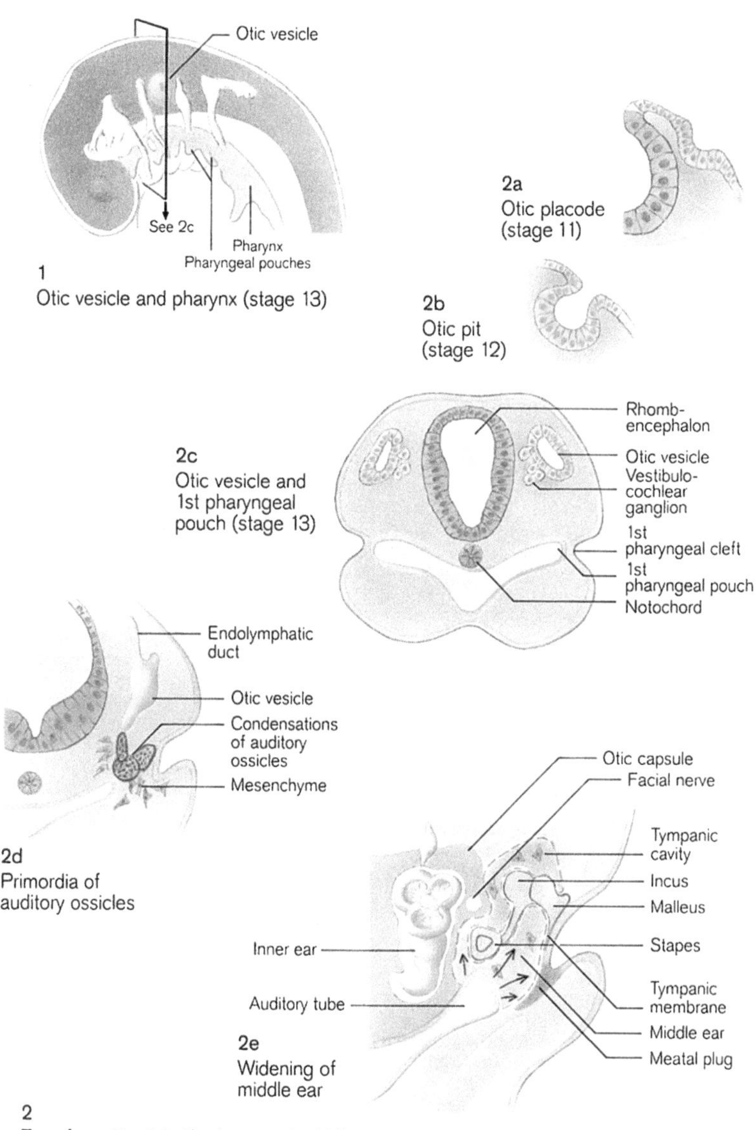


2
Transformation into the inner and middle ear

A. Development of the ear

## 5.9 Inner Ear

### B. Transformation of the Otic Vesicle into the Labyrinth

**1. Otic Vesicle (stage 15).** In stage 15 (9mm), the otic vesicle is characterized by relatively large extension of the endolymphatic duct. The vesicle is subdivided into a superior, club-shaped segment that will give rise to the *vestibular apparatus,* and an inferior process that will develop into the *cochlea.* The neuroblasts migrating from the otic vesicle form the *vestibulo-cochlear ganglion*, the subdivision of which is already indicated by the separation of the *cochlear* and *vestibular nerves*.

**2. Origin of the Semicircular Ducts (stage 16).** In the developing vestibular apparatus, the *utriculus* with the semicircular ducts (above) and the *saccule* (below) become delineated. The *semicircular ducts* originate as flat, crescent-shaped outpocketings of the otic vesicle, whose central wall segments coalesce and disappear (insets).

The vestibular apparatus (vestibule = entrance of the cochlea) is found in all vertebrates. An outpocketing of the labyrinth, which enables the perception of sound waves in the air arose in the transition to life on land (lagena in amphibians and birds, 5.10 D1c).

**3. Development of the Cochlea (stage 23).** The *cochlea*, together with the auditory ossicles, first developed in mammals. The cochlea grows out downward from the saccule and is ultimately connected with the saccule only by a narrow duct (*ductus reuniens*).

### C. Differentiation of Sensory Cells

The sensory cells in the wall of the otic vesicle project apically into the *endolymph,* filling the otic vesicle. Initially, this space communicates with the outside world, corresponding to the canal system of the lateral line organs of fish (→ 5.4). After the otic vesicle has internalized, its cavity corresponds to the ventricular space in the cerebral vesicles.

The **sensory cells** are located on the sensory crest in the ampullary dilatations of the *semicircular ducts* (**1a**) at the exit of the utricle, as well as in the macula of the utricle and saccule. In the *cochlea* (**2a**), sensory cells form the external and internal *hair cells* on the basilar membrane of the *organ of Corti* (**2b**). The sensory cells possess a *kinocilium* and up to 100 *stereocilia*, which are anchored to the cell surface by actin filaments (**1b**, inset). Movement of the stereocilia relative to the kinocilium induces a depolarization of the sensory cells proportional to the direction and strength of the deviation. The cilia are anchored in the *cuticular plate* (**1b**), which consists of intracellular microfilaments extending between the cell junctions. A firm, extracellular, gelatinous substance surrounds the cilia. It is formed by the glycocalix of adjacent supporting cells. This substance synchronizes and amplifies the mechanical stimulus caused by movement of the endolymph. On the *ampullary crests* of the semicircular ducts, the gelatinous substance forms the *cupula* (**1b**), which can move in "saddle-fashion" relative to the sensory cells on the *crest.* In the maculae of the utricle and saccule, *otoliths* of calcium salts are deposited in the gelatinous statoconial membrane in which the cilia of the sensory cells are inserted. In the organ of Corti, the supporting cells at the limbus produce a corresponding gelatinous structure with similar function, the *tectorial membrane* (**2b**).

**Perilymphatic Space.** The labyrinth formed by the otic vesicle is enclosed by a cartilaginous otic capsule that later ossifies (**1a**), leaving a narrow margin of loose mesenchyme between the otic capsule and the basement membrane of the membranous labyrinth. The intercellular spaces in the mesenchyme coalesce, forming the *perilymphatic space.* This space communicates with the cerebrospinal fluid in the subarachnoid space via a canal system. In the cochlea, the perilymphatic space forms the *scala vestibuli* and *scala tympani* (**2b**), which are continuous with each other at the apex of the cochlea (helicotrema).

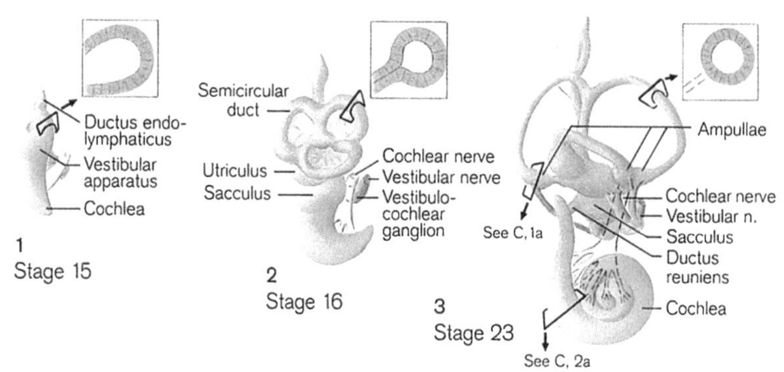


B. Transformation of the otic vesicle into the labyrinth

Cartilaginous capsule
Perilymph
Endolymph
Sensory cell

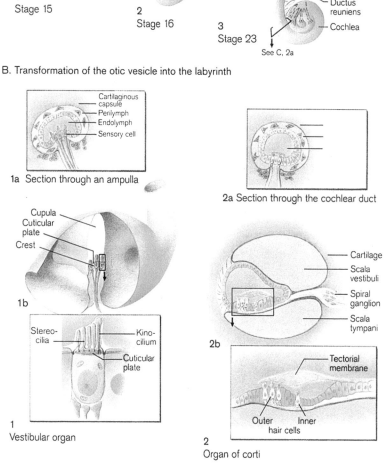

1a Section through an ampulla

2a Section through the cochlear duct

Cupula
Cuticular plate
Crest
1b

Stereo-cilia
Kino-cilium
Cuticular plate

1
Vestibular organ

Cartilage
Scala vestibuli
Spiral ganglion
Scala tympani
2b

Tectorial membrane
Outer
Inner
hair cells

2
Organ of corti

C. Differentiation of sensory cells

## 5.10 Displacement of Primary Jaw Joint

### D. Displacement into the Chain of Auditory Ossicles

#### 1. Derivation of the Primary Jaw Joint from the Pharyngeal Arches

**a Primordial Pharynx.** In jawless vertebrates (Agnatha), the primordial pharynx is supported by cartilaginous pharyngeal arches, which lie between the gill clefts. Each pharyngeal arch contains two cartilaginous skeletal elements connected by joints.

**b Fusion of Anterior Bridges of Cartilage into the Jaws.** The primary upper and lower jaw of vertebrates arises by the fusion of cartilaginous elements of the three or four pharyngeal arches. The *primary jaw articulation* between the primary upper jaw (*palatoquadratum*) and the primary *lower jaw* (Meckels cartilage) is produced by the articulation of the upper and lower pharyngeal arch elements. With the development of the primary jaws, the first pharyngeal cleft is displaced upward and becomes the *spiracle* in fish. The upper skeletal element of the second pharyngeal arch, the *hyomandibular*, becomes a support for the primary jaw joint, which movably connects the mandibular bone with the base of the skull.

**c Development of the Columella.** In the transition to life on land, the primary upper jaw (palatoquadratum) becomes fused with the *base of the skull*. The spiracle (first pharyngeal cleft), becomes closed by the *tympanic membrane*. The function of sound transmission between the tympanic membrane and the *labyrinth* is taken over by the upper element of the hyoid arch (hyomandibular). It gives rise to the *columella* of amphibians and birds, which conducts sound from the tympanic membrane to the inner ear through the air-filled tympanic cavity.

**d The Secondary Jaw Joint in Mammals.** Development of a *secondary jaw articulation* in mammals permits the closure of the oral fissure and thus enables sucking movements. It forms between the phylogenetically young desmally ossifying bones of the viscerocranium. The primary jaw articulation is retained between the *malleus* and the *incus*, while the columella persists as the *stapes*. The auditory ossicles allow the sensitivity of sound conduction to be regulated by variation in the tension of the stapedius muscle and the auditory tube muscle.

#### 2. Pharyngeal Arch Cartilage and Auditory Ossicles in Man

The joint between the *malleus* and *incus* corresponds to the primary jaw joint. The original connection to the skull base (hyomandibular, columella) is the *stapes*, which now links the *incus* with the otic capsule and the inner ear. The *secondary jaw articulation* arises between the dermally ossified mandible and the temporal bone. The auditory ossicles lose their connection to the pharyngeal arches.

The *facial nerve (VII)* is the nerve of the second pharyngeal arch. Its main branch passes between the inner ear and the middle ear and leaves the bony skull parallel to and behind the styloid process (the remnant of the hyoid arch). The branch of this cranial nerve passing in front of the pharyngeal cleft is called the *chorda tympani* (→ 5.4 A2, pink). It contains sympathetic fibers for the submandibular ganglion and taste fibers from the anterior two-thirds of the tongue.

### E. Development of the Auricle

The differentiation of the chain of auditory ossicles and the expansion of the tympanic cavity are accompanied by an elongation and deepening of the external auditory meatus (development of the meatal plug) and the development of the external ear. The auricle develops from six **auricular hillocks** organized around the first pharyngeal cleft (→ 2.25). The *tragus* and *helix* develop from the anterior three hillocks; the *antitragus* and *antihelix* from the posterior three.

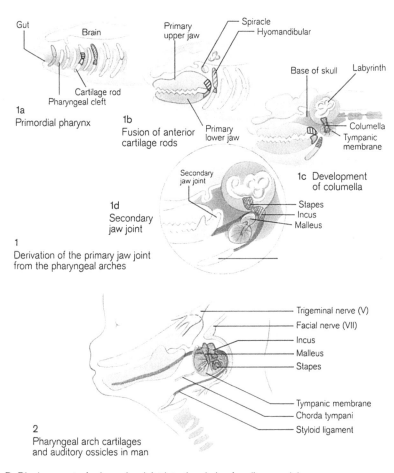

Gut
Brain
Cartilage rod
Pharyngeal cleft

1a
Primordial pharynx

Primary upper jaw
Spiracle
Hyomandibular
Primary lower jaw

1b
Fusion of anterior cartilage rods

Base of skull
Labyrinth
Columella
Tympanic membrane

1c Development of columella

Secondary jaw joint
Stapes
Incus
Malleus

1d
Secondary jaw joint

1
Derivation of the primary jaw joint from the pharyngeal arches

Trigeminal nerve (V)
Facial nerve (VII)
Incus
Malleus
Stapes
Tympanic membrane
Chorda tympani
Styloid ligament

2
Pharyngeal arch cartilages and auditory ossicles in man

D. Displacement of primary jaw joint into the chain of auditory ossicles

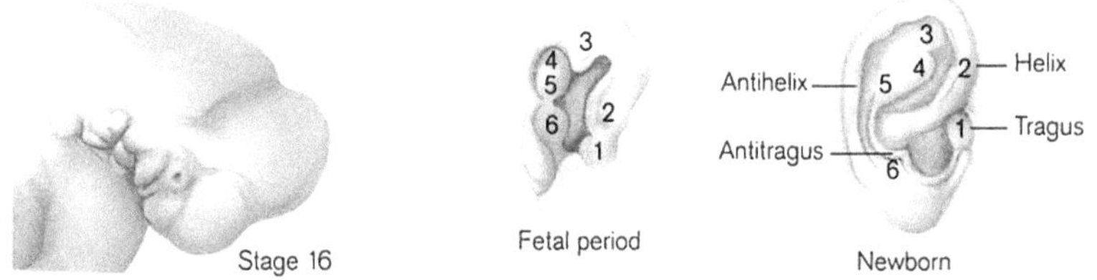


E. Development of the auricle

# Chapter 6: Heart and Vessels

## Introduction

This chapter, which covers the development of the circulatory system, should facilitate an understanding of the anatomy of the definitive heart and of its anomalies. By following the development of the heart from its origin as a **pulsating cardiac loop** with a pulsation wave propagating from the inflow tract to the outflow tract, the real three-dimensional anatomy of the heart and its anomalies are easier to comprehend than by the concept of a fourchambered valve pump.

**6.1 Circulatory Systems in the Embryo.** Embryos, like aquatic vertebrates, possess a simple circulation without lungs. In the latter, oxygen replenishment takes place in the region of the pharyngeal arches, where the gill apparatus develops. The pharyngeal arteries are incorporated as the aortic arches in the *systemic circulation*. In embryos with a large yolk sac, nutrition and respiration is fulfilled by the yolk sac, and correspondingly, a *vitelline circulation* develops. In the mammalian embryo this function is taken over by the placenta (*placental circulation*).

The yolk sac is derived from the gut. Nutrients resorbed from the yolk sac or the gut are metabolized in the liver. The liver is inserted into venous blood flow from the yolk sac or the intestine to the heart. During ontogeny, the **vitelline circulation** is transformed into the portal circulation as the adult form develops.

The yolk sac as nutritional and respiratory organ is followed by formation of a chorioallantois in birds and an allantois placenta in mammals. The main blood flow in the embryo is channeled from the vitelline circulation into the **placental circulation**. In human development, a placental circulation is established via the connecting (allantoic) stalk before a vitelline circulation has formed.

In the simple circulation of the embryo, the blood passes only once through the heart for each circuit through the body, whereas after birth when **the pulmonary circulation** has started, the blood must go twice through the heart for each trip. During embryonic life, the pulmonary circulation is established as a parallel bloodstream without hemodynamic effects on the simple embryonic circulation. It is switched on only after birth. It arises from an insignificant pharyngeal capillary area and is fed by the sixth pharyngeal arch arteries. Its blood returns directly into the atrial segment of the embryonic heart.

**6.2 Cardiac Tube.** The heart develops below the pharynx and bulges into the body cavity. For functional reasons, the anterior segment of the body cavity—the pericardial cavity—is sealed off from the peritoneal cavity. If development proceeds via an embryonic disc, the cardiac blastema is separated into a right and left primordium as the embryo spreads out on the yolk. The two parts are joined when the intestinal tube folds and closes, forming the cardiac loop below the foregut. The underlying morphogenetic movement is readily apparent in the folding-off process of the chick embryo.

**6.3 Cardiac Tube in Humans.** Due to the precocious development of a placental circulation, the cardiac primordium forms outside of the embryo as an unpaired primordium in front of the head fold. After the cardiac primordium has shifted beneath the foregut, the segments of the outflow tract (ventral aorta) and of the inflow tract (sinus venosus) elongate from paired primordia. In the human, a ventral mesocardium is not formed.

The description of the position of the cardiac tube in stage 11 is based on a computer-generated, schematic three-dimensional reconstruction, in which the classic ventral view (Davis, 1927) was modified by inclining the position and adding positional information gained from the "Mizuguti embryo" (1990) by computer-based analysis of the course of vessels and their relation to the digestive tract (Th. Bruhns).

**6.4 Overview.** In the classic didactic approach, definitive parts of the heart are traced back to the respective parts of the cardiac loop. Correspondingly, the bloodstreams for the left and the right heart are projected back to the cardiac loop. Although this approach has received vehement criticism (Steding and Seidel, 1990), it may provide a useful framework for understanding details of embryonic heart anatomy in humans and cardiac physiology in the chick. In phylogeny, the laminar current principle was initiated with the appearance of the pulmonary circulation. In amphibians, after metamorphosis and the transition to pulmonary respiration, the right and left hearts are functionally separated due to the laminar current, even though septa are still not present. The many different malformations of the heart can also be best explained in terms of hemodynamics in the embryo.

**6.5 Sinus and Atrium.** Classical descriptions of the heart become difficult to understand when the incorporation of veins in the atria and the formation of septa are discussed because the heart is shown first from behind and then from the front. The transformation of the sinus venosus, the septation of the atrium, and the outflow tract are therefore always represented ventrally, using three frontal sections through the same (fictitious) heart model, as illustrated in (→ 6.5 A2). Incorporation of veins into the atrium causes a steepening of the bloodstream from the inferior vena cava. During this process, a second opening arises in the septum primum dorsal to the first opening. The septum primum can be closed below, while on the right side, the septum secundum grows downward to the base of the bloodstream in preparation for closure at birth.

**6.6 Outflow Tract.** The involution and new formation of the bulboventricular fold (→ 6.6 A1) is central to the separation of the pulmonary and systemic circulation. The schematic illustrations of blood flow and of the valve planes of the heart are based on computer-generated three-dimensional models. From the ventral and superior side, the spiral septum meets the underside of the valve plane lying obliquely in the atrioventricular canal. The remaining wedge-shaped opening is closed by the inferior endocardial cushion during the formation of the membranous ventricular septum.

**6.7 Arteries.** As the brain increases in size, the vertebral column and neural tube ascend (→ 8.2) and the heart descends anterior to the gastrointestinal tract. With the descent of the heart, the intervertebral arteries in the cervical region are released from their origins at the dorsal aorta and anastomose into a single, long vertebral artery. The first intervertebral artery, which lies between the atlas and skull base, is retained; it connects the basilar artery to the vertebral artery.

**6.8 Veins.** The transformation of the venous system is classically represented in an anteroposterior projection. In such representations, it is not clear that the straight course of the portal vein through the U-shaped duodenum is brought about by anastomoses between the vitelline veins. The three-dimensional reconstructions of the venous system used here should clarify such points. The bloodstream shifts from the inferior cardinal vein to the subcardinal vein as a result of the return of blood from the mesonephros and later from the metanephros. Dorsally, where there is no connection to the vena cava system, the supracardinal veins ensure a return of blood from the posterior body wall behind the heart. Caudally, the sacrocardinal veins in the dorsal posterior body wall similarly collect blood from the legs and the lesser pelvis at the level of the original inferior cardinal veins, transporting it forward to the subcardinal veins in a more ventral plane. As a result of these developments, the renal veins course in front of the aorta; and the iliac vein, emerging from the sacrocardinal vein, passes behind the femoral artery.

**6.9 Changes in the Circulation at Birth.** The illustration provided here is modified somewhat from the classic description with respect to the hepatic circulation. The isthmus of the aorta is included. The isthmus may function in regulating blood flow to the brain; defects in its development can lead to *coarctation of the aorta*.

**6.10 Malformations.** Several representative anomalies are illustrated using modifications of the schematic three-dimensional reconstruction shown in 6.6B.

## 6.1 Overview: Circulatory Systems

### A. Systemic, Vitelline, Placental, and Pulmonary Circulation in the Embryo

**1. Systemic Circulation.** Initially, the vertebrate systemic circulation is a simple circulating system. Oxygen saturation takes place in the pharyngeal arches, which have been transformed into gills. The heart lies ventrally in front of the foregut. Blood flows from the pulsating *cardiac loop* via the *ventral aorta* into the *aortic arches* surrounding the pharynx. From the aortic arches, the blood travels to the descending *dorsal aorta*, which branches into the *segmental arteries* that supply the musculature and the organs of the body. Venous return is via the cardinal veins. The *anterior* and the *posterior cardinal veins* join into a *common trunk* that carries the blood ventrally into the inflow tract of the heart. This common trunk opens laterally into the *sinus venosus* and the atrium without flowing through the liver. The cardinal veins later give rise to the superior and inferior vena cava systems.

**2. Vitelline Circulation.** The yolk sac arises by the proliferation and enlargement of yolk-rich cells in the endoderm of vertebrate embryos. Ultimately, the nutrients in the yolk sac can no longer be resorbed directly by the endodermal lining of the intestinal tract. Blood vessels arise in the visceral mesoderm of the yolk sac and transport the nutrient-rich blood via the *vitelline veins* to the *liver*. From here, liver veins carry the blood to the *sinus venosus* in the inflow tract of the heart. The vitelline circulation is supplied by segmental arteries from the ventrally situated aorta. These arteries join into a *vitelline artery* that later gives rise to the superior mesenteric artery. In the vascular plexus of the yolk sac, the stem cells of the blood and the primordial germ cells arise. The capillary network in the yolk sac is responsible for the nutrition, as well as the respiration of the embryo prior to the development of a chorioallantois (→ 3.11) or a placenta (→ 3.13). The vitelline veins later give rise to the adult portal circulation.

**3. Placental Circulation.** In mammalian embryos, the placental circulation takes over the nutritional and respiratory functions. The still paired *dorsal aortae* give rise to segmental arteries, which in turn branch into *umbilical arteries* that lie within the visceral mesoderm on both sides of the intestinal tube. Since the placenta develops from the *allantois*, the umbilical arteries pass together with the allantois via the body stalk to the placenta. Blood flows back to the embryo via the umbilical veins. The *umbilical veins* enter through the body stalk into the parietal mesodermal layer of the lateral body wall, passing beyond the yolk sac to the anterior intestinal portal. From here, blood flows through the sinusoids of the liver—where nutrients transported from the placenta are metabolized—to the sinus venosus, the inflow tract of the heart. Toward the end of pregnancy, the bulk of the blood is channeled into the *ductus venosus*, bypassing the capillary network of the liver. Although the placental circulation arises last in phylogeny, it is first to arise in mammalian ontogeny, since it is a prerequisite for embryonic development.

**4. Pulmonary Circulation.** Although the pulmonary circulation is required only after birth, it is already established during embryonic development. *Lung buds* arise in the lower pharyngeal segment. The lung diverticulum is supplied arterially by small branches of the *sixth aortic arch*. The *pulmonary veins* arise from a small venous plexus that drains the lower part of the pharynx and opens directly into the *atrial segment* of the cardiac loop. The septation of the heart proceeds parallel to the development of the pulmonary circulation. This development allows a sudden transition at birth from the simple embryonic circulatory system into separate systemic and pulmonary circulations.

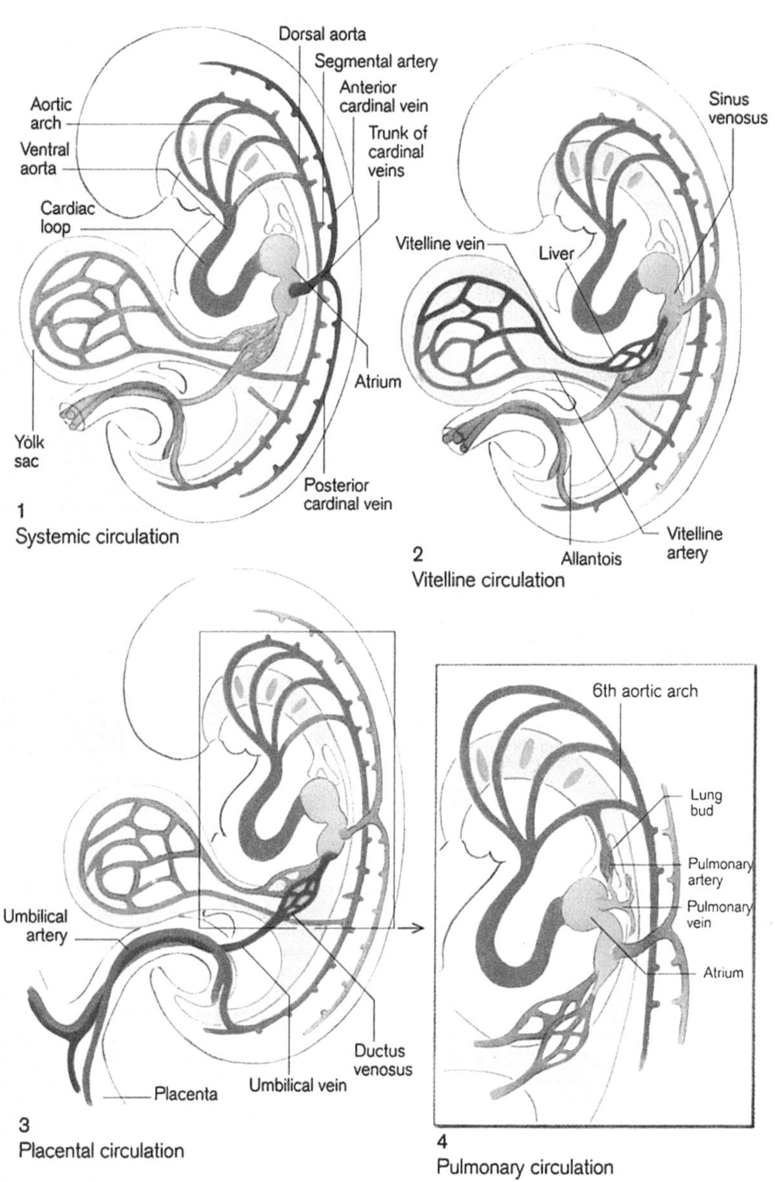
Dorsal aorta
Segmental artery
Anterior cardinal vein
Trunk of cardinal veins
Aortic arch
Ventral aorta
Cardiac loop
Atrium
Yolk sac
Posterior cardinal vein
1
Systemic circulation
Sinus venosus
Vitelline vein
Liver
Vitelline artery
Allantois
2
Vitelline circulation
6th aortic arch
Lung bud
Pulmonary artery
Pulmonary vein
Atrium
Umbilical artery
Ductus venosus
Placenta
Umbilical vein
3
Placental circulation
4
Pulmonary circulation

A. Circulatory systems in the embryo

# Heart Tube and Heart Loop

# 6.2 Formation of the Heart Tube

## A. Origin of the Heart Tube in the Visceral Mesoderm

**1. Location of the Heart Tube**

In a transverse section through the vertebrate embryo, the heart tube lies below the foregut. The heart tube begins caudally with the fusion of the paired vitelline veins and continues cranially into the paired aortic arches (→ 6.3 C3).

**2. Cardiac Blastema at Folding**

**a Embryonic disc.** In vertebrates with yolk-rich eggs, the *cardiac blastema* lies in the visceral mesoderm of the embryonic disc covering the yolk sac (**2a**). Capillary islands arise bilaterally between the mesodermal layer and the yolk sac endoderm and fuse into continuous *endocardial tubes*.

**b Folding.** As the embryonic body folds off, the right and left portions of the heart fuse in the midline and the endodermal layer in the fusion zone disappears.

**c Fusion of Right and Left Primordia.** The paired *endothelial tubes* fuse into a single endocardial tube. The visceral mesoderm that lies above the endocardial tube differentiates into cardiac muscle (*myocardium*). As the cardiac musculature begins to pulse, the cardiac tube detaches first from the yolk sac and then from the pharynx. The *dorsal* and the *ventral mesocardium* disintegrate.

## B. Development of the Chick Heart during Embryonic Folding

In the chick embryo, heart formation begins with the folding off of the embryonic body from the yolk sac, a process that progresses from cranial to caudal (→ 3.9).

**1. Cardiac Primordium in the 2-Day Old Chick Embryo.** The young chick embryo possesses a vitelline circulation. Blood from the capillaries in the yolk sac mesoderm is transported through the vitelline veins to the heart, where it is accelerated by pulsations of the cardiac tube and discharged into the aortic arches. The cardiac tube arises during the folding process below the foregut. This folding is driven by the thickened visceral mesodermal layer. The mesodermal cells form on both sides palisade-like structures that rise and fuse in the midline in a zipper fashion, bringing together the endodermal lips at the anterior intestinal portal. Fusion of these lips forms the floor of the foregut. The endoderm recedes between the mesodermal palisades, causing the endocardial tubes located between the endoderm and the *mesodermal palisades* to fuse with one another. After fusing above and below the endocardial tube, the mesodermal palisades lose their palisade-like structure. In a cranial transverse section (**1a**), fusion takes place on both sides of the endocardial tube, while further caudally (**1b**), the mesodermal palisades are still raised. In the lower portion of the body, the embryonic disc is still spread out flat (**1c**).

The **pericardial cavity** is the cranial part of the coelomic cavity between the parietal and visceral layers of the mesoderm. In the chick embryo, it becomes delimited from the extraembryonic coelom in the cranial region by the the amniotic folds. Caudally, it communicates with the remaining coelom via the coelomic canals.

**2. Differentiation of the Myocardial Mantle.** After folding has taken place, the mesodermal palisades disintegrate and the mesodermal cells differentiate into cardiac muscle cells. The myocardium is separated from the pericardial cavity by a thin mesothelial-like cell layer (epicardium). The heart begins to beat. Contraction waves originate in the inflow tract at the junction of the vitelline veins and progress cranially toward the outflow tract at the transition to the aortic arches. The myocardium and the endocardium are separated by a space filled with gelatinous fluid (*cardiac jelly*). This stage is reached in the human embryo at stage 10 (→ 2.17).

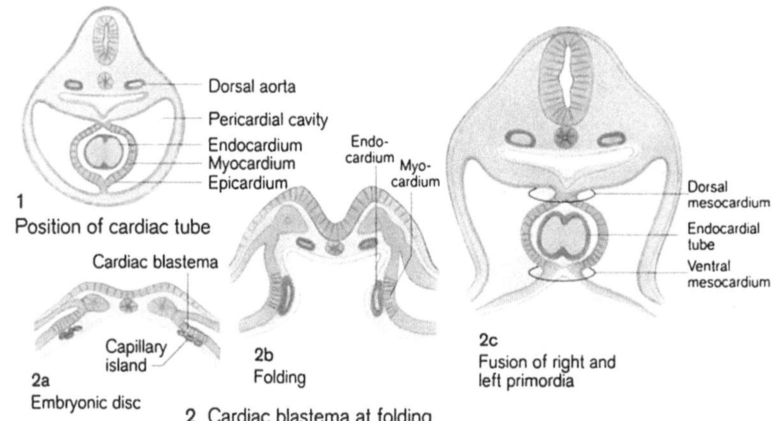


A. Origin of cardiac tube in the visceral mesoderm

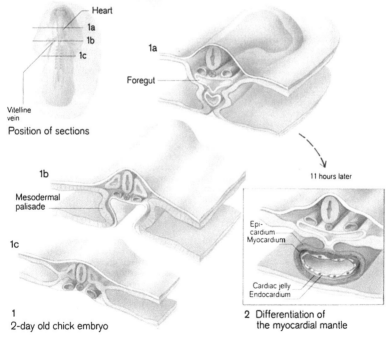

Heart
1a
1b
1c
Vitelline
vein
Position of sections

1a
Foregut

11 hours later

1b
Mesodermal
palisade

1c

1
2-day old chick embryo

Epi-
cardium
Myocardium
Cardiac jelly
Endocardium

2 Differentiation of
the myocardial mantle

B. Development of the chick heart during embryonic folding

## 6.3 The Cardiac Tube in the Human

*Background*

The **heart** is the first functional organ to develop in the human embryo. Pulsation of the cardiac tube drives the placental circulation. The vitelline circulation, which is established at the same time, is hemodynamically insignificant. The need for a placental circulation is probably the reason why the human heart arises before embryonic folding takes place.

### C. Cardiogenic Plate and Cardiac Tube in the Human

**1. Position of the Cardiogenic Plate**

The cardiac blastema in the human forms a U-shape in front of the *head fold*. The parietal and visceral layers of the mesoderm separate, giving rise to the pericardial cavity, the most anterior portion of the embryonic coelom. Caudally, the pericardial cavity opens into the chorionic cavity (extraembryonic coelom) via the *coelomic canals*. The visceral mesoderm at the floor of the pericardial cavity, known as the *cardiogenic plate*, gives rise to the myocardium. Between this plate and the endoderm, capillaries sprout and fuse to form the *endocardium* (**2a**, inset).

**2. Displacement of the Cardiac Primordium below the Foregut**

As the head fold rises and the foregut invaginates, the cardiac primordium is displaced below the foregut (**2a**). In this process, it becomes rotated 180 degrees with respect to the embryonic body, the axis of rotation lying in a transverse plane at the level of the foregut. As a result of this rotation, the cardiogenic plate (future myocardium) comes to lie directly under the foregut and is covered below by the pericardial cavity (**2b**). Fusion of capillary sprouts below the foregut gives rise to the *endocardial tube*, around which the cardiogenic plate differentiates into the myocardial mantle (**2c**). A dorsal mesocardium thus transitorily develops between the cardiac tube and the foregut. In humans, a ventral mesocardium does not form.

The origin of the cardiac tube in human embryos is speculative: It may be the result of a modified folding movement, or development may be based on a morphogenetic program found in amphibians (→ 3.18), in which an undivided cardiac primordium arises directly in the visceral mesoderm.

**3. Position of the Cardiac Tube**

**Venous Inflow Tract.** Three pairs of veins converge in the inflow tract of the heart: the *vitelline veins* from the visceral mesoderm of the yolk sac, the *umbilical veins* from the parietal mesoderm of the (not yet folded) body wall, and the stems of the *cardinal veins*, which transport blood from the cardinal veins (lying dorsal to the aorta) past the foregut into the ventral direction. These venous trunks merge into the transversely coursing sinus venosus. The sinus venosus lies between the *anterior intestinal portal* and the pericardial cavity in a plate of visceral mesoderm termed the *septum transversum*.

**Arterial Outflow Tract.** Cranially, the cardiac tube continues into the paired first aortic arch and the *dorsal aorta*. Below the first aortic arch, the capillary sprouts for the *second aortic arch* arise.

**Pericardial Cavity and Coelomic Canals.** The epicardium covering the heart tube is continuous with the lining of the pericardial cavity in transition zones at the outflow tract and the inflow tract of the heart. The regression of the dorsal mesocardium gives rise to the *transverse sinus* of the pericardial cavity (arrow behind the cardiac loop). The transverse sinus is located between the two transition sites of epicardium into pericardium and is still recognizable as an opening between the inflow and outflow tracts of the adult heart. The *oblique sinus* (not yet formed) of the pericardial cavity arises by displacement of the venous inflow tract in a superior and rightward direction relative to the leftward-pointing apex of the heart (→ 6.4 B1). In the embryo, the pericardial cavity opens into the chorionic cavity via two coelomic canals situated dorsally to the horns of the sinus venosus (arrow pointing downward) (→ 2.19).

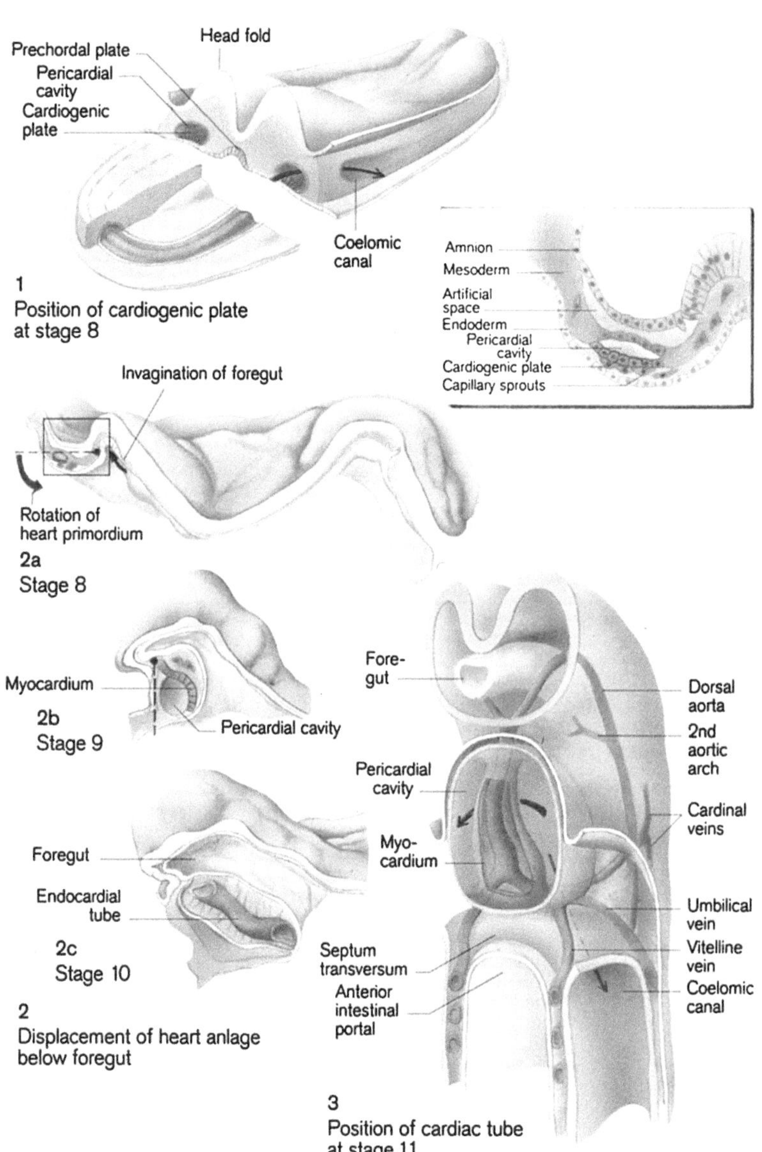
Prechordal plate
Head fold
Pericardial cavity
Cardiogenic plate
Coelomic canal
1
Position of cardiogenic plate at stage 8
Amnion
Mesoderm
Artificial space
Endoderm
Pericardial cavity
Cardiogenic plate
Capillary sprouts
Invagination of foregut
Rotation of heart primordium
2a
Stage 8
Myocardium
2b
Stage 9
Pericardial cavity
Foregut
Endocardial tube
2c
Stage 10
2
Displacement of heart anlage below foregut
Fore-gut
Pericardial cavity
Myo-cardium
Septum transversum
Anterior intestinal portal
Dorsal aorta
2nd aortic arch
Cardinal veins
Umbilical vein
Vitelline vein
Coelomic canal
3
Position of cardiac tube at stage 11

C. Cardiogenic plate and cardiac tube in the human

## Formation of Cardiac Septa

## 6.4 Overview: Transformation of the Heart Loop into the Definitive Heart

### A. Segments of the Cardiac Loop

Elongation of the cardiac tube, which is fixed in the *pericardial cavity* at the *inflow tract* and at the *outflow tract*, gives rise to the **cardiac loop** (**A1**). In this process, the **inflow tract** is shifted dorsally and superiorly (arrows in **A2**), as the atrial segment and a part of the sinus venosus are taken up into the pericardial cavity. During the embryonic period, the cardiac loop is transformed into a four-chambered heart without interrupting its function as the driving force for the simple placental circulation.

In the **cardiac loop** (**A3**), the **segments of the definitive heart** (**A4**) can already be recognized. The *sinus venosus* forms the *sinus cordis*. The *descending limb* of the cardiac loop gives rise to the *left ventricle* and the *ascending limb* to the right ventricle of the definitive heart. The *truncus* becomes subdivided by a spiral septum into the trunk of the *aorta* and the trunk of the *pulmonary artery*.

### B. Transformation of the Cardiac Loop into the Definitive Heart

**1. Cardiac Loop.** The cardiac loop first bulges ventrally in the midline and then becomes inclined *toward the right*. The *apex* of the definitive heart, in contrast, is directed *toward the left*. This repositioning is the result of the enlargement of the left ventricle in the descending limb of the cardiac loop. Ultimately, the apex of the cardiac loop—originally directed toward the right—is shifted into the lower segment of the right ventricle and the right ventricle comes to lie ventrally on the large left ventricle.

**2. Parallel Laminar Bloodstreams.** Asymmetries in the development of the cardiac loop result in the formation of two laminar streams, which functionally precede a subdivision into a right and left heart. The inflow tract of the heart becomes shifted toward the right. The **main bloodstream** (red) from the umbilical vein enters the right *atrial segment* of the heart through the *inferior vena cava*, flows from the right atrium through the opening in the atrial septum into the *left atrium*, and then enters the *left ventricle*, which discharges the blood into the trunk of the *aorta*. An **accessory bloodstream** (purple) enters the heart from above through the *superior vena cava*. It crosses under the main bloodstream in the *right atrium*, passing through into the *right ventricle*, and leaving the heart via the *pulmonary trunk*. The accessory bloodstream flows through the *ductus arteriosus* (→ 6.9 A1) and rejoins the main bloodstream in the descending aorta.

**3. Compartmentalization of the Bloodstreams by Septa and Valves.** The two bloodstreams are separated from each other by an *atrial septum* and by a *ventricular septum*. The atrial septum consists of two layers with staggered openings for the main bloodstream from the inferior vena cava. They are arranged in such a way that they can close like a valve when the pressure in the left atrium rises after birth (→ 6.9). The *ventricular septum* is composed of two parts: a muscular portion, which arises from the infolding of the myocardium between the left ventricle in the descending limb of the cardiac loop and the right ventricle in the ascending limb; and a *membranous portion* that connects the muscular ventricular septum with the atrioventricular plane (*valve plane*) and the base of the atrial septum.

The *atrioventricular valves* originate in the *valve plane*. On account of the shape of the cardiac loop, the *aortic* and *pulmonary valves* in the outflow tract of the heart come to lie ventral to the atrioventricular valves.

Above the muscular ventricular septum, the laminar streams spiral around each other. The two streams are delimited from one another by a *spiraling septum* that separates the trunk of the aorta from that of the pulmonary artery.

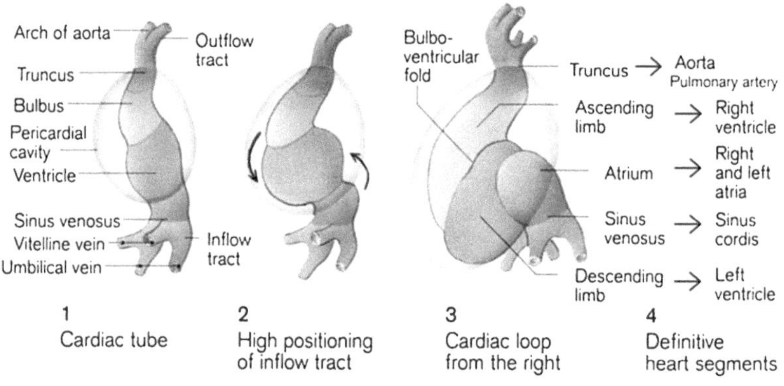


1
Cardiac tube

2
High positioning of inflow tract

3
Cardiac loop from the right

4
Definitive heart segments

A. Segments of the cardiac loop

Plane of aortic and pulmonary valves
Cardiac loop toward the right
Atrium
Atrioventricular plane
Apex of the heart toward the left

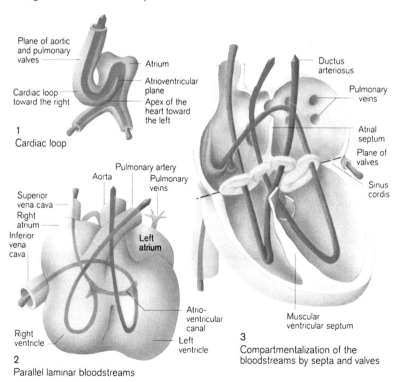

1
Cardiac loop

Pulmonary artery
Aorta
Pulmonary veins
Superior vena cava
Right atrium
Inferior vena cava
Left atrium
Atrio-ventricular canal
Right ventricle
Left ventricle

2
Parallel laminar bloodstreams

Ductus arteriosus
Pulmonary veins
Atrial septum
Plane of valves
Sinus cordis
Muscular ventricular septum

3
Compartmentalization of the bloodstreams by septa and valves

B. Transformation of the cardiac loop into the definitive heart

## 6.5 Sinus and Atrium

### A. Transformation of the Sinus Venosus

**1. Shifting of the Inflow Tract toward the Right.** The trunks of the *cardinal veins*, the *vitelline vein*, and the *umbilical vein* merge on each side into a right and left *sinus horn* of the *sinus venosus*. The originally symmetrical venous opening is shifted entirely to the right side. Changes in the venous inflow tract begin in stage 13 (→ 2.22) with the formation of a large, unpaired umbilical vein. Blood from the placenta enters the *left umbilical vein*, crosses over to the right side in the liver as the *ductus venosus*, and arrives at the heart via the trunk of the right vitelline vein (*bloodstream of the inferior vena cava*). Blood from the systemic circulation passes into the sinus horn from above, via the trunk of the right cardinal vein (*bloodstream of the superior vena cava*).

**2. Venous Openings of the Heart.** The *inferior vena cava* arises from the right sinus horn, while the *superior vena cava* originates from the right trunk of the cardinal veins and the right superior cardinal vein. The inferior cardinal vein now opens into the superior vena cava; its opening persists as the entrance of the *azygos vein*. The *coronary sinus*, which returns blood from the heart itself, is formed from the transversely coursing, central segment of the sinus venosus. The extracardial venous openings of the left side disappear.

### B. Septation in the Atrium

**1. Septum primum and Septum Secundum.** The right sinus horn opens into the right atrium through a slit-like orifice (**A2**). This orifice is guarded by two *venous valves*, which are continuous above with the transient ridge of the *septum spurium*. The main bloodstream, carried by the umbilical vein and entering obliquely from below, is guided across into the left atrium by the *venous valves*. Division of the simple atrial segment of the heart loop into a right and a left atrium is accomplished by the downward growth of the *septum primum* and the *septum secundum*, both of which leave an opening for the main blood flow.

**2. Incorporation of Veins.** During further development, the opening between the sinus and atrium expands until the entire right sinus horn is incorporated in the right atrium as the *venous wall* of the atrium. The upper segment of the venous valve and the septum spurium disappear. The lower remnant of the valve is subdivided into a *valve of the inferior vena cava* and a *valve of the coronary sinus*. On the left side, the trunk of the *pulmonary vein* (**B1**) is incorporated into the atrial wall in analogous fashion. The pulmonary veins develop via a pharyngeal venous plexus, which opens directly into the atrium (→ 6.1). The region of incorporation extends beyond the first ramifications of the trunk of the pulmonary vein so that four separate venous openings arise. Both atria are greatly expanded by the incorporation of the veins. The original trabecular atrial wall is displaced on both sides into the *auricle of the heart*.

**3. Development of Valve Function.** Before the veins are incorporated into the atrial walls, blood from the inferior vena cava passes through an opening (*foramen primum*) in the *septum primum* close to the atrioventricular plane (**B1** and **3a**). The *septum secundum* forms to the right of the *septum primum*. After the incorporation of the veins, the main bloodstream changes its direction of flow. Blood from the vena cava ascends more steeply upward and forces the formation of a new passage—the *foramen secundum*—in the upper segment of the *septum primum* (**3b**). After the shift of the main bloodstream, the primary opening in the septum primum near the AV canal (Foramen primum) is closed. Until birth, the bloodstream from the inferior vena cava passes through the atrial septal wall by means of a slit (**oval foramen**) between the staggered, curtain-like septa (**B2**).

At birth, when the pulmonary circulation begins and the pressure in the right heart falls relative to the left, the septum primum is pressed against the septum secundum and the oval foramen is closed.

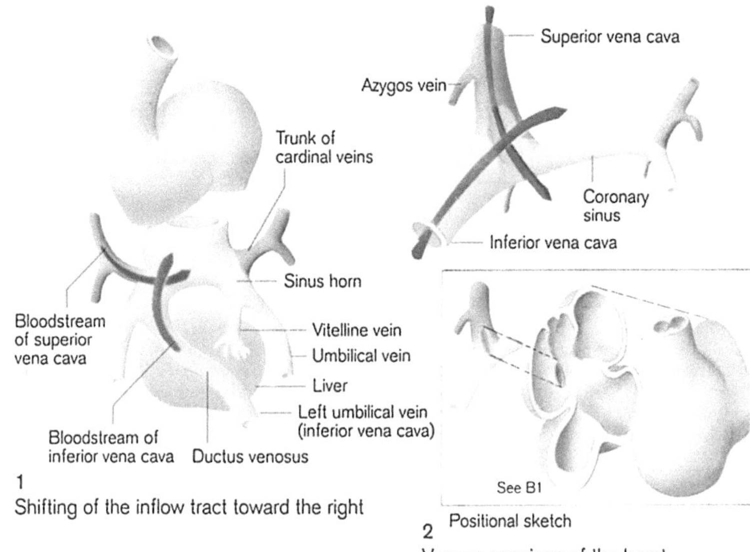


1
Shifting of the inflow tract toward the right

Positional sketch
2
Venous openings of the heart

A. Transformation of the sinus venosus

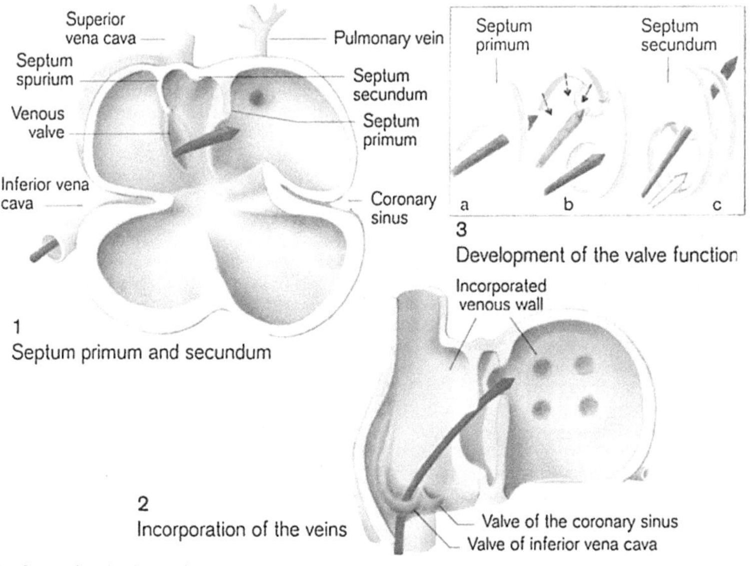


1
Septum primum and secundum

3
Development of the valve function

2
Incorporation of the veins

B. Septation in the atrium

## 6.6 Ventricles and Outflow Tract

### A. Septation in the Ventricle and Outflow Tract

**1. Displacement of the Bulboventricular Fold.** The *bulboventricular fold* divides the embryonic (left) ventricle in the descending limb from the bulbus (future right ventricle) in the ascending limb of the **cardiac loop (1a)**. The undivided bloodstream in the cardiac loop enters from the atrial segment into the embryonic ventricle via the atrioventricular canal and passes the *bulboventricular fold*, which is located on the left side of the outflow tract. When the bloodstreams separate, the original bulboventricular fold regresses and a new fold arises between the two bloodstreams (**1b**), dividing the atrioventricular canal (AV canal) into two compartments. Anteriorly, this fold merges with the myocardium that later forms the *muscular ventricular septum* and thus separates the right and left ventricles.

**2. Endocardial Cushions in the AV Canal.** The transverse opening of the AV canal is bounded by an *upper* and a *lower endocardial cushion* and laterally by two smaller cushions. These endocardial cushions consist of mesenchymal pads that push the endocardial endothelium into the bloodstream. The mesenchymal pads are formed by neural crest cells that migrate into the cardiac primordium. The hollowing out of the endocardial cushions by the bloodstream gives rise to the *atrioventricular valves*. The *chordae tendinae* are trabeculae of the ventricular wall, in which the cardiac myocytes have disappeared (not shown). At the convergence of the atrial septum and the membranous ventricular septum in the atrioventricular plane, the AV canal is divided into a *tricuspid* and a *mitral orifice*. In both orifices, the *septal cusps* originate by a fusion of portions of the upper and lower endocardial cushions.

**3. Spiral Septum in the Truncus and Conus.** In the outflow tract of the heart, the two bloodstreams are separated from each other by a spiral septum. This septum arises by the fusion of two swellings that form the *aorticopulmonary septum* in the truncus segment of the cardiac loop. The aorticopulmonary septum is continuous with the *upper* and *lower conus swellings*, which project inferiorly into the funnel-shaped initial segment of the outflow tract, the conus cordis. The conus swellings grow into the direction of the AV plane and form the anterior segment of the *membranous ventricular septum* (**A4**).

**4. Closure of the Interventricular Foramen.** Although the laminar bloodstreams of the right and left heart are already functionally separated, the two chambers communicate via an opening bordered above by the newly formed *bulboventricular fold* and below by the infolding of the *muscular ventricular septum* (**1b**). Both ventricles enlarge by appositional growth at the outer surface of the myocardium while simultaneously undergoing cavitation and trabecular formation at the inner surface. These processes lead to an expansion and deepening of the muscular ventricular septum.

The still-open segment of the ventricular septum becomes closed by the *membranous ventricular septum*, which is formed by the *lower endocardial cushion* (**A2**) and the *lower and upper conus swellings* (**A3**). The upper and lower conus swellings fuse with the upper and lower endocardial cushions in the AV canal. In the process, the lower endocardial cushion grows forward, contributing about one-third of the material used in forming the membranous ventricular septum (**A4**).

The closure of the *interventricular foramen* by the membranous ventricular septum is the final step in the septation of the heart. At the upper edge of the septum, the septum primum in the atrium, the cardiac skeleton in the *atrioventricular canal* (AV canal) and the spiral septum (**A3**) abut. Anomalous development of this junction causes heart defects with poor prognosis.

The **semilunar valves** in the outflow tracts of the aorta and the pulmonary artery, like the atrioventricular valves in the AV canal, arise from pads of mesenchyme beneath the endothelium. The mesenchyme cells for the formation of the endocardial cushion are derived from neural crest cells that have migrated from the rhombencephalic region to the cardiac primordium.

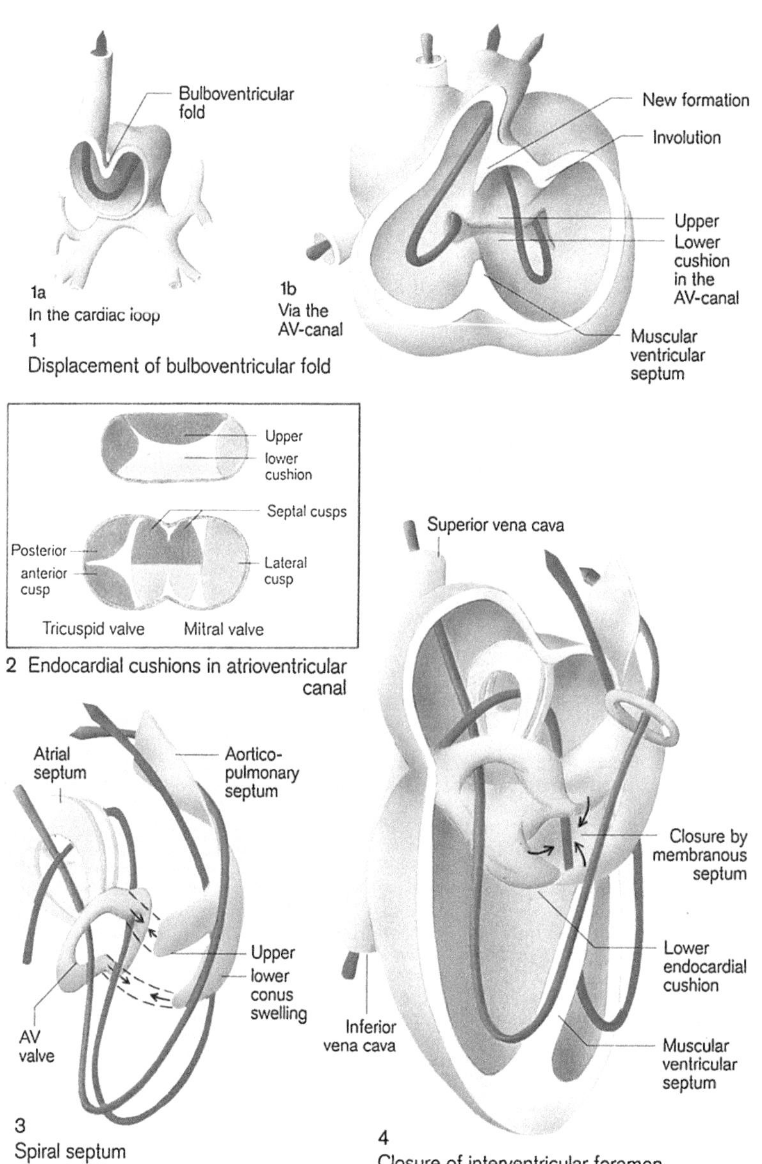
Bulboventricular fold
1a
In the cardiac loop
1b
Via the AV-canal
New formation
Involution
Upper
Lower
cushion
in the
AV-canal
Muscular ventricular septum
1
Displacement of bulboventricular fold
Upper
lower
cushion
Septal cusps
Posterior
anterior
cusp
Lateral
cusp
Tricuspid valve
Mitral valve
2 Endocardial cushions in atrioventricular canal
Superior vena cava
Atrial septum
Aortico-pulmonary septum
Upper
lower
conus
swelling
AV valve
3
Spiral septum
Closure by membranous septum
Lower endocardial cushion
Inferior vena cava
Muscular ventricular septum
4
Closure of interventricular foramen

A. Septation in the ventricle and outflow tract

# Vascular System
# 6.7 Arteries

## A. Development of Large Arteries

**1. Vascular Pathways in the Embryo.** In the **third week (1a)**, the vascular system is still symmetrical. For the **systemic circulation**, the segmental arteries exit dorsally from the paired dorsal aortae. Venous return to the *sinus venosus* is via the cardinal veins, of which only the anterior (upper) is illustrated. The **vitelline circulation** arises from segmental, ventral branches (*vitelline arteries*) that later form the superior mesenteric artery (→ 7.6 A2). Venous return is by the *vitelline veins*. The main bloodstream flows to the placenta via the *umbilical arteries* and returns to the heart by way of the *umbilical veins* in the lateral body wall (**placental circulation**). The two dorsal aortae later fuse to form the definitive dorsal aorta.

In the **fourth week (1b)**, the register of *aortic arches* forms. These arteries, connected in series, carry the blood from the ventral to the dorsal aorta. As the fourth arch arises, the first arch is already beginning to regress. Elongation of the ventral aorta forms the *external carotid artery*, while the extension of the dorsal aorta forms the *internal carotid artery*.

**2. Descent of the Heart.** In **stage 19 (2a)**, the heart lies at the level of the cervical flexure. By **stage 23 (2b)**, the heart, together with the aortic arches, has descended into the thorax. The descent of the heart accompanies the elongation of the pharynx into the esophagus (→ 7.1) and the descent of the entire viscera relative to the vertebral column and the neural tube (→ 8.2). The spinal cord is supplied by branches of the dorsal intersegmental arteries that pass through the intervertebral foramina and unite into a longitudinal anastomosis, forming the *anterior spinal artery*. During the descent of the heart, the segments of the first to seventh *intersegmental arteries* that are connected with the neural tube retain their original position. They become detached from the dorsal aorta and give rise to the longitudinal anastomosis of the *vertebral artery*, which passes through openings in the transverse processes of the vertebrae (**2a**).

In the brainstem, the anterior spinal artery continues as the *basilar artery* (**2b**). With the enormous growth of the brain, this vessel takes over the arterial supply of the posterior half of the brain and is anteriorly connected to the vascular region of the *internal carotid artery*. The unpaired *basilar artery* is supplied with blood by the two *vertebral arteries* via an anastomosis formed by the uppermost intersegmental arteries.

The stem of the *seventh intersegmental artery* lies at the level of the fourth (definitive) aortic arch. It persists and becomes the *subclavian artery* (**2b**), which on the right side also supplies the *vertebral artery*.

**3. Aortic Arch Derivatives.** In the vertebrate embryo, six aortic arches are formed in series (**3a**). In humans, the **first and second arches** disappear. The second arch gives rise to the *stapedial artery*, which as the second pharyngeal artery, initially extends between the *external* and *internal carotid arteries* (**2b**), but then loses its connection to the internal carotid artery.

The **third arch** gives rise to the arterial bifurcation between the *external* and *internal carotid arteries* (**3b** and **c**). The *common carotid artery* (**3b**) originates from the paired trunk of the ventral aorta, which continues anteriorly into the *external carotid artery*, coursing ventrally. The *internal carotid artery* corresponds to the paired, dorsal aorta.

The **fourth aortic arch** on the left side gives rise to the definitive arch of the aorta. On the right side, the fourth arch (together with a segment of the right dorsal aorta) persists up to the exit of the seventh intersegmental artery and gives rise to the *right subclavian artery*.

The **fifth aortic arch** does not develop in humans. The **sixth aortic arch** gives rise to the trunk of the pulmonary artery and the *ductus arteriosus*.

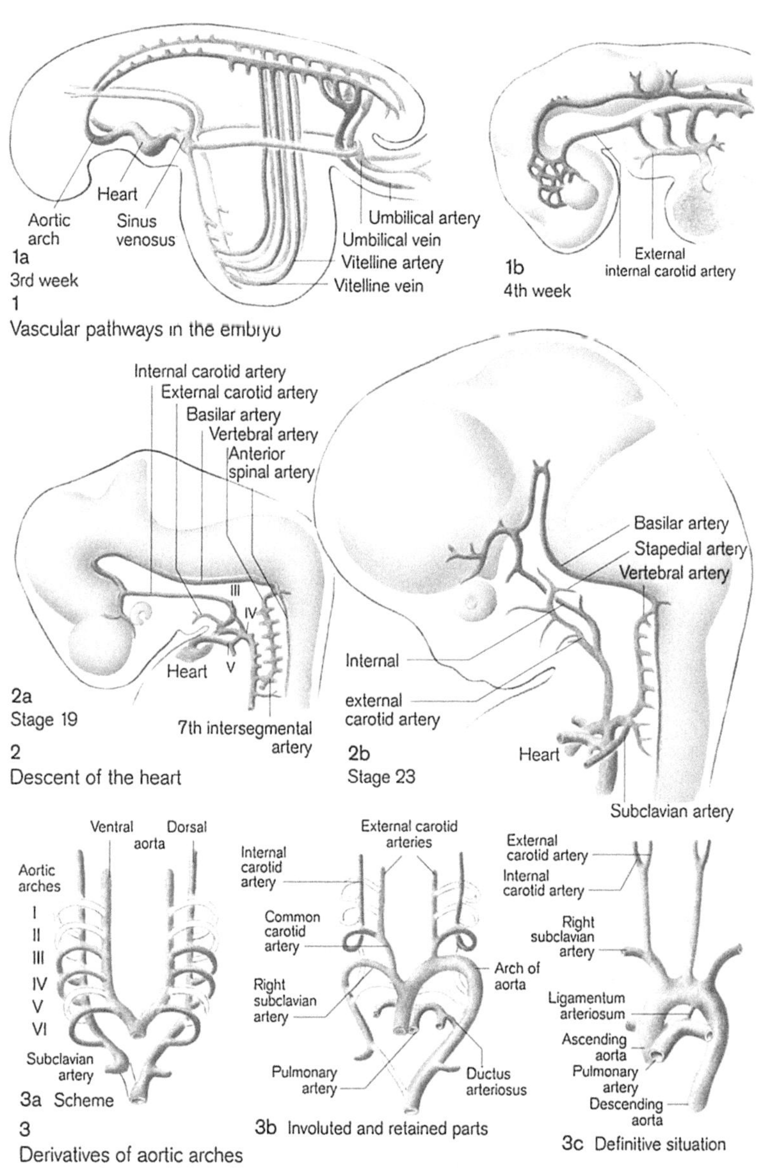


1 Vascular pathways in the embryo

2 Descent of the heart

3 Derivatives of aortic arches

A. Development of arteries

## 6.8 Veins

### A. Transformation of Vitelline, Umbilical and Cardinal Veins

**1. Large Veins in the 3rd Week**

Three large pairs of veins are found in the embryo: the **vitelline veins**, which conduct blood from the yolk sac to the sinus venosus; the **umbilical veins**, which carry oxygen-rich blood from the chorionic villi to the embryo; and the **cardinal veins**, which return the blood from the embryonic body. The vitelline and umbilical veins lie ventrally in the region of the intestinal tract and liver, while the cardinal veins course in the dorsal body wall.

**2. Vitelline and Umbilical Veins**

Both the **vitelline veins** and the vitelline arteries arise in the visceral mesoderm of the yolk sac (→ 6.1 and 2.16). Before the vitelline veins enter the sinus venosus, they flow through the liver primordium.

During the formation of the umbilical loop, the vitelline veins become transformed into the **portal vein.** The bloodstream of the future portal vein drains the *umbilical loop* and passes through the U-shaped loop of the duodenum before arriving at the liver. The main bloodstream in the *right vitelline vein* crosses over the lower crus of the duodenum by means of an *anterior anastomosis* between the right and left vitelline vein and then crosses under the upper crus of the duodenum, entering the *liver* via the trunk of the right vitelline vein by means of a *posterior anastomosis* between the vitelline veins.

The **umbilical veins** lie in the parietal mesoderm of the ventral body wall, in contrast to the umbilical arteries, which lie in the visceral mesoderm and reach the body stalk with the allantois (→ 6.1 and 2.16). Initially, the umbilical veins pass on both sides of the liver into the sinus venosus, but they soon contact the liver sinusoids. The right umbilical vein and the proximal segment of both umbilical veins recede, so that only the left umbilical vein remains to transport blood from the placenta to the liver. During the fetal period, the **ductus venosus**, a direct connection bypassing the network of the liver sinusoids, arises between the (left) *umbilical vein* and the stem of the right vitelline vein (portal vein) The main bloodstream from the placenta is thus channeled to the right side of the heart.

**3. Cardinal Veins**

The system of cardinal veins consists of the **superior cardinal veins** in the cranial segment of the embryonic body and the **inferior cardinal veins,** which return the blood from the rest of the embryonic body including the mesonephros. On each side, the superior and inferior cardinal veins merge into a *common stem* of the cardinal veins that opens into either the right or the left sinus horn, close beside the umbilical veins.

In the second half of the embryonic period, additional venous systems develop: 1. The **subcardinal veins** form for the drainage of the mesonephros (**3a**). 2. The **supracardinal veins** receive the blood from the intercostal veins of the body wall, thus taking over the interrupted function of the inferior cardinal veins in the region of the heart (**3b**). 3. The **sacrocardinal veins** arise in the developing lower limbs as continuations of the inferior cardinal veins that have atrophied at the level of the kidneys (**3b**).

**Transverse Anastomoses.** As the **definitive venous system of the vena cava (3c)** develops, transverse anastomoses appear and transport blood from the left side to the right side of the body toward the inflow tract of the heart.

The **anastomosis between the anterior cardinal veins** develops into the *left brachiocephalic vein*. The **anastomosis between the subcardinal veins** becomes the *left renal vein*. The distal segment of the left subcardinal vein persists as the gonadal vein. The right subcardinal vein becomes the *inferior vena cava*. Via a secondary connection with the liver, it opens directly into the heart (*liver segment of the inferior vena cava)*. The **anastomosis between the sacrocardinal veins** becomes the *left common iliac vein*. After the obliteration of the inferior cardinal veins behind the heart, the **supracardinal veins** form the *azygos vein* and the *hemiazygos vein*, linked by a **transverse anastomosis**. The trunk of the receded venous system of the left half of the body becomes the **sinus cordis.**

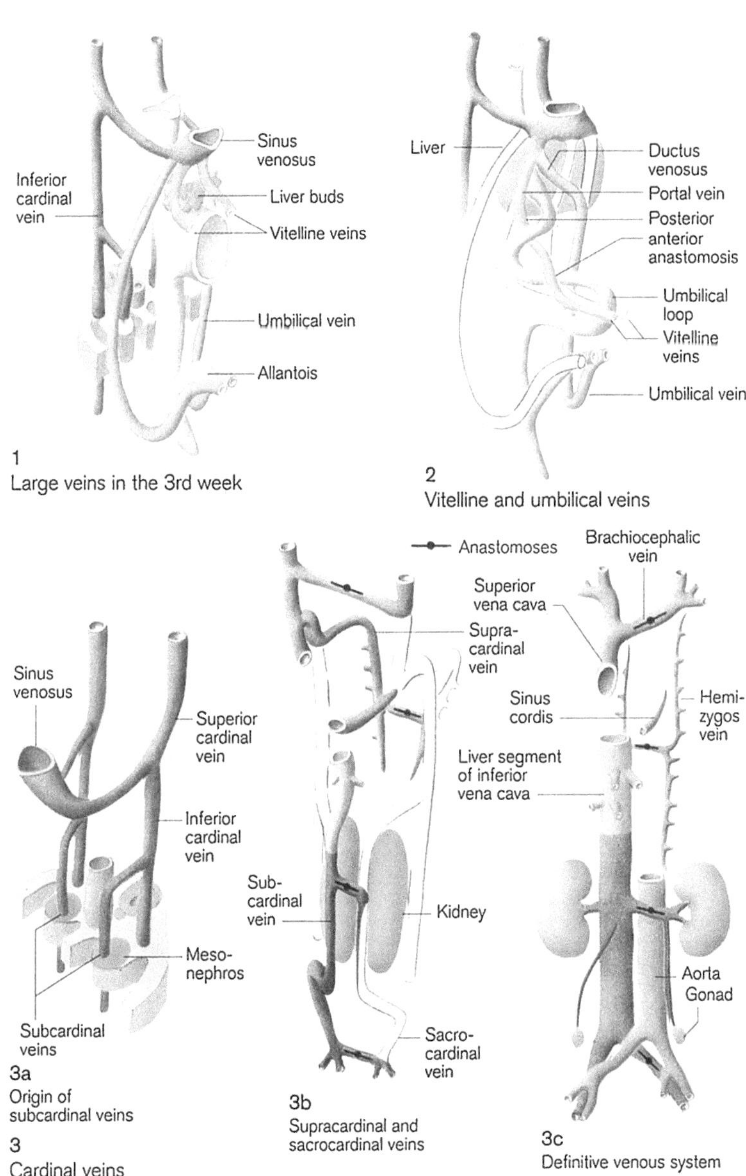


1
Large veins in the 3rd week

2
Vitelline and umbilical veins

3a
Origin of
subcardinal veins

3b
Supracardinal and
sacrocardinal veins

3c
Definitive venous system

3
Cardinal veins

A. Development of veins

## 6.9 Changes at Birth

### A. Changes in the Circulation at Birth

#### 1. Fetal Circulation

**Oxygen-rich blood** (red) from the *placenta* flows through the (left) *umbilical vein* to the liver where it is conducted via the *ductus venosus* towards the right side of the embryo into the *inferior vena cava*. From the inferior vena cava, the main bloodstream flows through the open *foramen ovale* into the *left atrium* and the *left ventricle*. The blood is then discharged into the arch of the aorta and passes directly into the large arteries of the head (i.e., the common carotid artery and the vertebral artery arising from the subclavian artery). Before the junction of the *ductus arteriosus,* lies a constriction of the aorta (*isthmus aortae*), which ensures that only a small amount of oxygen-rich blood from the left heart reaches the descending aorta, and thus only a little is supplied to organ systems that take up their function after birth only (movement apparatus, intestinal tract, kidneys, genital organs).

The **venous blood** (purple) from the upper half of the body is collected in the *superior vena cava* and crosses under the main bloodstream into the right atrium, forming an accessory bloodstream for the right heart. It is discharged from the *right ventricle* into the *descending aorta* via the *ductus arteriosus* and reaches the placenta through the *umbilical arteries*.

#### 2. Changes at Birth

In the fetal circulation, the right and left heart are about equally strong. Most organs receive mixed blood, whose composition is determined by pads in the *ductus venosus* (blood flow from the liver) and the *isthmus* of the aorta, as well as by the valve function at the *foramen ovale*.

At birth, a pressure difference between the right and left heart arises and causes the circulation to be redirected. Due to the onset of the pulmonary circulation and the interruption of blood flow from the placenta, the pressure in the right heart decreases while the pressure in the left heart rises. Compression of the thorax during parturition causes the amniotic fluid in the bronchial tree to be replaced by air. Respiration begins with the child's "first cry," which opens the pulmonary circuit.

**a Closure of Foramen ovale.** As the pressure in the left atrium rises and the pressure on the right side falls, the *septum primum* becomes pressed against the *septum secundum*. In the first postnatal days, this closure is still reversible: the neonate's crying can produce a right-left shunt and cause cyanotic phases. During the first postnatal year, the two septa fuse; however, in 20–25% of all cases, the closure is not anatomically complete (i.e., it is functionally closed but opens when probed with an instrument).

**b Constriction of Umbilical Arteries.** Several minutes after birth, the arteries are functionally closed by contraction of the smooth musculature in the wall of the vessels. However, the actual obliteration of the lumen by fibrous proliferation may require 2 to 3 months. The distal portions of the umbilical arteries on both sides form the **medial umbilical ligament**, while the proximal portions—the superior vesical arteries—remain patent(→ 7.6).

**c Closure of Umbilical Vein and Ductus Venosus.** The umbilical vein closes only after the umbilical arteries have closed. This means that blood can still flow from the placenta to the neonate until the placental circulation ceases. After the obliteration, the umbilical vein becomes the **round ligament of the liver** in the lower margin of the falciform ligament. The ductus venosus obliterates and becomes the **ligamentum venosum**. A dilatation remains at the former opening of the umbilical vein (umbilical recess, → 7.9).

**d Contraction of Ductus Arteriosus.** Contraction of the wall musculature commences immediately after parturition. In the first days after birth, a left-right shunt is not unusual. The complete anatomical obliteration by intimal proliferation takes about 1 to 3 months. In the adult, the obliterated ductus arteriosus becomes the **ligamentum arteriosum.**

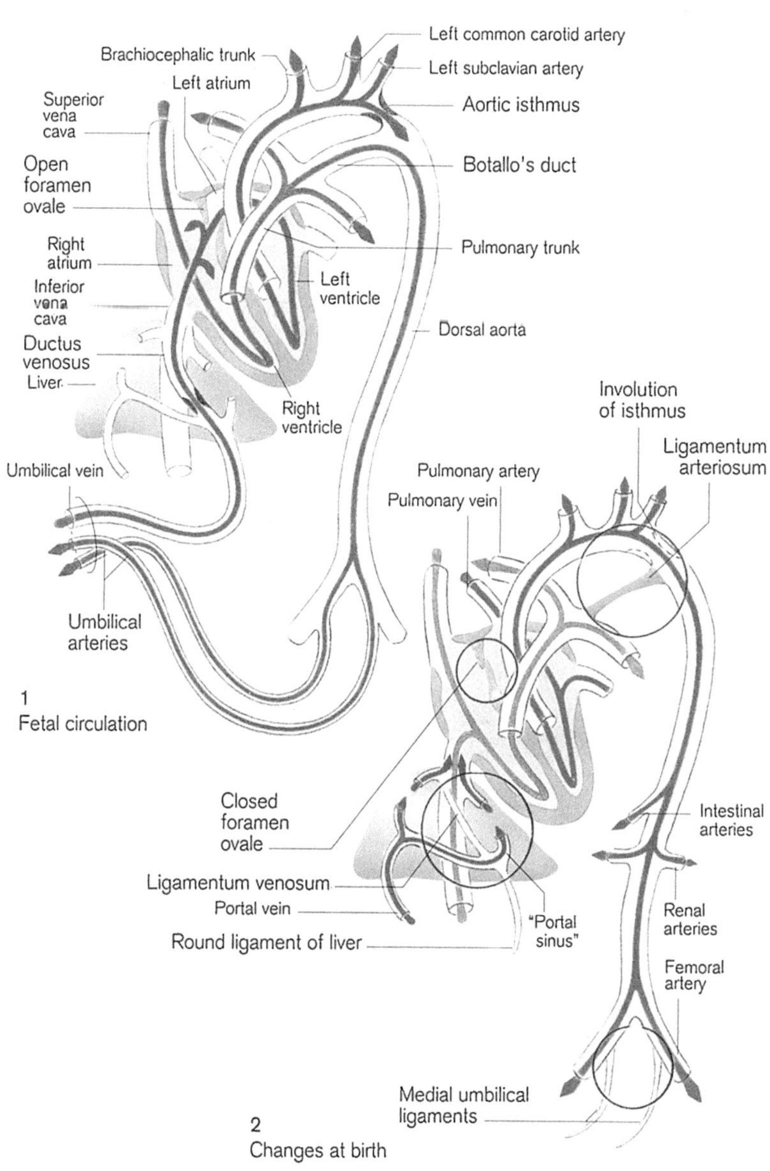
Left common carotid artery
Brachiocephalic trunk
Left subclavian artery
Left atrium
Superior vena cava
Aortic isthmus
Open foramen ovale
Botallo's duct
Right atrium
Pulmonary trunk
Inferior vena cava
Left ventricle
Ductus venosus
Dorsal aorta
Liver
Right ventricle
Umbilical vein
Umbilical arteries
1
Fetal circulation
Involution of isthmus
Ligamentum arteriosum
Pulmonary artery
Pulmonary vein
Closed foramen ovale
Ligamentum venosum
Portal vein
Round ligament of liver
"Portal sinus"
Intestinal arteries
Renal arteries
Femoral artery
Medial umbilical ligaments
2
Changes at birth

A. Changes in the circulation at birth

## 6.10 Malformations

### A. Malformations of the Heart

**1. Normal Separation of the Systemic and Pulmonary Circulation.** After birth, the blood pressure in the left heart rises while it falls in the right heart. The foramen ovale closes and the ductus arteriosus is obliterated, so that the systemic and pulmonary circulation are separated from each other. If the separation is incomplete, each heart contraction forces the blood to switch ("shunt") from one circulation into the other in accordance with the pressure difference.

**Septum Secundum Defect.** The septum secundum is incomplete, resulting in a completely or partially open foramen ovale. This defect can be repaired by applying a patch from the venous wall. The operation is uncomplicated; in simple cases, it can be carried out with a cardiac catheter.

**Septum Primum Defect.** The septum primum does not grow completely downward into the atrioventricular plane. The defect is in the AV canal; it is frequently associated with a disturbance in the subdivision of the AV canal. An operation is therefore difficult and has a poorer prognosis than an operation performed for a septum secundum defect.

**Ventricular Septum Defect.** This defect always resides in the membranous part of the ventricular septum and is caused by an incomplete fusion of the upper and lower conus swellings in the AV canal. A ventricular septal defect is frequently combined with other malformations.

**Hemodynamics.** In the case of simple atrial and ventricular septal defects, the shunt volume flows from left to right and strains the pulmonary circulation. The result is an acyanotic cardiac defect: With each shunt volume, oxygen-rich blood is recirculated through the lungs. The additional volume in the pulmonary circulation forces the right heart to work harder and eventually causes a right heart hypertrophy. The pulmonary vessels subsequently undergo pulmonary sclerosis, thus requiring even more output from the right heart (a classical "vicious circle").

**Shunt Reversal.** Ultimately, the effective pressure is higher in the right heart than in the left. The shunt volume reverses its direction and flows from right to left, so that venous blood is now recirculated through the systemic circulation. The acyanotic cardiac defect becomes cyanotic: the child turns blue. Since the lungs have been damaged by sclerosis, they can no longer attain the essential working pressure for sufficient oxygen saturation of the blood. The condition is thus preterminal; an operation is no longer feasible.

**3. Transposition of the Great Vessels.** The spiral septum in the outflow tract of the heart fails to spiral as it grows, so that the bloodstreams do not cross. The aorta originates from the right and the pulmonary artery from the left heart.

**Hemodynamics.** Survival is possible only if the foramen ovale is patent and the ductus arteriosus persists, so that mixed blood can form in the right heart and in the descending aorta.

**4. Tetralogy of Fallot.** This malformation is characterized by four symptoms: *Overriding aorta*, *pulmonic stenosis*, *ventricular septal defect*, and *right-heart hypertrophy*. The etiology is an incomplete rotation of the spiral septum. The outflow tract of the aorta is wide and lies above (overrides) the muscular ventricular septum. The outflow tract of the pulmonary artery is constricted. The interruption in the downward growth of the conus swellings, combined with the overriding aorta, is necessarily associated with a defect in the membranous ventricular septum.

**Hemodynamics.** The overriding aorta receives blood from the right and from the left ventricle, so that venous blood is mixed into the aortic stream (primary cyanotic cardiac anomaly). Depending on the individual pressure situation, the shunt volume of the ventricular septal defect flows from left to right or from right to left.

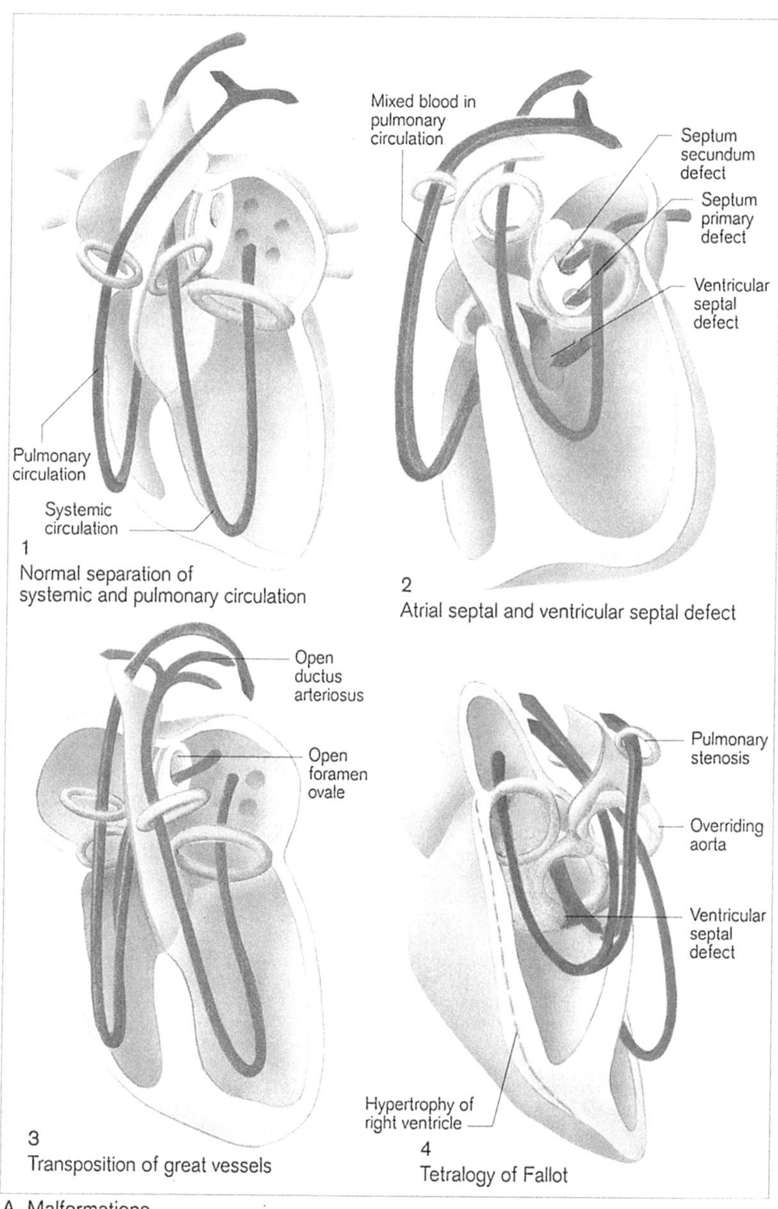


1
Normal separation of systemic and pulmonary circulation

2
Atrial septal and ventricular septal defect

3
Transposition of great vessels

4
Tetralogy of Fallot

A. Malformations

# Chapter 7: Gastrointestinal Tract

## Introduction

**7.1 Overview.** The schematic sagittal sections summarize the development of the digestive tube from the stage of folding of the embryo up to the end of the embryonic period. The staging data refer to Chapter 2, in which the formation of the digestive tract and its relation to the body cavities can be followed in detail.

**7.2 Pharynx.** The pharyngeal arches and pharyngeal pouches are basic, metameric structures of vertebrate embryos that possess homology to the elements of a prevertebrate primordial pharynx (→3.19 and 3.20). In fish, they differentiate into the gill apparatus. In humans, the pharyngeal pouches give rise to the branchiogenic organs, the tonsils, thyroid gland, and thymus. The upper half of the plate compares the pharyngeal pouches in stage 13, when they are most distinctly delineated, to the transformed pharynx at the end of the embryonic period.

The pharynx extends in an arch above the cardiac swelling. The pharyngeal pouches lie between the aortic arches. The descent of the pharyngeal arch derivatives, the thymus, and thyroid gland, is coupled with the descent of the heart (→6.7). This is evidenced by the displacement of the outflow tract of the heart and of the aortic arches. The lower half of the plate contains a schematic, three-dimensional representation of the pharyngeal pouches and shows how the definitive positions of the branchiogenic organs arise.

**7.3 Cervical Sinus and Cervical Cysts.** The plate illustrates the pharynx in classic, schematic frontal sections according to Kollmann (1907). These sections clearly show the origin of the cervical sinus from the elaboration of the cervical relief and its relationship to the cervical cysts and fistulae. The pharyngeal arches can be best understood on the basis of their derivation from the primordial pharyngeal gut, discussed in chapter 3 (→3.20). For systematic reasons, the cranial nerves (→4.12), the cranial arteries (→6.7), the visceral skeleton (→9.12), and the formation of the auditory organ are discussed separately.

**7.4 Lung Buds.** Paired lung primordia in the form of outpocketings of the pharynx are already present in certain primitive fish. Such fish could change from respiration through gills to pulmonary respiration and thus survive periods of drought by living in the mud. This way of life is highly developed in the lungfish, which is still found today in Africa and Australia. Four-footed terrestrial vertebrates (tetrapods) are derived from primitive fish with lung primordia. In the tetrapods, the lungs have developed into a highly differentiated organ system. The swim bladder of highly developed fish species is a specialized form of lung used for gravity adjustment in deep water.

In stage 10, the coelomic canals extend the unpaired pericardial cavity in the caudal direction and open into the chorionic cavity (→2.19). After the folding process, they connect the pericardial cavity and the peritoneal cavity.

In stage 14 (→2.21), the lung buds grow into the coelomic canals from dorsal. In stage 20 (→2.23), the coelomic canals separate as pleural cavities from the pericardium and from the peritoneal cavity. The pleuropericardial membrane interrupts the connection to the pericardial cavity, and the pleuroperitoneal membrane delimits the pleural cavities from the peritoneal cavity.

**7.5 Differentiation of the Lungs.** The branching pattern of the lung buds reflects the topography of the lung segments. On the left side, the heart lies in place of the seventh segment. The fourth and fifth segments of the middle lobe fuse with the upper lobe and form the lingula of the upper lobe. The less steeply descending course of the left main bronchus and of the overriding pulmonary artery on the left side are also determined by the position of the heart.

The structure of the lung corresponds to a gland that was modified for respiration. In lung differentiation, it is not the formation of alveoli but rather the functional arrangement of the septa and the optimization of the diffusion distance that plays a decisive role. In humans, the lung is in principle capable of functioning at the beginning of the alveolar phase in the 23rd week of pregnancy—that is, even before the growth phase has ended. Whether it can actually function depends on whether the type II alveolar epithelial cells, which produce surfactants, are adequately differentiated. Surfactants reduce the surface tension and thereby prevent lung collapse. According to Duncker (1990), the extraordinarily early potential of the lungs to function indicates that human pregnancy is prolonged relative to pregnancy in other primates because of the time required for the maturation of the brain.

**7.6 Overview: Mesenteries.** The presentation aims to clarify the relationships of mesenteries in their definitive locations. The courses of the ligaments and folds emanating from the umbilicus result from the position of the umbilical vessels in the embryo. The schematic transverse section A1b illustrates the arrangement of the arterial trunks of the gut in the dorsal mesentery. Venous blood is collected in the portal vein. The venous trunks pass from the dorsal into the ventral mesentery in the duodenal U and form the portal vein, which proceeds to the liver in the lower margin of the lesser omentum. At birth, when the circulation is redirected (→ 6.9), the portal circulation takes over the function of the placental circulation.

**7.7 Gastrointestinal Rotation.** The rotation of the stomach and intestine is not a true morphogenetic movement but results from differential relative growth. It serves as a didactic concept to explain the complicated mesenteric relations in the adult. It is presented here with the help of a three-dimensional computer model generated by the construction and animation program "Softimage." (This is a part of the "Anatü Tutor" computer teaching program, which allows the picture to be rotated in space on the computer screen.)

**7.8 Situs.** Kollmann's *Handatlas der Entwicklungsgeschichte ("Atlas of Embryology")*, published in 1907, was the first to give the classic embryological description of peritoneal relationships. The course of vessels in the upper abdomen can be understood by analyzing their courses between the peritoneal layers before the parts become fused. The celiac trunk, for example, arises in the dorsal aorta, and after the lienal artery branches off in the dorsal mesogaster, turns ventrally at the cardia of the stomach, and sends out branches for the liver and for the lesser curvature in the ventral mesentery.

**7.9 Liver.** The liver is the last of the organs to arise from the hypobranchial groove of the pharynx during embryonic folding and intestinal tube closure. In the actively deforming mesodermal palisades, a muscarinic cholinergic system is active; this activity can be localized by cholinesterase histochemistry. The muscarinic system appears in actively moving cells and tissues and disappears after the conclusion of the morphogenetic phase. Plate 3.28 indicates the significance of neurotransmitters for the regulation of cell movements.

The glandular structure of the liver acinus and the organization of venous lobules around the central vein are the two structural principles intermingled in the liver. Embryologically, it is interesting that the functionally important venous lobules arise earlier than the phylogenetically older glandular lobules containing biliary capillaries and biliary ducts.

The asymmetry of the liver hilus is due to the displacement of the umbilical vein on the right side and the displacement of the vitelline vein (the future portal vein) on the left side. Consequently, in the liver hilus the round ligament of the liver (umbilical vein) and the the falciform ligament (ventral mesentery) lie on the right side, whereas the portal vein with the hepatic artery and hepatic duct lies on the left side.

**7.10 Anomalies.** Since the closure of the intestinal tube and of the body wall are closely linked, developmental anomalies of both processes are illustrated in the plate. However, of the malformations of the body wall and the intestinal tract that could be derived from morphological development, only few examples can be given.

## 7.1 Overview: Digestive Tube

*Background*

The **digestive tube** is lined by endoderm that generally functions in the digestion and resorption food. During embryonic life, nutrition is provided by the yolk sac and the placenta; thus the gastrointestinal tract only takes up its function after birth. The **yolk sac** is an outpocketing of the midgut in which the yolk from the egg is initially stored during embryonic development. The yolk sac is replaced by the placenta, which arises from the allantois (→ 3.14). The **allantois** is an evagination of the cloaca that originally functioned in the storage of waste substances produced by embryos developing within an egg. In mammals, the endodermal component of the placenta is reduced to an *allantoic diverticulum*, since excretion of wastes is taken over by the placental circulation.

### A. Development and Organization of the Digestive Tube

**1. Folding off from the Yolk Sac.** The digestive tube arises by the folding process of the embryonic body (→ 2.15). The head and tail folds of the embryo are raised from the yolk sac. The *foregut* projects into the *head fold* and the *hindgut* projects into the *tail fold*.

**2. Intestinal Portals.** The future anterior and posterior intestinal openings are delineated by the *pharyngeal membrane* and the *cloacal membrane*. At these sites, the endoderm abuts directly against the ectoderm. During the folding process, the *anterior* and the *posterior intestinal portals* migrate inward toward each other, compressing the region in which the intestinal canal is open.

**3. Closure of the Intestinal Tube.** As the intestinal tube closes, the *yolk sac* and *body stalk* are joined with the umbilical cord (→ 2.14). In the foregut, the *thyroid gland*, the *liver*, and between the two, the *lung buds* develop (**A4**). The hindgut widens to form the *cloaca*.

**4. Intestinal Tube.** The future oral cavity with the outpocketing of the pituitary rudiment (→ 4.24) is of ectodermal origin. The **foregut** (**A2**) extends caudally up to the *primordia of the liver and pancreas*. The upper segment of the foregut takes a horizontal course (pharynx) and extends up to the origin of the *lung buds*. The caudal segment descends behind the heart and contains the prospective *esophagus* and *stomach* (**A5**).

**5. Umbilical Loop.** The midgut elongates into the umbilical loop. At the apex of the umbilical loop is the *vitelline duct* (**A4**), which recedes with the yolk sac when the chorionic cavity becomes obliterated (→ 2.32). It can persist as **Meckel's diverticulum**, in which case it frequently contains ectopic gastric mucosa.

The upward-turned limb of the umbilical loop contains the prospective colonic structures and ileum; the downward-turned limb contains the prospective jejunum. The border between the colon and small intestine is indicated by the small bulge of the *cecum*.

**6. Intestinal Rotation.** After stage 16, the umbilical loop lies outside of the body cavity in the *umbilical coelom* (**physiological umbilical hernia**), where the rotation of the umbilical loop takes place. The intestinal loop returns to the body cavity in the 11th week of pregnancy.

The **cloaca** (**A3**) is divided into the **urogenital sinus** (**A5**), which gives rise to the **bladder**, and the **rectum** (**A6**). The exit of the *allantoic diverticulum* comes to lie at the apex of the bladder.

During the entire embryonic period, the **border of the diaphragm** between the *pericardium* and the *liver* is continuously shifted further caudad. This is due to the disproportionate growth of the anterior half of the embryo containing the brain, the heart, and the liver. The size of the heart is determined by the placental circulation, that of the liver by hemopoiesis and by its function as a filter organ between the placenta and the embryo. The downward shift of the diaphragmatic plane creates space behind the heart and the liver for the development of the lungs and the esophagus and stomach.

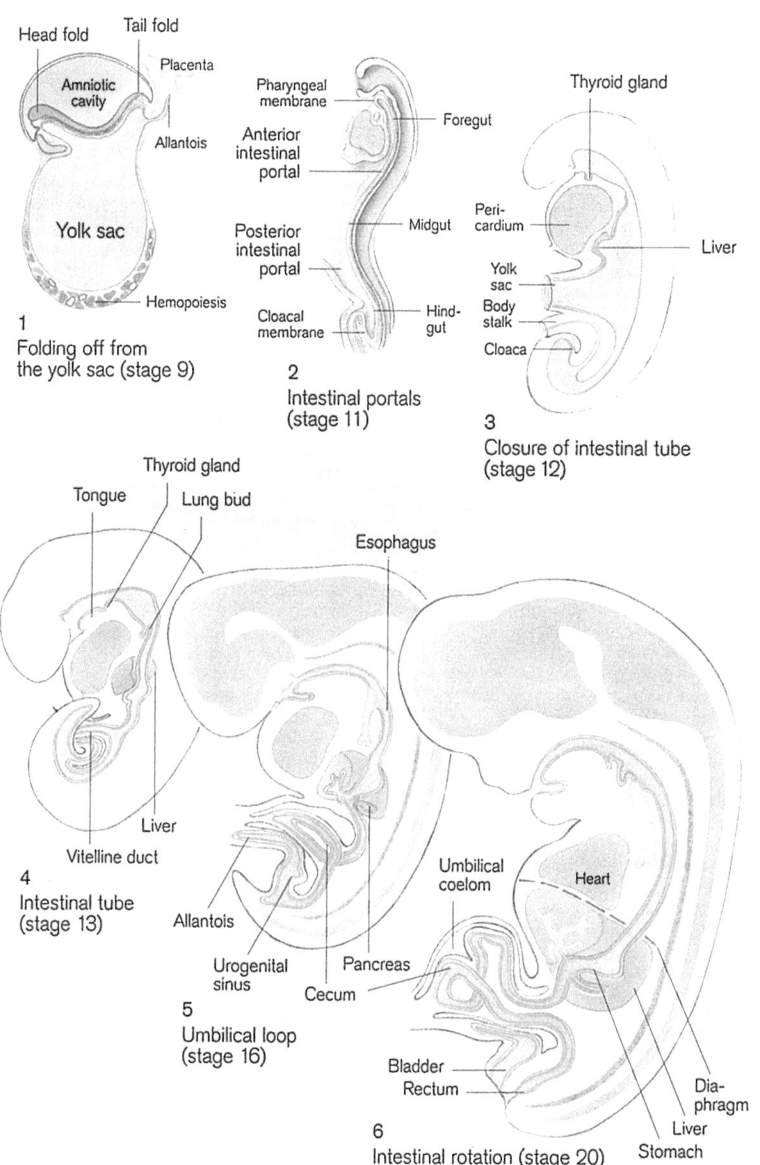
Head fold
Tail fold
Placenta
Amniotic cavity
Allantois
Yolk sac
Hemopoiesis
1
Folding off from the yolk sac (stage 9)
Pharyngeal membrane
Foregut
Anterior intestinal portal
Midgut
Posterior intestinal portal
Cloacal membrane
Hind-gut
2
Intestinal portals (stage 11)
Thyroid gland
Peri-cardium
Liver
Yolk sac
Body stalk
Cloaca
3
Closure of intestinal tube (stage 12)
Thyroid gland
Tongue
Lung bud
Liver
Vitelline duct
4
Intestinal tube (stage 13)
Esophagus
Allantois
Urogenital sinus
Pancreas
Cecum
5
Umbilical loop (stage 16)
Umbilical coelom
Heart
Bladder
Rectum
Dia-phragm
Liver
Stomach
6
Intestinal rotation (stage 20)

A. Development and organization of the digestive tube

## Pharynx

# 7.2 Entodermal Derivatives

## A. Auditory Tube, Thyroid Gland, Tonsils, and Thymus

### 1. Pharyngeal Pouches in Stage 13

In human embryos, the first three *pharyngeal pouches* are well developed. The endodermal outpocketings of the pharyngeal pouches are directly apposed to the ectoderm at the floor of the pharyngeal clefts. The fourth pharyngeal pouch is smaller and does not reach the ectoderm. A questionable fifth pharyngeal pouch has been described as an appendage of the fourth. A sixth pharyngeal pouch does not arise.

### 2. Pharynx in Stage 21

At the end of the embryonic period, the pharynx is transformed into the *definitive pharynx* and the *larynx*, so that the definitive anatomy is already recognizable. The organs developing from the pharynx—the *thyroid gland, parathyroid glands,* and the *thymus*—descend in front of the trachea into the cervical and thoracic regions.

### 3. Derivatives of the Pharynx

In cross section, the pharynx has a triangular shape. The groove at the floor of the pharynx—which in the case of filter-feeders is occupied by cilia—is called the **hypobranchial groove.** From it sprout the unpaired derivatives of the pharynx located in the median plane: the *thyroid gland*, the *lung diverticulum*, and, further down in the foregut, the *liver primordium*. The laterally situated pharyngeal pouches give rise to the *auditory tube*, the *tonsils*, the *thymus,* and the *parathyroid glands*.

**Thyroid Gland.** The buds of the *thyroid gland* arise at the floor of the pharynx at the level of the *first pharyngeal pouch*. The epithelial bud grows caudally in front of the lung buds and comes to lie below the larynx. It then breaks down into cords and epithelial buds, which develop into follicles. The site of origin of the thyroid gland is at the base of the tongue and can be recognized as the *foramen caecum* (→ 7.3). Remnants of the original epithelial connection between the base of the tongue and the thyroid gland (*thyroglossal duct*) can persist as the *pyramidal lobe* of the thyroid gland or as thyroid nests and cysts along the course of the thyroglossal duct.

**First Pharyngeal Pouch.** With the development of the palate (→ 9.1), the first pharyngeal pouch is shifted cranially into the epipharynx and forms the **auditory tube**. Its endoderm ultimately lines the entire middle ear and the air cells of the mastoid process (→ 5.8).

**Second Pharyngeal Pouch.** The second pharyngeal pouch is preserved as a fossa for the *tonsils*. The endoderm forms crypts in which the epithelium loosens into a netlike (reticular) structure. The lymphocytes of the tonsils settle within this endodermal reticulum.

**Third Pharyngeal Pouch.** This pouch gives rise to the **thymus**. The thymus, in the form of two epithelial cones, grows downward on both sides into the mediastinum behind the anlage of the thyroid gland and in front of the stem of the ventral aorta, ultimately coming to lie above the pericardium. The epithelial connection between the third pharyngeal pouch and the thymus disappears; however, epithelial nests may remain along the path and become colonized by lymphocytes, forming **thymus nests.**

Besides the thymus, the third pharyngeal pouch gives rise to the two **inferior parathyroid glands**. Together with the thymus, they are shifted caudally, passing the superior parathyroid glands and coming to rest in the inferior pole of the lobe of the thyroid gland.

**Fourth Pharyngeal Pouch.** The fourth pharyngeal pouch gives rise to the **superior parathyroid glands,** which attach posteriorly at the superior pole of the thyroid gland. A caudal outpocketing of the fourth pharyngeal pouch, designated the **ultimobranchial body**, was thought to give rise to the *calcitonin-* and *somatostatin*-producing parafollicular cells of the thyroid gland (*C cells*). Observations with chick/quail chimeras (→ 3.12), however, have shown that the C cells of the thyroid gland are derived from the neural crest.

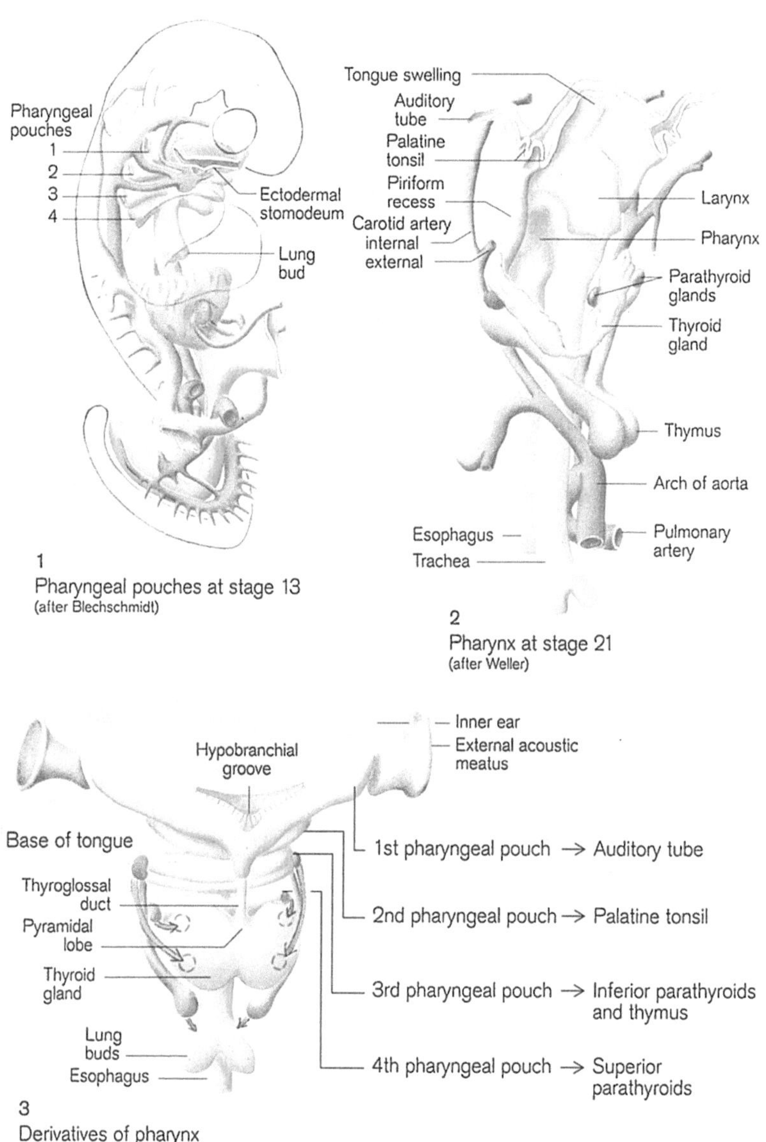


1
Pharyngeal pouches at stage 13
(after Blechschmidt)

2
Pharynx at stage 21
(after Weller)

3
Derivatives of pharynx

A. Pharyngeal gut

## 7.3 Cervical Sinus and Cervical Cysts

*Background*

The development of the tongue and the cervical sinus involves all components of the **pharyngeal arches** represented three-dimensionally in plate 3.20 and takes place at the same time as the development of the pharyngeal arch nerves (→ 4.12), the aortic arches (→ 6.7), and the visceral skeleton (→ 9.3).

### A. Tongue and Cervical Sinus

**1. Development of the Tongue**

The developing tongue bulges at the floor of the pharynx behind the *pharyngeal membrane* and grows anteriorly into the *oral cavity* (**1a**). It consists of parts of the first, second, and third pharyngeal arches. The site of origin of the thyroid gland (*foramen caecum*) at the base of the tongue marks the boundary between the first and second arches (**1b**).

The relation of the tongue to the pharyngeal arches is still apparent in the arrangement and the attachment of the **tongue musculature** (not illustrated). The genioglossus muscle originates at the genu of the mandible, which is derived from the first pharyngeal arch. The styloglossus muscle arises from the styloid process, a part of the second pharyngeal arch. The hyoglossus originates from the hyoid bone, which arises from the second and third arches. The tongue musculature is derived from myoblasts of the occipital myotome that migrate into the tongue in broad tracts. They receive their motor innervation from the hypoglossal nerve (→ 4.12).

The relations to the three pharyngeal arches are also apparent in the **sensory innervation**. The nerve of the first pharyngeal arch (trigeminal nerve with its second branch, the *mandibular nerve*) provides general sensory innervation for the anterior two-thirds of the tongue via the lingual nerve. The nerve of the second pharyngeal arch, the *facial nerve*, supplies this region of the tongue with sensory fibers for taste via the chorda tympani. The posterior third of the tongue is supplied with fibers for general sensibility and for taste by the nerve of the third pharyngeal arch, the *glossopharyngeal nerve*.

**2. Formation of the Cervical Sinus**

In stage 14, the pharyngeal arches still lie directly upon the cardiac swelling (**2a**). The neck is still absent. As the embryo elongates and the neck develops, the first two *pharyngeal arches* form the prominent viscerocranium (**2b**). The floor of the mouth and the tongue extend between the mandible and the hyoid bone. The third and fourth pharyngeal arches are incorporated in the slender neck and participate in the formation of a *laryngeal skeleton*. The lower margin of the second arch forms an **operculum**, which grows over the much smaller third and fourth arches. These are thus shifted to the interior, where they lie temporarily in an ectodermally-covered fossa, the **cervical sinus**, which is closed by the operculum. At the floor of the cervical sinus, the third and fourth pharyngeal arches disappear and the sinus loses its connection with the surface, finally disappearing entirely.

The deeply invaginated ectoderm of the cervical sinus takes part in the formation of the **thymus** (→ 7.2). It forms the epithelial portion of the cortical region and is important in the selection of T-lymphocytes (→ 3.35). The ectodermal components of the thymus are later found in the keratin-producing epithelial cells of Hassall's corpuscles.

### B. Malformations: Cervical Cysts

Remnants of the pharyngeal clefts and pouches that open into the cervical sinus and remnants of the sinus itself can persist as cysts and fistulae. Situated at the anterior margin of the *sternocleidomastoid muscle*, they may be connected to the ectodermal side (**external branchiogenic fistula**) or to the pharynx (**internal branchiogenic fistula**). As a rule, the lateral cervical cysts are associated with lymphatic tissue, so that they have also been interpreted as dystopic tissue from the tonsils (second pharyngeal pouch). **Median cervical cysts** are remnants of the thyroglossal duct (→ 7.2).

**Preotic fistulae** lie in front of the external auditory meatus. They are believed to arise by a defect in the fusion of the auricular hillocks (→ 5.10).

Hypophysis
Pharyngeal membrane
Oral cavity
See 1b
Lung bud

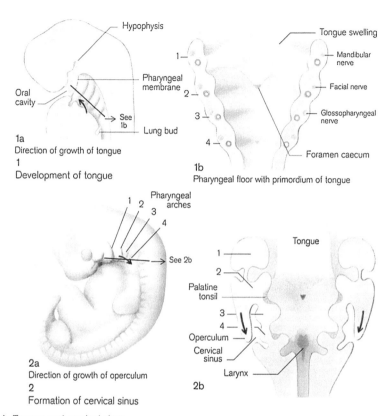

1a
Direction of growth of tongue

1
Development of tongue

Tongue swelling
1
Mandibular nerve
2
Facial nerve
3
Glossopharyngeal nerve
4
Foramen caecum

1b
Pharyngeal floor with primordium of tongue

Pharyngeal arches
1 2 3 4
See 2b

2a
Direction of growth of operculum

2
Formation of cervical sinus

Tongue
1
2
Palatine tonsil
3
4
Operculum
Cervical sinus
Larynx

2b

A. Tongue and cervical sinus

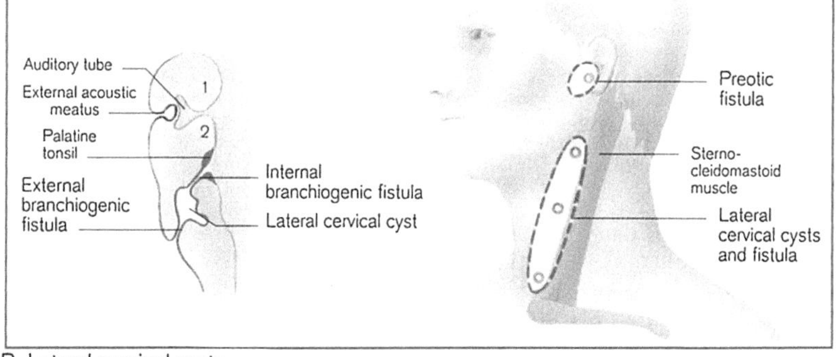


B. Lateral cervical cysts

# Respiratory System

# 7.4 Lung Buds

## A. Formation of Trachea and Lung Buds

### 1. Lung Buds in Stage 12

The lung and the air passages, the larynx, and trachea, arise from an evagination of the median groove of the pharynx (*hypobranchial groove*) between the fourth pharyngeal pouch and the *hepatic sinus* (→ 2.15). The esophagus, trachea, and stomach can develop only after the foregut has extended, which occurs with the descent of the heart (→ 6.7). In this process, space is also created behind the heart for the development of the lung.

### 2. Abscission of the Trachea from the Esophagus

The lung buds are bilobed from the outset and contain the material for the right and left lungs, but not for the trachea. The trachea arises by progressive detachment from the foregut as it elongates into the esophagus. The *esophagotracheal septum* is a transient structure formed during the abscission.

### 3. Malformation: Esophageal Atresia and Esophagotracheal Fistula

In the developing foregut, the prospective esophagus dorsally forms a thin epithelial groove, while ventrally the prospective trachea consists of thick epithelium (**A2**). This explains why a disturbance in the abscission process causes an atresia of the esophagus and not of the trachea. *Esophageal atresia* can be associated with the development of a fistular canal into the trachea between the upper or the lower blind esophageal segment. In the case of an *upper fistula* (arrow), milk or other food can enter the lung and lead to a deleterious pulmonary inflammation.

## B. Growth of the Lungs into the Coelomic Canals

### 1. Demarcation of the Pleural Cavities

The lung buds grow medially and dorsally into the **coelomic canals** (→ 2.21). The peritoneal covering over the lung buds becomes the *visceral* and the lining of the coelomic canal the *parietal pleura* (**B2**). Negative pressure can be generated in the pleural cavity only if it is completely separated from the pericardial and peritoneal cavities.

**Separation from the pericardial cavity** occurs by the growth of the **pleuropericardial fold** in the frontal plane. The fold contains the stem of the *cardinal veins*, which passes medially from the lateral body wall to the inflow tract of the heart. Initially, this entry into the heart lies in the extension of the septum transversum behind the liver primordium. As the inflow tract of the heart is displaced cranially (→ 6.2), the stem of the cardinal vein is also shifted cranially. In this process, the *pleuropericardial fold* is extended upward and ultimately separates the pericardial from the pleural cavity.

**Separation of the pleural cavity from the peritoneal cavity** occurs by the development of the **diaphragm**. The diaphragm originates by the outgrowth of the **pleuroperitoneal fold** from the dorsal body wall toward the *septum transversum* lying above the *liver* (**B1**). Fusion of the pleuroperitoneal fold and the septum closes the coelomic canal from below. Myoblasts for the **skeletal musculature of the diaphragm** migrate in from the cervical myotomes. Innervation is supplied by the *phrenic nerve* (**B2**) from C4, which passes to the diaphragm in the *pleuropericardial fold* (**B1**) below the stem of the cardinal vein.

### 2. Hilus of the Lung

The hilus of the lung arises at the border between the *visceral* and the *parietal pleura*. The bifurcated *trachea* is situated behind the heart and in front of the esophagus. In the hilus, the main bronchi thus lie dorsally and the vessels coming from the heart ventrally. The *pulmonary artery* courses dorsally with the arch of the aorta. The pulmonary arteries (red) are closely apposed to the main bronchus and follow the bronchi. As the heart is shifted toward the left, the left pulmonary artery is pushed upward and rides on the left main bronchus. The *pulmonary veins* (blue) lie in the hilus in front of the arteries and course in the lung along the boundaries of the segments.

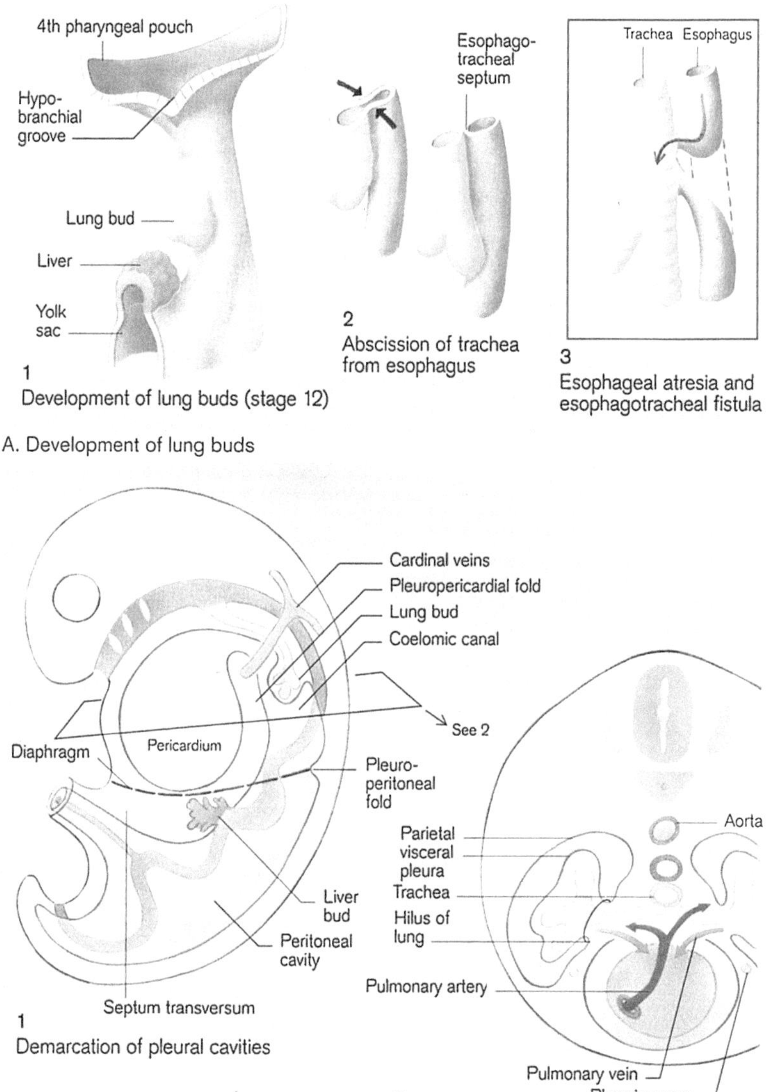


1
Development of lung buds (stage 12)

2
Abscission of trachea from esophagus

3
Esophageal atresia and esophagotracheal fistula

A. Development of lung buds

1
Demarcation of pleural cavities

2
Development of hilus of lung

B. Growth of lungs into the coelomic canals

## 7.5 Differentiation of the Lungs

### C. Formation of Bronchial Tree, Alveoli, and Septa

#### 1. Embryonic Phase: Lobules and Segments of the Lung

The lobules and segments of the lungs are formed with the branching of the lung buds in the embryonic period. The asymmetry between the right and left lung is due to the position of the *heart* on the left side. The *left main bronchus* takes a horizontal course, whereas the right descends steeply. Invagination of the visceral pleura between the lobar bronchi gives rise to three lung lobes on the right side, while on the left side the segments of the *middle lobe* are incorporated into the upper lobe. Ten segments are established on the right side; on the left side, segment seven is absent in the region of the heart. The left pulmonary artery is shifted upward and rides above the left main bronchus.

#### 2. Pseudoglandular Phase: Gland-like Outgrowth of the Duct System

The lung primordium now grows like an exocrine gland into the surrounding mesenchyme. *Dichotomous branchings* (arrows) are induced by the mesenchyme, which forms a thick cap over each epithelial bud. In the 19th week of pregnancy, after about 15–20 branchings, the gland-like growth of the ducts is arrested by the formation of sac-like or canal-shaped, broad terminal ramifications. The canaliculi correspond to the terminal parts of a gland. While the tall columnar epithelium in the bronchial branches differentiates into ciliated epithelium, the cuboidal epithelium of the canaliculi is capable of forming alveoli.

#### 3. Canalicular Phase: Development of Terminal Branches

In the 15th to 28th week of pregnancy, the canaliculi again branch out 5–10 times, thereby greatly increasing the amount of tissue capable of forming alveoli.

#### 4. Alveolar Phase: Sprouting of Alveoli

Differentiation of alveoli begins in the 23rd week of pregnancy, while the canaliculi are branching. The canaliculi and their branches are surrounded by collagenous and elastic fibers. The cuboidal epithelium of the canaliculi differentiates into regions of flat alveolar cells (**5a**), while the cuboidal epithelium at the periphery and in the proximal wall segments between the canaliculi continues to form buds. The thin wall segments form *alveoli* that bulge like berries from the wall of the canaliculi (**5c**). In a three-dimensional representation, the bulges of the alveoli squeeze through the meshwork of collagen and elastic fibers. In the stem canaliculi at the terminal branchings of the bronchial tree, segments of cuboidal epithelium persist. They become the *respiratory bronchioles,* while the duct branchings arising from them are transformed into *alveolar ducts*.

#### 5. Formation of Septa

During the differentiation of the canaliculi into alveoli, the gland-like structure disappears and is replaced by a lung-specific structure characterized by the differentiation of septa between the alveolar ducts and alveoli.

The cuboidal *alveolar stem cells* differentiate into flat *Type I alveolar epithelial cells* and cuboidal *Type II alveolar epithelial cells,* which produce *surfactant* in the lamellar corpuscles. The canaliculi widen, pressing the wall segments of adjacent canaliculi together. Loose mesenchyme rich in capillaries fills the regions in between. In the connective tissue layer between adjacent alveoli, the capillary networks meet, forming a double layer of capillaries (*primary septum*). After birth, the primary septum is transformed into a single thin layer of capillaries characteristic of the mature lung (*secondary septum*). This transformation is completed by the 7th day after birth.

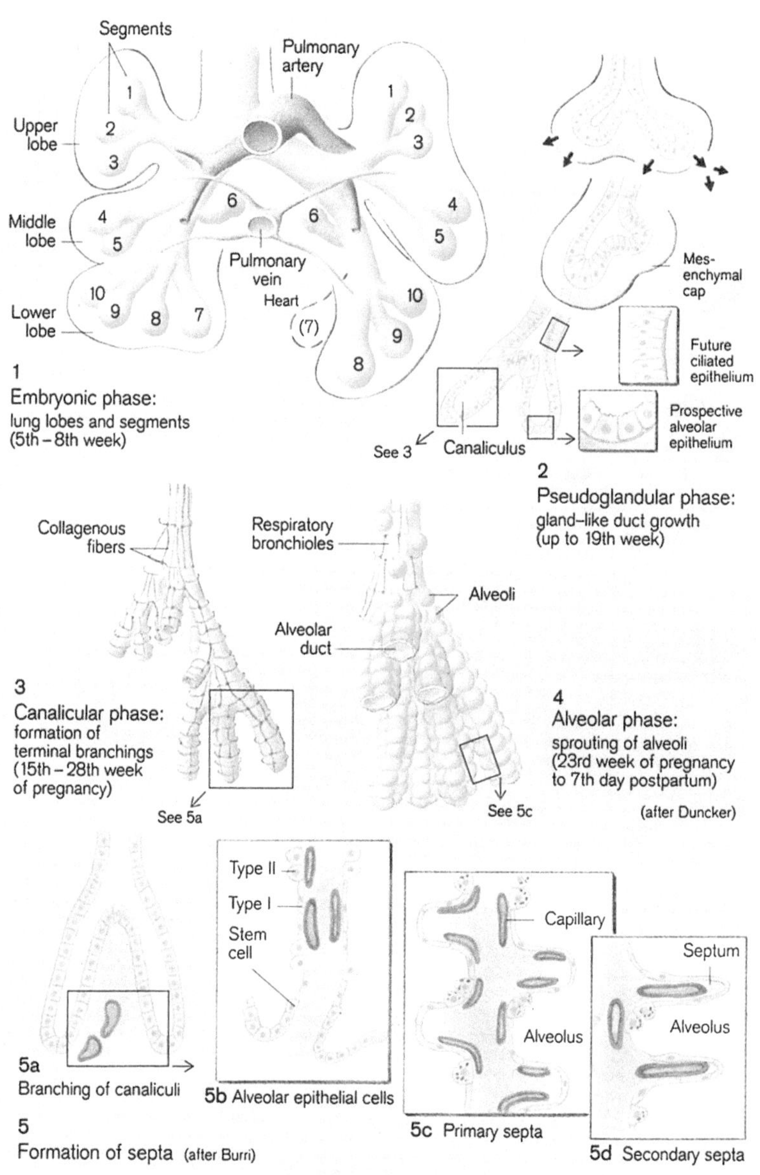
Segments
Pulmonary artery
Upper lobe
Middle lobe
Lower lobe
1 2 3 4 5 6 7 8 9 10
Pulmonary vein
Heart
(7)
1
Embryonic phase:
lung lobes and segments
(5th – 8th week)
Mes-enchymal cap
Future ciliated epithelium
Prospective alveolar epithelium
See 3
Canaliculus
2
Pseudoglandular phase:
gland–like duct growth
(up to 19th week)
Collagenous fibers
Respiratory bronchioles
Alveoli
Alveolar duct
3
Canalicular phase:
formation of terminal branchings
(15th – 28th week of pregnancy)
See 5a
4
Alveolar phase:
sprouting of alveoli
(23rd week of pregnancy to 7th day postpartum)
See 5c
(after Duncker)
Type II
Type I
Stem cell
Capillary
Septum
Alveolus
Alveolus
5a
Branching of canaliculi
5b Alveolar epithelial cells
5c Primary septa
5d Secondary septa
5
Formation of septa (after Burri)

C. Differentiation of lungs

# Umbilical Loop and Mesenteries

## 7.6 Overview

*Background*

**Mesenteries** are the routes by which vessels and nerves reach the gastrointestinal tract. The arterial trunks originate from the aorta and lie in the dorsal mesentery. The veins travel to the liver along the ventral mesentery. The vitelline and placental circulations (→ 6.1) arise from the vessels of the yolk sac and allantois associated with the intestinal tract. The vitelline vessels give rise to the superior mesenteric artery (→ 6.7) and the portal vein (→ 6.8); the umbilical vessels obliterate.

### A. Mesenteries and Large Vessels

#### 1. Dorsal and Ventral Mesentery

**a Mesenteries in the Upper Abdomen.** In the upper abdomen, the intestinal tube is attached to the body wall by a *dorsal* and a *ventral mesentery*. Before the stomach has rotated, its greater curvature is directed dorsally and the lesser curvature ventrally **(A1)**. The *spleen* arises in the dorsal mesentery of the stomach, and the *dorsal pancreas* grows into this mesentery from the duodenum. The ventral mesentery contains the *liver*, with the *gallbladder* and the buds for the *ventral pancreas*. The ventral mesentery lying between the liver and body wall becomes the *falciform ligament*, and the ventral mesentery between the liver and stomach becomes the lesser omentum.

**b Mesentery of the Umbilical Loop.** At the level of the *umbilical loop*, only a *dorsal mesentery* is present. The vitelline duct passes from the apex of the umbilical loop to the remains of the yolk sac in the chorionic cavity (→ 2.14). The *allantoic diverticulum* extends to the umbilical ring from the apex of the future bladder in the ventral body wall.

#### 2. Course of Vessels

**Umbilical Vessels.** During embryonic life, the main bloodstream flows from the heart to the placenta via the *aorta* and *umbilical arteries*. Beyond the bifurcation of the aorta, the umbilical arteries exit from the *femoral artery* and course in the medial body wall with the allantois to the umbilicus. The unpaired *umbilical vein* passes from the umbilical cord directly to the liver. It lies in the lower margin of the ventral mesentery, which extends from the umbilicus to the liver hilus.

**Arterial Trunks.** The intestinal tract in the body cavity is supplied directly with blood from the aorta via three arterial trunks. The *celiac trunk* supplies the organs of the upper abdomen. The branches for the liver and the lesser curvature of the stomach cross over from the dorsal mesentery into the ventral mesentery behind the pylorus of the stomach. The *superior mesenteric artery* is the axis for the rotation of the umbilical loop. The *inferior mesenteric artery* supplies the lower segment of the colon ( i.e., the segment from the left end of the transverse colon to the lower end of the rectum).

**Portal Vein.** The blood from the gastrointestinal tract is collected in the portal vein. The intestinal veins course together with the arteries in the dorsal mesentery. Ahead of the entrance of the arteries into the aorta, the venous trunks exit from the dorsal mesentery and pass behind the duodenum into the ventral mesentery. They join the *portal vein*, which arrives in the liver through the *hepatoduodenal ligament* **(A3)**. The lower edge of the ventral mesentery is thereby separated into two portions: into the *hepatoduodenal ligament*, the lower margin of the lesser omentum between the duodenum and hilus of the liver, and into the *round ligament of the liver* between the liver hilus and the umbilicus, which contains the *umbilical vein* **(A2)**. The *round ligament* is the lower margin of the *falciform ligament*.

#### 3. Mesenteric Relations after Birth

After birth, nutrients are transported to the liver by the portal vein rather than by the umbilical vein. The umbilical vein in the *round ligament of the liver* obliterates. The umbilical arteries give rise to the medial umbilical folds, while the obliterated allantois becomes concealed exactly in the midline in the *median umbilical fold*. The *lateral umbilical folds* contain the inferior epigastric arteries.

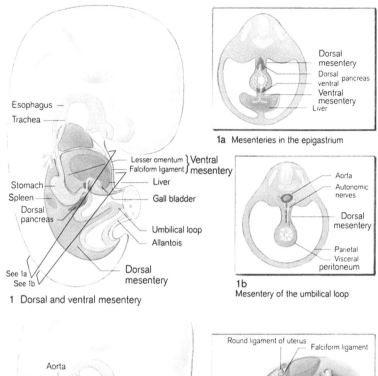

Esophagus
Trachea
Lesser omentum
Falciform ligament
Ventral mesentery
Stomach
Spleen
Dorsal pancreas
Liver
Gall bladder
Umbilical loop
Allantois
See 1a
See 1b
Dorsal mesentery

1 Dorsal and ventral mesentery

Dorsal mesentery
Dorsal
ventral
pancreas
Ventral mesentery
Liver

1a Mesenteries in the epigastrium

Aorta
Autonomic nerves
Dorsal mesentery
Parietal
Visceral
peritoneum

1b
Mesentery of the umbilical loop

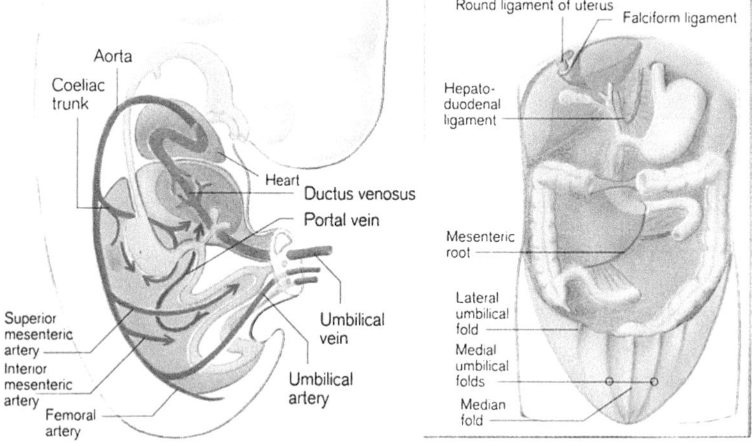


2 Course of vessels

3 Mesenteric relations after birth

A. Mesenteries and large vessels

## 7.7 Gastrointestinal Rotation

*Background*

The embryological movement referred to as the "**rotation of the stomach and intestine**" is caused by the elongation of the intestinal tube up to a length many times that of the body. This movement includes the rotation and tilting of the stomach and the counterclockwise rotation of the intestinal loop. In fact, the so-called "rotation" does not actually entail movement, but is due to increased growth of individual intestinal segments relative to the body wall. The impression of a developmental movement arises because (for didactic reasons) the definitive gastrointestinal tract is projected back upon the embryonic state in which the digestive tube is situated in the midline—without taking into account the size difference between the embryonic and definitive state.

### A. Rotation of the Stomach and Intestine

**1. Initial Position.** The dorsal mesentery is attached to the greater curvature of the stomach, whereas the ventral mesentery is attached to the lesser curvature. The greater curvature faces dorsally, the lesser curvature ventrally. Emanating from the duodenum, the bile duct with the *gallbladder* and the *liver* extends into the ventral mesentery, while the pancreas extends into the dorsal mesentery.

**2. Rotation of the Stomach.** The stomach rotates clockwise 90 degrees around its longitudinal axis. In this process, the greater curvature (with the spleen) is displaced toward the left and the lesser curvature (with the liver and gallbladder) toward the right. The outpocketing of the dorsal mesentery behind the stomach forms the *omental bursa*. The ventral mesentery gives rise to the *lesser omentum* between the lesser curvature and the liver hilus, as well as the *falciform ligament* anchored in the midline between the liver and the body wall.

**3. Rotation of the Umbilical Loop.** The umbilical loop lies in the median plane (**A1**). It rotates counterclockwise 180 degrees around an axis defined by the superior mesenteric artery, so that the lower limb of the umbilical loop comes to lie upward. The apex of the loop is formed by the vitelline duct. The proximal segment of the loop—now lying inferiorly—forms the coils of the small intestine, while the distal segment gives rise to the part of the large intestine extending from the left side of the transverse colon to the rectum.

Rotation of the umbilical loop occurs outside of the body cavity in the physiological umbilical hernia (→ 2.28). The return into the body cavity begins with the shifting of the intestinal coils and ends with the formation of the large intestine. In this process, the colon, led by the cecum, rotates counterclockwise (**A4**), again around the axis of the superior mesenteric artery.

**4. Tilting of the Stomach.** Besides rotating, the stomach also tilts around an axis located in the midpoint of the lesser curvature, so that the greater curvature comes to lie horizontally over the transverse colon. The pancreas, located in the dorsal mesentery, now lies behind the stomach and its apex points to the hilus of the spleen.

**5. Displacement of the Ventral Pancreas.** In front of the opening of the bile duct into the duodenum, an additional pancreatic bud arises and projects into the ventral mesentery (*ventral pancreas*). As the stomach rotates, the opening of the bile duct migrates behind the duodenum to the left side, taking the ventral pancreas with it. Between the ventral pancreas (*uncinate process*, **A6**) and the dorsal pancreas lies the *superior mesenteric artery*.

**6. Fusion of the Bile and Pancreatic Ducts.** The bile duct crosses under the pancreatic duct. The ventral pancreas fuses with the dorsal pancreas from behind. Fusion of the crossed ducts gives rise to a common opening for the pancreatic and bile ducts (*greater duodenal papilla*). The original duct of the dorsal pancreas may persist as an accessory opening (*lesser duodenal papilla*).

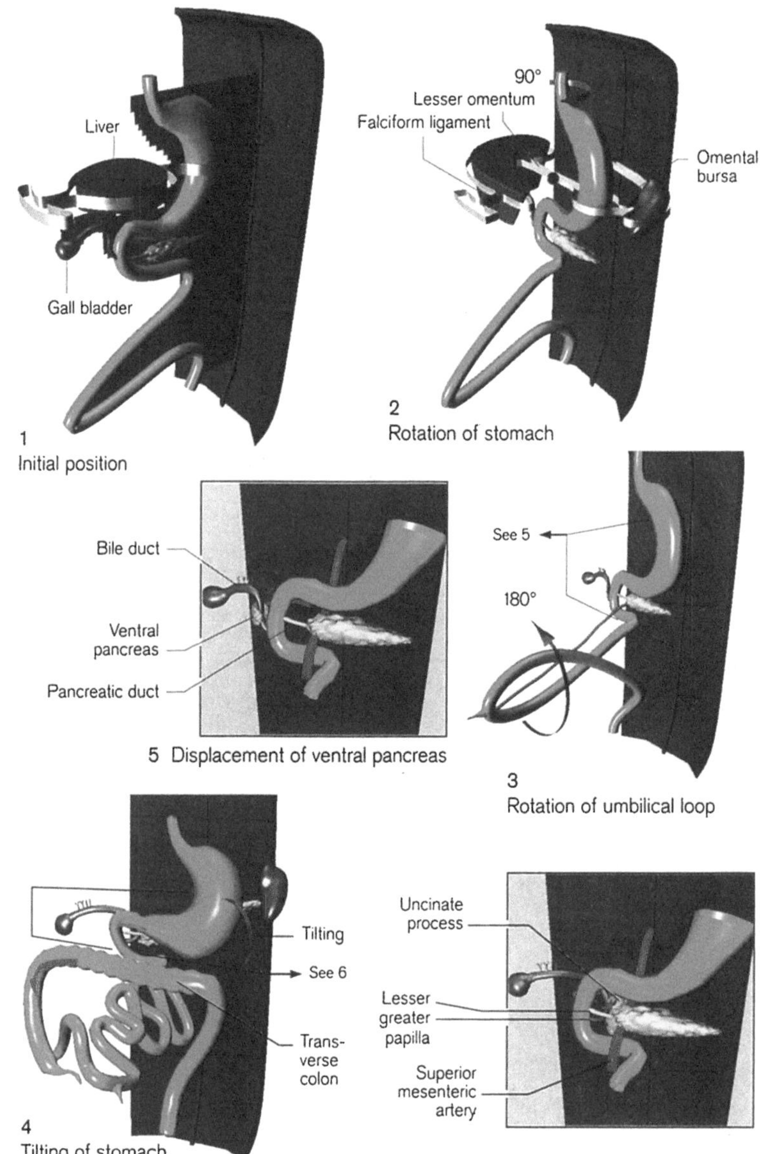


1 Initial position

2 Rotation of stomach

5 Displacement of ventral pancreas

3 Rotation of umbilical loop

4 Tilting of stomach

## 7.8 Derivation of Situs

### A. Primary Course of Mesenteries and Fusion with Body Wall

#### 1. Outpocketings of the Mesenteries

As the stomach rotates toward the left, its greater curvature takes the *dorsal mesogastrium* along with it. Behind the stomach, arises the **omental bursa** (arrow), which terminates on the left at the hilus of the spleen. Its natural opening is the *epiploic foramen* below the hepatoduodenal ligament.

An outpocketing of the dorsal mesogaster at the greater curvature of the stomach gives rise to the **greater omentum**. The tilting of the stomach causes this outpocketing to drop, so that it comes to lie over the transverse colon (**3a**).

The *mesentery of the colon* and the *mesentery of the intestinal loop* (mesentery in the narrower sense) arise from the **mesentery of the umbilical loop**.

#### 2. Course of Vessels

The **arteries** travel from the dorsal body wall to their target organs via the mesenteries. Their definitive positions can thus be deduced from the original course of the mesenteries (i.e., prior to the definitive fusions).

The **celiac trunk** arises in the dorsal mesogastrium on the right side of the stomach cardia. The *lienal artery* travels to the spleen in the dorsal mesogastrium behind the stomach. The *hepatic artery* passes from the dorsal mesogastrium into the ventral mesogastrium and then travels in the lesser omentum to the liver. The *left* and *right gastric artery* course in the ventral mesogastrium in the lesser curvature. The *left gastric artery* enters the ventral mesogastrium directly at the stomach cardia, while the *right gastric artery* branches off from the hepatic artery in the ventral mesogastrium.

The *gastroduodenal artery* also branches from the hepatic artery. It courses steeply in the dorsal direction via the dorsal mesogastrium to its target region behind the pylorus. The gastroduodenal artery, which passes into the dorsal region, and the *right gastric artery*, which remains ventral, are superimposed in an anteroposterior view. The *gastroepiploic arteries* travel in the dorsal mesogastrium along the greater curvature of the stomach. The left originates from the lienal artery, the right from the gastroduodenal artery.

The **superior mesenteric artery** originates from the aorta in the duodenal U, passes the horizontal part of the duodenum below the transverse colon, and enters directly into the mesenteric root of the intestinal convolutions. Apart from the small intestine, it also supplies the ascending and transverse colon.

The branches of the **inferior mesenteric artery** lie flat at the dorsal body wall and supply the descending colon, the sigmoid, and the upper part of the rectum (for the development of the portal vein → 6.8).

#### 3. Fusion with the Body Wall

The **dorsal mesogastrium** fuses with the body wall at the posterior wall of the *omental bursa*. Due to the tilting of the stomach, the *pancreas* comes to lie behind the stomach (→ 7.7 A4), passing obliquely upward in the dorsal mesoduodenum into the dorsal mesogastrium. A sagittal section (**3a**) therefore cuts the pancreas transversely at the floor of the omental bursa. An outpocketing of the dorsal mesogastrium at the greater curvature of the *stomach* forms the *greater omentum* and fuses with the *transverse colon* and the *transverse mesocolon*. As shown in the ventral view (**3b**), only the intraperitoneally situated *spleen* does not become fused with the dorsal body wall. The ligaments of the spleen, the *lienorenal* and *gastrolienal ligaments*, are derived from the dorsal mesogastrium.

The **duodenum** is a fixed point for the rotation of the stomach (occurring above) and for the rotation of the umbilical loop (occurring below). The mesoduodenum fuses with the posterior body wall. The duodenum itself is crossed by the transverse colon and is shifted completely into a retroperitoneal position.

The **mesentery in the narrower sense** serves in the attachment of the coils of the small intestine. The *root of the mesentery* extends from the *duodenojejunal flexure* to the *ileocolic flexure*. The **mesentery of the colon** fuses with the posterior body wall except for the *transverse mesocolon* and the *sigmoid mesocolon*.

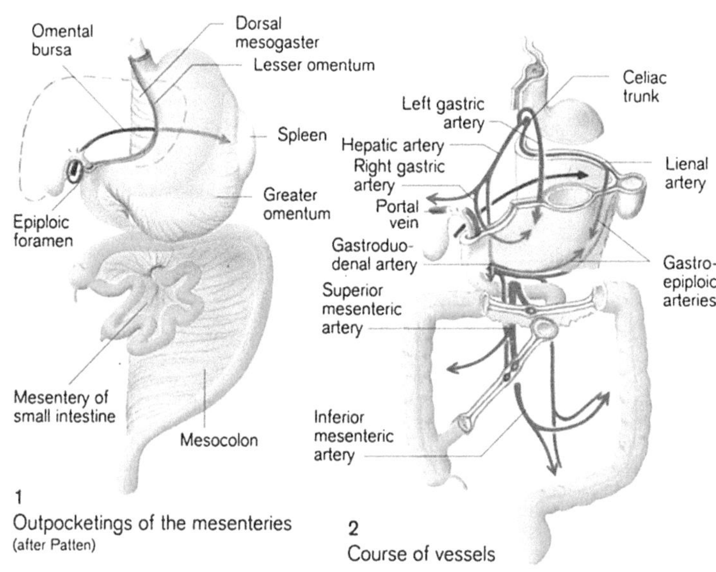


1
Outpocketings of the mesenteries
(after Patten)

2
Course of vessels

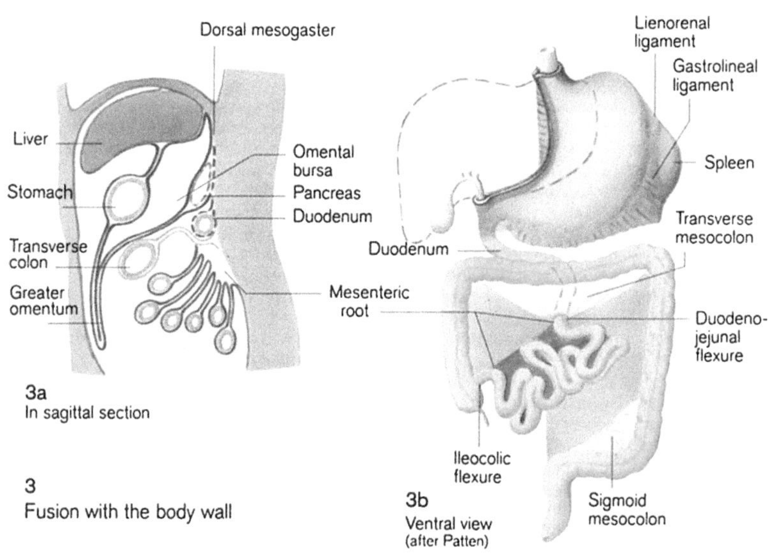


3a
In sagittal section

3
Fusion with the body wall

3b
Ventral view
(after Patten)

A. Derivation of definitive situs

## 7.9 Liver

*Background*

Already in embryonic life, the **liver** is inserted between the nutrient-supplying veins and the main circulation as a filter and a metabolic organ. Nutrients are transported initially by the vitelline veins, then by the umbilical vein, and finally by the portal vein.

### A. Differentiation of the Liver

**1. Abscission of the Liver Buds**

The liver arises in the endoderm of the **liver recess (1a)** at the transition between the foregut and the yolk sac. During the folding process, the endodermal material for the liver becomes delimited as the anterior intestinal portal migrates caudally (→ 2.15). The upper region of the liver diverticulum contains the cranial liver bud, from which hepatic cylinders sprout. The lower segment of the diverticulum gives rise to the gallbladder with the bile duct and two caudal buds.

**Abscission (1b)** is driven by the cells of the visceral mesoderm, which are organized into *epithelial plates*. The abscission progresses from cranial to caudal; at its completion, the epithelial plates disintegrate. The mesodermal cells form a loose *mesenchymal network* into which the liver cylinders grow. On the other side, the *vitelline veins* invade the epithelial network, unite into the sinus venosus, and form the *sinusoids* of the liver (**A2**). During the abscission and the development of hepatic cylinders, the mesodermal cells exhibit a *cholinesterase (ChE) activity* (→ 3.28), which indicates that they represent the morphogenetically active component in liver development.

**2. Outgrowth of Hepatic Plates.** The liver is an exocrine gland; its cells function not only in the production of bile but also in metabolic processes requiring an active exchange of substances with the blood. Since the metabolic function is important already in embryonic life, it develops first. The *hepatic plates* sprout into the current carried by the *vitelline veins* and the sinus venosus. A three-dimensional network of liver plates arises which, like a sponge, is perfused by inflowing blood from the vitelline veins. The visceral mesoderm functions simultaneously as the mesodermal component of the hepatic cylinders and as the *endothelium of the sinusoids*. The duct system for bile secretion forms later by the development of biliary capillaries and the transformation of liver plates into *bile ducts*.

**3. Secretory and Venous Lobules of the Liver.** The *secretory lobule* corresponds to the *acinus* of an exocrine gland, in which the terminal buds are formed by the hepatic cylinders with the bile capillaries. The *hepatic artery* and the *portal vein* enter the liver hilus with the bile duct and ramify with the biliary ducts. Blood from the portal vein and the hepatic arteries flows through the acinus and collects in the *central veins* located in the periphery of the secretory lobule. The central veins converge into the *hepatic veins* that empty into the inferior vena cava. Each central vein collects blood from segments of adjacent acini. The hepatic tissue centered around a central vein forms a *venous liver lobule*.

**4. Organization into Lobes.** The development of the lobes of the liver can be traced back to the course of the veins in the fetal period. In the **neonate (4a)**, the *umbilical vein* still possesses a direct connection to the *inferior vena cava* (*ductus venosus*). Since the definitive umbilical vein originates from the left umbilical vein, it lies to the left. The trunk of the *portal vein*, on the other hand, arises from the right vitelline vein and therefore lies on the right. This arrangement gives rise to the typical H structure in the organization of liver lobes seen in the **infant (4b)**. The central region of the H bounded on the right side by the *hilus* and the gallbladder, and on the left side by the remnant of the umbilical veins and the ductus venosus (*round ligament of the liver* and *ligamentum venosum*) contains the *caudate lobe* in the upper portion and the *quadrate lobe* in the lower. The widening of the portal vein at the former opening of the umbilical vein is known as the *umbilical recess*.

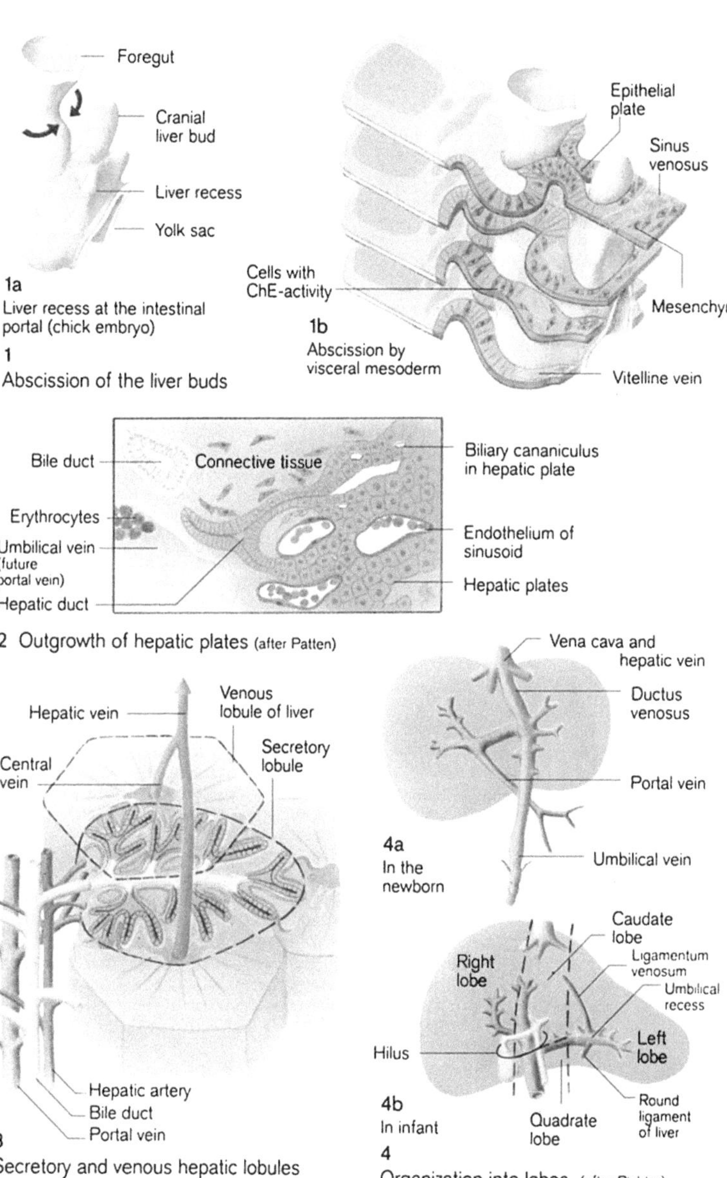


1a
Liver recess at the intestinal portal (chick embryo)

1b
Abscission by visceral mesoderm

1
Abscission of the liver buds

2 Outgrowth of hepatic plates (after Patten)

3
Secretory and venous hepatic lobules

4a
In the newborn

4b
In infant

4
Organization into lobes (after Richter)

A. Differentiation of liver

## 7.10 Malformations

### A. Anomalies and Malformations of the Gastrointestinal Tract

**1. Congenital Diaphragmatic Hernia.** Incomplete closure of the diaphragm by the **pleuroperitoneal fold** (→ 7.4) can result in the displacement of intestinal loops and of a part of the stomach into the left pleural cavity. This leads to a compression of the left lung and shifts the heart and the mediastinum toward the right.

**2. Defects in the Body Wall.** In the final stages of the folding process, the **lateral folds** (→ 2.15) fuse in the midline and close the body wall. A disturbance in this process can cause the heart (**ectopia cordis**) or the abdominal viscera to lie outside of the body cavity.

**3. Persistence of the Physiological Umbilical Hernia.** If the intestinal loops do not reenter the body cavity after the physiological hernia, a hernial sac persists in the umbilical cord. Since the umbilical cord is covered by amniotic epithelium (→ 2.14), the hernial sac is composed of amnion. In an acquired hernia, on the other hand, the hernial sac consists of layers of the body wall.

**4. Malrotation.** A disturbance in the rotation of the intestine can cause positional anomalies due either to a reversal in the direction of rotation of the umbilical loop (**4a**) or to an incomplete rotation during the return of the intestinal loops into the body cavity (**4b**). The different forms of "malrotation" can be considered cases of incomplete **situs inversus**. In a total situs inversus, all viscera are arranged as a mirror image. In embryonic development, right–left asymmetry of the viscera begins when the cardiac loop turns toward the right (→ 2.21 and 6.4). Partial forms of situs inversus lead to malformations of the heart (for example, the transposition of the great vessels, → 6.10) or to malpositions of the abdominal viscera that can be recognized as deviations from the normal developmental movements.

**5. Annular Pancreas.** The pancreas encircles and constricts the duodenum. This anomaly results from a disturbance in the migration of the ventral pancreas and in its fusion with the dorsal pancreas (→ 7.7).

**6. Stenoses and Atresia.** In the normal development of the mucous membrane, proliferation of the endodermal epithelium leads to a physiological closure of the gastrointestinal canal at stage 17 (→ 2.26) before the mucosal folds form. At this point, the lumen is completely filled by stratified layers of endodermal cells. During recanalization, lumens form throughout the tissue so that the intestine becomes filled with epithelial follicles and sponge-like clumps of tissue. After reorganization into a mucosa with folds and villi, local **septa** (**6a**) and **cysts** (**6b**) from the epithelial proliferation can remain in the mucous membrane. Disturbances in the recanalization process are possibly also the cause for **stenoses** (**6c**), in which short segments of the small intestine are constricted. This hypothesis, however, cannot be reconciled with the early time of damage observed in cases of thalidomide embryopathy (→ 10.1). The most common site for such anomalies is the duodenum, but anomalies can also arise in the **bile duct** (ductus choledochus) (**6d**) and in the gallbladder, where the mucosa develops in the same manner as in the intestinal canal. Stenoses in the small intestine (**6c**) lead to a prestenotic widening of the intestine, while stenoses in the bile duct (**6d**) cause a dilatation of the intrahepatic biliary ducts. A stenosis or obliteration of the bile duct leads to a deleterious jaundice if not operated early.

**Total Bile Duct Atresia.** In the case of total atresia of the bile duct, biliary ducts do not form in the liver. This anomaly can be interpreted as a disturbance in the second phase of liver development, when the biliary channels are formed secondarily from the hepatic cylinders (→ 7.9).

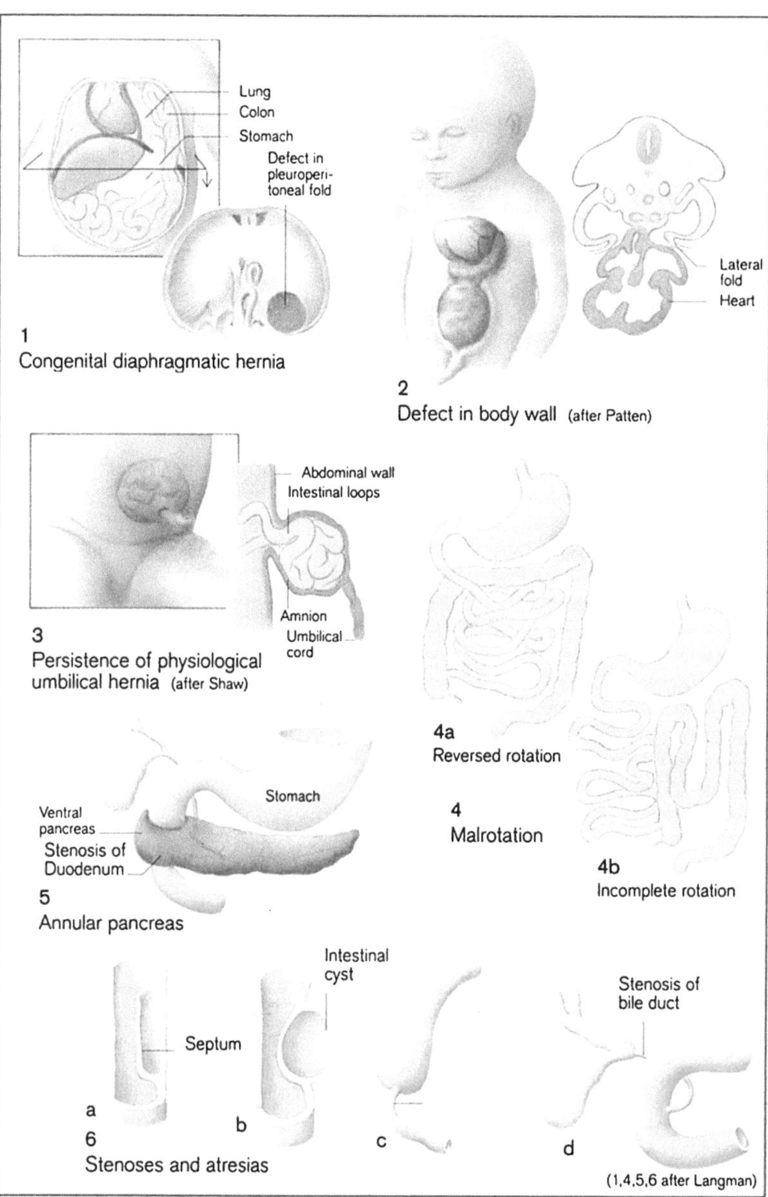
Lung
Colon
Stomach
Defect in pleuroperitoneal fold
1
Congenital diaphragmatic hernia
Lateral fold
Heart
2
Defect in body wall (after Patten)
Abdominal wall
Intestinal loops
Amnion
Umbilical cord
3
Persistence of physiological umbilical hernia (after Shaw)
4a
Reversed rotation
4
Malrotation
4b
Incomplete rotation
Stomach
Ventral pancreas
Stenosis of Duodenum
5
Annular pancreas
Intestinal cyst
Septum
Stenosis of bile duct
a
b
c
d
6
Stenoses and atresias
(1,4,5,6 after Langman)

A. Malformations of the gastrointestinal tract

# Chapter 8: Urogenital System

## Introduction

**8.1 Overview.** The use of segmental excretory tubules as efferent ducts for the germ cells is a phylogenetically old mechanism, conserved from simple, metameric organisms such as earthworms up to mammals. In mammals, the oviduct takes up the egg by means of a ciliated funnel opened to the body cavity. The system of egg transport through the body cavity, although primitive at first glance, is optimized to the smallest detail for each species. An example is the finely tuned, cyclic hormonal regulation of Fallopian tube movement in humans (→ 1.12).

The development of the embryonic urinary system through the **pronephros**, **mesonephros**, and **metanephros** stages reflects the phylogenetic development of this system in vertebrates. The pronephros is the primordial segmental form of the kidney. The mesonephros is the dominant excretory organ in fish. Development of the metanephros in tetrapods is associated with the enlargement of the nephron around Henle's loop. This enables water to be resorbed and urine to be concentrated, essential functions for life on dry land.

Separation of the metanephros from the mesonephros is accompanied by the separation of the kidneys from the genital ducts. The principle of the pronephros is reserved for the female genital ducts, that of the mesonephros for the male genital ducts. The separation takes place by translocation of the ureteric openings from the mesonephric (Wolffian) ducts into the bladder. In female mammals, the downward growth of the vagina ultimately leads to a complete separation, whereas in male mammals, the urethra is preserved as a common excretory duct. The complete separation in female organisms permits internal fertilization and intrauterine development of the embryo.

The term "paramesonephric duct" is based on the assumption that humans have no pronephros. However, pronephric structures can be observed in the human embryo (Jacob, 1990) and thus the paramesonephric duct (Mullerian duct) may well be derived from a pronephric tubule, which instead of entering into the common excretory duct of pronephros and mesonephros (Wolffian duct, mesonephric duct) grows down to the urogenital sinus inside the basal lamina of the latter.

The downward growth of the mesonephric duct to the cloaca was first observed by Caspar Friedrich Wolff in the living chick embryo in 1759. Wolff interpreted his observation as clear proof that new structures arise during embryogenesis (**epigenesis**). He therefore rejected the homunculus theory (**preformation**), according to which the embryo is already preformed in the sperm or in the egg and must simply grow. With this, he questioned the creationist belief and initiated the scientist-creationist controversy persisting to this day. In his treatise on the "Developmental History of the Genital Organs ..." (1830), Johannes Müller did not directly describe the müllerian duct. However, he recognized the development of the male and female genital ducts from a common indifferent stage and the general homology of these structures in the mammalian embryo, including the human.

**8.2 Ascent of the Kidney.** The true-to-scale reconstruction of the mesonephros, metanephros, and intestinal tract by James Didusch, the artist of the Carnegie Laboratories of Embryology of the Carnegie Institution of Washington, in the work by Shikinami (1926) shows not only the ascent of the metanephros but also the relative displacements of all large organ systems during the embryonic period. This displacement is due to growth spurts at different times in embryonic development: the initially disproportionately large heart is overtaken in growth by the brain and spinal cord, which leads to the descent of the heart. The growth of the brain and spinal cord then lags behind that of the vertebral column and the axial skeleton. This leads to the caudal outgrowth of the vertebral column and to the descent of the extremities, as well as the ascent of the conus medullaris relative to the vertebral column (→ 4.4). The retroperitoneally situated metanephros ascends together with the conus medullaris. Both arise below S1 and ascend up into the lumbar segments. The bifurcation of the aorta descends with the vertebral column. The intraperitoneally situated mesonephros descends below the liver, together with the intestinal coils.

**8.3 Differentiation of the Kidney.** Branching of the ureteric bud is induced by the metanephrogenic blastema, and the renal tubules are induced by the ureteric bud, a classic example of an **epithelial–mesenchymal interaction**. This interaction was studied in organ culture by combining epithelial and mesenchymal components, focusing on the question of specificity (chorda tissue can replace the ureteric bud as an inductor) and on the question of whether direct cell contact or a diffusible molecule is responsible for the induction. Recent investigations suggest that induction is mediated by growth factors and cell adhesion molecules of the cadherin type (→ 3.28).

**8.4 Malformations of the Kidney.** Defects in the separation of the genital ducts from the urinary tract, a phylogenetically recent development, can cause clinically important syndromes. During embryonic life, such defects can lead to disturbances in the development of the metanephros (aberration of the ureteric bud); and after birth, they can lead to the secondary loss of the kidneys due to ascending infection (reflux of urine into the ureter).

**8.5 Sex Determination.** In mammals, a regulatory sequence on the Y chromosome, Sry, induces the cascade of sex determination. The dominance of Sry relative to the sex hormones in the induction of the gonads is a mammalian specialization that apparently prevents maternal hormones from interfering with sex determination in the embryo. In certain fish, the development of a testis can be induced by testosterone and that of an ovary by estradiol. In birds, the female sex is heterogametic (ZW/ZZ). Ovarian development is induced by the W-chromosome. The testis originates constitutively; it can be transformed into an ovary by estradiol.

**8.6 Differentiation of the Gonads.** The migration of primordial germ cells from the yolk sac to the gonads is the central event in the germ line. The term "germ line" was coined in 1880 by Nussbaum, who observed the migration of yolk-rich primordial germ cells in lower vertebrates and thus refuted the concept that germ cells originate in the "germinal epithelium," the thickened coelomic epithelium over the gonadal ridge.

The gonadal primordium is organized into a medulla and a cortex; the medulla gives rise to the testicular tubules, while ovarian structures develop in the cortex. Thus the ovotestis of true hermaphrodites has interior testicular tubules surrounded by external ovarian structures.

**8.7 Genital Ducts.** The organization of the female genitalia, with a transverse plate structure between the rectum and the bladder, resembles the arrangement in the indifferent anlage. Male genital development is determined by the descent of the testis. The coverings of the spermatic cord can be perceived as outpocketings of the body wall that bulge into the scrotum, an outpocketing of the skin.

**8.8 Downward Growth of the Vagina.** The downward growth of the vagina is a continuation of the caudal growth of the mesonephric and paramesonephric ducts. Defects in this process can lead to many malformations in this region, such as an aberrant ureter.

**8.9 External Genitalia.** The glans of the clitoris and penis develop from the genital tubercle. Secondary canalization of the glans of the penis causes the cavernous body at the apex of the genital tubercle (phallus) to detach from the cavernous bodies of the genital tubercle (corpora cavernosa) and unite secondarily with the cavernous body of the urethral folds (corpus spongiosum).

**8.10 Malformations of the Sexual Organs**. The sex organs are not essential for the viability of the embryo. Thus, all conceivable disturbances in the determination cascade shown in plate 8.5 are encountered as malformations in patients because they are compatible with life after birth.

## 8.1 Overview: Urogenital System

*Background*

The urinary and genital organs are grouped together as the **urogenital system,** since the genital ducts are derived from the renal tubules.

### A. Renal Tubules and Genital Ducts

**1. Renal Tubules of a Ringworm.** In simple, metamerically organized organisms, the *renal tubules* are segmentally arranged. In ringworms (→ 3.1), the tubules form *ciliated funnels* that project into the coelomic cavity of each segment, perforating the segmental border and opening into the body cavity at the level of the following coelomic segment. The ciliated funnels thus collect metabolic end products from the coelomic fluid. In sexual segments they serve for the transport of mature germ cells to the exterior.

**2. External and Internal Glomeruli in the Vertebrate Embryo.** In vertebrate embryos, the primordial material for the renal tubules lies between the somites and the lateral plates (intermediate mesoderm, → 3.24). The nephrogenic material of a segment is a **nephrotome**. Cranial nephrotomes give rise to renal tubules that open into the coelomic cavity through a ciliated funnel. Associated with each ciliated funnel, is a vascular tuft (*glomerulus*) that protrudes into the body cavity (*external glomerulus*). Waste products are released by the glomerulus into the body cavity, from where they are taken up by the ciliated funnel. Afferent vessels come from the aorta; efferent vessels open into the cardinal vein. In the further development of this functional unit, the vascular tuft invaginates directly into the renal tubules (*internal glomerulus*). An excretory tubule with its glomerulus is a **nephron**.

**3. Transformation of the Pronephros and Mesonephros into Genital Ducts.** Three **renal systems** develop from cranial to caudal (**3a**): *pronephros*, *mesonephros*, and *metanephros*. The **pronephros** includes the cranial nephrons, which still open into the body cavity through a *ciliated funnel* (**A2**) and possess an external glomerulus. In the human embryo, a rudimentary pronephros with sporadically appearing external glomeruli forms, but recedes during the embryonic period.

The pronephros merges into the **mesonephros** without a clear boundary. The tubules of the mesonephros possess internal glomeruli and open into a common excretory duct known as the *mesonephric (Wolffian) duct*.

The **metanephros** (definitive kidney) arises from fused nephrotomes lying caudally to the mesonephros (metanephrogenic blastema). This blastema has no direct connection to the mesonephric duct, since the duct diverges medially toward the cloaca. Outgrowth of the *ureteric bud* later links the metanephros to the mesonephric duct.

By incorporation of ducts into the bladder(→ 8.8), the ureter separates from the mesonephric duct. The mesonephric duct becomes the male genital duct, while the female genital ducts arise from the paramesonephric duct (**indifferent stage**). The paramesonephric duct is formed by an invagination of the coelomic epithelium that grows downward toward the cloaca within the basement membrane of the mesonephric duct. Although the paramesonephric duct develops after the pronephros has regressed, it can be perceived as a derivative of the pronephros, since it opens through a ciliated funnel above the mesonephros into the body cavity. In the indifferent stage, mesonephric and paramesonephric ducts are laid down in identical manner in both sexes.

The **female genital ducts** (**3b**) arise from the *paramesonephric ducts*. These ducts give rise to the *Fallopian tubes* . The paramesonephric ducts cross over the mesonephric ducts in the lower third and fuse with each other in the midline. The fused paramesonephric ducts give rise to the *uterus* and the *vagina*. The mesonephric ducts recede (→ 1.10).

The **male genital ducts** (**3c**) are formed by the fusion of the upper mesonephric tubules with the testis to form the *efferent ductules* and the differentiation of the mesonephric duct into the convoluted *duct of the epididymis* and the *vas deferens*. The paramesonephric duct degenerates (→ 1.7).

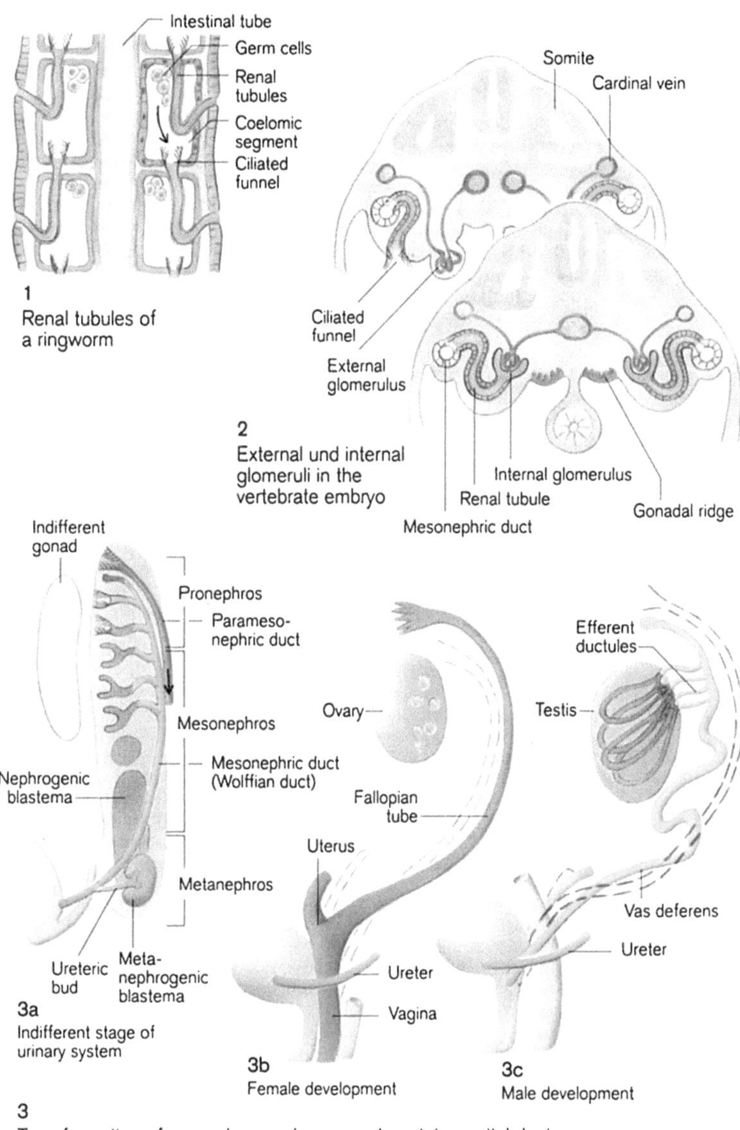


1
Renal tubules of a ringworm

2
External und internal glomeruli in the vertebrate embryo

3a
Indifferent stage of urinary system

3b
Female development

3c
Male development

3
Transformation of pronephros and mesonephros into genital ducts

A. Relation between renal tubules and genital ducts

## Urinary System

# 8.2 Ascent of the Kidney

*Background*

The definitive kidney, the **metanephros,** originates in the sacral segments below S1 and the bifurcation of the aorta, and the exits of the umbilical arteries. In the adult, it lies in the lumbar region and is projected onto the twelfth rib. The repositioning is known as the ascent of the kidney. If the kidney fails to ascend, it remains in the lesser pelvis below the bifurcation even after birth (→ 8.6). The ascent of the kidney is not an active migration but occurs as a result of the differential growth of the various organ systems.

## A. Ascent of the Kidney

**1. Position of the Segments of Origin.** At stage 14, the organs emerging from the somitic segments still lie at the level of their segments of origin: the *upper limb buds* between C4 and T1, the *lower limb buds* between L2 and S3, and the *metanephros* between S1 and S3.

**2. Ascent of the Kidney Relative to the Vertebral Column.** The first half of the embryonic period is characterized by the enormous growth of the central nervous system and the entire upper half of the body (green arrow above L1). The cervical segments of the vertebral column, together with the exits of the brachial plexus and phrenic nerve (C4), are pushed upward. The upper limb buds and the heart and liver undergo a relative descent. In the second half of the embryonic period, the growth of the spinal cord slows as the vertebral column elongates caudally. The growth of the lumbar and sacral segments causes the lower end of the body to "unroll" (Jacob, 1990), creating space for the pelvic organs (arrow below L1). By this unrolling, the body wall is shifted downward behind the kidney, and the kidney undergoes a relative ascent from the sacral region into the lumbar region. The ascent of the kidney occurs at the same time as the ascent of the conus medullaris (→ 4.4), which is also due to the unrolling of the lower end of the body. The bifurcation of the aorta remains at the level of S1. It now lies below the kidney.

**3. Descent of the Viscera.** In stage 14, the mesonephros extends into the cervical segments. While the metanephros ascends in the retroperitoneal space and grows to its definitive size, the size of the mesonephros does not change. The mesonephros (in contrast to the retroperitoneally situated metanephros) is situated intraabdominally and participates in the descent of the gastrointestinal canal. This involves the caudal displacement of the stomach and the withdrawal of the intestinal loops into the umbilical cord. Ultimately, the mesonephros, together with the gonadal primordia (→ 2.30 and 2.34), comes to lie at the lower pole of the metanephros at the entrance into the lesser pelvis.

**Insets: Development of the Urogenital Sinus.** In stage 14, the intestinal canal and the urogenital tract open into a common terminal segment termed the *cloaca*. The termination of the cloaca is marked by the *cloacal membrane* (**1a**). The *postanal gut* at the caudal end of the cloacal membrane recedes. The cloaca is divided by a tissue bridge, the *urorectal septum*, into a ventral *urogenital sinus* and a dorsal *rectum* (**2a**). Unrolling of the lower end of the body creates room for the development of the pelvic organs and permits the extension of the urogenital sinus. The upper portion of the urogenital sinus gives rise to the *bladder* and the middle segment to the *urethra* (**3a**). The lower segment, which opens into the cloaca (*urogenital sinus in the narrow sense*), is transformed into either the penile urethra or the vestibule of the vagina (→ 8.9). The metanephros (**1a**), lying caudally to the mesonephros, ascends to the level of the fundus of the stomach (**A3** and **3a**). The ureter gains a separate opening into the bladder, while the mesonephric ducts descend further. The paramesonephric duct, descending along the mesonephric duct, has not yet reached the urethra.

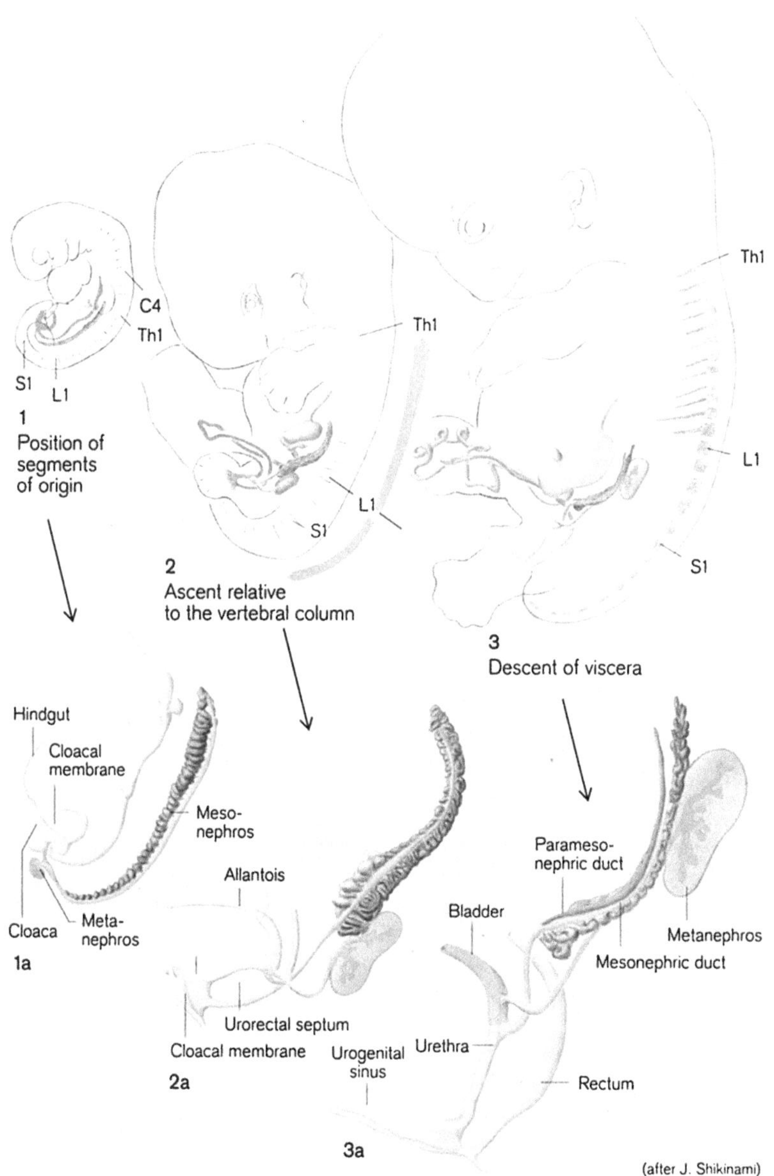
C4
Th1
S1
L1
1
Position of segments of origin
Th1
L1
S1
2
Ascent relative to the vertebral column
Th1
L1
S1
3
Descent of viscera
Hindgut
Cloacal membrane
Meso-nephros
Cloaca
Meta-nephros
1a
Allantois
Urorectal septum
Cloacal membrane
2a
Urogenital sinus
Parameso-nephric duct
Bladder
Metanephros
Mesonephric duct
Urethra
Rectum
3a
(after J. Shikinami)

A. Ascent of kidneys

## 8.3 Differentiation of the Kidney

### A. Branching of Ureteric Bud and Differentiation of Nephrons

**1. Branching of the Ureteric Bud.** The metanephros develops from two components: the *ureteric bud*, which emanates from the mesonephric duct, and the *metanephrogenic blastema*, into which the buds grow (**1a**). The ureteric bud induces the mesenchymal blastema to form an epithelial-type condensation that in turn induces the ureteric bud to branch dichotomously. This branching gives rise to the renal pelvis, renal calices, and the collecting ducts. In the metanephrogenic blastema, nephrons differentiate.

Branches of the ureteric bud directed toward the poles of the renal primordium grow slightly longer than those in the middle, giving the organ its typical kidney shape (**1b**). The tubules of the third to fifth generation of branching fuse into the renal pelvis (**insect**). In the *zones of fusion*, folds remain behind; these later fill with urine and form the *renal pelvis* (**A2**).

**2. Arrangement of Lobes.** After about the sixth division of the ureteric bud, division slows and the renal pelvis becomes separated into *major calices*. The branchings of the seventh to eleventh generation fuse with one another to form the *minor calices*, into which the *collecting ducts* open. The basic unit of the mammalian kidney is the renal calix into which projects a *medullary papilla* with parallel *collecting ducts*. The *unipapillary kidney* of the rodent (**2a**) consists of only one basic unit, whereas the kidneys of large mammals contain several such units (*renal lobes*). In humans, the organization into lobes is apparent only during fetal life. In the adult kidney, the *cortical zones* of the basic units fuse with one another, giving rise to a kidney with several papillae.

**3. Collecting Ducts and Nephron Arcades.** The branching of the collecting ducts can be divided into three phases. In the **first phase** (**3a**), the ampullary endpieces of the ureteric bud divide dichotomously. Each branching develops into a nephron and an ampullary bud that again divides dichotomously. In the **second phase** (16–24th week of pregnancy, **3b**), at the transition to the collecting duct of each newly formed nephron a new nephron is induced, so that arcade-type chains of nephrons are formed. In the **third phase** (22–38th week of pregnancy) (**3c**), the two ampullary endpieces of the ureteric bud each continue to grow further into the blastema of the cortex. Each branching again gives rise to a nephron and an ampullary dilatation. After four to seven divisions (toward the end of the fetal period), the ampullary dilatations disappear so that new nephrons can no longer arise. The kidney now increases in size only by interstitial growth.

**4. Differentiation of Nephrons.** Each terminal ramification of the ureteric bud possesses an *ampullary dilatation* with a cap of *metanephrogenic blastema*. In the differentiation phase, each branching gives rise to a growing bud with an ampullary dilatation and a nephron. On the nephron side, the ureteric bud induces a cellular condensation in the nephrogenic blastema that is transformed into an epithelial *renal vesicle*. The vesicle grows out into an S-shaped, convoluted tubule, at the base of which lies the hook-shaped Bowman's capsule. In the concave indentation of the "hook," a *capillary tuft* (the *glomerulus)* develops and becomes linked to the vascular system. The nephron arising from the renal vesicle fuses with the terminal branching of the ureteric bud and becomes linked to the collecting duct. The apex of the upper loop of the nephric tubule differentiates into the *macula densa*, which becomes applied against the vascular pole of the glomerulus. The lower limb of the S-shaped curvature grows out to form the *proximal tubule*; the upper limb forms the *distal tubule* and Henle's loop.

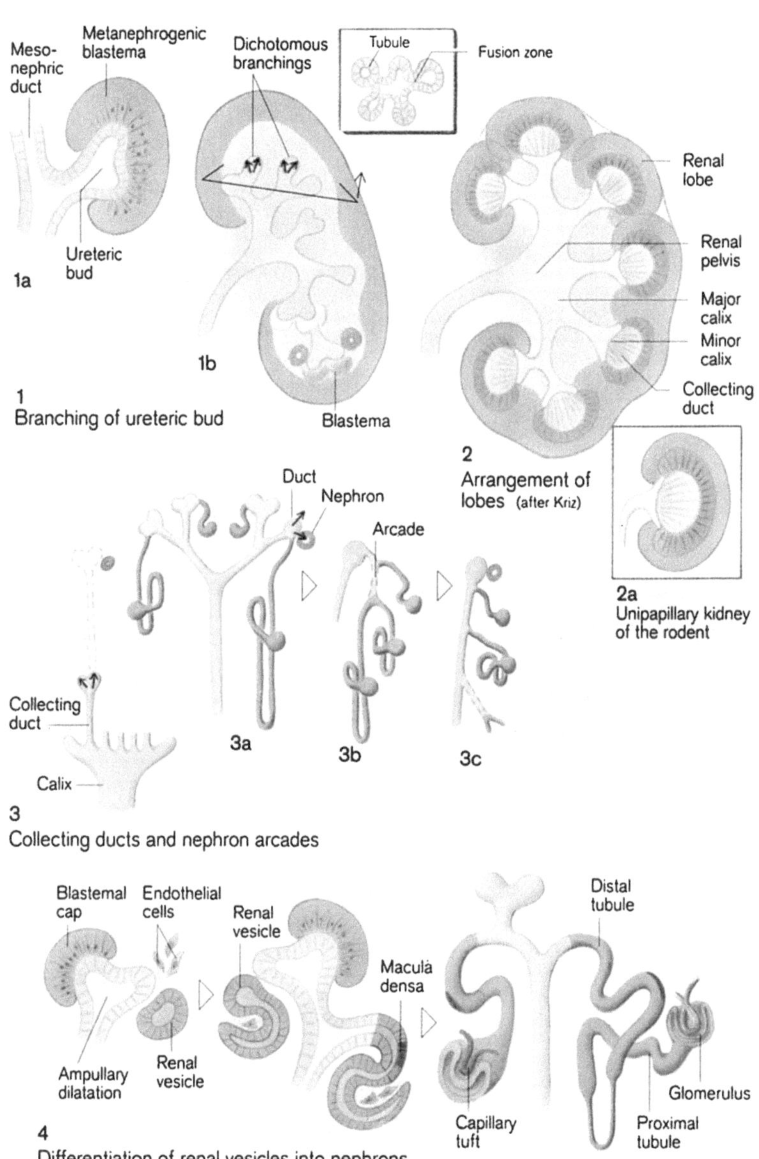

Meso-
nephric
duct
Metanephrogenic
blastema
Ureteric
bud
1a
Dichotomous
branchings
Tubule
Fusion zone
1b
Blastema
1
Branching of ureteric bud
Renal
lobe
Renal
pelvis
Major
calix
Minor
calix
Collecting
duct
2
Arrangement of
lobes (after Kriz)
2a
Unipapillary kidney
of the rodent
Duct
Nephron
Arcade
Collecting
duct
Calix
3a
3b
3c
3
Collecting ducts and nephron arcades
Blastemal
cap
Endothelial
cells
Renal
vesicle
Ampullary
dilatation
Renal
vesicle
Macula
densa
Distal
tubule
Glomerulus
Capillary
tuft
Proximal
tubule
4
Differentiation of renal vesicles into nephrons

A. Differentiation of the metanephros

## 8.4 Malformations of the Urinary System

### A. Renal Cysts, Pelvic Kidney, and Supernumerary Ureters

**1. Congenital Renal Cysts.** Cystic illnesses of the kidney, classified on the basis of morphology according to *Potter*, have a number of different causes. In the case of **autosomal recessive polycystic nephropathy (1a** ) (Potter I), the collecting ducts widen into tubular cysts. Prenatally, both kidneys enlarge and show a striped pattern of fibrotic condensations in the medullary zone. Additionally, the liver is afflicted with a periportal fibrosis and with cysts in the biliary duct system. This indicates a general disorder of duct development. In the **autosomal dominant inherited form (1b)** (Potter III), the disease first becomes manifest between the 30th and 50th year of life. Cysts are formed throughout the region of the collecting ducts and the nephrons, so that a functional renal aplasia may develop. The nonhereditary **multicystic nephropathy (1c)** (Potter II) originates in a disturbance in the development of the ureteric bud. Depending on the time and place of injury, the cysts may be confined to one side or limited to one segment. Cyst development begins in the calices of the renal pelvis; the clinical picture resembles an engorged kidney.

Bilateral or unilateral **renal aplasia** probably results from early degeneration of the ureteric bud. If the metanephrogenic blastema is not induced by a ureteric bud, it cannot develop further. Unilateral renal aplasia occurs with a frequency of 1:1500. Bilateral renal aplasia, on the other hand, is rare. A neonate with total renal aplasia dies shortly after birth.

**2. Pelvic and Horseshoe Kidneys.** During development, the kidneys are shifted from their original position in the pelvis into the lumbar region. In this **ascent** they are turned from the sagittal to the frontal plane **(2a)**. Occasionally, a kidney remains lying in the pelvis, close to the common iliac artery. This phenomenon, known as a **pelvic kidney (2b)**, is thought to be caused by the kidney becoming caught in the aortic bifurcation. While passing the aortic bifurcation, the two kidneys may become pressed so close to one another that their lower poles grow together and form a **horseshoe kidney (2c)**. This form of kidney lies in the region of the lower lumbar vertebrae, since its ascent is hindered by the exit of the *inferior mesenteric artery*. The descending ureters cross over on the ventral side of the isthmus. Horseshoe kidneys occur relatively frequently (about 1:600).

**3. Supernumerary Ureters.** A precocious division of the ureteric bud can lead to partial or complete **ureteric duplication (3a)**. The metanephrogenic blastema can be separated into two primordia with separate renal pelvis and ureter. A **supernumerary ureter (3b)** generally crosses over the normal ureter and opens further caudally into the *bladder*, the *urethra*, the *vagina*, or the vas deferens. The supernumerary bud arises cranially to the normal position. After the mesonephric duct has been incorporated into the bladder up to the exit of the normally situated bud, the second ureteric bud migrates further caudally with the mesonephric duct (→ 8.8). Reflux symptoms always arise at the opening of an aberrant ureter.

**4. Urethral Valve.** The urethral valve is an obstructing mucosal fold that, in boys, develops at the opening of the regressing paramesonephric ducts, expanding in sail-fashion on both sides toward the base of the bladder. The development of a urethral valve is probably associated with the caudal migration of the mesonephric and paramesonephric ducts. It leads to a balloon-like dilatation of the urethra into the *prostate*, to a *hypertrophy of the bladder wall* with the formation of *bladder diverticula*, and to an engorged kidney.

**5. Urachal Fistulae and Cysts.** If the lumen is preserved in the entire allantoic segment between the bladder and the umbilicus, urine can flow from the umbilicus (**urachal fistula, 5a**). If only a portion of the intraembryonic allantois persists, the secretion of fluid can lead to a cystic dilatation (**urachal cyst, 5b**).

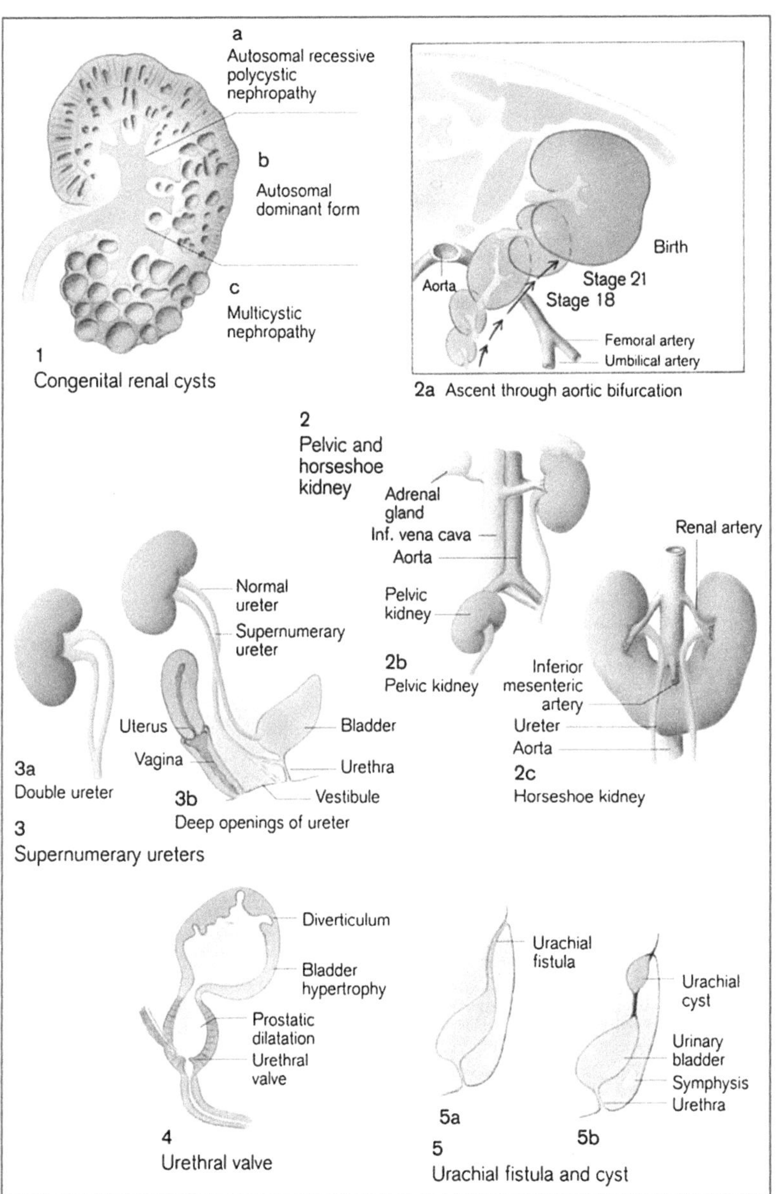

a
Autosomal recessive polycystic nephropathy
b
Autosomal dominant form
c
Multicystic nephropathy
1
Congenital renal cysts
Aorta
Birth
Stage 21
Stage 18
Femoral artery
Umbilical artery
2a Ascent through aortic bifurcation
2
Pelvic and horseshoe kidney
Adrenal gland
Inf. vena cava
Aorta
Pelvic kidney
2b
Pelvic kidney
Renal artery
Inferior mesenteric artery
Ureter
Aorta
2c
Horseshoe kidney
Normal ureter
Supernumerary ureter
Uterus
Vagina
Bladder
Urethra
Vestibule
3a
Double ureter
3b
Deep openings of ureter
3
Supernumerary ureters
Diverticulum
Bladder hypertrophy
Prostatic dilatation
Urethral valve
4
Urethral valve
Urachial fistula
Urachial cyst
Urinary bladder
Symphysis
Urethra
5a
5b
5
Urachial fistula and cyst

A. Malformations of kidney and urinary passages

# Sexual Organs

## 8.5 Sex Determination

### A. Stages of Sex Determination

**1. Chromosomal Sex.** Chromosomal sex is determined at fertilization. It depends on whether the haploid sperm contributes a Y or an X chromosome to the new organism.

**2. Gonadal Sex.** If a Y chromosome is present, the indifferent gonad in stage 18 begins to differentiate into a testis. If no Y chromosome is present, an ovary is formed.

**3. Somatic Sex.** The transformation of the indifferent genital ducts into a male or female genital tract is determined by the gonads. The *Sertoli cells* of the testis produce AMH and the *Leydig cells* produce testosterone. **AMH** (antimüllerian hormone) induces the involution of the müllerian (paramesonephric) duct. **Testosterone** transforms the mesonephric duct into the epididymis and induces the male sexual organs. In the cytoplasm of the target cells, the enzyme **5α-reductase** reduces testosterone to *dihydrotestosterone* (**DHT**), which binds to the cytoplasmic **androgen receptor** (→ 3.29) and is transported as a receptor-ligand complex to binding sites in the nucleus. The female sex organs arise constitutively: in the absence of testosterone, the mesonephric duct regresses; and in the absence of AMH, the paramesonephric ducts persist and develop into the tubes, the uterus, and the vagina.

**4. Sex Determination of the Brain.** In mammals, the male or female determination of the brain is also dependent on testosterone. Treatment of experimental animals with testosterone at the end of the fetal period leads to a masculine imprinting even in the case of female animals. The treated animals tonically secrete LH and FSH at the onset of puberty and exhibit male sexual behavior. Without testosterone, LH and FSH are secreted cyclically, and female sexual behavior develops constitutively. In the case of male imprinting, testosterone is transformed in the neurons of the brain into estradiol by the enzyme complex **aromatase**. Inside the neurons, estradiol binds to the cytoplasmic estrogen receptor and is transported to the nucleus.

### B. Mechanisms of Regulation

**1. Expression of Sry.** The regulatory gene *Sry* on the Y chromosome ("**s**ex determining **r**egion of **Y**") encodes a transcription factor. It is activated for a short time in the somatic cells of the germinal cords (→ 3.16), causing them to differentiate into Sertoli cells and secrete AMH.

**2. AMH and Testosterone. AMH** diffuses from the germinal cords into the adjacent mesonephric body and induces the degeneration of the paramesonephric duct. It acts on the mesenchyme and leads to the contraction of the cells arranged circularly around the duct. AMH is a glycoprotein and belongs to the TGF-β-family (→ 3.28). **Testosterone** has a trophic effect for the mesonephric duct; in female development, the duct degenerates because testosterone is absent. (The mechanism of degeneration is different, however, from that observed in the directly adjacent paramesonephric duct. In the epithelium of the mesonephric duct, necrosis occurs without the morphological involvement of mesenchyme).

**3. Phase-Specific Action of Testosterone.** Testosterone also determines whether a vagina or a prostate and seminal vesicle arise. In the indifferent stage, the cytoplasmic *androgen receptor protein* (→ 3.29) appears simultaneously with the embryonic muscarinic system (→ 3.23) in the *mesenchymal cells* at the opening of the genital ducts into the urethra. If testosterone is present, the *seminal vesicle* sprouts out from the *mesonephric duct* and the *prostatic buds* develop from the *urethra*. Without testosterone, the genital ducts descend further caudally as vaginal buds (→ 8.8). After birth, the androgen receptor disappears from the mesenchyme and is expressed in the epithelial component of the organs. Testosterone stimulates further growth and secretory function of the glands.

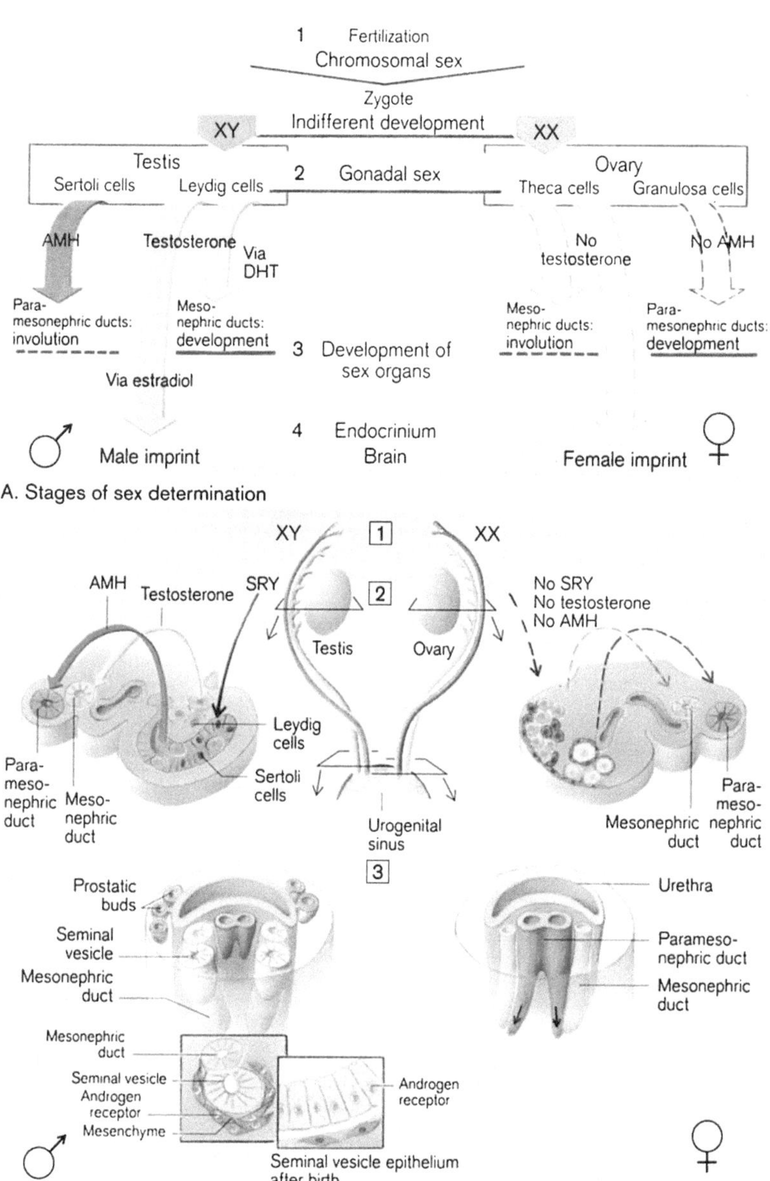


A. Stages of sex determination

B. Mechanisms of regulation

# 8.6 Gonads

## A. Differentiation of the Gonads

**1. Migration of Primordial Germ Cells.** Beginning in stage 11, human *primordial germ cells* can be distinguished from somatic cells on the basis of their size and chromatin structure (**1a**). They are located caudally in the wall of the *yolk sac* in front of the exit of the *allantois*. In stage 13, they migrate by amoeboid movements from the yolk sac to the *gonadal ridge* via the *dorsal mesentery* (**1b**).

**2. Indifferent Gonadal Primordium.** The gonadal primordium arises from a thickening of the coelomic epithelium (**2a**) in the coelomic angle between the *root of the mesentery* and the *mesonephros*. The *thickened coelomic epithelium* produces a chemotactic factor from the TGF-β -family (→ 3.28) that attracts the primordial germ cells and simultaneously stimulates them to proliferate. The coelomic epithelium grows by means of ramifying epithelial cords (*germinal cords*, **2b**) into the underlying mesenchyme and forms a genital ridge that protrudes into the body cavity. Its ever-narrowing connection to the mesonephros is the prospective root of the gonadal *mesentery*. Up to stage 18, no sexual differences are apparent.

**3. Differentiation of the Testis.** In male development, the *germinal cords* (**2b**) become distinctly delineated in the center (*medulla*) of the gonadal primordium, forming the *testicular cords*. Germ cells enclosed by these cords become the *spermatogonia*. They stop proliferating and remain in a resting stage until puberty. *Leydig cells* differentiate in the gonadal mesenchyme between the seminiferous tubules. Separating the testicular cords from the coelomic epithelium is a vascularized connective tissue layer that develops into the *tunica albuginea* of the testis. Germ cells lying within the coelomic epithelium die; the epithelium becomes the peritoneal covering of the testis. The testicular cords form horseshoe-shaped loops connected at their ends to the *rete testis* at the hilus of the testis. Each loop gives rise to a seminiferous tubule of a testicular lobule (→ 1.7). The rete testis connects the seminiferous tubules with the *efferent ductules* that arise from the mesonephric tubules. The lumen of the seminiferous tubules first appears with the onset of spermatogenesis at puberty (→ 1.8).

**4. Differentiation of the Ovary.** In female development, the connection between the coelomic epithelium and the germinal cords is preserved. The germ cells continue to proliferate in the germinal cords of the cortical zone, forming cords and nests of proliferating oogonia (oospheres). The germinal cords of the medullary zone become pressed against the hilus and regress. The oogonia at the corticomedullary border ultimately enter prophase of the first meiotic division. They become surrounded by a single layer of follicular epithelial cells arising from the epithelial cells of the germinal cords (*primordial follicle*). The follicular epithelial cells synthesize a factor that arrests meiosis in prophase I (→ 1.2). The oocytes in the primordial follicles thus enter a resting stage (dictyotene), in which they remain until puberty. Proliferating oogonia and oocytes that begin meiosis without becoming enclosed in primordial follicles die (→ 1.11). The coelomic epithelium becomes the peritoneal covering of the ovary and the connective tissue beneath it becomes the tunica albuginea of the ovary (→ 1.12).

**Homology between the Testis and Ovary.** The somatic cells of the germinal cords become the **Sertoli cells** (supporting cells) of the seminiferous tubules. They nourish the spermatogonia and determine their development (→ 1.8). The corresponding nourishing cells of the oogonia are the **follicular epithelial cells,** which become the granulosa cells of the follicle (→ 1.11).

The **Leydig cells** originate in the mesenchyme of the testis and already produce testosterone during embryonic life. Testosterone induces the male sex organs and a masculine phenotype (→ 1.8). The **theca cells** and the interstitial cells of the ovary correspond to the Leydig cells of the testis. They produce estradiol only after puberty.

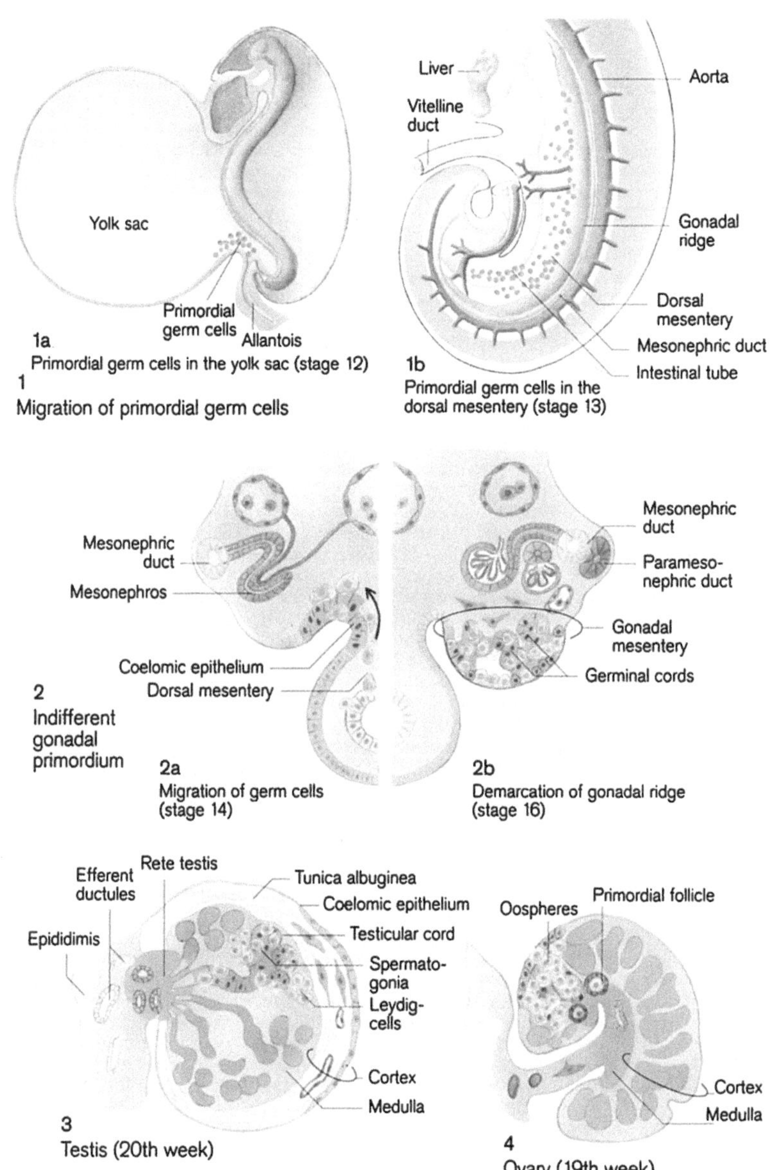
Yolk sac
Primordial germ cells
Allantois
1a
Primordial germ cells in the yolk sac (stage 12)
1
Migration of primordial germ cells
Liver
Vitelline duct
Aorta
Gonadal ridge
Dorsal mesentery
Mesonephric duct
Intestinal tube
1b
Primordial germ cells in the dorsal mesentery (stage 13)
Mesonephric duct
Mesonephros
Coelomic epithelium
Dorsal mesentery
2
Indifferent gonadal primordium
2a
Migration of germ cells (stage 14)
Mesonephric duct
Paramesonephric duct
Gonadal mesentery
Germinal cords
2b
Demarcation of gonadal ridge (stage 16)
Efferent ductules
Rete testis
Tunica albuginea
Coelomic epithelium
Epididimis
Testicular cord
Spermatogonia
Leydig-cells
Cortex
Medulla
3
Testis (20th week)
Oospheres
Primordial follicle
Cortex
Medulla
4
Ovary (19th week)

A. Differentiation of the gonads

## 8.7 Genital Ducts

### A. Development of the Female and Male Genital Tract

**1. Course of the Genital Ducts.** The *gonadal ridge* develops on the surface of the *mesonephros*. The *mesonephric duct* lies in a ridge laterally attached to the mesonephros. The *paramesonephric duct* descends in the ductal ridge between the mesonephric duct and the coelomic epithelium; in the lower third of the common ventral and medial course, the paramesonephric duct crosses over the mesonephric duct and unites with the paramesonephric duct of the opposite side. The *metanephros* ascends cranially in the retroperitoneal space behind the mesonephros (→ 8.2). The *ureters* cross under the genital ducts in order to open into the *urogenital sinus*, situated ventrally in front of the *rectum*.

**2. Rounding Off of the Gonads.** The mesonephros, with the gonad and the excretory duct, detaches from the body wall and develops its own mesentery, through which vessels from the aorta travel to the mesonephros (**A1**). The *gonadal ridge*, like the mesonephros, rounds off into an oval organ. The laterally attached *ductal ridge* takes a medial course below the gonad and mesonephros and fuses with the ridge of the other side. A broad *transverse plate* is formed between the bladder and rectum (**A2**). It contains the fused paramesonephric ducts (the prospective uterus and tubes) and the mesonephric duct (the prospective vas deferens). The plate itself is formed by the mesentery of the ductal ridge and is the prospective **broad ligament of the uterus**. The mesonephros extends caudally into a ligamentous tract that lies in the mesentery of the mesonephros and radiates into the body wall. After the regression of the mesonephros and the enlargement of the gonadal primordium, this ligamentous tract becomes the *inferior gonadal ligament*. It crosses under the genital ducts and ends in an outpocketing of the ventral body wall. This outpocketing in turn passes into a cutaneous swelling known as the *labioscrotal swelling* (→ 8.9), which later gives rise to the scrotum or the labia majora. The vessels to the gonad lie in a corresponding superior ligamentous tract, the *superior gonadal ligament* (**A3**).

**3. Female Development.** The paramesonephric ducts differentiate into the *uterine tubes* and the *uterus*. The *broad ligament* arises directly from the fusion of the two ridges containing the genital ducts. The *superior gonadal ligament* becomes the *suspensory ligament of the ovary*, carrying the ovarian artery and vein. The upper portion of the *inferior gonadal ligament* forms the the *proper ovarian ligament*, which passes from the ovary to the junction of the uterus and the Fallopian tube. The lower portion becomes the *round ligament of the uterus* (inferior gonadal ligament), which passes into the inguinal canal from the junction of the uterus and the Fallopian tube and radiates out into the labia majora.

**4. Male Development.** The mesonephric ducts differentiate into the *duct of the epididymis* and the *vas deferens*. They are connected with the *testis* through the *efferent ductules*, which develop from the *mesonephric tubules* (**A1**). Only the *utricle* remains from the fused paramesonephric ducts (→ 1.6); it ultimately comes to lie in the prostate. The *inferior gonadal ligament* (**A2**) becomes the **gubernaculum testis**, the guiding structure for the **descent of the testis.** While the gubernaculum contracts, the testis and epididymis glide downward along the dorsal body wall beneath the peritoneum and enter the *scrotum* . The peritoneum forms an outpocketing in the *inguinal canal*, the *processus vaginalis*, which extends into the scrotum and comes to lie above the testis and epididymis. The testis lies in an outpocketing of the body wall that extends into the cutaneous pocket of the scrotum; thus the *covering* of the *spermatic cord* has the same structure as the *body wall*. The aponeurosis of the external oblique is continuous with the *external spermatic fascia*; the musculature of the body wall, with the *cremaster muscle*; and the transversalis fascia, with the *internal spermatic fascia*.

**Congenital Inguinal Hernia.** The stalk of the *processus vaginalis* obliterates after birth so that the *tunica vaginalis testis* loses its connection to the body cavity. If the obliteration does not take place, loops of the intestine may enter the scrotum.

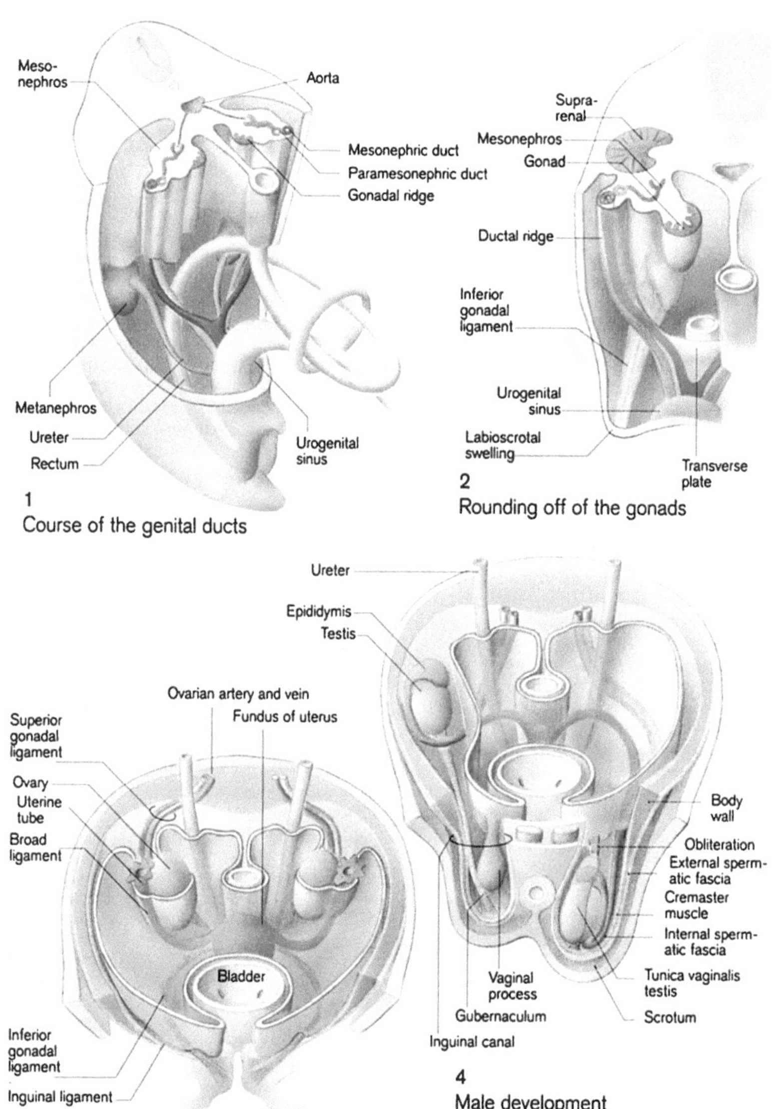


1
Course of the genital ducts

2
Rounding off of the gonads

3
Female development

4
Male development

A. Development of the internal genital organs

# 8.8 Downward Growth of Vagina

## A. Separation of the Ureter from the Mesonephric Duct

**Incorporation of the Duct Openings into the Bladder.** The functional transformation of the mesonephric duct from a urinary conduit of the mesonephros (**A1**, stage 10) into a genital duct (→8.1) involves the separation of the genital duct from the definitive kidney. The lower segments of the mesonephric ducts are incorporated into the wall of the bladder during its expansion (**A2**, stage 14), so that these ducts are separated from the openings of the ureters (**A3**, stage 21). The entrance site of the mesonephric duct migrates further downward in the midline of the dorsal wall of the bladder (**A4**). The paramesonephric duct grows down along the mesonephric duct and reaches the sinus only after the ureters have detached (→8.2).

**Position of Supernumerary Ureters.** A cranially situated supernumerary ureter generally crosses over the normal ureter and opens further caudad into the bladder, urethra, or vagina (→8.4). In the case of two *ureteric buds* (**A1**), the cranially situated ureter does not gain a separate opening into the bladder (**A2**) but remains connected to the mesonephric duct. It is drawn downward as the mesonephric duct migrates caudally (**A3**). In female development, the opening of the cranial ureter can thus be drawn into the vagina or the vulva (**A4**).

## B. Downward Growth of the Vaginal Anlage

From reconstructions of the vaginal primordium in human embryos of the Carnegie Collection, Koff (1933) concluded that the vagina grows upward as a compact plate emanating from sinus swellings, whereas Witschi (1970), studying the same material, concluded that the vagina arises by the downward growth of the paramesonephric ducts. Our experiments with mice carrying the mutation for testicular feminization have confirmed the hypothesis advanced by Witschi: The vagina develops by downward growth of the paramesonephric ducts. In this process, the mesonephric ducts and the sinus swellings function as guiding structures.

**1. Indifferent Stage.** The *mesonephric ducts* are situated below the neck of the bladder on two *swellings* of the *urogenital sinus*. The *paramesonephric ducts* form compact epithelial buds that push the sinus wall between the mesonephric ducts into the sinus lumen (without breaking through).

**2. Male Development**. *Testosterone* from the testis stimulates the sprouting of *seminal vesicles* from the mesonephric ducts and the sprouting of a corona of *prostatic buds* from the sinus epithelium ( →8.8). AMH, also produced by the testis, induces the progressive degeneration of the paramesonephric duct from cranial to caudal, until only a small remnant is left between the prostatic buds.

**3. Female Development.** *Without testosterone*, the fusion of the downward-growing paramesonephric ducts with the mesonephric ducts is preserved. The fusion zone migrates downward along the urogenital sinus, forming paired vaginal buds. Cranially, the mesonephric and paramesonephric ducts are again separated. The paramesonephric ducts fuse with each other in the midline and form the uterus and vagina. Since the dorsally situated mesonephric ducts fail to receive trophic support in the form of testosterone, they degenerate.

**4. Testicular Feminization.** The X-linked mutation causing testicular feminization (→8.10) involves a defect in the *androgen receptor protein*. This mutation occurs in mice and in humans with the same pattern of inheritance and the same effect. Mice or humans having the genotype $X^{Tfm}$/Y develop a testis that produces testosterone and AMH. Since the androgen receptor is defective, the testosterone cannot exert an effect and the vaginal buds grow down constitutively. Cranially, the paramesonephric ducts degenerate under the influence of AMH. The mesonephric ducts degenerate because they cannot respond to the trophic stimulus of testosterone. A short vagina forms; its extent depends on the amount of AMH produced by the intraabdominally located testes.

Mesonephric duct
Ureteric bud
1
Separation from the kidney
Posterior wall of bladder
Ureter
2
Incorporation into the bladder
Parameso-nephric duct
Mesonephric duct
3
Downward growth of ducts
4
Supernumerary ureter

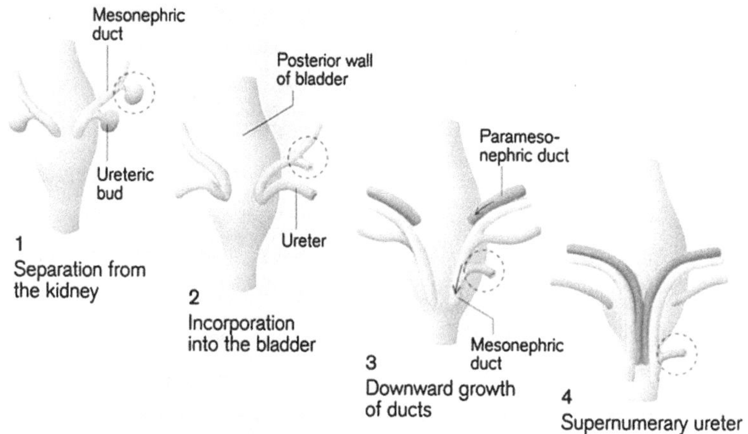

A. Separation of the ureter from the mesonephric duct

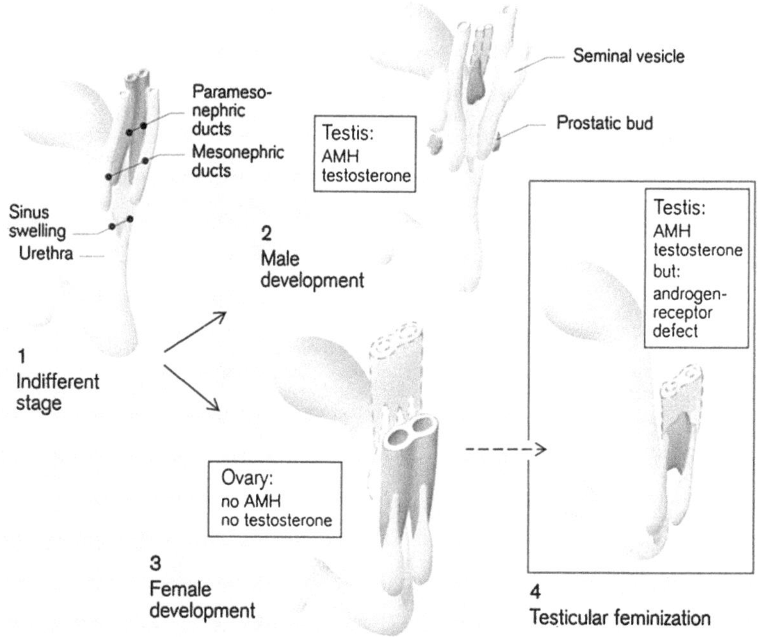

Parameso-nephric ducts
Mesonephric ducts
Sinus swelling
Urethra
1
Indifferent stage
Testis:
AMH
testosterone
2
Male development
Seminal vesicle
Prostatic bud
Ovary:
no AMH
no testosterone
3
Female development
Testis:
AMH
testosterone
but:
androgen-receptor defect
4
Testicular feminization

B. Downward growth of the vaginal anlage

## 8.9 External Genitalia

*Background*

Phylogenetically, the **phallus** (the copulatory organ) is formed from a mucosal fold of the cloaca that can be evaginated (amphibians, birds). The evagination is driven by muscles originating from the muscle layer of the cloaca. In mammals, they are conserved as striated muscles on the cavernous bodies (corpora cavernosa and corpus spongiosum). The cavernous bodies are related to the submucosal venous plexuses that develop as closing mechanisms at the anus and in the urethra.

### A. Development of the External Genitalia

**1. Indifferent Anlage.** In stage 16, the rectum and urogenital sinus have still not separated. The cloaca is closed to the exterior by the **cloacal membrane** (→ 7.1). The cloacal membrane is bordered anteriorly by the *genital tubercle* and laterally by the *urethral folds*, which in turn are bounded laterally by the *labioscrotal swellings*. The genital tubercle, as well as the folds and swellings, contain undifferentiated mesodermal tissue. In stage 18, the urorectal septum reaches the cloaca and separates the anus from the urethral groove (→ 8.2). Endodermal sinus epithelium beneath the (still closed) urogenital membrane grows in at the underside of the genital tubercle and forms an **urethral plate**. When the cloacal membrane disintegrates at stage 19, the urethral plate is transformed to the **urethral groove** on the underside of the genital tubercle, which lateron in **male development (1a)** forms the **penile urethra**. In the female, the externally open urogenital sinus (→ 8.2) is essentially preserved and becomes the *vestibule of the vagina*, which receives the openings of the urethra and vagina (**3a** and **3b**).

**2. Male Development.** Sexual differences in the external genitalia are readily apparent in the 13th week of pregnancy and completely developed by the 16th week. In male embryos, the fusion zone of the urethral folds advances from the anus to the apex of the phallus (**2a**). A raphe arises on the underside of the penis (**2b**). The *labioscrotal swellings* (**A1**) become the *scrotum* (**2b**).

**Differentiation of the Cavernous Bodies.** The mesenchyme of the urethral folds differentiates into the cavernous bodies of the *corpus spongiosum*, ending in the *bulb* behind the urethral groove (**2a1**). The overlying mesenchyme of the genital tubercle gives rise to the *corpora cavernosa*, which attach by crura to both sides of the pubic ramus. Above the cavernous bodies lie the associated striated muscles.

**Canalization of the Glans.** The apex of the genital tubercle becomes the glans of the penis or the clitoris. A compact ectodermal epithelial plate grows into the penile glans and fuses with the endodermal urethra (**2a1** and **2**). After the urethral groove has closed completely, it becomes canalized. In this process, the orifice of the urethra is secondarily shifted to the apex of the glans. The spongiose tissue in the glans fuses with the *corpus spongiosum urethrae*, thus losing its connection to the *corpora cavernosa*.

**Preputium.** The preputium (prepuce) is formed by the margins of the urethral folds, which grow anteriorly over the *coronary sulcus* (**2a1**). During this process, a circular *compact epithelial plate* invaginates between the folds and the glans (**2a2**); this plate disintegrates only in early childhood.

**3. Female Development.** After the 10th week of pregnancy, the urethral groove in the female fetus is shorter than in the male (**3a**). The genital tubercle curves ventrally and becomes the clitoris. The labioscrotal swellings become the *labia majora* and the urethral folds the *labia minora*. The vagina develops as a compact epithelial bud from the fused paramesonephric ducts. It descends at the dorsal wall of the sinus and opens into the lower portion of the urogenital sinus. The urogenital sinus is preserved as the *vestibule of the vagina*. The vaginal lumen forms secondarily in the compact vaginal primordium. The hymenal membrane is preserved at the entrance into the sinus.

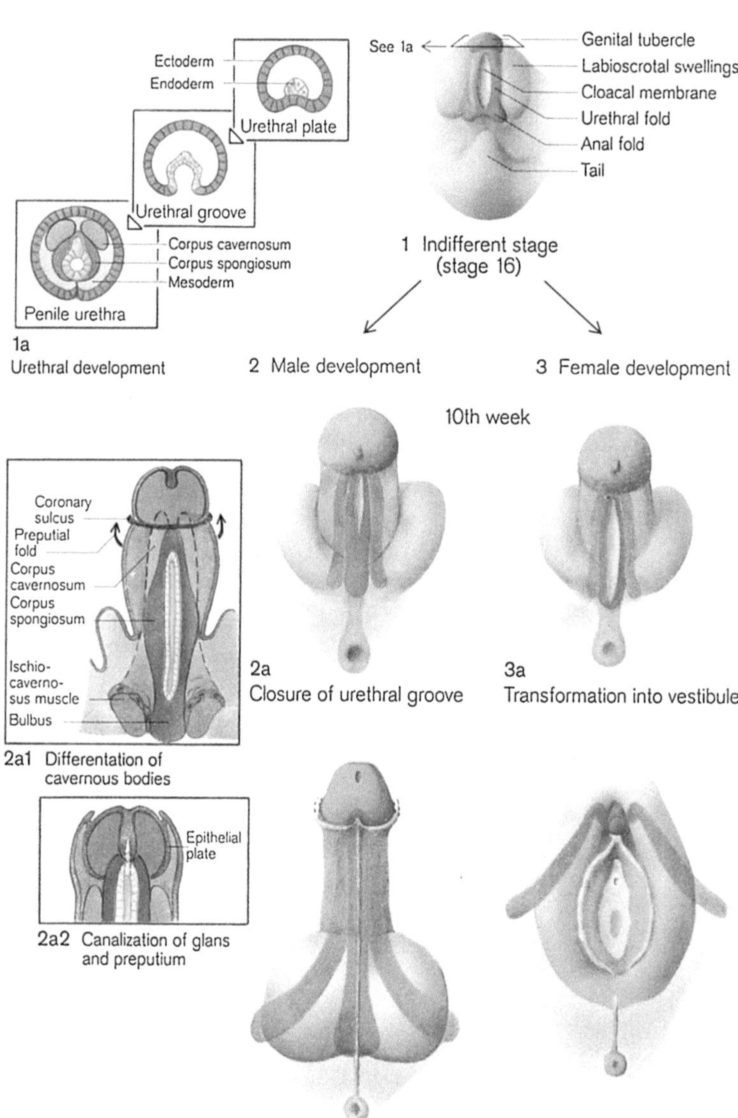


1a Urethral development

2 Male development

3 Female development

2a Closure of urethral groove

3a Transformation into vestibule

2a1 Differentation of cavernous bodies

2a2 Canalization of glans and preputium

2b Penis and scrotum

3b Clitoris and vulva

A. Development of the external genitalia

## 8.10 Intersexuality

*Background*

**Hermaphrodites** are defined clinically by their *gonadal sex*. According to this definition, only individuals with an **ovotestis** are *true hermaphrodites*. Hermaphrodites possessing testes are referred to as *male pseudohermaphrodites*; those with ovaries, as *female pseudohermaphrodites*. A true hermaphrodite with an ovotestis can arise by an XY/XO mosaic or by a disturbance in gonadal induction. Regardless of the cause for hermaphroditic development, the **somatic sex** that is expressed depends on the amounts of AMH and testosterone present during fetal life.

### A. Disturbances in Sexual Development

Somatic sex (**B III**) is determined by the **effects of AMH and testosterone** (**A1**). Presence of both factors leads to male and absence to female development. Testosterone in female development (e.g. in AGS, **B III 2a**) or lack of AMH in male development (**B III 1a**) leads to male differentiation of mesonephric ducts and external genitalia and inhibition of downward growth of the female genital ducts, the regression of which is not induced in both cases due to lack of AMH. Lack of testosterone in a male embryo (*hypoplasia of testes*, **B III 1b**), or *5α-reductase deficiency* (**B III 1c**), in which the conversion of testosterone to DHT in the external genitalia is insufficient, or the genetic androgen receptor defect (**B III 1d**), lead to partial or total feminization in patients, which carry testes but possess no female internal organs due to the presence of AMH.

**Intersexual development of the external genitalia** (**A2**) arises in female fetuses if androgens are present during pregnancy (*AGS*, **III**, **2**), and in male fetuses as a result of testosterone deficiency (**III**, **1b**). It comprises all transitional states between the male and the female phenotyp with an intermediate size of the phallus, hypospadia, and scrotal development of the labia majora. If closure of the urethral groove and canalization of the glans fail to occur, the urethra opens on the underside of the penis (**Hypospadia**).

### B. Tabular Overview

**I. Chromosomal Sex**

a) Defective distribution of sex chromosomes:
   - XXX ovary.
   - XXY testis (Klinefelter).
   - XYY testis (spermatogenic defect).

b) Mosaics due to fusion of blastocysts in early stages of development:
   - XX/XY testis or ovotestis.

c) Loss of a Y chromosome in cleavage divisions:
   - XO/XY testis or streak gonads.
   - XO streak gonads (Turner).

d) Translocation of the testis-determining sequence onto an an X chromosome:
   - XX males.

e) Mutation in the testis-determining sequence (SRY) on the Y chromosome:
   - XY females.

**II. Gonadal Sex**

True hermaphrodites with an **ovotestis**. Gradual masculinization or normal male or female development, depending on the amount of functional testicular tissue.

**III. Somatic sex**

**1. Male Pseudohermaphrodites**

a) *Selective AMH defect*: The uterus and tubes descend with the testis and epididymis of one side into the scrotum.

b) *Hypoplastic testis*: AMH and testosterone deficiency. Remnants of the uterus and tubes; hypospadia.

c) *5α-reductase deficiency*: gradual feminization (autosomal inheritance).

d) *Androgen receptor defect (testicular feminization, Tfm)*: total feminization, no paramesonephric derivatives (X-linked inheritance).

**2. Female Pseudohermaphrodites**

a) Endogenous androgen formation in the fetal adrenal: adrenogenital syndrome (AGS); ovaries and female internal genitalia, masculinization of external genitalia.

b) Exogenous androgens, e.g., progestogen with androgenic effects during pregnancy.

**IV. Disturbance in Central Sex Determination**

a) Discordant sexual identity (transsexuality).

b) Rhythm disturbances, centrally based infertility.

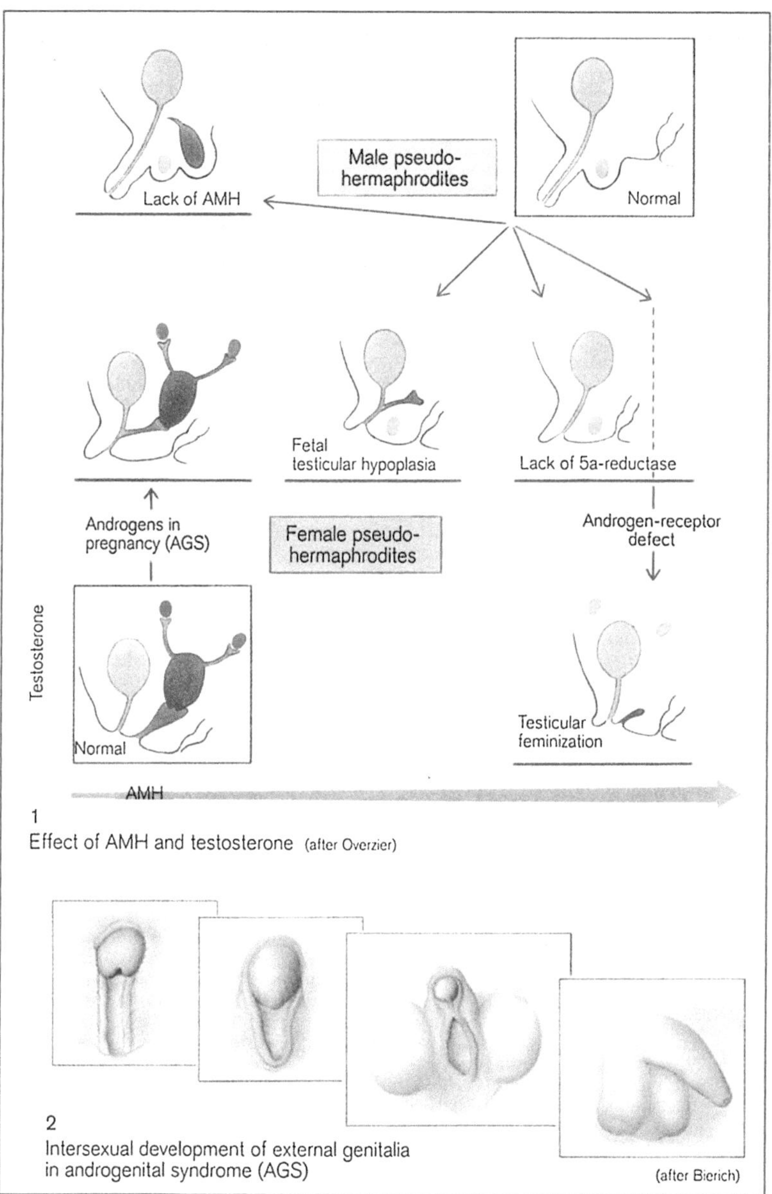


1
Effect of AMH and testosterone (after Overzier)

2
Intersexual development of external genitalia in androgenital syndrome (AGS)

(after Bierich)

A. Disturbances in sexual development

# Chapter 9: Head

## Introduction

Chapter 9 deals with the medically relevant aspects of head development. The fusion of the **facial swellings** (→ **9.1**) and the formation of the secondary palate are the basis for an understanding of phenomena such as cleft lips, jaw, or palate. Analysis of the cartilaginous elements of the embryonic **chondrocranium** (→ **9.2**) clarifies the functional organization of the definitive skull. The membranously ossified **neurocranium** forms over the chondrocranium. The **viscerocranium** (→ **9.3**) arises from the pharyngeal arch cartilages and undergoes secondary ossification into the definitive facial skeleton. In stage 15 (→ 2.24), the arteries and veins of the head still course together along the base of the skull. As the trigeminal ganglion and the otic capsule form, the **cranial veins** (→ **9.4**) are displaced to the surface of the brain. The expanding cerebral hemispheres then compress the venous plexuses between the two layers of the dura to form the venous sinuses. Malformations due to **defective neural tube closure** (→ **9.5**), ranging from anencephaly to "cleft spine" (rachischisis) and spina bifida, are analyzed with reference to the sagittal section of a fetus in the 14th week of pregnancy. Stage 10 (→ 2.16) is the sensitive phase (→ 10.1) for disturbances in neural tube closure. Disturbances in the architecture of the cerebral cortex can arise at the beginning of the fetal period ("inside-out layering" - → 2.17). The functional differentiation of the brain can be impaired even during the second half of the fetal period, e.g., in fetal alcohol syndrome.

### The "Head Problem"

The "head problem" in embryology concerns the question of whether the organization of the head is fundamentally metameric (Starck, 1978). The answer to this question has been influenced by changing concepts in developmental and evolutionary biology. Darwin's theory of evolution and its extension into the fundamental law of ontogeny by Haeckel (→ 3.0) left no doubt that the basic head design is metamerically organized. Considerable discussion has focused on the question of whether the entire body is derived from a basic unit whose prototype is the somitic segment, or whether the metamerism of the axial organs and the metamerism of the pharynx represents two different principles. Important arguments in favor of metamerism in the head are the existence of neuromeres in the brain vesicle portion of the neural tube, the formation of a part of the skull base from occipital sclerotomes (→ 9.2), and the observation that lower vertebrates possess preotic myotomes that give rise to the extrinsic eye muscles in evolution. Arguments against the metamerism of the head include the development of nonsegmental brain vesicles in vertebrate embryos and the replacement of the neuromere concept by the concept of brain vesicles as major organizational unit, the absence of somitic segmentation in the primordial pharynx, and the interpretation of somitic segments in vertebrates as functional units required for swimming movements, being independent of the metamerism in other phyla of the animal kingdom. In contrast to Anglo-Saxon authors, Starck and his students ultimately reject the concept of metameric organization of the head.

The demonstration that a Hox-cluster (Hox 2) is expressed in the rhombomeres of the chick and mouse (Nieto et al., 1992) (→ 4.7) sheds new light on the question. Hox 2 is a vertebrate homologue to antennapedia in Drosophila (→ 3.17). Does this observation imply that segmentation in Drosophila and in vertebrates is homologous according to the classical definition of homology? The term **homology** is classically defined morphologically: homologous structures are derived from the same element of a common fundamental body plan. The hand of a human, the wing of a bat, and the fin of a dolphin are homologous structures that develop from the five-rayed vertebrate limb bud. On the other hand, the bat wing and the insect wing are **analogous** structures that have developed the same function from different basic elements as a result of evolutionary pressure (examples from Starck, 1978).

Homology and analogy are tools of comparative anatomy. Molecular biology has now opened a new dimension with the analysis of homologous DNA sequences. In the course of evolution, gene families and supergene families, as well as clusters of Hox regulator genes, have arisen by reduplication and recombination in the genome. Genetic analysis reveals more common features between animal phyla than can be demonstrated by the classic methods of evolutionary theory.

In the Atlas of Embryology, the head problem arises in several places. Chapter 2 gives a morphologically **descriptive presentation** of skull and face development in the human (→ 2.30 to 2.38).

In chapter 3, the **fundamental structure of the vertebrate body** is discussed by comparing the structure of the visceral pharyngeal region and of the somatic trunk region of the vertebrate body (→ 3.19 and 3.20). The metameric arrangement of the pharyngeal region into pharyngeal arches can be traced back to the structure of the primordial pharynx of filter feeders, while the organization of the trunk region into somites can be traced back to serially arranged muscle and skeletal elements required for swimming movements. During the development from the jawless vertebrates with pharyngeal arches to the shark embryo with a primary upper and lower jaw, the first pharyngeal arch elements fuse with one another. The primary jaw articulation between the maxilla and the mandible corresponds to a hinge-like connection between the upper and lower elements of the original two-part pharyngeal arch. The upper element functions as a connecting piece (copula) to the axial skeleton of the head. Fusion of the copula elements gave rise to the upper jaw of fish, which in turn became united with the base of the skull and formed the **palatoquadrate**. In the mammalian skull, the palatoquadrate can no longer be distinguished as a separate skeletal element. The definitive **pharyngeal arches** thus consist only of the lower skeletal elements of the original pharyngeal arches, which form a typical U-shape by fusion in the midline (at the chin). The prototype is the mandibular arch (Meckel's cartilage), now designated the first arch. The hyoid arch (Reichert's cartilage) is the second arch. In mammals, the primary jaw articulation is shifted into the auditory ossicle chain and a secondary jaw articulation forms. These developments, discussed in relation to the development of the ear (→ 5.10), are also put into evolutionary perspective.

The **association of the central sense organs with the cerebral vesicles** is an important didactic principle in the study of brain development. This principle is illustrated by the fictitious **phylontotractus** (→ 4.1). In the discussion of skull development, this principle is again used by correlating the central elements of the chondrocranium with the laterally associated capsules for the central sense organs (9.3).

**Head mesoderm** originates not from the primitive streak but from the prechordal plate, the foregut diverticulum (→ 3.8), and the neural crest (→ 4.7). The derivation of the blastema for the pharyngeal arch cartilage from the cephalic neural crest—and thus from ectoderm—is frequently used as an argument against the universal validity of the germ layer theory. The terms "mesectoderm" and "head mesenchyme" are used in place of "head mesoderm" to emphasize this distinction. If mesoderm is not defined as originating from the primitive streak, but rather as the tissue lying as a middle germ layer between the ectodermal and endodermal epithelium, one can speak loosely of head mesoderm. Individual mesenchymal cells migrating from the head neural crest and placodes correspond to the droplet cells that leave the ectoderm of the early germinal disc and become mesodermal cells independently of the primitive streak. (→ 3.7). In general, the neural crest and placodes, and even the optic vesicle (→ 5.4) at an early developmental stage, form head mesoderm, which is distinct from the neural ectoderm that gives rise to neurons and sensory cells.

## 9.1 Facial Swellings

### A. Development of Face and Palate and Causes of Cleft Formation

**1. Development of the Face.** In stage 13, the embryo is curved in such a way that the facial swellings and the stomodeum lie on the heart swelling and are thus not visible in intact embryo specimens (→ 2.22). Only if the head is lifted from the heart swelling can the **stomodeum (1a)** be seen. In a frontal view, the *olfactory placodes* situated above the *prosencephalon*, the ventral aspect of the *pharyngeal arches*, and the *stomodeum*, with the remains of the *pharyngeal membrane*, can be distinguished.

As the brain grows anteriorly up to stage 16 (→ 2.25), head mesoderm proliferates between the cerebral vesicles and the surface ectoderm and gives rise to the **facial swellings (1b)**. The bulge above the prosencephalon is called the *frontal prominence*. With the invagination of the olfactory placode, a *medial* and a *lateral nasal swelling* form.

The original mouth opening between the base of the skull and the mandibular arch narrows and is closed laterally by the **maxillary process (1c)** growing in from behind. Lateral closure of the oral cleft is a phylogenetically recent development occuring in mammals. The maxillary process is composed of tissue from the first pharyngeal arch that migrates in between the mandible and the cranial base. The *medial nasal swellings* (**1b**) fuse in the midline into the *primary palate*. An epithelial margin ("Epithelmauer" from Hofstetter) is transiently formed in the fusion zone between the medial and lateral nasal swellings and the maxillary process. In the deeper regions, this epithelial margin courses between the primary palate (*intermaxillary bone*, **A4**) and the secondary palate.

The fusion zone between the lateral nasal swelling and the maxillary process extends to the medial angle of the eye, forming the **nasolacrimal furrow (1d)**. By the 10th week of pregnancy, a compact, epithelial duct has grown down between the two swellings and shortly before birth becomes patent (**nasolacrimal duct**).

**2. Primary and Secondary Palates**
The ectoderm of the *stomodeum* and the endoderm of the pharynx together form the **pharyngeal membrane (2a)**, which disintegrates in stage 13 (**1a**). The olfactory placodes invaginate to form the **olfactory pits (2b)**. These contain the olfactory epithelium, from which *olfactory fibers* pass to the prosencephalon (→ 5.5). The floor of the olfactory pit and the roof of the oral cavity form the *bucconasal membrane*. It lies anterior to the former pharyngeal membrane and to the *pituitary gland* (hypophysis) (→ 4.24). The olfactory pits open into the oral cavity as the *primary choanae*.

Behind the **primary palate (2c)** and extending to the skull base lies an undivided pharyngeal space that is occupied by the tongue. Growth of the **secondary palate** divides this space into the definitive nasal passage and the oral cavity. In this process, the transition between the nasal and oral spaces is shifted posteriorly (*definitive choanae*).

**3. Rise of the Palatine Plates.** The *palatine shelfs* are inwardly directed portions of the *maxillary processes* (**1c**). Initially, they lie below the tongue on both sides. In stage 19, they rise above the tongue and fuse with each other and with the *nasal septum*. The erection of the palatine plates or shelfs is an active process that occurs within a few hours. At the boundary between the primary palate (intermaxillary bone) and the secondary palate formed by the palatine shelfs, the *incisive foramen* (**A4**) remains and is visible in the definitive skeleton. Neither nerves nor blood vessels pass through this opening.

**4. Cleft Formations.** Defective fusion of the maxillary process and the medial nasal swelling causes **cleft lips** (harelip) and, in severe cases, **maxillary clefts**, which may be accompanied by a **cleft palate**. Cleft palates arise as a result of disturbances in the erection and fusion of the palatineshelfs. **Oblique facial clefts** can arise along the nasolacrimal furrow (**1c** and **d**).

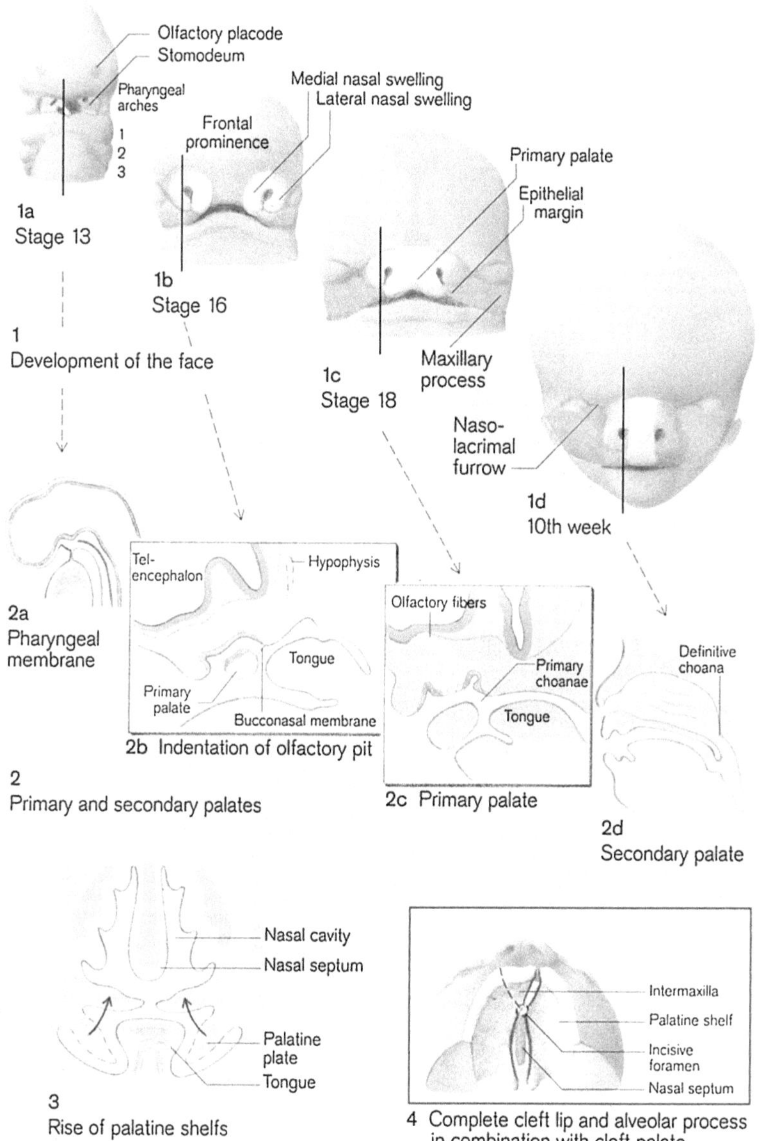
Olfactory placode
Stomodeum
Pharyngeal arches
1
2
3
1a
Stage 13
Medial nasal swelling
Lateral nasal swelling
Frontal prominence
1b
Stage 16
Primary palate
Epithelial margin
Maxillary process
1c
Stage 18
Naso-lacrimal furrow
1d
10th week
1
Development of the face
2a
Pharyngeal membrane
Tel-encephalon
Hypophysis
Tongue
Primary palate
Bucconasal membrane
2b Indentation of olfactory pit
Olfactory fibers
Primary choanae
Tongue
2c Primary palate
Definitive choana
2d
Secondary palate
2
Primary and secondary palates
Nasal cavity
Nasal septum
Palatine plate
Tongue
3
Rise of palatine shelfs
Intermaxilla
Palatine shelf
Incisive foramen
Nasal septum
4 Complete cleft lip and alveolar process in combination with cleft palate

A. Facial swellings and palates

## 9.2 Skull Base

*Background*

In the course of evolution, the **skull** was formed from two components: the extension of the axial skeleton into the region of the cerebral vesicles, with the laterally attached capsules for the central sense organs (**A1**); and the pharyngeal skeleton formed by the pharyngeal arches (**9.3, B1**). The two components fuse with the **chondrocranium,** the cartilaginous skull base. In further development, a membranously ossified skull cap (**neurocranium**) is built up over the base of the skull. The facial skeleton (**viscerocranium**) originates from the cartilaginous pharyngeal arch elements below the skull base (**9.3, B2**). With the development of a separate air passage for respiration, the **maxillary floor** becomes inserted between the skull base and the alimentary tract. The primary jaw articulation is shifted into the chain of auditory ossicles. This leads to a fundamental reconstruction of the facial skeleton by membranous ossification.

### A. Development of the Skull: Chondrocranium

**1. Basal Plate and Capsules for the Sense Organs.** In stage 18, the notochord terminates at the *pituitary gland* (hypophysis), which arises from an evagination of the roof of the stomodeum (Rathke's pouch). The cervical vertebral column around the *notochord* is extended by formation of a contiguous cartilaginous plate, the *basal plate*. This structure, which later gives rise to the basilar part of the occipital bone, is bent at a right angle to the *cervical vertebrae* at the cervical flexure. In front of the hypophysis, the basal plate continues into two fused cartilage rods (*trabeculae cranii*, future ethmoid plates, **A2**) that slope down between the roof of the pharynx and the floor of the prosencephalon.

The invaginated *olfactory pit* becomes enclosed by a shell-shaped, inferiorly open cartilaginous *nasal capsule* that arises below the trabeculae cranii on both sides. Around the eyeballs, which are still situated laterally, the *orbit* of the eye is formed by the cartilaginous models of the greater and lesser wings of the sphenoid (**A2**). The inner ear, arising from the otic vesicle lateral to the rhombencephalon, is enclosed by the cartilaginous *otic capsule* (→ 5.8).

**2. Relationships between Cartilage Elements and the Definitive Skull Base.** The functional components of the skull base are easier to recognize in the cartilaginous chondrocranium than in the definitive bones, which (after endochondral ossification) are delimited from each other only by bony sutures.

The basal plate elongates caudally through the fusion of three *occipital sclerotomes*. The roots of the associated spinal nerves are united into the *hypoglossal nerve* (*XII*). The vertebral arches of the occipital sclerotomes encircle the neural tube and fuse behind the *foramen magnum* (**2b**), forming the cartilaginous segment of the *occipital bone*, which is later completed by the membranously ossifying occipital squama. The *basal plate* itself becomes the *clivus*.

The cartilaginous *otic capsule*—the future petrous part of the temporal bone—surrounds the inner ear (derived from the otic vesicle), leaving openings only for the passage of the endolymphatic duct, as well as for the *statoacoustic* (*VIII*) and *facial* (*VII*) *nerves*.

The body of the *sphenoid bone* arises from paired *hypophysial cartilages*. The *lesser wing* (*orbital part*) and the *greater wing* (*temporal part*) of the sphenoid bone bound the *orbit* of the eye and provide access openings from the cranium (*optic canal* and *superior orbital fissure*). The greater wing arises from of a small cartilaginous model. The lateral part has already undergone membranous ossification, leaving open the *foramen rotundum* and the *foramen ovale*, the openings for the branches of the *trigeminal nerve* (*V*).

The *trabeculae cranii* give rise to the cartilaginous nasal septum, to which the conchae of the nasal capsule attach laterally on both sides. The cartilaginous nasal skeleton is closed off at the top by the *ethmoidal plate* (ethmoid bone), through which the olfactory filaments (I) pass.

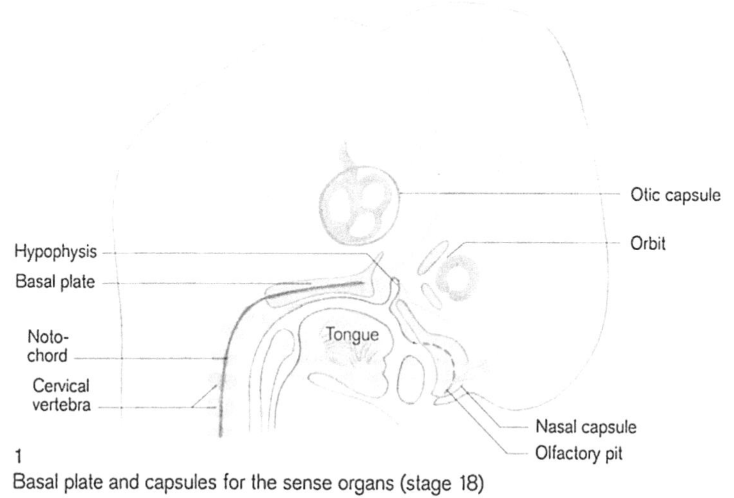


1
Basal plate and capsules for the sense organs (stage 18)

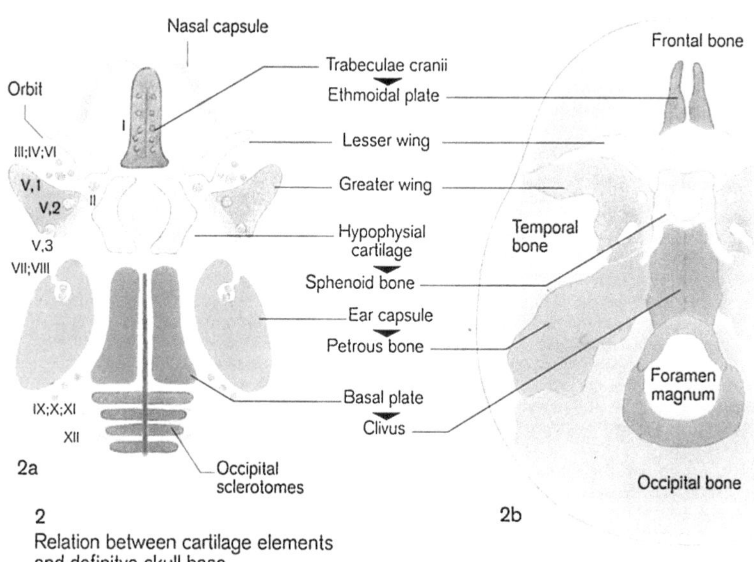


2
Relation between cartilage elements and definitve skull base

A. Development of the skull: chondrocranium

## 9.3 Braincase and Facial Skeleton

### B. Neurocranium and Viscerocranium

**1. Chondrocranium and Pharyngeal Arch Cartilages.**

The *chondrocranium*, a cartilaginous model for the skull base, is an extension of the vertebral column in the head region providing skeletal support for the developing brain. The central sense organs are encapsulated by skeletal elements apposed on both sides: the *nasal capsule*, the *orbit*, and the *otic capsule*.

Below the chondrocranium lies the pharynx, the entrance into the gastrointestinal tract. The skeletal elements of the pharynx are the cartilaginous rods in the pharyngeal arches. The *pharyngeal arch cartilages* initially consist of a proximal and a distal element connected with each other by joints (→ 3.19). The upper (proximal) elements are movably attached to the primordial axial skeleton around the chorda skeleton, allowing a scissor-like opening of the pharynx. As the head develops, the proximal elements fuse with each other to form the primary maxilla, a square bony element called the *palatoquadrate*. It is tightly joined to the skull base.

The distal, lower elements of the original pharyngeal arch cartilages fuse to form the primary mandibular element (*mandibular arch, Meckel's cartilage*), which is now designated the first pharyngeal arch. The palatoquadrate forms the base for the primary jaw articulation between the mandibular arch and the skull base. In the ontogeny of the mammalian skull, the palatoquadrate becomes integrated into the chondrocranium and can no longer be recognized as an individual cartilage model. It is incorporated into the petrous (temporal) and sphenoid bones.

**2. Expansion of the Chondrocranium by Membranous Ossification**

**a Neurocranium.** The endochondrally ossifying elements of the braincase are supplemented by membranously ossifying portions, forming the skull cap, which completely encloses the brain (*neurocranium*). The endochondrally ossifying part of the occipital bone (→ 9.2 **A2**) enlarges around the membranously ossifying *occipital squama*. The membranous *temporal squama* completes the otic capsule to form the temporal bone. The membranous extension of the *greater wing* completes the sphenoid bone. The *frontal bone* is formed as a separate membranous bone above the endochondrally ossifying ethmoid plate. The two *parietal bones* arise by membranous ossification and have no direct connection to the cartilaginous skull base.

**b Viscerocranium.** In mammals, the separation of the air passage from the alimentary tract leads to a complete transformation of the facial skeleton (*viscerocranium*). This separation, like the creation of the secondary jaw joint, is necessary for sucking. Between the skull base and the oral cavity, an additional element, the hard palate, is formed. The additional bony elements arise by membranous ossification of the tissue from the medial and lateral nasal swellings and from the maxillary process. They are the *intermaxillary segment* (*primary palate*), the *maxilla* with the *zygomatic bone*, and the downward-pointing *pterygoid process* of the sphenoid bone with the palatine bone. The nasal capsule is completed by the membranous *nasal* and *lacrimal bones*, as well as the osseous nasal septum. The boundaries of the definitive bones are formed by the sutures and fusion zones between the endochondral and membranous ossific centers and do not always coincide with the derivation of the bony elements (→ 2.35 and 2.38).

The shifting of the primary jaw articulation into the *chain of auditory ossicles* (→ 5.10) and the development of the secondary jaw joint are associated with the replacement of the cartilage rod of the first pharyngeal arch (Meckel's cartilage) by the membranously ossifying, definitive mandible. The cartilages of the second and third arches form the hyoid bone, which is connected to the middle ear by the *styloid process* and *stylohyoid ligament*. The fourth, fifth, and sixth arches fuse to form the laryngeal skeleton.

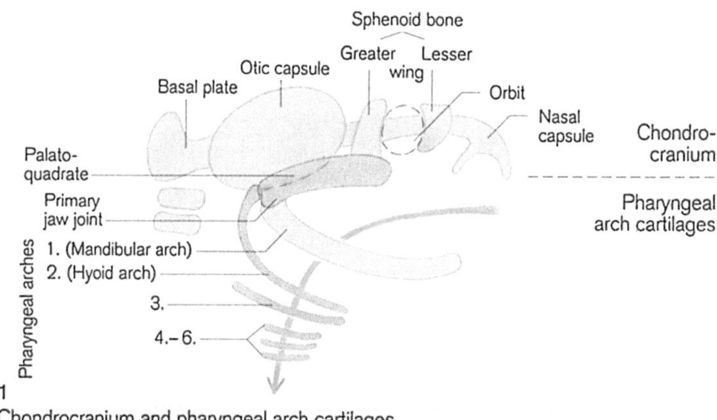


1
Chondrocranium and pharyngeal arch cartilages

Temporal squama
Parietal bone
Occipita squama

2a
Neurocranium

Membranously ossifying cover bones

Endo-chondrically ossifying skull base

Membranously ossifying facial skeleton

Frontal bone
Orbit
Airway
Pterygoid process
Intermediate maxillary segment
Food path
Maxilla
Zygomatic bone
Hyoid bone

2b
Viscerocranium

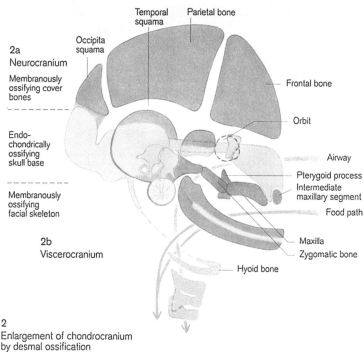

2
Enlargement of chondrocranium by desmal ossification

(after Hamilton, Boyd, Mossmann)

B. Neurocranium and viscerocranium

# 9.4 Cerebral Veins and Meninges

## A. Development of the Cerebral Veins

**1. Three Venous Trunks.** Venous drainage of the head takes place via the *anterior cardinal veins* (→ 6.1), which later develop into the *internal jugular vein* (**A3**). Three venous plexuses are formed over the cerebral vesicles; their trunks empty into the cardinal veins. The anterior plexus (**I**) lies in front of the ganglion of the *trigeminal nerve* and drains the prosencephalic and mesencephalic vesicles. The middle plexus (**II**) lies in front; the posterior plexus (**III**) behind the *otic vesicle*. Both drain the rhombencephalon (→ 2.24).

**2. Interruption of the Cardinal Vein.** As the cephalic flexure develops, an anastomosis forms above the *trigeminal ganglion* between the anterior and middle plexus and now transports the bulk of the blood. Development of the *otic capsule* leads to a further interruption in the course of the anterior cardinal vein. The middle and the posterior plexus anastomose into the *sigmoid sinus*, which courses over the future petrous bone. The *cavernous sinus* arises from the anterior segment of the interrupted cardinal vein.

**3. Fusion of the Venous Plexuses.** As the cerebral hemispheres expand posteriorly, they compress the anterior venous plexus into the *superior and inferior sagittal sinuses* (only visible in a frontal section, **B1**). At the posterior pole, they push the middle venous plexus back to the tentorium cerebelli, between the cerebrum and the cerebellum. The branches of this plexus fuse into the *confluence of the sinuses*; its trunk gives rise to the *transverse sinus*.

While the venous drainage of the brain becomes displaced to the brain surface (through the interruption of the cardinal vein), the arterial inflow continues to come from the skull base. The veins at the surface of the brain transport blood into the venous sinuses of the dura, which empty via the *sigmoid sinus* into the *jugular vein*, the original anterior cardinal vein.

## B. Derivation of the Meninges

**1. Subarachnoid Space.** The meninges arise from the mesenchyme surrounding the neural tube (→ 2.30). As the skull cap develops (→ 2.36), the loose tissue forms the *subarachnoid space* lined by **meningeal cells.** These cells give rise to the **arachnoid** between the veinous plexus at the brain surface (**pia mater**) and the **dura mater** covering the inner surface of the skull.

Below the dura, the meningeal cells arrange to the external layer of the *arachnoid*, a thin epithelioid layer that forms an external boundary to the fluid-filled space. Although the arachnoid merges into the dura without a basement membrane, it forms a functional barrier between the blood and the dura (blood-brain barrier). The cells of the arachnoid extend throughout the *subarachnoid space* (arachnoid space) like a spiderweb. At the brain surface they form the internal layer of the arachnoid, covering the vascular connective tissue (the **pia mater**) and enveloping the *bridging veins* that conduct the blood from the pial cerebral veins to the venous sinuses.

The **dura mater** consists of an *external* and an *internal layer*, between which lie the veins of the *epidural venous plexus*. The external layer is identical to the periosteum of the *braincase*. The internal layer of the dura becomes compressed toward the skull cap by the cerebral hemispheres and fuses with the external layer. Only in the regions where the venous plexuses open into large venous blood conduits do the two layers remain separate; here they bound the venous sinuses (*sagittal sinus*, *cavernous sinus*). In the midline between the two brain hemispheres, the inner layers of the dura fuse into the *falx cerebri*. The lower margin of the falx cerebri bounds the *inferior sagittal sinus*.

**2. Dura Mater and Epidural Venous Plexus**. In the spinal cord, the *epidural venous plexus* is completely preserved. The *periosteum* of the vertebral canal and the *dural sac* of the spinal cord do not fuse with one another.

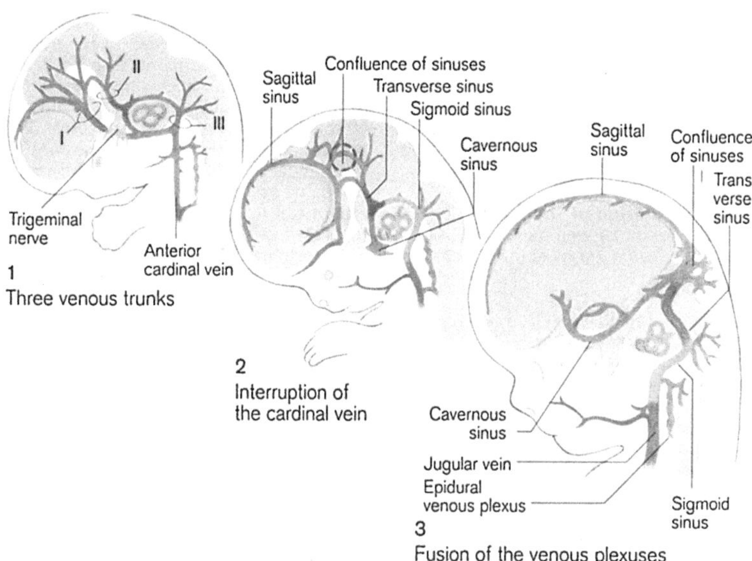


A. Development of the cerebral veins

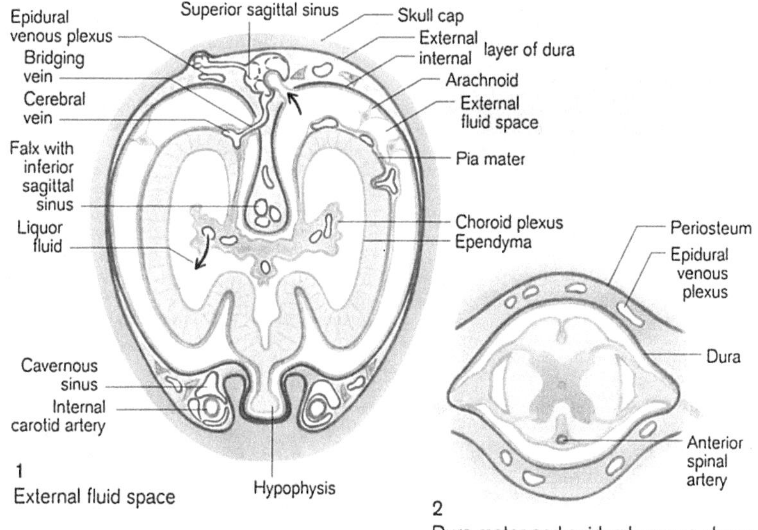


B. Derivation of meninges

## 9.5 Malformations

### A. Malformations of the Head and Central Nervous System

Potential anomalies are projected on the outline of a fetus in the 14th week of pregnancy (→ 2.36).

**1. Cleft Formation of the Face.** Cleft lip, jaw, and palate, as well as facial fissures, arise in the fusion zones of the facial swellings (→ 9.1).

**2. Cyclopia and Proboscis.** Fusion of the optic primordia (cyclopia) is the result of defective development of the prosencephalic vesicle, whereas a proboscis (a deformation in the region of the nose) results from defective development of the olfactory placodes.

A **disturbance in neural tube closure** is presumed to be the cause for the following anomalies (**nos 3–5**). In severe cases, the neural tube itself is affected; in milder forms, only the meninges, the bony spinal canal, or the brain capsule are involved, or there may be an anomaly only in the covering skin. Malformations located in the dorsal "body suture" may be collectively termed **dysraphia.**

**3. Anencephaly.** The cerebral portion of the neural tube does not close. *Extraversion of the neuroepithelium* (**3a**) results and the brain consists only of a degenerating tissue mass lying exposed at the surface. The skull roof is absent. Since the fetus lacks reflex mechanisms for swallowing, hydramnios results.

**4. Encephalocele**. A disturbance in the closure of the neural tube in the cervical region causes a defect in the occipital bone that may extend into the *foramen magnum*. A balloon-like swelling forms beneath the skin; it may contain an arachnoidal cyst connected to the subarachnoidal space (**meningocele**) or in addition brain tissue (**encephalomeningocele**).

**5. Myelocele**. Disturbances in neural tube closure at the level of the spinal cord characteristically lie in the lower lumbar region. In severe cases, the neural tube is not closed and the nervous tissue of the spinal cord is exposed to the surface as a neural plate (**rachischisis**). In the **meningomyelocele**, the arachnoid space dilates beneath the skin enclosing spinal cord tissue, occasionally with cystic dilatations of the neural canal (**syringocele**). In a **meningocele,** the arachnoid cyst does not contain nervous tissue. In **spina bifida occulta** , no cyst is formed, but the vertebral arches fail to close. In still milder forms, the skin has fused with the spiny process of a vertebra, forming an indentation, a pigmentation anomaly, or a characteristic tuft of hair over the lumbar region.

**6. "Tethered Cord."** This syndrome, in which the spinal cord is anchored ("tethered") in the sacral canal, is classically caused by a thickened, inflexible *filum terminale*. The conus medullaris cannot ascend into the lumbar region (→ 4.4). As growth occurs, there is progressive loss of function due to hyperextension of the spinal cord (micturition difficulties, paresthesias, and paralyses). The syndrome is also caused by the different forms of spina bifida and can lead to a downward herniation of the cerebellum and medulla oblongata, accompanied by the development of an external hydrocephalus (**Arnold–Chiari syndrome**).

**7. Internal Hydrocephalus.** In internal hydrocephalus, the cerebrospinal fluid located in the cerebral ventricles increases, causing the ventricular system to enlarge. This leads to distension of the cranial sutures, expansion of the skull cap, and ultimately to the atrophy of the cerebral cortex as a result of excess pressure. The fluid produced in the choroid plexus cannot flow out into the subarachnoid space via the aqueduct and the fourth ventricle. A frequent cause is the closure of the *cerebral aqueduct*, which can arise by an intrauterine encephalitis.

**8. External Hydrocephalus.** An external hydrocephalus is caused by an increase in the cerebrospinal fluid located in the subarachnoid space. This may be caused by the interruption of fluid circulation due to entrapment of the brainstem and the cerebellum in the foramen magnum.

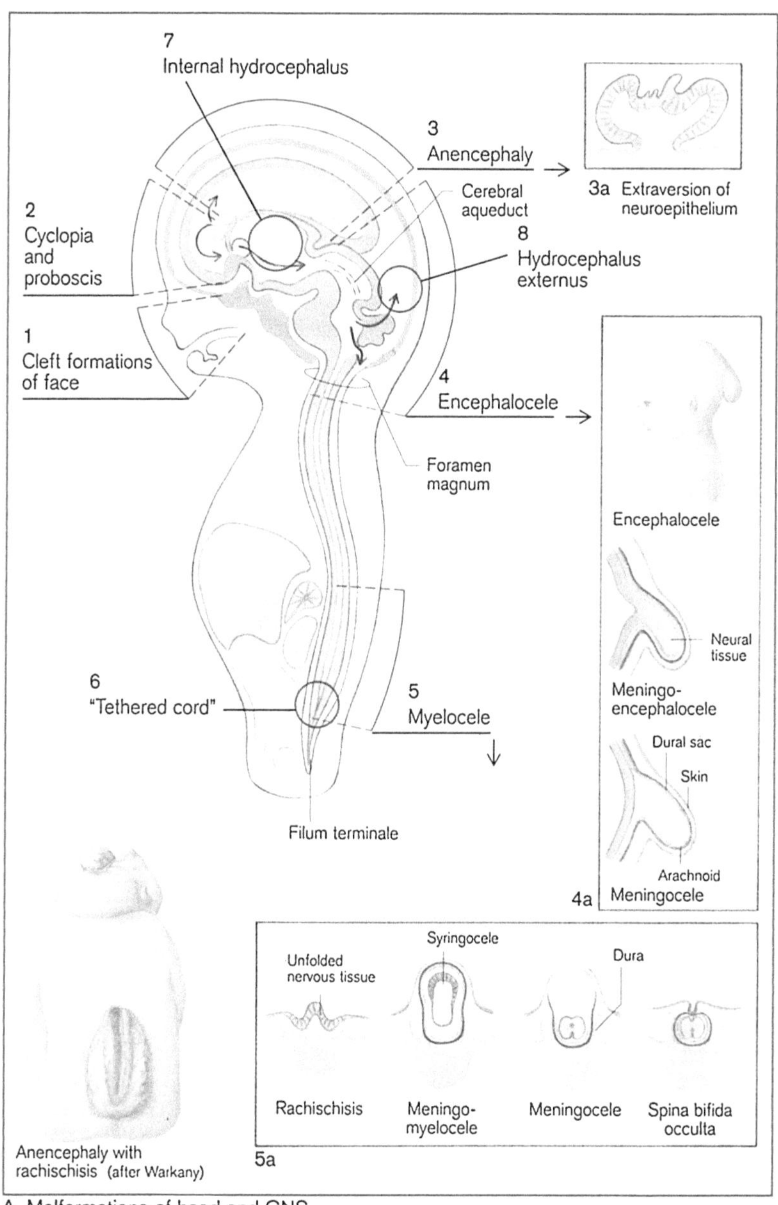
7
Internal hydrocephalus
3
Anencephaly
3a Extraversion of neuroepithelium
Cerebral aqueduct
2
Cyclopia and proboscis
8
Hydrocephalus externus
1
Cleft formations of face
4
Encephalocele
Foramen magnum
Encephalocele
Neural tissue
Meningo-encephalocele
Dural sac
Skin
Arachnoid
4a Meningocele
6
"Tethered cord"
5
Myelocele
Filum terminale
Syringocele
Unfolded nervous tissue
Dura
Rachischisis
Meningo-myelocele
Meningocele
Spina bifida occulta
5a
Anencephaly with rachischisis (after Warkany)

A. Malformations of head and CNS

# Chapter 10: Causes of Malformations

## A. Definition of Congenital Malformations

Congenital malformations are conspicuous morphological defects apparent at birth. In contrast to many other diseases, congenital malformations are principally irreversible. They are caused by disturbances in the genomic determination of an embryonic blastema or by disturbances in morphogenetic movements occurring during specific phases of embryonic development.

Malformations can have genetic causes, or they may arise due to exogenous factors acting on the embryo. Defects that can only be demonstrated biochemically are generally a consequence of mutations in structural genes. They are classified as inherited diseases.

**Medical Implications.** From a medical viewpoint, malformations are diseases requiring treatment. Possible medical approaches include: (1) social integration measures, (2) surgical intervention, (3) prevention by identification and avoidance of teratogens, (4) prenatal diagnosis.

**Morphological Derivation.** The morphological aspect of many malformations can be understood with reference to normal development. For this reason, some characteristic anomalies were presented in the chapters dealing with the normal development of individual organs. For example, a spinal cord that is exposed to the surface indicates a *disturbance in neural tube closure* (→9.5). *Esophagotracheal fistulae* arise during the abscission of the tracheobronchial groove (→7.4).

*Recklinghausen's neurofibromatosis* is associated with pigment spots in the skin (birthmarks) and neurofibromas (benign proliferations of Schwann cells), clear indications that the disease is due to a disturbance in the migration of *neural crest* cells.

Experiments with chick/quail chimeras (→3.12) have shown that mesenchymal cells from the *neural crest* migrate into the endocardial cushion. Manipulation of the neural crest in the rhombencephalic vesicle leads to disturbances in the formation of the spiral septum in the outflow tract of the heart. Thus, an observed *heart defect* can be traced back to a preceding disturbance in the migration of neural crest cells. However, recognizing a developmental anomaly as a defect in morphogenesis is not equivalent to identifying its cause. In the following sections, some genetic and exogenous causes of human malformations are discussed.

## B. Genetic Causes of Malformations

The simplest theoretical origin for a malformation is a gene mutation. Most genes are necessary for the viability of cells or embryos; thus most gene mutations are deleterious. Critical genes are highly conserved: they do not give rise to malformations since mutations at these genetic loci prevent the development of gametes or cause the death of the zygote. Only relatively few genetic loci exist in which a mutation leads to a morphological or biochemical alteration that is compatible with life. In a given population, mutations at a gene locus occur with a certain frequency per generation, the spontaneous mutation rate (about $10^{-6}$). When the frequency of a genetically caused malformation is higher than the spontaneous mutation rate, one or more heritable variants of the responsible gene must exist.

**Dominant Inheritance**. In general, morphological or biochemical malformations greatly reduce the reproductive potential of the affected individual. As a result, dominantly inherited diseases are frequently expressed only after the 40th year of life, i.e., at the end of the individual's reproductive period (e.g., *Huntington's chorea*). Other dominantly inherited malformations occur with the frequency of the spontaneous mutation rate or have only weak penetrance.

**Recessive Inheritance.** Recessively inherited defects appear with high frequency in small, isolated populations (e.g., thesaurismosis). In genetically mixed (highly heterozygous) populations, the frequency of such gene variants approaches the frequency of the spontaneous mutation rate. In a number of severe diseases, such as cystic fibrosis (mucoviscidosis), in which a single protein (here, an ion channel) is affected by a mutation, prenatal diagnosis is available, enabling parents with an afflicted child to monitor further pregnancies (family planning).

Certain defects that can be treated with diet therapy (e.g., phenylketonuria) or hormone therapy (adrenogenital syndrome, → 8.10) can be diagnosed immediately after birth.

**Chromosomal Anomalies.** Monosomy, i.e., the absence of a chromosome, and trisomy, i.e., the occurrence of three homologous chromosomes, is a relatively frequent occurrence resulting from “nondisjunction” of a chromosome pair during meiosis (generally in the oocyte). Nondisjunction occurs with roughly equal frequency for all chromosomes. However, such chromosomal defects are generally lethal, leading to spontaneous abortion of the fetus. Only for chromosomes 13, 18, and 21 (Down's Syndrome) are trisomies compatible with life.

**Homeotic Genes.** Segmentation genes were discovered and characterized in the fruit fly *Drosophila*. (Fruit flies are suitable for such studies because they have a short generation time and thousands of offspring.) Radiation treatment of these flies induces random mutations, some which cause segmental transformations and are heterozygously transmitted. These can be selected and analyzed using molecular biological techniques. Corresponding genes were identified in the mouse and the human genomes by DNA hybridization techniques. In the mouse, mutations in these genes lead to characteristic malformations, for example, in the vertebrae. From this it may be concluded that analogous malformations in the human are similarly caused by mutations in homeotic genes.

**Malformation Syndromes.** Characteristic combinations of defects in different organ systems are termed syndromes and are named after the authors who first described them. An example is *Marfan's syndrome*, associated with a slender, tall stature, arachnodactyly, scoliosis (lateral curvature of the vertebral column), lens luxation, and aortic anomalies. For certain syndromes, the underlying mutations or chromosomal aberrations are known. Since the aberrations affect a variety of organ systems, the characteristic syndrome results. Examples are *Down's syndrome* (trisomy 21), *Turner's syndrome* (XO, absence of the Y-chromosome), and *Klinefelter's syndrome* (genotype XXY). Generally, a causal analysis is only possible by analysis of corresponding mutations in the mouse (e.g., *testicular feminization*, androgen receptor defect, → 8.8).

**Fragile X Syndrome.** The fragile X syndrome is the most frequent genetic cause of mental retardation. Its origin is an unstable locus on the long arm of the X chromosome at which the chromosome is easily broken. This site can be identified with an appropriate DNA probe. The mode of inheritance resembles the pseudoautosomal dominant pattern with obligatory cross-over between the X and Y chromosomes that was observed in the Sxr-factor (→ 3.16). During meiosis, chromosomal exchanges occur between the X and Y chromosomes as they undergo end-to-end pairing. In this process, a part of the X chromosome may be transferred to the Y chromosome and later be again transferred to the X chromosome. A male carrier can transmit the trait to a daughter who is not affected but has afflicted male and female children. Development of the disease is apparently associated with increased DNA methylation at the fragile site of the X chromosome.

## C. Exogenous Causes

The fetus is naturally protected from mechanical injuries by the formation of the fetal membranes, and from medications by the development of the placenta (placental barrier). Thus, a causal relationship between a malformation and specific external influences that may have disturbed the pregnancy can rarely be demonstrated. However, certain medications have been shown to cause specific damage to the embryo. It is therefore advisable to refrain from taking medications during pregnancy.

## 1. Sensitive Phases for Teratogens

The effect of an exogenous teratogenic factor on a pregnancy depends on the developmental age of the embryo. During **early development**, the reaction is "all or none": either the pregnancy is terminated by a spontaneous abortion, or the damage is repaired by the still pluripotent cells. In the **embryonic period**, the action of a teratogen that does not lead to the death of the embryo can cause typical malformations of organs that are in their sensitive (susceptible) phase at the time of exposure to the teratogen. In the **fetal period**, morphogenesis of the organ primordia has concluded, so that gross morphological malformations no longer arise. An exception is the cerebral cortex, which is in its sensitive phase (e.g., to radiation damage) between the 8th and 15th week of pregnancy.

**Reactions during Early Development.** Interruption of the implantation process in cases of chromosomal or genetic defects appears to be a physiological event. A high percentage of spontaneous abortions possess chromosomal anomalies. Similarly, a high percentage of early implantations investigated by Hertig and Rock (→ 2.0) had defects. Hertig and Rock suggested that these implantations—as yet unnoticed by the mother—would not have been carried to term. Chorionic biopsy in the 4th week yields a higher frequency of pathological findings than are found by later methods of prenatal diagnosis. From this observation, it may be concluded that many of the documented pregnancies would have been terminated naturally without medical intervention.

*Identical twins* arise during early development (→ 2.45) by an unknown process that is not associated with exogenous factors. Twins are formed when the zygote or the germinal disc divides in half and each half develops into an equivalent embryo. The division may be incomplete and development may proceed asymmetrically so that one twin is linked to the other (Siamese twins). **Duplications** range from a dulpication of the body axis in the primitive streak stage to a duplication or anomaly of the axial organs in the blastema of the tail bud.

In **teratomas**, pluripotent embryonic cells form variably differentiated, unorganized tissue masses. Teratomas may be derived from dispersed, pluripotent embryonic tissue or may be caused by parthenogenesis, i.e., embryonic development of unfertilized germ cells (ectopic primordial germ cells, germ cells in the ovary or in the testis).

In the **hydatidiform mole** (chorionic epithelioma), the embryo dies as the result of a chromosomal anomaly or from other causes, but the trophoblast alone continues to proliferate without the development of embryonic vessels. If the growth is malignant, it is called a **chorionic carcinoma**.

**Reactions in the Embryonic Period.** The "sensitive phase" (or "susceptible phase") of an organ primordium is the time window during development in which exogenous factors can cause organotypic malformations. Most organ systems have sensitive phases in the embryonic period. The type of malformation that occurs depends on the time of injury and on the developmental stage of the primordium. Data on the sensitive phases of organs in human development (**10.1**) are based on retrospective analyses of rubella embryopathy and of the thalidomide disaster, as well as on correlations between the time of exposure and the type of anomaly induced by other known noxious agents. If the teratogenic factor is based on cell destruction in the blastema produced by cytostatic agents, radiation, or viral infection, the sensitive phase is equivalent to the blastemal phase. However, the sensitive phase may also precede the development of the blastema. A plausible explanation for this observation is a disturbance in cell determination during the expression of early segmentation genes.

**Reactions in the Fetal Period**. Disturbances in the fetal period no longer influence morphogenesis, but affect the cellular differentiation of the brain, kidneys, and intestinal tract, as well as the sex-specific development of the external genitalia. In the cerebral cortex, proliferation occurs in the matrix zone and progresses by "inside-out layering" (→ 4.17, 16th week of pregnancy). The axons of the pyramidal cells grow into the nuclear regions of the brainstem and spinal cord. Anomalies arising in the embryonic pe-

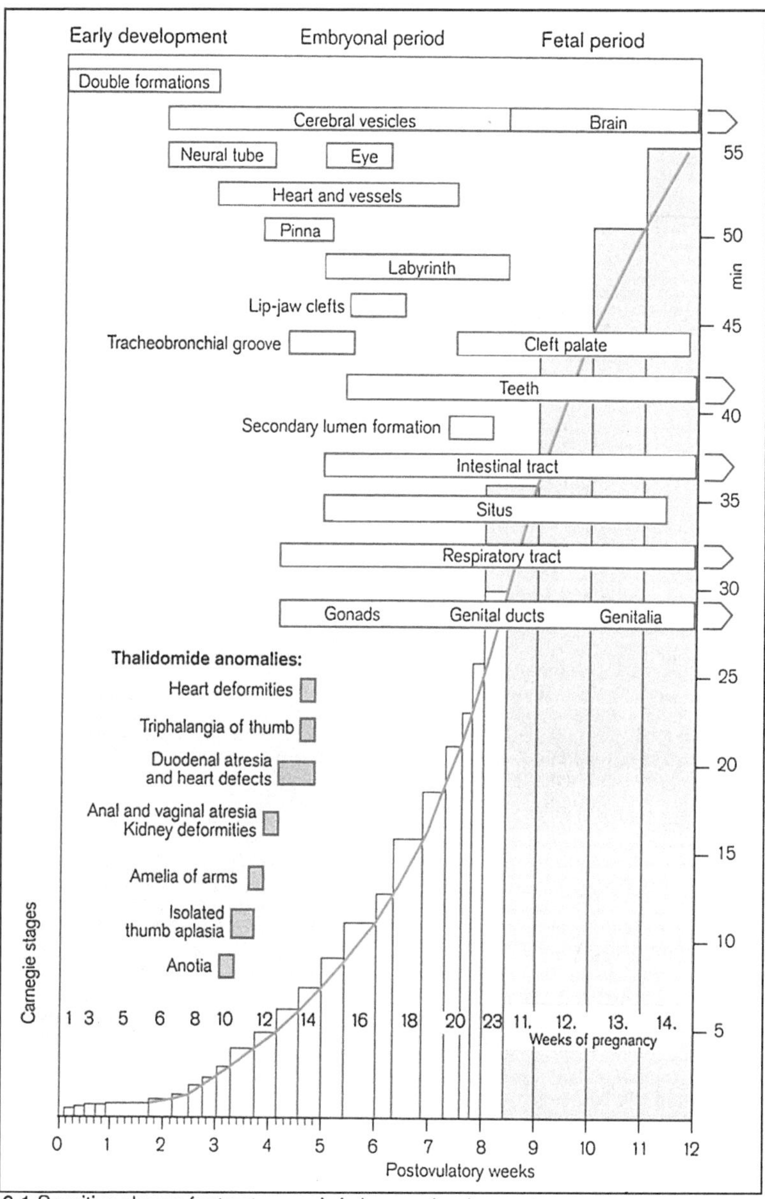


10.1 Sensitive phases for teratogenesis in human development

(after Hinrichsen, Schumacher and Lenz)

riod, like anencephaly and encephalocele, are replaced in the fetal period by anomalies such as microcephaly, hydrocephalus, mental retardation, hypokinesis, and paralyses with secondary defects in the positions of the extremities. Hydrocephalus internus (→ 9.5) can arise either by primary loss of cortical substance with associated primary widening of the ventricles or by obstruction of the flow of the cerebrospinal fluid through the cerebral aqueduct or the fourth ventricle due to intrauterine infections or malformations of the brain vesicles. In the second half of a pregnancy, brain damage is caused by fetal pathologies, like encephalomeningitis after intrauterine infection, with concomitant cell destruction, scar formation, and calcification.

## 2. Intrauterine Infections

**Rubella (German measles).** In a primary infection with rubella virus during pregnancy, the lack of immunity in the mother may lead to transmittance of the virus to the embryo resulting in spontaneous abortion or stillbirth. An infection during the embryonic period can cause a typical syndrome with stage-specific malformations. An infection in the fetal period can be associated with inflammation of sensitive organ systems, such as the eye (chorioretinitis) or the brain (encephalomeningitis). These inflammations leave calcification foci in the meninges that can be demonstrated radiographically. Scar formation in the choroid plexus and in the cerebral aqueduct can cause an internal hydrocephalus, while a general disturbance in the growth of the brain results in microcephaly. Infection of the infant during delivery causes the characteristic clinical picture of early childhood infection.

Intrauterine infection with rubella virus, first described in 1941, was the first recognized cause of teratogenic damage to the embryo. Malformations of the eye correlate with an infection around the 6th week of pregnancy, deafness with an infection around the 9th week, and heart defects and anomalies of the central nervous system with infections between the 5th and 10th week of pregnancy. Abnormalities of the teeth are observed after infection between the 6th and 9th week of pregnancy. A centrally based deafness can be caused by an infection after the 12th week of pregnancy. The risk of malformations as a consequence of intrauterine infection is 30% up to the 12th week and decreases continuously up to the 20th week. A vaccination program in girls during childhood is carried out as a prophylactic measure.

**Cytomegalovirus.** Infection with cytomegalovirus causes no symptoms in the mother. The risk of intrauterine infection increases to 40% up to the 3rd trimester. Observed effects include hepatosplenomegaly, microcephaly, and symptomatic hydrocephalus, progressive calcification of the brain vessels, psychomotor and mental retardation, and cerebral paralyses.

**Herpes Simplex Virus.** If the mother has genital herpes, she can infect the child with herpes at birth. In the neonate, the virus can cause brain damage and mental retardation or death. For this reason, delivery by cesarean section is recommended for women infected with genital herpes.

**Chickenpox (Varicella).** Among pregnant women, the frequency of infection with chickenpox is slight, amounting to only 5 in 10 000. The resulting characteristic malformation syndrome involves an inflammatory disorder of brain development, anomalies in the urogenital system, and heart defects. Its stage specificity corresponds to that of rubella.

**AIDS Virus.** The AIDS virus can be transmitted prenatally and perinatally. It causes a dysmorphic syndrome involving growth retardation and microcephaly, as well as hypertelorism with characteristic facial features.

**Syphilis.** An intrauterine infection with syphilis can lead to spontaneous abortion, stillbirth, or congenital syphilis with associated neurological disturbances, mental retardation, cardiovascular defects, and craniofacial anomalies.

**Toxoplasmosis.** Infection with the intracellular protozoon Toxoplasma gondii can result from the consumption of raw meat or contact with cats. In the case of a first infection of the mother, the fetus may be afflicted. Toxoplasmosis causes hydrocephalus, chorioretinitis, hepatosplenomegaly, and mental retardation.

## 3. Damage from Medications

**Thalidomide Embryopathy.** Thalidomide, a hypnotic and sedative drug sold by a German firm under the trademark Contergan from 1957 to 1962, provides the best example of a causal link between drug intake and fetal malformations. Typical anomalies were symmetrical amelia (absence of arms or legs), micromelia (shortened limbs), phocomelia (attachment of fingers or toes directly to the trunk), and hypoplasia of the radius (underdeveloped radius). Apart from defects in the extremities, other disturbances were observed, including anotia (absence of ears), microphthalmia (small eyes), persistence of coloboma (→ 5.6), as well as defects of the inner organs, the heart, the urinary excretory pathways, and the gastrointestinal tract. The connection between the malformation syndrome and thalidomide use during pregnancy was recognized and published in 1961 by Lenz in Germany and by McBride in Australia. Intrauterine mortality due to thalidomide amounted to about 40%. A study published in 1988 by Lenz describes 3049 live-born infants with malformations. In some cases, thalidomide had been prescribed during hospital stays, so that the time of medication intake and the type of resulting defect could be exactly correlated. These data are included in 10.1. For example, damage to the limbs takes place even before the limb buds have appeared. This suggests that thalidomide does not act like a classic teratogen (e.g., a cytostatic agent) by destroying cells in the progression zone of the limb bud, but acts in an earlier stage, possibly by influencing homeotic genes during segmental determination.

The failure of thalidomide to be recognized as a teratogen prior to its registration is frequently taken as an indication that this was not possible and that teratogenicity tests in animals in general were useless. In 1957, animal tests for teratogenicity were not yet required by law. A sedative such as thalidomide was not a suspected teratogen. The typical thalidomide embryopathy can be observed both in rabbits and in primates. Taking into account the complex pharmacokinetics of thalidomide, a corresponding malformation syndrome can also be demonstrated in the mouse (Kocher et al., 1992).

**Hormones.** Steroid hormones with androgenic action can cause masculinization in female fetuses, whereas steroid hormones with antiandrogenic action induce female development in male fetuses. The sensitive phase begins at the end of the indifferent stage of the sexual organs in stage 18 –20, when androgen receptors first appear in the mesenchyme of the genital ducts (→ 8.5). Described malformations have resulted from the treatment of pregnant women with synthetic progestogens to prevent an abortion. Progestogens can have an androgenic or antiandrogenic effect. Female fetuses showed masculinization in the form of fused labia; male fetuses showed disturbances in the canalization of the glans penis with development of hypospadia, evidence of antiandrogenic effects. The synthetic estradiol diethylstilbestrol (DES) used to prevent imminent abortions, has been reported to cause adenomas of the vagina in female infants after puberty. The risk of a vaginal adenoma is between 0.14 and 1.4 per thousand children born to mothers treated with DES (data according to Persaud, 1992). In early pregnancy, the use of hormonal contraceptives or related substances does not increase the risk of malformations.

**Fetal Alcohol Syndrome.** Children born to alcoholic mothers may suffer from fetal alcohol syndrome, characterized by mental retardation, diminished prenatal and postnatal growth, microcephaly, and a characteristic face with short palpebral fissures, flat nose bridge, and hypoplastic upper and lower jaws.

**Nicotine.** Heavy smoking during pregnancy has been reported to cause intrauterine growth retardation. This is attributed to fetal hypoxia resulting from maternal vasoconstriction and a concomitant deficiency in placental blood supply.

**Ionizing Radiation.** After the explosion of atomic bombs over Hiroshima and Nagasaki in 1945, the rate of miscarriages in radiation-exposed pregnant women increased by 28%. Twenty-five percent of the children died in their first year of life and 25% of the surviving children exhibited malformations in the central nervous system (data according to Persaud, 1992). The natural cosmic radiation load is about 1 cGy. A radiation exposure below 5 cGy carries very little risk for the embryo. Still, X-rays in the pelvic region—which have an energy of about 2 cGy—should, if possible, be carried out within the first 10 days post menstruation, a time at which pregnancy is least likely, or should be postponed until after the 24th week of pregnancy.

## D. Teratology

Teratology is a branch of experimental embryology dealing with the causes of malformations. One aspect of this research is the testing of new drugs for teratogenic effects in animal models.

In animal experiments, the sensitive phases of the organs can be precisely determined by systematic treatment with teratogens. The severity of a malformation depends less on the type of teratogen than on the time of application. For dose-response data and for statistical analyses, inbred strains of experimental animals with large litter sizes (mice, rats, rabbits) are used. The results are essentially transferable to humans. However, because of different gestation periods, information on the exact times at which drugs act cannot be transferred.

### 1. Site of Action of Teratogens

The methods of comparative embryology and experimental teratology allow a drug to be classified as teratogenic or nonteratogenic with reasonable certainty. Every new drug is therefore now routinely tested for teratogenicity in animals before it is approved for human use. These teratological studies provide a statistical analysis of morphological effects, but allow no conclusions regarding the site of action of a teratogen. Teratogens generally act on DNA or interfere with the embryonic transduction chain (-› 3.29).

### 2. Action at the DNA level

Cytostatic agents are drugs that form adducts with DNA or interfere with DNA replication. In **proliferating cell populations,** they cause the death of daughter cells. Radiation, which induces the breakage of DNA strands, has the same effect. Both cytostatic agents and radiation are used in tumor therapy to destroy proliferating cell populations. Exposure to these agents during pregnancy leads to the death of the embryo or to phase-specific damage of organ primordia proliferating at the time of exposure.

In smaller doses, cytostatic agents and radiation cause an **increase in the mutation rate** of proliferating cell populations (in differentiated cells, which have permanently exited from the cell cycle, the mutations have no consequence, since still only a small portion of the genome is transcriptionally active and the damage is lost with the death of the cell). In proliferating cell populations, mutations compatible with the survival of the daughter cells are subjected to a selection process. Mutations that switch on embryonic transduction chains and stimulate proliferation (oncogenes →3.29) have a selective advantage and can give rise to malignant tumors. In embryonic blastemas, such mutations appear to have no selective advantage. This is indicated by the experimental observation that a malignantly growing teratoma cell implanted into the blastocyst of a mouse can participate in the formation of normal embryonic structures and can even differentiate into a normal germ cell. During the passage through embryonic development, the oncogenes switched on in the teratoma cell are apparently switched off, so that the cell can be integrated into the normal life cycle.

Irradiation is used to increase the **mutation rate in the germ line** of animal species with high rates of reproduction (e.g., *Drosophila* and mice). A multitude of mutations result; those of interest for specific studies (and having suitable heritability) can then be selected. Mutations generated as models for human diseases (e.g., testicular feminization in the mouse, → 8.8) are maintained on an appropriate genetic background or held as an inbred strain. The manipulations thus do not interfere with the genomes of natural populations, but may rather be thought of as a special form of domestication, a process that has been practiced by mankind time after time.

After the explosions of atomic bombs in Hiroshima and Nagasaki, pregnant women surviving the explosion experienced miscarriages and gave birth to children with malformations. However, under normal circumstances, an increase in the mutation rate above the spontaneous mutation rate is difficult to demonstrate statistically in humans, since the reproduction rate is very low and genetic variability is very high.

### 3. Action on Embryonic Transduction Chains

The teratogenic effect of **vitamin A deficiency** has been known for a long time. This effect is due to the function of retinoic acid as a ligand in the induction of regulatory genes, which are switched on during embryonic development (→ 3.23, B4).

Many **hormones,** such as *thyroid hormone* and the *sex steroids,* are embryonic inductors that can cause malformations when present in excess or when deficient. *Cortisone* and *insulin* are essential for the differentiation of all organs investigated to date. High doses of cortisone induce cleft palates in mice. In humans, cortisone is probably nonteratogenic on account of the modulatory action of the steroid hormone metabolism in the placenta and the fetal adrenal cortex (→ 1.17). Insulin is a growth factor of the short glycoproteins type. Diabetes can cause abnormally large infants and increase in the incidence of other malformations, such as caudal malformation syndrome.

A number of **neuropharmacological drugs** are teratogenic. Included in this category are thalidomide and *antiepileptic drugs* (e.g., diphenylhydantoin, trimethadione, and valproic acid). *Neurotransmitters* play a role in cellular interaction during embryonic development; these primitive functions may be forerunners of the differentiated functions in the adult central nervous system. However, the mechanism of action of neuropharmacological drugs including thalidomide is still speculative.

### 4. Phenocopy

The imitation of a genetically determined malformation by treatment with teratogens is called a phenocopy. The *thalidomide embryopathy* initially appeared as an increased occurrence of the already known but rare phocomelia and thus was an example of a phenocopy. A phenocopy phenomenon can be further clarified in animal experiments. Polydactyly (appearance of supernumerary finger or toe rays) is caused in mice by a recessive mutation. The expression of this mutation, i.e., the frequency of its manifestation and the type of defects expressed in an inbred strain homozygous for the polydactyly depends on the genetic "background." The genetic background refers to the total number of genes that influence the expression of the mutation in question. By changing successively the genetic background, the expression of polydactyly can be strengthened, so that instead of supernumerary phalanges, hypoplasia of the radius and ulna and finally hypoplasia of the humerus appear. In a typical phenocopy experiment, the influence of the genetic background on the expression of a mutation could be mimicked by a low dose of the cytostatic agent triethylenemelamine (TEM), which alone caused no malformation in a nonselected animal strain. Genetic background and the exogenous teratogen had additive effects on the expression of the malformation. The appearance of an anomaly is thus not caused by disturbance of a single factor, but is influenced by a multiplicity of factors. In this aspect, the primary role of the genetic information in the determination of an individual becomes questionable. In embryonic development, the genetic information is embedded in a network of external factors, feedback mechanisms, mutual modulation, mutations, and repair mechanisms. Thus the countless individual factors and miniature regulatory circuits together produce an organism that is far more complex than the sum of its morphological and biochemical aspects.

# Further Reading and References

## Textbooks

(1) Alberts, B., D. Bray, J. Lewis, M. Raff, K. Roberts und J. D. Watson: Übers. von L. Jaenicke: Molekularbiologie der Zelle. Weinheim; Deerfield Beach, FL: VCH, 1986.

(2) Arey, L. B.: Developmental Anatomy. A Textbook and Laboratory Manual of Embryology. Saunders Company, Philadelphia 1965

(3) Balinsky, B. I.: An Introduction to Embryology. 5th Edition. Saunders, Philadelphia 1981

(4) Blechschmidt, E.: Der menschliche Embryo (Totalrekonstruktionen). Schattauer, Stuttgart 1963

(5) Blechschmidt, E.: Die pränatalen Organsysteme des Menschen. Hippokrates, Stuttgart 1973

(6) Boyd, J. D. and W. J. Hamilton: The Human Placenta. Cambridge W. Heffer & Sons Ltd 1970

(7) Darnell, J. E., H. Lodish, and D. Baltimore: Molecular cell biology. 2nd Edition. Scientific American Books, Inc. 1990

(8) Hamilton, W. J., J. D. Boyd and H. W. Mossmann: Human Embryology. Prenatal development of form and function. 4th Edition. Heffer, Cambridge 1972

(9) Hinrichsen, K. V. (Hrsg.): Humanembryologie. Lehrbuch und Atlas der vorgeburtlichen Entwicklung des Menschen. Springer, Berlin 1990

(10) Johnson, M. H. and B. J. Everitt: Essential Reproduction. 2nd Edition. Blackwell Scientific Publications. 1984

(11) Kleinig, H. und P. Sitte: Zellbiologie. Ein Lehrbuch. 3rd Edition. Gustav Fischer 1992

(12) Kollmann, J.: Handatlas der Entwicklungsgeschichte des Menschen. In zwei Bänden. Gustav Fischer Jena 1907

(13) Langman, M. D.: Medizinische Embryologie. 8th Edition. Thieme, Stuttgart 1991

(14) O'Rahilly, R. and F. Müller: Developmental Stages in Human Embryos. Carnegie Institution of Washington Publication 637, 1987

(15) O'Rahilly, R. and F. Müller: Human Embryology and Teratology. Wiley-Liss, New York 1992

(16) Patten, B. M.: Human Embryology. New York: McGraw-Hill 3, 1968

(17) Romer, A. S. und T. S. Parsons: Vergleichende Anatomie der Wirbeltiere. 5th Edition. Verlag Paul Parey Hamburg und Berlin 1983

(18) Starck, D.: Embryologie. 3rd Edition. Thieme, Stuttgart 1975

(19) Tuchmann-Duplessis, H., P. Haegel: Illustrated Human Embryology. Masson, Paris 1972

## References

Behind the plate and figure number, the source is given. Numbers in brackets refer to the above-cited text books. The data of the human specimens of the Carnegie collection (characterized by their C number) are found in (14).

Chapter 1: Reproduction

1.8A2 Schulze W, Rheder U (1984) Cell Tiss Res 237:395. 1.11A Baker TG (1963) Proc roy Soc Lond B 158:417. 1.15C Pschyrembel Praktische Geburtshilfe. DeGruyter 1965 1.16A Döring GK (1962) Geburtsh und Frauenh 22:1191. 1.17A (10)

Chapter 2: Human Development

2.0 und 2.1A (14). 2.6B Hertig AT et al (1954) Contr Embryol 35:199. 2.6C Heuser CH; Streeter GL (1941) Contr Embryol 29:15. 2.8A Vögler H (1987) Bibliotheca Anatomica No 30. Luckett WP (1975) Am J Anat 144:149. 2.9A1 C7700, 2.9A2

C7802. 2.10A1 C7950, 2.10A2 C9250, 2.10A3 C7801. Luckett (1978) Am J Anat 152:59. 2.11A C7801, 2.11B C7802. 2.12A C5960, (14). 2.13A Ludwig E (1928) Morph Jahrb 59:41. 2.14A2 Ortmann R (1938) Z Anat Entwicklungsgesch 108:450. 2.15 (16). 2.16A Ingalls NW (1920) Contrib Embryol 11:61. 2-16B Payne F (1925) Contrib to Embryol 16:115. 2.17 und 2.18 Corner GW (1929) Contrib to Embryol 20:81. 2.19A3 Davis CL (1923) Contr Embryol 15:1. 2.20 bis 2.27 (5). 2.28A (4). 2.29, 2.31 und 2.32A (5), 2.32B (6), 2.34 und 2.35 (5). 2.37A (5). 2.40 und 2.41 (6). 2.42A1 (16), 2.42A2 (8). 2.43 (19), 2.44A (6) 2.44B (19), 2.44C (13)

Chapter 3: General Embryology

3.5 (18). 3.6A Niewkoop (1969) Spemann H Mangold H (1938); 3.6B Smith JP et al (1990) Nature 345:729. 3.12A Le Douarin N (1969) Bull Biol Belg 103:435, 3.12B Le Douarin N (1982) The Neural Crest. Univ Press Cambridge. 3.14 (8). 3.15B Mossmann HW. (1937 Contr Embryol 26:129) 3.15C (18). 3.16A (7), 316.B McLaren (1991) Nature 351:96, Koopman P et al (1991) Nature 351:117. 3.17A (7). 3.19B (17). 3.22B2 Christ B in (9). 3.23A Drews U, Drews U (1973) Wilh RouxArch 173:208, 3.23B2 (1). 3.23B3 Tickle C Nature 358:188. 3.24A Mizoguti H (1989) Adv Anat Embryol 116. 3.25 (7). 3.27A1 (11), 3.27A3 Tabin C, Laufer E (1993) Nature 361:692. 3.29 Berridge MJ (1993) Nature 361:315. 3.30 (16) 3.31 (1). 3.31B3 (10). 3.33A1a Hughes SM (1992) Nature 360:536. 334A1 Pardanaud L Dieterlen-Lièvre F (1993) Anat Embryol 187:107, 3.34A2 v Gaudecker B (1990) in (9). 3.35 Ohno S in Genetic Markers ed Haseltine FP et al Plenum Press 1987

Chapter 4: Nervous System

4.2A s. 2.16B. 4.2B1 (19). 4.4B (8). 4.5A1 (5). 4.5A2 (13). 4.7B2 Lumsden A Keynes R 1993 Nature 337:424. 4.12 (16). 4.15A1b (14). 4.17 Rakic J (1972) Comp Neur 145:61. 4.18A Wiedersheim R Vergleichende Anatomie. Gustav Fischer Jena 1906. 4.18B Kahle W Neurology Series Bd1 Springer-Verlag 1969. 4.21A1 (5). 4.22A1b (12). 4.23A1 s. 4.18A 4.23A2 Vollrath L, Oksche A (1981) Handb Mikr Anat Bd VI, 7. Teil

Chapter 5: Sense Organs

5.1A Kühn A Grundriß der allgem Zool Thieme 1969. 5.4A Boeke J in Handb der vgl Anat der Wirbeltiere. Ed Bolk et al Urban und Schwarzenberg 1934, 5.4B (16). 5.5A (16). 5.6 und 5.7 (8). 5.9B Streeter GL (1906) Amer J Anat 6:139. 5.10D (17)

Chapter 6: Heart and Vessels

6.0 Steding G, Seidel W (1990) in (9). Davis (1927) Contr Embryol 19:245. 6.7A1 (2), 6.7A2 Padget DH (1948) Contr Embryol 32:205

Chapter 7: Gastrointestinal Tract

7.1A (2). 7.2A1 (5), 7.2A2 Weller GL Jr. (1933) Contrib Embryol 24, 93:140. 7.3A (12), 7.3B (13). 7.5C3 Duncker HR in (9), 7.5C5 Burri PH (1984) Ann Rev Phyisol 46:617. 7.8 (12) und (16). 7.9A1 Drews U (1975) Pr Histochem Cytochem 3, 7.9A4 Richter E (1976) RöFo 124:552. 7.10 (16) und (13)

Chapter 8: Urogenital System

3.0 Jacob (1990) in (9). 8.1A1 s. 5.1A. 8.2 Shikinami J (1926) Contrib Embryol 18:49. 8.3A2 Kriz in Benninghoff Bd2. 8.6A2 (16). 8.5A Drews U in Klinik der Frauenh und Geburtsh Eds Wulf Schmidt-Matthiesen Bd13 Urban und Schwarzenberg 1987. 8.6A1 Witschi E (1948) Contrib Embryol 32:67. 8.8 s. 8.5. 8.10 Overzier C Die Intersexualität. Thieme 1961. A2 Bierich JR in Overzier

Chapter 9: Head

9.1A (13). 9.2A1 (8), 9.2A2 (13). 9.3B (8). 9.4A Stoeter P, Drews U (1983) Radiologie 23:273. 9.5 (8) und Warkany J Congen Malformations. Year Book Med Pub Chicago 1971

Chapter 10: Causes of Malformations

Persaud D T Umweltteratologie. In Schumacher et al Teratologie Gustav Fischer 1992. Lenz W (1988) Teratology 38:203

## Index

Chief references to an item and references to whole plates are printed in bold type.

**H**

**Q**